OF

ENTARY

TIVE

E

ESSENTIALS OF

COMPLEMENTARY AND

ALTERNATIVE

MEDICINE

Edited by

WAYNE B. JONAS

Department of Family Practice
Uniformed Services University of the Health
　Sciences
Bethesda, Maryland

Director (1995–1998)
Office of Alternative Medicine
National Institutes of Health
Bethesda, Maryland

JEFFREY S. LEVIN

Senior Research Fellow
National Institute for Healthcare Research
Rockville, Maryland

President (1997–1998)
International Society for the Study of Subtle
　Energies and Energy Medicine (ISSSEEM)
Golden, Colorado

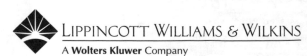

LIPPINCOTT WILLIAMS & WILKINS
A **Wolters Kluwer** Company
Philadelphia · Baltimore · New York · London
Buenos Aires · Hong Kong · Sydney · Tokyo

ASSOCIATE EDITORS

Editor: Timothy Hiscock
Managing Editor: Joyce Murphy
Marketing Manager: Kathy Neely
Project Editor: Kathleen Gilbert

351 West Camden Street
Baltimore, Maryland 21201-2436 USA

227 East Washington Square
Philadelphia, PA 19106

Printed in Canada

Library of Congress Cataloging-in-Publication Data

Essentials of complementary and alternative medicine / editors, Wayne B. Jonas, Jeffrey S. Levin.
    p.   cm.
   Includes bibliographical references and index.
   ISBN 0-683-30674-X
   1. Alternative medicine.   I. Jonas, Wayne B.   II. Levin, Jeffrey S.
   [DNLM: 1. Alternative Medicine.   WB 890 E78 1999]
R733.E87   1999
615.5—dc21
DNLM/DLC
for Library of Congress   98-22365
                                               CIP

To purchase additional copies of this book call our customer service department at **(800) 638-3030** or fax orders to **(301) 824-7390**. International customers should call **(301) 714-2324**.

                                    99 00 01 02
                     1 2 3 4 5 6 7 8 9 10

This book is dedicated to my wife, Susan Cunningham Jonas, whose love, wisdom, and service to others is an example for us all.

WBJ

For Lea Steele Levin, my beloved wife and partner.

JSL

FOREWORD

The publication of *Essentials of Complementary and Alternative Medicine*, the first comprehensive textbook for physicians about these increasingly popular forms of medical treatment, is very timely. For the first time, information about the foundations of complementary and alternative medicine (CAM), the safety of CAM products and practices, and overviews of nearly two dozen CAM systems are available in one place.

The purpose of this textbook is to provide mainstream medical professionals useful and balanced information about CAM. The development of this type of book is an ambitious and difficult goal for several reasons. Many CAM systems are claimed to have special patient benefits not met by either conventional medicine or other CAM approaches. There are few unifying themes across these systems (other than the belief that there are unmet patient benefits outside of conventional medicine). Faced with these problems, the editors have sought the best individuals in these diverse areas and worked with them to produce a balanced and useful book developed specifically for physicians. In many areas of CAM, there is a history of long-term and vigorous antagonism with conventional medicine, as well as different educational standards, training, and practices. Also, the basic concepts of what constitutes sufficient evidence of safety and efficacy vary among CAM systems. Ultimately, the usefulness of this book will depend on its success in addressing these issues in an objective, pragmatic, and convincing way.

Why is it important to publish this textbook? The main reason is the compelling evidence that medicine has been changing both scientifically and culturally for several decades. Let us start with the changes in conventional medicine since World War II.

The medicine of my childhood in a small rural town in Virginia was very different from the conventional medicine of today. For example, my 80-year-old sister who had a heart attack was treated by removal of the clot and insertion of a stent; both she and her husband viewed the procedure on television, and she was up and walking the next day. In contrast, when my 59-year-old father suffered a heart attack over 50 years ago, medicine really had little to offer.

Although there are many reasons for these dramatic changes in medicine, the dominant force has been the emergence of exact sciences underlying medicine (whereas once they were viewed as "soft sciences"). The rewarding results have been an ever-increasing understanding of basic life processes. This understanding, in turn, has allowed novel and successful approaches to disease control.

However, the advancement of science-based medicine has a downside: science-based specialty medicine has become less personal and more costly. And, cost-containment efforts pay for procedures done, rather than time spent with patients. For these and other reasons, patients seek to augment the benefits of modern conventional medicine with CAM.

The initial striking evidence of the widespread use of CAM in the United States was reported by David Eisenberg and colleagues in the *New England Journal of Medicine* in 1993. According to Eisenberg's report, one in three Americans saw an alternative health care practitioner in 1990 (constituting more visits than to conventional primary care physicians), and they paid more than 10 billion dollars in out-of-pocket expenses for this care. In addition, patients did not tell their physicians of their use of CAM because they assumed the physicians would not be interested or would not approve. In a follow-up study now completed, the evidence of even greater use of CAM has been confirmed and is most striking: more than 40% of Americans currently use CAM (approaching European and Australian rates), and as much out-of-pocket money is spent for CAM care as is out-of-pocket money spent for all of conventional medicine. These facts confirm the need for readily available information to help physicians understand, evaluate, and address CAM treatments that their patients are receiving. This textbook will help them do that.

A significant change occurred when the United States Congress mandated the opening of the Office of Alternative Medicine (OAM) at the National Institutes of Health (NIH). Medical schools are now seeking research support from this source. Research findings supported by the OAM can be expected to meet the familiar standards of NIH. In addition to research, more than 70 medical schools have (or are planning) courses in CAM for their medical student curriculum. And, although future physicians and other conventional health care workers will be versed in the advantages and disadvantages of CAM, most of those now in practice need accurate information.

Both conventional medicine and CAM share similar concerns in several important areas. Both systems need always to be committed to eliminating fraudulent practice or practitioners who severely misguide desperately ill patients. Therefore, a complete section on safety is provided in this book. However, information about efficacy is likely the most needed. Over the last few decades, conventional medicine has relied increasing on highly disciplined experimental methods to arrive at the most reasonable conclusions about effective treatments. Even with complex, large-scale, double-blind, controlled clinical trials, the goal always is both to increase our understanding of life processes and to demonstrate a difference in health outcomes. NIH-supported studies of CAM share this approach. Yet, there is also interest in developing other methods for testing effectiveness. For example, in Germany and elsewhere, efforts are being made to collect and use carefully evidence of symptomatic and clinical improvement in patients with long-term problems. Demonstrating well-documented alleviation of troublesome chronic symptoms, improved function, and better quality of life in satisfied patients using CAM would interest both the CAM and conventional medical communities.

In summary, CAM is being used by large numbers of people who derive benefits they have not received from conventional medicine. NIH-sponsored research is exploring the underlying scientific mechanisms of these approaches as well as their clinical efficacy. Medical students are being educated in the advantages and disadvantages of CAM systems and modalities. This textbook has been crafted to serve the growing communities of professionals who need thorough and accurate information about CAM. A majority of the authors are MDs or PhDs who have taught in medical schools. Only time will tell how useful any new textbook will be, but this goal is timely and the effort is to be commended.

Emotions and opinions range widely on the subject of CAM, yet at such times it is well to remember the words of Thomas Jefferson: "We are not afraid to follow the truth wherever it may lead, nor to tolerate any error so long as reason is left free to combat it."

Robert Marston, M.D.
Director, National Institutes of Health (1968–1973)

PREFACE

The publication of a medical textbook for a new or emerging field always signals a turning point—a shift toward greater awareness of theories, basic science research, and modes of clinical practice at the cutting edge of medicine. *Essentials of Complementary and Alternative Medicine* represents just such a coming of age for an important new clinical and scientific field. With this book and the forthcoming and comprehensive *Textbook of Complementary and Alternative Medicine*, information is available in one place on the social and scientific foundations of complementary and alternative medicine (CAM) and the safety of CAM products and practices, and providing detailed overviews of most CAM systems and modalities.

The primary purpose of these books is to provide medical and health care professionals with useful and balanced information about CAM in general and about particular CAM systems and practices. This is an ambitious and difficult task for several reasons. For one, the CAM systems detailed here offer benefits to patients not entirely available from mainstream medicine and not easily described in conventional terms. Further, the unifying themes or concepts across these systems are still undifferentiated from the dominant perception that unmet patient needs can be addressed outside of conventional medicine. In addition, CAM is characterized by a long-term history of vigorous antagonism; differing standards of education, training, and practice; and lack of consensus as to what constitutes sufficient evidence of safety and efficacy. Faced with these challenges, we have sought the leading experts in these diverse areas to contribute to this textbook, and have worked with them to provide balanced information for the conventional practitioner.

This book is designed to be a companion volume to the forthcoming *Textbook of Complementary and Alternative Medicine* and to serve as a clinical resource for practicing physicians and health care professionals and for medical and health professions students and postgraduates enrolled in courses on CAM. Although originally envisioned as a condensed version of the *Textbook*, it quickly became apparent that this objective would be served better by including profiles of only the most popular complementary therapies and by focusing the first two parts of the book on safety, patient management issues, and social and scientific foundations of CAM. With the clinical reader clearly in mind, this book provides an entire section detailing the safety information needed in addressing CAM products and practices. The book also includes an Indications and Precautions Chart (IPC), which provides information-at-a-glance along with chapter references on CAM systems or modalities most highly supported by empirical evidence and most likely to be efficacious in the treatment of the most common conditions presented to primary care providers.

Part I, "The Social and Scientific Foundations of Complementary and Alternative Medicine," includes five chapters outlining the history and utilization patterns of CAM, issues related to professional ethics and evaluation of efficacy claims, and how to practice in an evidence-based context. Part II, "The Safety of Complementary and Alternative Products and Practices," includes five chapters reviewing the safety of herbal and animal products, dietary and nutrient products, and homeopathy, as well as the adverse effects of acupuncture and manipulative therapies. Part III, "Overviews of Complementary and Alternative Medicine Systems," provides thorough summary overviews of key issues such as history, principal concepts, patient assessment and diagnostic procedures, therapeutic options and treatment evaluation, indications and contraindications, training, quality assurance, and future prospects for 20 major systems of CAM. These include osteopathy, naturopathy, homeopathy, chiropractic medicine, traditional Chinese medicine, biofeedback, behavioral medicine, medical acupuncture, and a dozen other systems of therapy.

It is our hope that *Essentials of Complementary and Alternative Medicine* will provide a useful resource for clinicians and clinicians-in-training. We also hope that this book will serve to further the integration of safe, efficacious complementary and alternative therapies into the mainstream of primary care practice.

Wayne B. Jonas, M.D.
Jeffrey S. Levin, Ph.D., M.P.H.

ACKNOWLEDGMENTS

This book is the result of many minds, hearts, and souls who have shared a vision of healing with me. It would not exist without them. It began when Lance Sholdt, then at the Uniformed Services University of the Health Sciences, asked if I would work with him to put together a course in complementary and alternative medicine for the medical students. His careful construction of this course helped us outline the contents of the book. This book is the brainchild of Jeff Levin. He was the first to suggest that a textbook like this was needed and could be written. His heartfelt work and attention to detail kept things moving when I was bogged down. Janette Carlucci is the soul of the book, managing both the special features and the day-to-day contact with the many authors. To her, a special thanks on this journey. Ron Chez provided a much needed balance for the book. He was always ready and willing to assist with a critical eye and keep us anchored to how this book could be of benefit for patients. I would also like to thank the editors, Jane Velker, Beth Goldner, and Joyce Murphy, for understanding the complexity of the topic and for a commitment to quality over deadlines. And Tim Hiscock for finally saying that we were going to press—ready or not. I would just as soon have worked another three years on it as finish.

WBJ

Many thanks are due to so many people whose hard work and dedication made this book possible. Wayne Jonas has already mentioned the staff at Lippincott Williams & Wilkins and his assistant, Janette Carlucci. My job would have been impossible without their tireless efforts. I must also thank Christine Boothroyd, my former secretary at Eastern Virginia Medical School. Christine coordinated all of my work on this book for nearly two years, and I am forever in her debt. My former department chairman, Dr. Terence C. Davies, also could not have been more supportive as I devoted considerable time to writing, editing, reviewing, and corresponding. Finally, thanks are due to Wayne for agreeing to tackle this project with me. At times, I imagine he, like me, must have wondered what in the world we had gotten ourselves into, but we somehow managed to complete our task. Wayne's breadth of clinical knowledge in complementary and alternative medicine and his wisdom and expertise in matters related to this field are what really made this book possible.

JSL

Contributors

VLADIMIR BADMAEV, M.D., PhD.
Staten Island, New York

MICHAEL J. BAIME, M.D.
Division Chief
Department of General Internal Medicine
The Graduate Hospital
Assistant Professor
University of Pennsylvania School of
Medicine
Philadelphia, Pennsylvania

DANIEL J. BENOR, M.D.
Author of Healing Research, Vols. I-IV
Vision Publications
Southfield, Michigan

KEITH I. BLOCK, M.D.
Medical Director
Institute of Integrative Cancer Care
Evanston, Illinois
Clinical Assistant Professor
College of Medicine
University of Illinois
Chicago, Illinois

HOWARD BRODY, M.D., PhD.
Professor
Departments of Family Practice and
Philosophy
Michigan State University
Director
Center for Ethics and Humanities in the Life
Sciences
East Lansing, Michigan

EDWARD H. CHAPMAN, M.D., PhD.
Clinical Instructor
Harvard University School of Medicine
Boston, Massachusetts

RONALD A. CHEZ, M.D.
Professor of Obstetrics and Gynecology
Professor of Community and Family Health
University of South Florida
Tampa, Florida

KENNETH S. COHEN, M.A., M.S.TH.
Adjunct Professor
Union Institute Graduate School
Cincinnati, Ohio

PETER A.G.M. DE SMET, PhD.
Pharmaceutical Care Unit
Scientific Institute of Dutch Pharmacists
The Hague, The Netherlands

BARBARA DOSSEY, R.N., M.S., F.A.A.N.
Director
Holistic Nursing Consultants
Santa Fe, New Mexico

DAVID EISENBERG, M.D.
Assistant Professor of Medicine
Harvard Medical School
Director Center for Alternative
Medicine Research and Education
Beth Israel Deaconess Medical Center
Boston, Massachusetts

EDZARD ERNST, M.D., PhD., F.R.C.P.
(EDIN)
Professor and Director
Department of Complementary Medicine
University of Exeter
Exeter, England

MICHAEL D. FETTERS, M.D., M.P.H.
Assistant Professor
Department of Family Medicine
University of Michigan Health System
Director
Japanese Family Health Program
University of Michigan Health System
Ann Arbor, Michigan

TIFFANY FIELD, PhD.
Director, Touch Research Institute
Nova/Southeastern University
Fort Lauderdale, Florida

ALAN R. GABY, M.D.
Professor of Nutrition
Bastyr University
Kenmore, Washington

HAROLD GOODMAN, D.O.
Private Practice
Silver Spring, Maryland

JUDITH A. GREEN, PhD.
Professor
Department of Psychology
Aims Community College
Co-director
Health Psychology Services, LLC
Greeley, Colorado

JOSEPH M. HELMS, M.D.
Private Practice
Berkeley, California
Chairman of Physician Acupuncture Training
Programs
UCLA School of Medicine
Los Angeles, California

WAYNE B. JONAS, M.D.
Department of Family Practice
Uniformed Services University of the Health
Sciences
Bethesda, Maryland
Director (1995–1998)
Office of Alternative Medicine
National Institutes of Health
Bethesda, Maryland

STANLEY KRIPPNER, PhD.
Professor of Psychology
Saybrook Graduate School
San Francisco, California

D. VASANT LAD, B.A.M.S., M.A.Sc.
The Ayurvedic Institute
Albuquerque, New Mexico

LIXING LAO, PhD., L.Ac
Assistant Professor and Clinical Director
Department of Complementary Medicine
University of Maryland School of
Medicine
Baltimore, Maryland
Clinic Director
MD Institute of Traditional Chinese
Medicine
Bethesda, Maryland

DANA J. LAWRENCE, D.C.
Professor of Chiropractic Practice
Director of Publications and Editorial
Review
National College of Chiropractic
Lombard, Illinois

CHING-TSE LEE, PhD.
Professor, Department of Psychology
Brooklyn College of the City
University of New York
Brooklyn, New York
Visiting Scholar
Institute of Ethnology
Academia Sinica
Taipei, Taiwan

TING LEI, PhD.
Assistant Professor
Department of Social Science
Borough of Manhattan Community
College of the City University of New York
New York, New York

JEFFREY S. LEVIN, PhD., M.P.H.
Senior Research Fellow
National Institute for Healthcare Research
Rockville, Maryland
President (1997–1998)
International Society for the Study of Subtle
Energies and Energy Medicine (ISSSEEM)
Golden, Colorado

GEORGE T. LEWITH, M.A., D.M., M.R.C.P., M.R.C.G.P.
Partner
The Centre for the Study of Complementary Medicine and
Senior Research Fellow
University Medicine
University of Southampton School of Medicine
Southampton, Hampshire, United Kingdom

KLAUS LINDE, M.D.
Muenchener
Modell-Research Center for Complementary Medicine
Department of Internal Medicine II
Technische Universitaet
Munich, Germany

TIERAONA LOW DOG, M.D., A.H.G.
Medical Director
Treehouse Center of Integrative Medicine
Medical Advisor
Quality Control & Standards
Materia Medica Group
Physician
Private Practice
Albuquerque, New Mexico

MICHAEL T. MURRAY, N.D.
Member, Board of Trustees and Faculty
Bastyr University
Kenmore, Washington

JOSEPH E. PIZZORNO, JR., N.D.
President
Bastyr University
Kenmore, Washington

JANIS M. RYGWELSKI, M.D.
Assistant Professor
Department of Family Practice
Michigan State University
East Lansing, Michigan

G. RANDOLPH SCHRODT, JR., M.D.
Associate Professor
Department of Psychiatry and Behavioral Sciences
University of Louisville School of Medicine
Medical Director
Behavioral Medicine Program
Norton Psychiatric Clinic
Louisville, Kentucky

ROBERT SHELLENBERGER, PhD.
Licensed Psychologist
Chair of Psychology
Aims Community College
Co-Director
Health Psychology Service LLC
Greeley, Colorado

ALLAN TASMAN, M.D.
Professor and Chairman
Department of Psychiatry and Behavioral Sciences
University of Louisville School of Medicine
Louisville, Kentucky

HARALD WALACH, PhD., DIPL. PSYCH.
Department of Psychology
University of Freiburg
Freiburg, Germany

JAMES C. WHORTON, PhD.
Professor
Department of Medical History and Ethics
University of Washington School of Medicine
Seattle, Washington

IAN WICKRAMASEKERA, PhD., A.B.P.P., A.B.P.H.
Consulting Professor of Psychiatry
Stanford Medical School
Stanford, California
Professor of Family Medicine
Eastern Virginia Medical School
Norfolk, Virginia

CONTENTS

PART I. THE SOCIAL AND SCIENTIFIC FOUNDATIONS OF COMPLEMENTARY AND ALTERNATIVE MEDICINE

PART II. THE SAFETY OF COMPLEMENTARY AND ALTERNATIVE MEDICINE PRODUCTS AND PRACTICES

PART III: OVERVIEWS OF COMPLEMENTARY AND ALTERNATIVE MEDICINE SYSTEMS

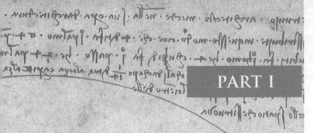

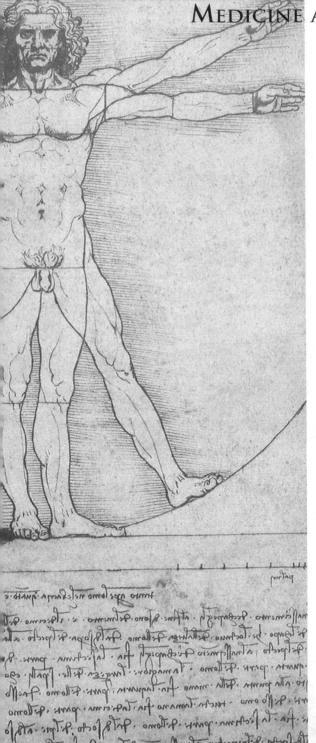

PART I

THE SOCIAL AND SCIENTIFIC
FOUNDATIONS OF COMPLEMENTARY
AND ALTERNATIVE MEDICINE

INTRODUCTION: MODELS OF MEDICINE AND HEALING

Wayne B. Jonas and Jeffrey S. Levin

PHYSICIANS ARE FACED DAILY WITH DISEASE, ILLNESS, SUFFERING, AND DEATH. THE MEDICAL PROFESSION AIMS TO HELP CURE, TREAT, COMFORT, AND SAVE THE LIVES OF THOSE WHO SEEK HELP. MOST PHYSICIANS MUST ALSO PERSONALLY FACE ILLNESS AT SOME TIME IN THEIR LIVES OR CARE FOR A LOVED ONE WHO IS ILL. WHETHER PROFESSIONALLY, PERSONALLY, OR WITH FAMILY, WHEN ILLNESS COMES ALL PRACTITIONERS WANT BASICALLY THE SAME THING—RAPID, GENTLE TREATMENT THAT CAN CURE US OR AT LEAST ALLAY OUR FEARS AND ALLEVIATE OUR SUFFERING. IN 1996, AN INTERNATIONAL GROUP OF HEALTH SCHOLARS AND PRACTITIONERS RECLARIFIED THE TRADITIONAL GOALS OF ALL MEDICINE (1). THESE GOALS ARE:

1. THE PREVENTION OF DISEASE AND INJURY AND PROMOTION AND MAINTENANCE OF HEALTH.

2. THE RELIEF OF PAIN AND SUFFERING CAUSED BY MALADIES.

3. THE CARE AND CURE OF THOSE WITH A MALADY, AND THE CARE OF THOSE WHO CANNOT BE CURED.

4. THE AVOIDANCE OF PREMATURE DEATH AND THE PURSUIT OF A PEACEFUL DEATH.

IT IS TOWARD THESE GOALS, THEY URGED, THAT
ALL MEDICAL EDUCATION, RESEARCH, PRACTICE
AND HEALTH CARE DELIVERY SHOULD BE AIMED.

Despite these common goals, practitioners'
responses to disease and illness are remarkably
varied, and opinions about these differences in
approach are often strongly held. Who we trust
to our care, what we decide is the best treatment,
how we evaluate success, and when we look
for alternatives depend on many factors. These
factors include how one understands the nature
of health and disease, what is believed to have
gone wrong and why, the type and strength of
the evidence supporting various treatments, and
who is consulted when obtaining help. In short,
our choice of medical modalities depends on
our *models* and perceptions of the world, the
preferences and *values* we share, and the believed
benefit that may come from a certain treatment,
system of practice, or individual. Even in an
age of modern science when medical decisions
can be made on a more objective basis than
ever before, these decisions are a complex social
process. To understand what shapes our behavior toward health care, we must carefully examine these social forces. The rise in interest and
use of complementary and alternative medicine
(CAM) reflects social changes in our models,
values, and perceived benefit from modern
health care practices in the last several decades.

THE RISING INTEREST
IN COMPLEMENTARY AND
ALTERNATIVE MEDICINE

Public and Professional Adoption
of CAM

Two identical surveys of unconventional medicine use in the United States, one done in 1990
and the other in 1997, showed that during that
time frame CAM use had increased from 34%
to 42%. Visits to CAM practitioners went from
400 million to more than 600 million visits per
year, and the amount spent on these practices
rose from $14 billion to $27 billion–most of
it not reimbursed (2). As increased use of the
phrase of "integrated medicine" for the CAM
field suggests, these practices are now being integrated into mainstream medicine. Over seventy-
five medical schools have courses on CAM (3),
hospitals are developing complementary and integrated medicine programs, health insurers are
offering "expanded" benefits packages that include alternative medicine services (4), and biomedical research organizations are investing
more into the investigation of these practices
(5). The American Medical Association recently
devoted an entire issue of each of their journals
to CAM.

This rising interest in CAM reflects not only
changing behaviors, but also changing needs
and values in modern society. This includes
changes in the psychosocial determinants of
CAM use; the "normalization" of users over
time; concepts of the body; the relationship
among the growing "fitness" movement, aging
"baby boomers," and CAM; and the nature of
both the therapeutic relationship and the health
care preferences. Many complementary health
care practices diffuse throughout society
through health "networks" that increasingly determine therapeutic choices (5a).

Of note is that CAM practices, like most
conventional practices, are adopted and normalized long before scientific evidence has established their safety and efficacy. A key difference
in how this occurs, however, is that in conventional practice, procedures are usually introduced by professionalized bodies or industries
rather than by the public (6). Adoption in complementary medicine has occurred in the opposite direction: the public adopts and seeks out
these practices first, and health care professions
and industries follow. This says something
about the changing nature of public preferences
and professional responsiveness to those preferences. It also predicts that new "unconventional" practices will arise in the future as
current CAM groups become more "professionalized" themselves and are adopted into the
mainstream. Thus, we will always need ways of
addressing alternative practices responsibly.

Responding to CAM

The prominence and definition of unorthodox practices varies from generation to generation. With the development of scientific medicine and advances in treatment of acute and infectious disease in this century, interest in alternatives largely subsided. As the limitations of conventional medicine have become more obvious, interest in alternatives has risen. The medical and scientific response to claims of efficacy outside official medicine has a distinct pattern (7). Initially, orthodox groups either ignore these practices or attempt to undermine and suppress them by making them hard to access, by labeling them as quackery or pseudo-scientific, and by disciplining those that use them (8–10). Later, if the influence of these practices grows, the mainstream community begins to examine them, find similarities with what they already do, and selectively adopt practices into conventional medicine that easily fit (8, 9) (see also Chapter 1). Once these concepts are "integrated," the groups that originally held them are then considered mainstream, and those left on the fringes are again ignored and persecuted until their influence rises. This pattern of wholesale marginalization, followed by rapid but selective adoption, results in almost continual conflict between differing "camps" and wide fluctuations in resources and attention devoted to these areas–producing what Thomas Kuhn called "revolutions" in science and medicine (10).

How can the mainstream scientific and medical community responsibly address the "unofficial," "unorthodox," "fringe," and "alternative" on a less erratic, more regular, and more rational basis? Any approach must not completely ignore or attempt to eliminate important values, concepts, and activities that alternatives have to offer. At the same time it must not throw open medicine to dangerous practices that compromise the desirable quality and ethical and scientific standards in the conventional world. Any such process must create a space and provide resources whereby unconventional concepts and claims can officially be explored, developed, and accommodated. Given the diversity of concepts, languages, and perceptions about reality that these various systems hold, this process must intentionally incorporate methods for conflict resolution, knowledge management, and transparency (11, 12). Such a process must first systematically explore the reasons for alternative practices. It must then seek out the common, underlying concepts upon which change in both alternative and conventional practices can be based.

WHY IS THERE INCREASING INTEREST IN CAM?

The Potential Benefits of CAM

Many CAM practices have value for the way their practitioners manage health and disease. However, most of what is known about these practices comes from small clinical trials. For example, there is research showing the benefit of herbal products such as *ginkgo biloba* for improving dementia due to circulation problems (13) and possibly Alzheimer's (14); saw palmetto and other herbal preparations for treating benign prostatic hypertrophy (15, 16); and garlic for preventing heart disease (17). Over 24 placebo-controlled trials have been done with hypericum (St. John's wort) and have shown that it effectively treats depression. For mild to moderate depression, hypericum appears to be equally effective as conventional antidepressants, yet produces fewer side effects and costs less (18). The scientific quality of many trials, however, is poor.

As credible research continues on CAM, expanded options for managing clinical conditions will arise. In arthritis, for example, there are controlled trials reporting improvement with homeopathy (19), acupuncture (20), vitamin and nutritional supplements (21), botanical products (22, 23), diet therapies (24), mind–body approaches (25), and manipulation (26). Collections of (mostly small) studies exist for many other conditions, such as heart disease, depression, asthma, and addictions. The Cochrane Collaboration (with assistance from the

Research Council for Complementary Medicine in the United Kingdom) provides a continually updated list of randomized controlled trials in CAM. A summary of the number of controlled trials currently in that database by condition and modality is in Appendix (B) of this book. The database in available online through the NCCAM webpage and through the Cochrane Collaboration (see Chapter 5). With increasingly better research, more options and more rational and optimal CAM treatments can be developed. A diversity of credible approaches to disease is something that the public increasingly seeks (5a, 7).

The Potential Risks of CAM

Safety concerns of unregulated products and practices are also an important area for concern. Despite the presence of potential benefits, the amount of research on CAM systems and practices is nonetheless quite small when compared with conventional medicine. For example, there are more than 20,000 randomized controlled trials cited in the National Library of Medicine's bibliographic database, MEDLINE, on conventional cancer treatments, but only about 50 on alternative cancer treatments. As public use of CAM increases, limited information on the safety and efficacy of most CAM treatments creates a potentially dangerous situation. Although practices such as acupuncture, homeopathy, and meditation are low-risk, they must be used by fully competent and licensed practitioners to avoid inappropriate application (27). Herbs, however, can contain powerful pharmacological substances that can be toxic and produce herb–drug interactions (28). Some of these products may be contaminated and made with poor quality control, especially if shipped from Asia and India (29).

Reasons for Supplementary Role of CAM

Patients use CAM practices for a variety of reasons. For example, use of alternative therapies may be normative behavior in their social networks; they may be dissatisfied with conven-

tional care; and they may be attracted to CAM philosophies and health beliefs (5a, 30, 31). The overwhelming majority of those who use unconventional practices do so along with conventional medicine (32), thus corresponding to the implicit ideal of the phrase "complementary medicine." CAM is truly "alternative"–that is, used exclusively–for less than 5% of the population (31). Further, contrary to some opinions within conventional medicine, studies have found that patients who use CAM do *not* generally do so because of antiscience or anticonventional-medicine sentiment, nor because they are disproportionately uneducated, poor, seriously ill, or neurotic (30, 31, 33, 34). Instead, several salient beliefs and attitudes motivating CAM and characterizing CAM users can be identified.

PRAGMATISM

For the majority of patients, the choice to use unorthodox methods is largely pragmatic. They have a chronic disease for which orthodox medicine has been incomplete or unsatisfactory. Thus, we see many patients with chronic pain syndromes (low back pain, fibromyalgia, arthritis) or chronic and frequently fatal diseases (cancer, AIDS) seeking out CAM for supportive care (2, 30, 30a). An underlying characteristic of all of these conditions is that a specific cause of the disease either is unknown or cannot be stopped. Medical approaches did not work well with these conditions. Many CAM systems offer supportive care under these circumstances rather than addressing specific causes.

HOLISM

CAM users are attracted to certain philosophies and health beliefs (31). In medicine, this philosophy is reflected in the desire for a "holistic" approach to the patient. In reality, all therapy, whether conventional or alternative, is holistic in the sense that the whole person always responds. Any intervention–drugs, surgery, psychotherapy, acupuncture, or herbal treatments–affects the entire body and mind. For patients, holism often means attending to the psychosocial aspects of illness. CAM practitioners spend more time addressing psychosocial issues, leaving patients more satisfied than with their visits to conventional practitioners (35). This perspective also emphasizes using health enhancement in the treatment of the disease, and being proactive in addressing early warning and life style factors that put patients at risk (36, 36a).

LIFE STYLE

The emphasis on health promotion as an integral part of disease treatment is part of almost all CAM systems. Most of these systems use similar health enhancement approaches that cover five basic areas. These five areas are: a) stress management; b) spirituality and meaning issues (37); c) dietary and nutritional counseling; d) exercise and fitness; and e) addiction or habit management (especially tobacco and alcohol use) (38, 38a). All major CAM systems (and increasingly conventional approaches) make these areas primary in disease treatment (see chapters in Part III). Many patients find that the more they incorporate these activities into their lives, the less difficulty they have in managing chronic disease no matter what the cultural orientation (38, 38a, 39).

SPIRITUALITY

There is a surge of interest in the role of religion and spirituality in medical practice, research, and education (39a). The concept of "holism" often takes on the language of spirituality, in which patients seek a greater meaning in their suffering than is offered in conventional medicine (39b). Most CAM systems address spirituality and the meaning of suffering directly. Often they have their own special concepts and terms for how healing relates to the inner and outer forces of the spirit. Tibetan medicine (Chapter 14) and Native American medicine (Chapter 13) illustrate this most clearly. In anthroposophically-extended medicine, physicians receive conventional training and then get special instruction aimed at developing intuitive and spiritual sensitivity.

HEALING

When a specific cause is the dominant factor in an illness, it makes sense to direct a therapy toward that factor and then attempt to minimize the side effects of therapy. If a patient has an upper respiratory tract infection (URI) that develops into bacterial meningitis, for example, the healing action of the body has been overwhelmed by the cause, and the only hope of recovery is to eliminate the bacteria with high-dose antibiotics. However, if the URI becomes a chronic sinus problem, in which the efforts of the body are the dominant factor in the illness complex, a drug must act on the person to enhance (by stimulation or support) those self-healing efforts. Approaches for stimulating the immune system (e.g., acupuncture or herbs) or supporting auto-regulatory mechanisms (e.g., rest, fluids, dietary changes, relaxation and imagery) may be preferred. Most CAM systems aim to enhance the body's healing efforts but may not address a known cause. This characteristic of CAM is attractive to patients (40).

ADVERSE EFFECTS OF CONVENTIONAL THERAPIES

Patients are also concerned about the side effects of conventional medicine. Approximately 10% of hospitalizations are due to iatrogenic factors (41), and properly delivered conventional treatments are the sixth leading cause of death in the West (42). There is a perception among patients that orthodox treatments are too harsh, especially when used over long periods for chronic disease (43) and that CAM treatments are safer. Some interest in CAM is based on the myth that "natural" is somehow inherently safer than conventional medicine—an idea that is certainly not true (44, 45). Another misconception is that avoiding "harsh" orthodox treatments will result in better quality of life. This is also not necessarily true. For example, Cassileth showed that patients who underwent chemotherapy compared with those who underwent a dietary and life style treatment for cancer actually had slightly better quality of life scores (46).

COSTS

Concern over the escalating costs of conventional health care is another reason for the interest in CAM. Control of health care costs by improving efficiency in delivery and management of health care services has reached a maximum, and costs are expected to double in the next 10 years (47). Many developing countries are realizing that access to and affordability of conventional medicine are impossible for their population and that lower-cost, "traditional" medical approaches need to be developed (47a). Approaches that attempt to induce auto-regulation and self-healing and that rely on life style and self-care approaches may reduce such costs (39, 48).

The Democratization of Medicine

Several other social factors also influence the increasing interest in CAM. These include the rising prevalence of chronic disease with aging; increased access to health information in the media and over the Internet; and a declining faith that scientific breakthroughs will have relevant benefits for personal health; (49). An especially salient factor has been the "democratization" and "consumerization" of medical decision making (12, 50). The explosion of readily available information for the consumer and the ability to experience diverse cultures around the world have accelerated this process. Increasingly, patients wish to be active participants in their health care decisions. This participation includes evaluating information about treatment options, accessing products and practices that enable them to explore those options, and engaging in activities that may help them remain healthy (5a).

CAM AND STANDARDS OF EVIDENCE

New standards may be needed for the examination of both unconventional and conventional medicine (51, 54). Historically, medical science has benefited from the development of new methodologies, such as blinding and randomization which are first applied to unorthodox practices before being adopted as standards for all medicine (51–53).

Humans seem to have an infinite capacity to fool themselves and are constantly making spurious claims of truth, postulating unfounded explanations, and ignoring or denying the reality of observations they cannot explain or do not like. Science is one of the most powerful

tools for mitigating this self-delusionary capacity. However, the complexity of disease and the powerful healing capacity of the body often make it difficult to apply science to clinical medicine, especially when evaluating chronic disease (55, 56). K. B. Thomas demonstrated that nearly 80% of those who seek out medical care get better no matter what hand-waving or pill-popping is provided (57). This is called the "80 Percent Rule," meaning that data collected on novel therapies delivered in an enthusiastic clinical environment typically yield positive outcomes in 70 to 80% of patients (58).

Nonspecific Effects

Oftentimes our most accepted treatments are shown to be nonspecific in nature (59, 60, 60a) or even harmful (61) when finally studied rigorously. Their apparent effectiveness in practice is due to a variety of factors unrelated to the treatment, such as the ability of the body to heal (often enhanced by expectation), statistical regression to the mean (a measurement problem), and self-delusion (sometimes called bias) (58). It is not surprising that for the majority of physicians and patients, many therapies, both orthodox and unorthodox, seem to work. The methods of clinical research—especially blinding and the randomized controlled trial—have emerged as powerful approaches for better identifying to what extent the outcome can be attributed to the treatment. These methods must be used rigorously, however, if we wish to examine both the social and statistical forces that shape our perception of reality. As sophistication in clinical trials methods improves in order to better control for these nonspecific effects, however, the rigorous evaluation of chronic disease prevention and treatment approaches become more difficult and expensive (62).

Methods for Examining Chronic Disease Treatments

For these and a variety of other ethical, economic, and scientific reasons, it is very unlikely that all CAM (or conventional) therapies can be examined using large, rigorous, randomized trials (see Chapter 4). There are now sophisticated scientific methods for applying basic-science information to clinical practice and highly effective approaches for the management of trauma and acute and infectious diseases. Current methods for examining chronic disease or practices that have no explanatory model in Western terms, however, are not adequately informed by science. CAM offers the opportunity to test new approaches for examining these areas as their presence in medicine increases. For example, the development of observational and outcome research methods is being explored in CAM as a new approach for obtaining acceptable evidence for the use of low-risk therapies for treatment of chronic disease (63–65).

SYNERGISTIC EFFECTS

Most research on plant products is done to identify single active chemicals for drug development. Many herbal products, however, contain multiple chemical agents that may operate synergistically, producing effects with low amounts of multiple agents and lower risk for adverse effects. Standardization and quality production of herbals (necessary for producing safe and reliable products) may allow us to develop low-cost therapies with reduced risk over pharmaceuticals (16, 18).

CONSCIOUSNESS

Another frontier area with potentially profound implications for science and medicine is the area of consciousness and its relationship to statistical events and biological outcomes. For example, extensive research has documented that intention can have an influence on chance events (75a, 76, 76a) and living systems (77, 78). Traditional and indigenous healing practices from around the world universally assume that this is true and claim to use these "forces" in practices such as shamanism, spiritual healing, and prayer. Science now has the experimental methodology, sophisticated technology, and statistical expertise to examine this question precisely. If changes in consciousness do have significant effects, what potential might this have for diagnosis and treatment (79, 80)? What implications would this have for our methods of experimentation and the notion of "objectivity?" Research on unorthodox medical practices

allows us to begin serious scientific investigation of such areas.

ANOMALOUS FINDINGS

The unconventional basic-science assumptions that underlie some CAM practices provide opportunities to explore some of the deepest and most difficult enigmas of modern biology and medicine. Acupuncture, for example, was largely ignored in the United States until brought to national attention by a prominent reporter traveling with President Nixon in 1972. This led to basic science research and the discovery of its pain-relieving mechanisms (66). Another current enigma is whether biologically active nonmolecular information can be stored and transmitted through water or over wires, as claimed in homeopathy and electrodermal diagnosis (40, 67–72). Most scientists are unaware of the research in this area and claim that the concept is impossible. If some version of this claim were true, however, its potential implications for biology, pharmacology, and medical care are enormous. Data from clinical research on homeopathy do not support the expected assumption that homeopathy operates entirely like placebo (73–75). Basic research on homeopathy can help examine the accumulating anomalous observations and experiments in this area (40).

CENTRAL MODELS OF ETIOLOGY AND TREATMENT IN MEDICINE

What can we make of the diversity of CAM approaches? Are they an unrelated, socially defined, and shifting group of disparate practices, or do they have common concepts and central themes that tie them together and to conventional medicine? If so, how are these approaches similar to and different from modern Western medicine? Historically and cross-culturally, different medical systems have exhibited different understandings of disease causation and of factors relevant to etiology. Alongside this diversity are different approaches to identifying etiological factors and to addressing them in clinical practice. These diverse perspectives can be classified into (a) those that focus on a specific cause, and (b) those that emphasize complex systems of causative or antecedent factors. Alongside these two central perspectives on disease etiology, most major medical systems emphasize one of three approaches in the treatment of disease. These are (a) a hygiene-oriented or health-promotion approach, (b) approaches that induce or stimulate endogenous healing responses, and (c) approaches that oppose, interfere with, or eliminate disease causes and biological responses to those causes.

Figure 1 illustrates these different models of etiology and approaches to treatment. The "specific cause model" (1, Figure 1) attempts to identify the most prominent linear etiological pathway of the headache. This usually leads to a therapy that interferes with that pathway directly (opposition approach—a, Figure 1). Thus, in a patient who presents with a headache, an understanding of the pathophysiology of the headache is traced to vasospasm, and medication or biofeedback is provided to interfere with that pathway. Treatment is offered for only

those aspects of the illness that cross a predefined diagnostic threshold. The "systems model" (2, Figure 1) attempts to identify the web of etiological influences that contribute to the headache and their relationships to other covert problems or risks. Intervention targets the most prominent of these factors on multiple levels. Thus, a chronic headache patient who has other less prominent problems (fatigue, borderline blood pressure, insomnia, etc.) is treated with lifestyle changes and behavioral therapy addressing diet, exercise, relaxation skills, and drug or medication abuse (hygiene approach—b, Figure 1). The "wholistic model" (3, Figure 1) examines the patient's reactions to etiological agents and influences. Treatment approaches focus on improving resistance, restoring homeostatic "balance," or stimulating self-healing processes in the patient (induction approach—c, Figure 1). Thus, the headache patient may be given acupuncture to restore the balance of *chi*, a vasospastic agent (e.g., caffeine or belladonna alkaloids) to adjust autonomic reactivity, or a specifically selected homeopathic drug to restore auto-regulatory processes.

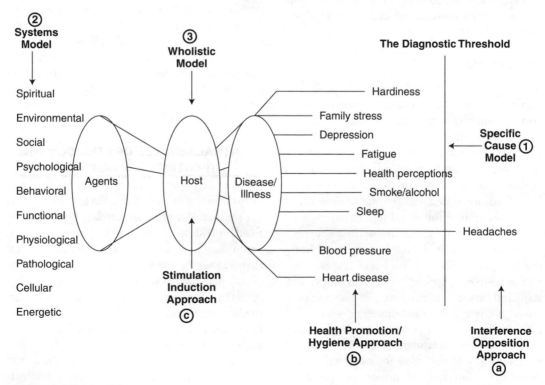

Figure 1. Models of disease treatment.

The Use and "Specialization" of Central Models in Medicine

The specific cause model, the systems model, and the wholistic models of etiology (and their frequently corresponding treatment approaches) allow us to better understand the relationship between various medical traditions. They help explain how quite varied interventions can produce restorative effects on similar diseases and how single interventions may affect a variety of conditions. In addition, they allow us to examine how different medical traditions have "specialized" in developing theories and interventions based around one or more aspects of agent/host interactions. All major medical systems use all three of these approaches when needed. Figure 1 illustrates how these common concepts of etiology and treatment can be used to "map" a particular medical system's emphasis. Conventional medicine frequently waits until a disease has crossed a certain diagnostic threshold before intervention is attempted. The treatment usually assumes a linear cause—effect pathway and uses a treatment designed to interfere with that specific pathway (combination 1.a in Figure 1). Many CAM (and some conventional) systems use the hygiene approach which intervenes prior to the diagnostic threshold and assumes that general multi-level support across systems is needed (combination 2.b in Figure 1). Many CAM systems assume complex etiologies may or may not wait until the diagnostic threshold is crossed. Finally, interventions may be aimed at altering the host response to multiple etiologies in a way that reestablishes homeostasis (combination 3.c in Figure 1).

While most major medical systems use all these etiological models and treatment approaches, some medical systems have developed approaches that emphasize particular levels as primary and have developed them extensively. In Native American and many indigenous medical systems, for example, the spiritual nature of the disease/healing complex is often emphasized. In these cultures, access to and interaction with patterns and forces in the spirit realms is considered a central focus for healing practices. Spirits are removed or opposed to stop a pathological process. In acupuncture and homeopathy, the "energetic" nature of disease/healing systems is emphasized. Patterns of "energy" assessed through history and physical examination are stimulated and balanced to induce a restorative response. In Ayurvedic medicine, the emphasis is on approaching illness through "consciousness," and entry into "pure consciousness" is the core of meditative and cleansing practices that support healing. Naturopathy, nutritional biotherapy, and orthomolecular medicine all contain elements that have their roots in the Greek "hygiene" approach, which used diet, plant remedies, baths, tonics, and other supplements as the central focus of intervention. Modern Western medicine addresses illness on the "naturalistic" level typically uses approaches that block a path in the disease/healing process or by removing a specific causal agent.

These central approaches are also used in conventional medicine today as since antiquity. If a person has an infection one is given an *anti*-biotic, a drug designed to kill the infecting agent. If one has inflammation and pain in the joints one is given an *anti*-inflammatory or analgesic (literally "against sensation"). These are examples of the "interference/opposition" approach as used in modern medicine. This approach has evolved tremendously over the last 50 years and is a very sophisticated component of modern medical treatment. This approach works well when a cause is simple, easily identified and dominates the disease/healing complex. Vaccination and allergy desensitization shots are examples of the "induction/stimulation" approach in modern medicine. Some drug treatments use the "induction" principle, too, such as Ritalin (a stimulant) for hyperactive (overstimulated) children and vaccines to induce resistance to disease. For the most part, modern drug therapy looks for chemicals that will stop or interfere with physiological processes involved in an illness and then try to manage the side effects separately. It is much easier to use the interference approach when a specific cause is known, which is one reason it is currently the dominant method. Finally, life style, diet, exercise, and other health promotion and support approaches were considered outside of mainstream medicine until the last 20 years or so, but have now become more accepted and widely used in modern medicine. These are examples of the "hygiene" approach that overlap conventional and complementary medicine.

THE INTEGRATION OF CAM AND CONVENTIONAL MEDICINE

If we, as health care practitioners, scientists, and educators, do not begin to examine more closely the social and scientific forces that shape medicine, then we are destined to relive much of the divisiveness that has characterized the past and current relationship between mainstream and nonmainstream medical care (81). To adopt CAM without developing quality standards for its practices, products, and research threatens to return us to a time in medicine when therapeutic confusion prevailed. Modern conventional medicine excels specifically in the provision of quality-controlled health care and the use of cutting-edge scientific findings. CAM must adopt similar standards. Conventional medicine is also the world's leader in the management of infectious, traumatic, and surgical diseases; in the study of pathology; and in biotechnology and drug development. All medical practices, conventional and unconventional alike, have the ethical obligation to retain these strengths for the benefit of patients (82).

At the same time, important characteristics of CAM are at risk of being lost in its "integration" with conventional care. The most important of these is an emphasis on self-healing as the lead approach for both improving wellness and treating disease. All of the major CAM systems approach illness by first trying to support and induce the self-healing processes of the patient. If this can stimulate recovery, then the likelihood of adverse effects and the need for high-impact/high-cost interventions are reduced. It is precisely this orientation toward self-healing and health promotion—what Antonovsky has termed salutogenesis as opposed to pathogenesis (84)—that makes CAM approaches to chronic disease especially attractive.

The rush to embrace a new integration of alternative and conventional medicine should be approached with great caution. Alternative medicine, like conventional medicine, has pros and cons, promotes bad ideas and good ones, and offers both benefits and risks. Without critical assessment of what should be integrated and what should not, we risk developing a health care system that costs more, is less safe, and fails to address the management of chronic disease in a publicly responsible manner. We must examine carefully the potential risks and benefits of CAM before we head into a new, but not necessarily better, health care world.

The Potential Risks of Integration

The potential risks of integration are easily identifiable, yet much resistance to their amelioration remains among CAM practitioners. These risks include issues related to quality of care, quality of products used in treatment, and quality of scientific research underlying CAM therapies.

QUALITY OF CARE

The formal components of medical doctor licensure are usually not required of various CAM providers. These requirements include the content and length of time of training, testing, and certification; a defined scope of practice; review and audit; and professional liability with regulatory protection and statutory authorization complete with codified disciplinary action (85). All 50 states provide licensure requirements for chiropractic, but only about half do so for acupuncture and massage therapy, and much fewer do for homeopathy and naturopathy. Many of these practitioners operate largely unmonitored (27) (see Chapter 2).

QUALITY OF PRODUCTS

The "natural" products used by CAM practitioners are largely unmonitored and their quality uncontrolled. These products are available on the market as "dietary supplements" and may be contaminated or vary tremendously in content, quality, and safety (86, 87). Garlic, for example, demonstrated to have cholesterol lowering effects for many years (17), may not produce such effects if processed in certain ways

(88). Thus, even if one product is proven safe and effective, other similar products on the market may have quite different effects that preclude consistent dosing. Fifteen million Americans are taking high-dose vitamins or herbs along with prescription drugs, thus risking adverse effects from unknown interactions (2) (see Part II, Chapters 6, 7, and 8).

Quality of Science

There is often no scientific foundation for a particular CAM practice—whether according to Western biomedicine or even to an alternative scientific world view (e.g., Ayurveda, traditional Chinese medicine). Most CAM systems have been around largely unchanged for hundreds or thousands of years. Many of these tenets originated from the teachings of a charismatic leader—tenets that have not been advanced with new observations, hypothesis-driven testing, innovation, and peer-review. Claiming that their practices are too "individual" or "holistic" to study scientifically, many CAM practitioners hide behind anecdotal, case-series, or outcomes research (89). To accept such views is to falsely label conventional medicine as "nonholistic" and to reject the hard fought gains made in the use of basic biological knowledge, randomized controlled clinical trials, and evidence-based medicine for health care decision making (90) (see Chapters 4 and 5).

The Potential Benefits of Integration

Among the potential benefits of integration, several in particular are especially valuable. The emergence of a truly integrated medicine promises to shift medicine's emphasis to the total healing process, to reduce unnecessary side effects, and to reduce the costs of care.

Emphasis on Healing

Most CAM systems carefully attend to the illness and suffering that accompanies all disease. Patients are often more satisfied with their interactions with unorthodox than orthodox medical practitioners (35). Patients require understanding, meaning, and self-care methods for managing their condition. Empowerment, participation in the healing process, time, and personal attention are essential elements of all medical care, yet these elements are easily lost in the subspecialization, technology, and economics of modern medicine. By increasingly being integrated into mainstream medical practice, CAM promises to restore to medicine a more focused emphasis on the healing process.

Reduction in Side Effects

In the eighteenth century, unconventional medical practices increased in popularity in part because they eschewed the use of severe treatments such as bloodletting, purging, and use of toxic metals—all staples of conventional medicine at one time (91). The popularity of CAM in this century is also driven by the perception that conventional treatments are too harsh to use for chronic and non-life-threatening diseases (30, 31). Iatrogenic disease from conventional medicine is a major cause of death and hospitalization in the United States (43). Although some CAM practices may introduce toxicity, many of them offer reduced potential for adverse effects when properly delivered (45). Unconventional medicine may help us "gentle" our approach by focusing on the patient's inherent capacity for self-healing (84).

Reduction in Costs

The skyrocketing costs of conventional medicine also drive the search for medical alternatives. Savings from managed care are now maximized, and health care costs are predicted to double within the next 10 years (47). If low-cost interventions, such as life style changes, diet and supplement therapy, and behavioral medicine, can be delivered as substitutes for high-cost drugs and technological interventions, true cost reductions and reductions in morbidity may be achieved (48).

Science and Healing

Today we have discovered more scientific ways of deciding how to counter and oppose disease causes, but very little research has been done on the support and induction of healing processes. This has made the interference/opposition approach (see Figure 1) much more useful than in the past, and is one of the reasons for the tremendous rise in the use of these kinds of therapies around the world. Technology has provided another impetus for this growth. Biotechnology allows for finer dissection of disease causes and for development of scientific methods to manipulate these causes. The usefulness of this approach, however, is limited to those diseases in which there are only a few causes and they have been clearly identified. For illnesses of multifactorial or unknown causation (as in most chronic diseases), this approach is not very useful for producing long-term healing. Unfortunately, application of the scientific method to the study of the induction and hygiene approaches is still in its early stages. As investigation of conventional practices (e.g., physical therapy, dietary therapy, and immunization) and of CAM systems (e.g., acupuncture, homeopathy, and manipulation) increases, a science of healing may emerge.

WHAT PHYSICIANS NEED TO KNOW ABOUT CAM

For physicians to be able to help their patients choose the most rapid, safest, and most effective long-term solutions for treating disease and alleviating suffering, certain basic knowledge and skills are needed. Understanding the fundamental assumptions of etiology and treatment of medical systems—both conventional and unconventional—is crucial. When specific causes are known and effective methods for intervention exist, approaches that can interfere with those causes are key to successful treatment. When specific causes are unknown or complex contributory influences are dominant in a disease, approaches that support health and induce healing become primary. Sometimes a combination of approaches is needed, whereby causes are blocked and healing mechanisms are stimulated and supported. An optimal practice makes flexible use of what best fits the clinical situation.

To respond appropriately, physicians and other health care practitioners must be able to obtain information about the history of self-treatment by their patients and must communicate to them the results of the best current research evidence. Practitioners need a variety of skills: communicating with patients, documenting patient encounters with alternative therapies, evaluating and applying modern principles of scientific evidence and medical ethics, and understanding the current quality and liability status of CAM medical treatments. Finally, practitioners should become familiar with the basic principles of treatment for specific CAM systems as well as the current evidence of benefit or harm from these systems. This information is required for the careful and thoughtful management of patients, many of whom have already visited alternative practitioners. This basic knowledge of common CAM practices will be an indispensable component of medical information in the twenty-first century.

REFERENCES

1. Hastings Center Report. The goals of medicine: setting new priorities. Briarcliff Manor, NY: The Hastings Center, 1996.
2. Eisenberg DM, Davis RB, Ettner S, et al. Trends in alternative medicine use in the United States 1990–1997: results of a follow-up national survey. JAMA 1998;280:1569–1575.
3. Wetzel MS, Eisenberg DM, Kaptchuk TJ. A survey of courses involving complementary and alternative medicine at United States medical schools. JAMA 1998;280:784–787.
4. Pelletier KR, Marie A, Krasner M, Haskell WL. Current trends in the integration and reimbursement of complementary and alternative medicine by managed care, insurance carriers, and hospital providers. Am J Health Prom 1997;12:112–123.
5. Marwick C. Alterations are ahead at the OAM. JAMA 1998;280:1553–1554.
5a. Kelner M, Wellman B, eds. Complementary and alternative medicine: challenge and change. Reading, England: Gordon & Breach. In press.
6. McKinlay JB. From "promising report" to "standard procedure": seven stages in the career of a medical innovation. Milbank Memorial Fund Quarterly/Health and Society 1981;59:374–411.
7. Hufford DJ. Cultural and social perspectives on alternative medicine: background and assumptions. Alt Therap Health Med 1995;1:53–61.

8. Gevitz N. Other healers: unorthodox medicine in America. Baltimore: The Johns Hopkins University Press, 1988.

9. Inglis B. The case for unorthodox medicine. New York: GP Putnam's Sons, 1965.

10. Kuhn TS. The structure of scientific revolutions. 2nd ed. Chicago: University of Chicago Press, 1962.

11. Hufford DJ. Authority, knowledge, and substituted judgement, part II. Alt Therap Health Med 1996;2:92–94.

12. Hufford DJ. Authority, knowledge, and substituted judgement, part II. Alt Therap Health Med 1997;3:86–89.

13. Kleijnen J, Knipschild P. Gingko biloba for cerebral insufficiency. Br J Clin Pharm 1992;34:352–358.

14. Le Bars PL, Katz MM, Berman N, et al. A placebo-controlled, double-blind, randomized trial of an extract of ginkgo biloba for dementia. JAMA 1997;278:1327–1332.

15. Di Silverio F, Flammia GP, Sciarra A, et al. Plant extracts in BPH. Minerva Urol Nefrol 1993;45:143–149.

16. Wilt TJ, Ishani A, Stark G, et al. Saw palmetto extracts for treatment of benign prostatic hyperplasia. JAMA 1998;280:1604–1609.

17. Neil A, Silagy C. Garlic: its cardio-protective properties. Curr Opin Lipidol 1994;5:6–10.

18. Linde K, Ramirez G, Mulrow CD, et al. St John's wort for depression—an overview and meta-analysis of randomised clinical trials. BMJ 1996;313:253–258.

19. Gibson RG, Gibson S, MacNeill AD, Watson BW. Homeopathic therapy in rheumatoid arthritis: evaluation by double-blind clinical therapeutical trial. Br J Clin Pharm 1980;9:453–459.

20. Berman BM, Lao L, Greene M, et al. Efficacy of traditional Chinese acupuncture in the treatment of symptomatic knee osteoarthritis: a pilot study. Osteoarthritis Cartilage 1995;3:139–142.

21. Jonas WB, Rapoza CP, Blair WF. The effect of niacinamide on osteoarthritis: a pilot study. Inflamm Res 1996;45:330–334.

22. Tao XL, Dong Y, Zhang NZ. [A double-blind study of T2 (tablets of polyglycosides of Tripterygium wilfodii hook) in the treatment of rheumatoid arthritis]. Chung-Hua Nei Ko Tsa Chih 1987;26:399–402, 444–445. Chinese.

23. Altman RD. Capsaicin cream 0.025% as monotherapy for osteoarthritis: a double-blind study. Semin Arthritis Rheum 1994;23:25–33.

24. Kjeldsen-Kragh J, Mellbye OJ, Haugen M, et al. Changes in laboratory variables in rheumatoid arthritis patients during a trial of fasting and one-year vegetarian diet. Scand J Rheumatol 1995;24:85–93.

25. Lavigne JV, Ross CK, Berry SL, et al. Evaluation of a psychological treatment package for treating pain in juvenile rheumatoid arthritis. Arthritis Care Res 1992;5:101–110.

26. Assendelft WJ, Koes BW, Knipschild PG, Bouter LM. The relationship between methodological quality and conclusions in reviews of spinal manipulation. JAMA 1995;274:1942–1948.

27. Boards FoSM. Report on Health Care Fraud from the Special Committee on Health Care Fraud. Austin, TX: Federation of State Medical Boards of the United States, Inc., 1997.

28. De Smet PAGM, Keller K, Hänsel R, Chandler RF. Adverse effects of herbal drugs. Heidelberg: Springer-Verlag, 1997.

29. Bensoussan A, Myers SP. Towards a safer choice. Victoria, Australia: University of Western Sydney Macarthur, 1996.

30. Furnham A, Forey J. The attitudes, behaviors and beliefs of patients of conventional vs. complementary (alternative) medicine. J Clin Psychol 1994;50:458–469.

30a. O'Connor BB. Healing traditions, alternative medicines and the health professions. Philadelphia: University of Philadelphia Press, 1995.

31. Astin JA. Why patients use alternative medicine: results of a national study. JAMA 1998;279:1548–1553.

32. Eisenberg DM, Kessler RC, Foster C, et al. Unconventional medicine in the United States—prevalence, costs, and patterns of use. N Engl J Med 1993;328:246–252.

33. Cassileth BR, Lussk EJ, Strouss TB, Bodenheimer BJ. Contemporary unorthodox treatments in cancer medicine: a study of patients, treatments, and practitioners. Ann Intern Med 1984;101:105–112.

34. Vincent C, Furnham A, Willsmore M. The perceived efficacy of complementary and orthodox medicine in complementary and general practice patients. Health Education: Theory and Practice 1995;10:395–405.

35. Ernst E, Resch KL, Hill S. Do complementary practitioners have a better bedside manner than physicians? [letter]. J R Soc Med 1997;90:118–119.

36. Chesworth J. The ecology of health: identifying issues and alternatives. Thousand Oaks, CA: Sage, 1996.

36a. Dacher ES. A systems theory approach to an expanded medical model: a challenge for biomedicine. J Altern Complement Med 1995;2:187–196.

37. Kleinman A, Eisenberg L, Good B. Culture, illness, and care: clinical lessons from anthropologic and cross-cultural research. Ann Intern Med 1978;88:251–258.

38. McCamy JC, Presley J. Human life styling—keeping whole in the 20th century. New York: Harper Colophon Books, 1975:191.

38a. Ornish D, Scherwitz LW, Billings JH, et al. Intensive lifestyle changes for reversal of coronary heart disease. JAMA 1998;280:2001–2007.

39. Orme-Johnson DW. An innovative approach to reducing medical care utilization and expenditures. Am J Man Care 1997;3:135–144.

39a. Levin JS, Larson DB, Puchalski CM. Religion and spirituality in medicine: research and education. JAMA 1997;278:792–793.

39b. Dossey L. Meaning and medicine. New York: Bantum Books, 1991.

40. Jonas WB, Jacobs J. Healing with homeopathy. New York: Warner, 1996.

41. Steel K, Gertman PM, Crescenzi C, Anderson J. Iatrogenic illness on a general medical service at a university hospital. N Engl J Med 1981;304:638–

42. Lazarou J, Pomeranz BH, Corey PN. Incidence of adverse drug reactions in hospitalized patients: a meta-analysis of prospective studies. JAMA 1998;279:1200–1205.

43. Vincent C, Furnham A. Why do patients turn to complementary medicine? An empirical study. Br J Clin Psychol 1996;35:37–48.

44. Ernst E. Bitter pills of nature: safety issues in complementary medicine. Pain 1995;60:237–238.

45. Jonas WB. Safety in complementary medicine. In: Ernst E, ed. Complementary medicine: an objective appraisal. Oxford: Butterworth-Heinemann, 1996:126–149.

46. Cassileth BR, Lusk EJ, Guerry D, et al. Survival and quality of life among patients on unproven versus conventional cancer therapy. N Engl J Med 1991;324:1180–1185.

47. Smith S, Freeland M, Heffler S, et al. The next ten years of health spending: what does the future hold? Health Affairs 1998;17:128–140.

47a. Panel on Traditional Medicine. Developing a research agenda for traditional medicine. Bodeker J, ed. Bethesda, MD: National Institutes of Health, 1997.

48. Sobel DS. Rethinking medicine: improving health outcomes with cost-effective psychosocial interventions. Psychosom Med 1995;57:234–44.

49. Fox E. Predominance of the curative model of medical care: a residual problem. JAMA 1997;278:761–763.

50. Starr P. The social transformation of American medicine. San Francisco: Basic Books (a division of Harper Collins Publishers), 1982:514.

51. Eddy DM. Should we change the rules for evaluating medical technologies. In: Gelijns AC, ed. Modern methods of clinical investigation. Washington, DC: National Academy Press, 1990:117–134.

52. Horton R. The rhetoric of research. BMJ 1995;310:985–987.

53. Kaptchuk TJ. Intentional ignorance: the history of blind assessment and placebo controls in medicine. Bull Hist Med 1998;72:389–433.

54. Leibrich J. Measurement of efficacy: a case for holistic research. Comp Med Res 1990;4:21–25.

55. Taylor JFN. Clinical trials and the acceptance of uncertainty. BMJ 1987;294:1111–1112.

56. Egger M, Smith GD. Misleading meta-analysis. BMJ 1995;310.

57. Thomas KB. The placebo in general practice. Lancet 1994;344:1066–1067.

58. Jonas WB. Therapeutic labeling and the 80% rule. Bridges 1994:5:1, 4–6.

59. Roberts AH, Kewman DG, Mercier L, Hovell M. The power of nonspecific effects in healing: implications for psychological and biological treatments. Clin Psychol Rev 1993;13:375–391.

60. Bowers TG, Clum GA. Relative contribution of specific and nonspecific treatment effects: meta-analysis of placebo-controlled behavior therapy research. Psychol Bull 1988;103:315–323.

60a. Kirsch I, Spirstein G. Listening to Prozac but hearing placebo: a meta-analysis of antidepressant medication. Prevention Treatment 1998;1:0002a.

61. Pratt CM. The cardiac arrhythmia suppression trial. Introduction: the aftermath of the CAST–a reconsideration of traditional concepts. Am J Cardiol 1990;65:1b–2b.

62. Colditz GA, Miller JN, Mosteller F. How study design affects outcomes in comparisons of therapy. I: Medical. Stat Med 1989;8:441–454.

63. Melchart D, Linde K, Liao JZ, et al. Systematic clinical auditing in complementary medicine: rationale, concept, and a pilot study. Alt Therap Health Med 1997;3:33–39.

64. Standish LJ, Calabrese C, Reeves C, et al. A scientific plan for the evaluation of alternative medicine in the treatment of HIV/AIDS. Alt Therap Health Med 1997;3:58–67.

65. Pincus T. Analyzing long-term outcomes of clinical care without randomized controlled clinical

trials: the consecutive patient questionnaire database. Advances 1997;13:3–31.

66. Pomeranz B. Acupuncture research related to pain, drug addiction and nerve regeneration. In: Pomeranz B, Stux G, eds. Scientific bases of acupuncture. Berlin, Heidelberg: Springer-Verlag, 1989:35–52.

67. Scofield AM. Experimental research in homoeopathy. Br Hom J 1984;73:161–181, 211–225.

68. Davenas E, Beauvais J, Oberbaum M, et al. Human basophil degranulation triggered by very dilute antiserum against IgE. Nature 1988;333: 816–818.

69. Ovelgonne JH, Bol AW, Hop WC, van Wijk R. Mechanical agitation of very dilute antiserum against IgE has no effect on basophil staining properties. Experientia 1992;48:504–508.

70. Linde K, Jonas WB, Melchart D, et al. Critical review and meta-analysis of serial agitated dilutions in experimental toxicology. Hum Exp Toxicol 1994;13:481–492.

71. Bellavite P, Signorini A. Homeopathy–a frontier in medical science. Berkeley, CA: North Atlantic Books, 1995:335.

72. van Wijk R, Wiegant FAC. The similia principle as a therapeutic strategy: a research program on stimulation of self-defense in disordered mammalian cells. Alt Therap Health Med 1997;3:33–38.

73. Kleijnen J, Knipschild P, Riet ter G. Clinical trials of homoeopathy. Br Med J 1991;302:316–323.

74. Linde K, Clausius N, Ramirez G, et al. Are the clinical effects of homeopathy all placebo effects? A meta-analysis of randomized, placebo controlled trials. Lancet 1997;350:834–843.

75. Boissel JP, Cucherat M, Haugh M, Gauthier E. Critical literature review on the effectiveness of homoeopathy: overview of data from homoeopathic medicine trials. Brussels: Homoeopathic Medicine Research Group. Report to the European Commission, 1996.

75a. Jahn RG, Dunne BJ. Margins of reality. The role of consciousness in the physical world. New York: Harcourt Brace Jovanovick, 1987.

76. Radin DI, Nelson RD. Evidence for consciousness-related anomalies in random physical systems. Foundations of Physics 1989;19:1499–1514.

76a. Radin DI. The conscious universe: the scientific truth behind psychic phenomena. San Francisco: HarperEdge, 1997.

77. Braud WG, Schlitz MJ. Consciousness interactions with remote biological systems: anomalous intentionality effects. Subtle Energies 1992;2:1–46.

78. Schlitz M, Braund W. Distant intentionality and healing: assessing the evidence. Alt Therap Health Med 1997;3:62–73.

79. Bem DJ, Honorton C. Does psi exist? Replicable evidence for and anomalous information transfer. Psychol Bull 1994;115:4–18.

80. Benor DJ. Intuitive diagnosis. Subtle Energies 1992;3:41–64.

81. Jonas WB. Alternative medicine–learning from the past, examining the present, advancing the future. JAMA 1998;280:1616–1618.

82. Chez RA, Jonas WB. The challenge of complementary and alternative medicine. Am J Obstet Gynecol 1997;177:1156–1161.

83. Deleted.

84. Antonovsky A. Unraveling the mystery of health: how people manage stress and stay well. San Francisco: Jossey-Bass, 1987.

85. Fund MM. Enhancing the accountability of alternative medicine. New York: Milbank Memorial Fund, 1998.

86. Ernst E. Harmless herbs? A review of recent literature. Am J Med 1998;104:170–178.

87. Angell M, Kassirer JP. Alternative medicine–the risks of untested and unregulated remedies. N Engl J Med 1998;339:839–841.

88. Berthold HK, Sudhop MD, von Bergmann K. Effect of a garlic oil preparation on serum lipoproteins and cholesterol metabolism. JAMA 1998; 279:1900–1902.

89. Coulter HL. The controlled clinical trial: an analysis. Washington, DC: Center for Empirical Medicine, 1991.

90. Jonas WB. Clinical trials for chronic disease: randomized, controlled clinical trials are essential. J NIH Res 1997;9:33–39.

91. Worton JC. The history of complementary and alternative medicine. In: Jonas WB, Levin JS, eds. Essentials of complementary and alternative medicine. Philadelphia: Lippincott Williams & Wilkins, 1999.

CHAPTER 1

The History of Complementary and Alternative Medicine

James C. Whorton

GENERAL CONSIDERATIONS

The notion of *complementary* medicine—the possibility that treatments not commonly employed or recognized by the allopathic medical profession might be combined with the conventional therapeutic armamentarium to balance and complete it—has appeared only recently. Before the 1990s, unconventional therapies were largely dismissed by the American medical profession as opposed to and incompatible with scientific medical practice. Even the term *alternative*, which has been used since the 1970s, would not have been acceptable to the allopathic practitioners of previous generations; it would have conferred too much respectability, implying that non-allopathic remedies might be an equal, if separate, option. Historically, the phrases preferred by mainstream physicians have been *irregular medicine, fringe medicine, sectarian medicine, medical cultism,* and *quackery*—all pejorative terms. To avoid such dismissive language as well as to maintain consistency, the term *alternative medicine* is used throughout this chapter.

However, if our present willingness to think of alternative medicine as complementary signifies the opening of a new era, we can hardly expect to make a clean break with the past. The story of complementary medicine's years as despised alternative medicine is one of unceasing conflict with the medical establishment, during which an untold amount of bad feeling accumulated on both sides. If alternative medicine is to be enfranchised scientifically and professionally, if it is to become complementary in fact and not just in aspiration, this historical legacy of mutual ill will must be addressed and overcome.

An awareness of the historical development of complementary medicine is essential for understanding the philosophical orientation that binds together many alternative systems of practice. Whether an alternative system proclaims itself to be natural healing (the favored description in nineteenth-century parlance), drugless healing (the term popular during the early twentieth century), or holistic healing (the label since the 1970s), alternative medicine has consistently, from its beginnings in the late 1700s, seen itself as offering a distinctive approach to therapy and to physician–patient interactions. That distinctive outlook is drawn, ironically, from the work of the very same physician whom orthodox practitioners revere as the "father" of their medicine—Hippocrates. Complementary medical philosophy might thus be thought of as the Hippocratic heresy.

ORIGINS OF ALTERNATIVE MEDICINE

I am stating only what everybody knows to be true, when I say that the general confidence which has heretofore existed in the science and art of medicine . . . has within the last few years been violently shaken and disturbed, and is now greatly lessened and impaired. The hold which medicine has so long had upon the popular mind is loosened; there is a widespread skepticism as to its power of curing diseases, and men are everywhere to be found who deny its pretensions as a science, and reject the benefits and blessings which it proffers them as an art (1).

This complaint sounds modern enough, something that might have appeared in last week's *JAMA*. In fact, it was issued in 1848. At that time (as with today), the clearest sign of erosion of public confidence in allopathic medicine was the rapid growth over the preceding two decades of rival healing systems that claimed to be safer and more effective than conventional medicine. Those systems began to appear at the turn of the century, largely as protests against the bleeding, purging, and other heroic measures practiced by physicians of the day; however, there were more reasons for revolt than dissatisfaction with standard therapies. There had been alternatives to conventional methods of cure before the 1800s: both folk medicine and quackery had been options for centuries. But the different versions of alternative medicine, as they were derisively labelled even through the early decades of the twentieth century, were a distinct departure. They were actual *systems* of care, the practitioners of each being bound together not just by their opposition to the medical establishment, but also by shared theoretical precepts and therapeutic regimens: by membership in local, state, even national societies and by publication of their own journals and operation of their own schools. Essentially, they were professionalized. And by the

end of the 1840s, this medical counterculture had cornered roughly 10% of the health care market (2–6).

Thomsonianism, Homeopathy, Hydropathy, and Mesmerism

Thomsonianism was the first alternative system to be developed in America. It involved a program of botanical healing formulated in the 1790s by Samuel Thomson, a New Hampshire farmer. His combinations of plant drugs that either evacuated or heated the body (e.g., the emetic lobelia, cayenne pepper enemas) were warmly received by the public of the 1820s and 1830s. However, the system quickly foundered after Thomson's death in 1843 (7). Homeopathy, the system formulated by the German physician Samuel Hahnemann in the 1790s, established a foothold in the United States in the 1830s. Derived from Greek roots meaning "like the disease," homeopathy treated constellations of symptoms with drugs that had been found to produce the very same symptoms in healthy people—i.e., like cured like. Homeopathic remedies were claimed to work most effectively after being carried through a series of dilutions that essentially removed all the matter of the original drug before the preparation was given to the patient; molecularly speaking, homeopathic remedies were "infinitesimals." Hahnemann also coined the term *allopathy*—"other than the disease"—to signify the orthodox philosophy of neutralizing complaints with therapies opposite to the symptoms. By the mid-1800s, all alternative medical groups had embraced *allopathic* as the standard term for orthodox medicine; only in recent years has the word shed its negative connotations. Homeopathy was easily the most popular alternative system by midcentury, and would remain so into the early 1900s (8–9).

The next most popular medical alternative at midcentury was hydropathy, an Austrian creation of the 1820s imported into the United States in the early 1840s. The water-cure, as Americans liked to call it, stimulated the body to rid itself of disease through a variety of baths (usually cold), supplemented with careful regulation of lifestyle (e.g., diet, exercise, sleep, dress). Hydropathy maintained a sizeable following into the 1860s, but steadily faded after the Civil War (10–12). During this time in America, the rise and fall of Mesmerism, or magnetic healing, occurred. The invention of eighteenth-century Austrian physician Franz Mesmer, magnetic therapy relied on hypnotism and the power of suggestion to relieve patients; Mary Baker Eddy, the founder of Christian Science in the 1870s, was highly influenced by this therapy (13). Finally, eclecticism, as its name implies, was an assortment of therapies selected from all schools of practice, allopathic and alternative, on the basis of clinical experience. Originated by New York practitioner Wooster Beach in the late 1820s, eclectic medicine lasted into the 1930s (14).

THE SECOND GENERATION OF ALTERNATIVE MEDICAL SYSTEMS

Less successful challengers of allopathic medicine—Baunscheidtism, chronothermalism, physiomedicalism, and other medical *isms*—might also be mentioned to complete the antebellum generation of alternative systems. A second wave appeared in the later nineteenth century, beginning with osteopathy, a technique of musculoskeletal manipulation originated by Andrew Taylor Still in the 1870s. However, the first osteopathic school would not begin operation until 1892 (15). The first school of chiropractic opened its doors in 1895, the same year that the manipulation method was discovered by Daniel David Palmer in Davenport, Iowa (16). During the last few years of the century, German emigre Benedict Lust blended the new manipulation procedures with hydropathic philosophy and treatments, herbal tradition, and other natural remedies to create naturopathy (17). By then, nearly 20% of all practitioners of medicine were alternative physicians, up from the estimated 10% of the 1850s; in 1900 in America, there were approximately 110,000 allopaths, 10,000 homeopaths, 5000 eclectics, and another 5000 practitioners of other alternative systems (18–19). Acupuncture

has more recently been rediscovered; there was some experimentation with acupuncture in Europe and America in the nineteenth century. Reports of its efficacy by travelers to China in 1970 triggered an explosion of interest not only in acupuncture, but also in all aspects of traditional Chinese medicine and in Ayurveda, the ancient healing system of India (20).

ALTERNATIVE MEDICINE'S CRITIQUE OF ALLOPATHIC MEDICINE

Despite the differences between Hahnemann's and Thomson's drug, or between Palmer's and Still's theories, the philosophy of healing and its implicit critique of allopathy was (and remains) the same for all alternative systems. That philosophy was presented in a cartoon published in 1834, in the first issue of *The Thomsonian Botanic Watchman*, at the very beginning of the clash between orthodoxy and the new medical heretics (Fig. 1.1). This Thomsonian cartoonist shows a man mired in the slough of disease, despite—actually, because of—the ministrations of an allopathic doctor. The physician is attempting to bludgeon the disease into submission with a club labelled *calomel*. Calomel (mercurous chloride) was the most popular purgative in nineteenth century medical practice; in fact, with the possible exception of opium, it was the most frequently prescribed drug. As a mercurial, it could (and often did) produce severe side effects: ulceration of the mouth, loss of teeth, necrosis of the jawbone, and, most typically, a profuse, thick, fetid salivation. In the cartoon, the MD is assuring his patient that, "You must be reduced, Sir!," intending that the disease will be reduced by calomel's cleansing of the intestinal tract. The patient, however, fears that he is being reduced to the grave: "The Doctor knows best," he moans facetiously, "but send for the Parson." In the middle of the picture, an objective observer attempts to get the doctor's attention, to show him there is a better way, the way of the Thomsonian healer to the right, who rescues the patient by pulling him up the steps of common sense (21).

By depicting the allopathic physician as

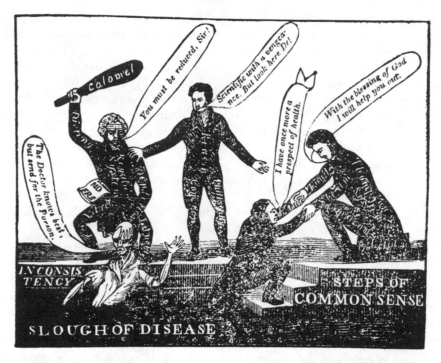

FIGURE 1.1. The Contrast; or an illustration of the difference between the regular and Thomsonian systems of practice in restoring the sick to health.

seemingly "holding his patient down," depicting calomel as a club, and having the patient call for the parson, the Thomsonian cartoonist is suggesting that allopathy attacks disease so brashly as to indiscriminately overwhelm the patient, too; its therapies are, in the language of a later day, invasive. However, Thomsonian remedies are indicated to be gentle and natural, and to support and enhance the body's own innate recuperative powers: "I will help you out," the Thomsonian doctor tells the patient, "with the blessing of God." He might as well say, "with the blessing of nature" because, in nineteenth century thought, God and nature were implicitly one. Thomsonians often stated the matter explicitly though, Thomson himself declaring that nature "ought to be aided in its cause, and treated as a friend; and not as an enemy, as is the practice of the physicians." His approach had "always been ... to learn the course pointed out by nature," then to administer "those things best calculated to aid her in restoring health" (22). He hardly stood alone. Most alternative practitioners, in his day and

the present, professed to consult and cooperate with the *vis medicatrix naturae*, the healing power of nature first described and praised by Hippocrates:

- "All healing power is inherent in the living system." (Russell Trall, hydropath, 1864) (23)
- "Naturopathy, with all its various methods of treatments, has always one end in view and one only: to increase the vital force." (Benedict Lust, naturopath, 1903) (24)
- Osteopathic manipulation removes obstacles to "the free flow of the blood ... and with the lifting of this embargo nature itself does the necessary work to restore the body to its normal state and even beyond it .... Osteopathy fights on the side of nature." (M. A. Lane, osteopath, 1925) (25)

In Figure 1.1, the diploma hanging from the physician's coat pocket is as prominent as his calomel club. Emblazoned with the MD, the diploma is emblematic to Thomsonians of the abstruse theoretical training the allopath has received and that dictates his practice. As the person in the middle of the figure observes, the allopathic physician is "scientific with a vengeance," hellbent on doing what theory tells him ought to work, oblivious to the common sense that would show him he is poisoning his patient. But the error of his allopathic way is not just that he makes the sick even sicker with misguided therapies; his devotion to theory, the cartoonist suggests, prevents him from even attempting a fair evaluation of alternate remedies, remedies that cannot be rationalized by, or that seem to conflict with, his science.

Hence, from the onset, homeopathic drugs were laughed at by allopaths because of what seemed the theoretical simple-mindedness of the "like cures like" principle and the impossibility of infinitesimals exerting any material action. Still's musculoskeletal manipulations were dismissed because of the perceived naivete of his "rule of the artery" theory; Palmer's chiropractic adjustments were dismissed because of the apparent silliness of the vertebral subluxation model; and acupuncture in the early 1970s was dismissed because of the alien concepts of *qi* and energy meridians. The recent response of a university medical scientist to reports of clinical trials showing that patients who are prayed for recover better than those who do not receive prayers is a wonderfully direct summary of this historical attitude: "That's the kind of crap I wouldn't believe," this scientist is reported to have said, "even if it were true." (L. Dossey, unpublished). Complementary physicians contend that the scientific medical establishment has always had a negative attitude about complementary methods—most allopaths refuse to believe them even if they are true because they make no sense in terms of conventional science. Like the doctor in the cartoon, MDs as a group are seen by alternative practitioners to be scientific with a vengeance.

Alternative Medicine's Emphasis on Empiricism

Alternative practitioners have never relied on purely theoretical determinants of practice, maintaining their methods have been derived largely from empirical bases. With the exception of Mesmerism, alternative medical systems originated from the founder's therapeutic experiences, initially untainted by the influence of speculative hypothesis. Hahnemann claimed for his *materia medica* that it was "free from all conjecture, fiction, or gratuitous assertion—it shall contain nothing but the pure language of nature, the results of a careful and faithful research" (26). Likewise, Thomson "had nothing to guide him but his own experience .... His mind was unshackled by the visionary theories ... of others; his whole studies have been in the great book of nature" (27). The power of musculoskeletal manipulation was discovered by Still through practical trials on his neighbors and by Palmer during an experiment on his janitor. Alternative systems have consistently started through what today would be described as observational, or outcome, studies.

Once a therapeutic method was determined to have positive outcomes, however, the temptation to explain it was almost never resisted, and theoretical rationalizations were soon forthcoming. Eclecticism alone was able to stand firm with an "it works, who cares how" attitude; all other systems quickly surrendered to the lure of conjecture and visionary theories. Hahnemann conjectured his infinitesimals operated through dynamic—i.e., spiritual—action. Thomson theorized his empirically demonstrated herbs worked by promoting the distribution of life-sustaining heat through the system. Still hypothesized a "rule of the artery" that restored the body to health as soon as skeletal pressures on blood vessels were relieved by manipulation. Palmer imagined that vertebral subluxations constricted nerves and impeded the flow of Innate Intelligence, a divine life force, through the body. Alternative practitioners, in other words, generally reversed the process attributed to allopathic physicians. Instead of formulating a theory, then deducing therapy from it—the allopathic model—they discovered a therapy, then deduced a theory. And invariably, the theoretical principle that followed was that the therapy in question worked by eliminating some obstacle to the free functioning of the body's innate healing power. Ultimately, it was nature that did the curing, not the manipulation or the infinitesimal similar or the cayenne in the enema. Those original theoretical formulations would eventually be recognized by adherents as unfounded and confining, and during the twentieth century they have been steadily abandoned for more sophisticated and demonstrable arguments (although nature remains the fundamental healing power). But the initial dedication of many alternative systems to a simple, all-inclusive theory gave alternative medicine the appearance of sectarian fanaticism in allopaths' eyes.

HOLISTIC MEDICINE IN THE NINETEENTH CENTURY

The Thomsonian in Figure 1.1 is extending a fraternal helping hand to the weak and harried patient, whereas the MD appears to be restraining him, even pushing the struggling man deeper into the slough of sickness and death. The Thomsonian practitioner's show of caring for his patient as a person is an expression of a holistic orientation—treat the whole patient and treat him as a unique human being. This cartoon shows holistic orientation nearly a century and a half before the word *holistic* came into vogue. Homeopathy went even farther, giving consideration to a patient's every little complaint, mental as well as physical, in the search for just the right drug to duplicate the sick person's full array of symptoms. Holism was exhibited in the teachings of other alternative schools of practice as well. From the beginning, practitioners of complementary medicine have claimed superior relations with patients, sometimes offending conventional physicians with an air of "holisticer than thou" condescension.

The holism of nineteenth-century alternative medicine, however, went well beyond the basic principle of paying heed to the emotional and spiritual side of patients. Today's definition of *holistic* has been expanded from "treatment of the whole patient" to include an emphasis on motivating patients to assume some responsibility for and participation in their care and recovery. Likewise, from its inception, alternative medicine aimed to give patients the power to help themselves. Thomsonianism took self-help most seriously, actually selling Family Right Certificates that gave purchasers the legal right to prescribe for and treat themselves botanically: "Every man his own physician" was the Thomsonian motto. But homeopaths encouraged people to be their own physicians, too, selling domestic kits of the most useful remedies, complete with instructions on how to use them for self-care; hydropaths published manuals of health advice and home water treatments; and in the early twentieth century, naturopaths also produced an extensive body of popular literature promoting a wide array of natural remedies for home use (28).

Our contemporary interpretation of holism has also embraced lifestyle regulation and the promotion of wellness as a major element of complementary care. This orientation, it can be argued, stems from American hydropathy in the 1850s, which drew on an earlier popular health reform movement to graft behaviors, such as abstinence from alcohol and tobacco, vegetarianism, regular exercise, fresh air, and sexual restraint, onto the original system of various cold water baths (29). The resulting hybrid was known as *hygeio-therapy,* a method that "restores the sick to health by the means which preserve health in well persons" (30). The hygeio-therapeutic tradition was preserved and carried on to the present by naturopathic medicine.

Other features of nineteenth-century alternative medicine have persisted to the present, such as objection to the medicalization of pregnancy and labor. Enough has been said, however, to make it clear that nineteenth-century alternative practitioners looked upon the allopaths as the true irregulars in medicine (31, 32).

ALLOPATHIC MEDICINE'S CRITICISM OF ALTERNATIVE MEDICINE

The first generation of allopathic doctors hardly turned the other cheek to such criticism. They gave as good as they got, putting forward a range of objections to alternative medicine. In the orthodox analysis, alternative practitioners were not simply ignoramuses and incompetents;

they were zealots, medical cultists obsessed with a single theoretical and therapeutic tenet, blind and deaf to the merits of any conflicting belief or practice, and determined to bend every case to their fundamentalist faith. The alternative doctor, a Baltimore medico declared, "circumscribes himself and practises a . . . *one-idea* system *only*, and is so tied down and limited to that . . . that he *denies* the usefulness of all known and honorable means of aiding the sick." Regular doctors resented the label *allopathy* because it was implied their medicine was just another -*pathy*, merely one more sect instead of open-minded science. "The title 'Allopathy'," it was objected, was an "insignificant misnomer . . . applied to us opprobriously . . . with sinister motives . . . . [I]t is both untrue and offensive." Hence, "when people ask you 'what school you practise,' you may very properly answer that you are simply a PHYSICIAN, that you belong to no sect," that you, "like the bee, take the honey of truth wherever you find it" (33).

Insinuation and derision were a game two could play. Homeopathy, Oliver Wendell Holmes declared, was "a mingled mass of perverse ingenuity, of tinsel erudition, of imbecile credulity" (34). Another doctor characterized it as "a confused mass of rubbish" (35). Other unorthodox schools of practice were accorded comparable respect. For example, osteopathy was denounced by an end-of-the-century physician as "a complete system of charlatanism . . . and quackery, calculated and designed to impose upon the credulous, superstitious, and ignorant" (36). Soon after, the editor of *JAMA* described naturopathy as "a medical cesspool" (37). Irregulars might protest all they wanted that their methods had empirical foundations, and therefore were scientific. However, allopaths believed that enslavement to simplistic "one-idea systems" resulted in biased interpretations of clinical experience. Hence, "this subterfuge cannot avail. Call himself by what name he will, a quack is still a quack—and even if the prince of darkness should assume the garb of heavenly innocence, the cloven hoof would still betray the real personage"(38).

Cloven-hooved or not, alternative prac-titioners did see most of their patients return to health. But those successes, mainstream physicians argued, could be accounted for entirely by the operations of nature. By the mid-1800s, allopathic philosophy acknowledged that most diseases are self-limited, and will resolve themselves under anyone's care. However, that explanation was much more frequently applied to alternative patients than to mainstream ones. Homeopathy in particular, with its immaterial doses of drugs, seemed to be explainable in no other way than as "placeboism etherealized" (39). Homeopaths, one physician laughed, would be just as successful "were the similars left out, and atoms of taffy or sawdust . . . substituted, to give their patients room to exercise their faith, and *nature* time and opportunity to do the work" (40).

MEDICAL LICENSING

The mutual hostility between allopathic and alternative practitioners was played out at both the political and the philosophical level. The context for the Thomsonian cartoon was that movement's assault on the state medical licensing laws that had been enacted throughout the country in the early 1800s. Although the laws were only casually enforced, they did confer the blessing of government on allopathic medicine. Alternative healers regarded this legislation as undemocratic violations of both their right to pursue the calling of their choice and the public's right to select whom they wanted as their doctors; they also regarded this legislation as transparent attempts by allopaths to corner the medical market. Denouncing the laws as elitist and monopolistic, alternative practitioners (Thomsonians, particularly) succeeded in getting virtually every state licensing law wiped from the statute books by mid-century. Licensing provisions for allopaths would be revived, however, in the 1880s and 1890s, as the impact of the germ theory renewed public respect for the power of allopathic medicine. Alternative physicians would then campaign for the passage of separate licensing laws to govern their systems too, and although they were generally successful in their quest, licensing was obtained only very gradually, and painfully, through vicious political struggles waged state by state (41). The first osteopathic licensing law, for example, was adopted in Vermont in 1895; by 1901, 14 other states had followed suit. Chiropractic, by contrast, did not win its first licensure battle until 1913 (Kansas), but then another 31 states passed chiropractic laws within a decade. Not until 1973, however, were osteopaths fully licensed in every state, and it was the following year before the same could be said of chiropractors. Naturopathic licensing has developed more slowly; presently only 12 states issue ND licenses (42, 43).

Until winning legislation in their individual states, alternative medicine practitioners were subject to fine or imprisonment for practicing medicine without a license. Not even the leaders of the major systems were exempt: Benedict Lust was arrested in 1899, and D. D. Palmer was jailed seven years later (44, 45). In the early part of this century, there was also a good bit of courtroom conflict between osteopaths and chiropractors, the former often succeeding in getting the latter prosecuted for practicing osteopathy without a license (46). Battles over the adoption or expansion of alternative medical licensing privileges continues to enliven the deliberations of state legislatures. Meanwhile, practitioners of therapeutic approaches that have not managed to achieve licensure status deplore (much like the alternative physicians of the 1830s did) the infringements on "medical freedom" practiced by the "medical/pharmaceutical complex" (47).

THE ISSUE OF CONSULTATION

State legislatures were one battleground, and the sickroom and hospital ward were another. War was declared in that arena in 1847, with the founding of the American Medical Association and the Association's adoption of a code of ethics. Although most of the code was taken verbatim from a noted English publication of half a century earlier, an innovation was intro-

duced in response to the emergence of alternative medicine during the interim. This consultation clause began by urging physicians to call in qualified colleagues when perplexed by a case. But it ended with the stricture that anyone "whose practice is based upon an exclusive dogma"—i.e., who is a sectarian, an irregular—could not be accepted as "a fit associate in consultation" (48). In other words, it would be unethical, a threat to the patient's health and not just the doctor's sense of decorum, for an allopathic physician to consult or agree to be consulted by a homeopath or other alternative "dogmatist." Thus, in one doctor's interpretation, one might ethically consult "with foreign physicians, doctresses [women physicians]," even "colored physicians . . . provided they are regular practitioners." But if the would-be consultant were a dogmatist, even a native-born white male one, "justly exclude him as unsuitable for fellowship with those who profess to love all truth." It would be as suitable for "a Jewish rabbi . . . to exchange pulpits with Christian ministers" as for allopathic doctors to consult with alternative ones (49). For the rest of the nineteenth century, the consultation clause would be used to oppose the admission of alternative practitioners to local and state medical societies, the staffs of public hospitals and the military medical corps, and the faculties of publicly funded medical schools. The original clause was dropped from the AMA code when it was revised in 1903, but the principles adopted in its stead maintained the understanding that ethical practitioners would not voluntarily associate with alternative healers; only in 1980 would the Association revise its ethical principles so as to remove all restrictions on consultation (50–52).

Official disdain for alternative medicine would only be intensified by the grand reformation of medical education that began in the later years of the nineteenth century, and culminated with the celebrated Flexner Report of 1910. That survey—rather exposé—of the miserable educational standards that prevailed at nearly all of America's medical schools was an acute embarrassment to the allopathic profession. But it catalyzed an educational housecleaning that drove many institutions out of business and forced the surviving ones to impose far more rigorous programs of training.

Flexner's report did not have so immediate an impact on alternative schools and practitioners. He did include homeopathic and osteopathic colleges in his survey, and had as scathing words for them as for any allopathic schools. The eight osteopathic educational facilities, for example, were condemned as "hopelessly meager," "utterly wretched," "intolerably foul" (53). Even Still's own college, osteopathy's flagship, was dismissed as "absurdly inadequate" (53). This ridicule solidified mainstream practitioners' conviction of the unscientific (and therefore unworthy) nature of alternative medicine, but it did not result in the wholesale closing of alternative medical schools. To be sure, the number of homeopathic colleges dropped precipitously, from a high of 22 in 1900 to only 2 by 1923; however, homeopathy was already weakened by internal dissension (54). Osteopathy, by contrast, lost only one school in the twenty years following the Flexner Report, and the number of chiropractic schools actually grew prolifically (55–56). Thus, as late as the mid-1920s, a Philadelphia physician could determine that alternative medicine was still flourishing, at least in his region: one third of his patients admitted they had also put themselves under the care of an alternative practitioner of some sort within the three months preceding their visit to him (57). Eisenberg's 1993 survey found also that one third of Americans rely on unconventional therapies (58). Public respect for alternative healers was already being undermined, however, by the compelling image of *scientific medicine*, the term insisted upon by allopathic doctors to distinguish the new medicine derived from the germ theory and the Flexnerian reformation of education.

The scientist-physician in shining lab coat armor confidently predicted endless triumphs over disease with the weapons of modern medical research; to the dazzled public, alternative systems appeared static and impotent by comparison. Alternative medicine fell lower in the popular estimation when sulfa drugs appeared in the 1930s; then the introduction of antibiotics the following decade made good on the promises of scientific medicine and made healing alternatives seem less necessary. As early as the 1930s, a survey of America's "healing cults" concluded that "homeopathy is past and gone," and that chiropractic was approaching its twilight, both because they could not compete with scientific medicine (59).

Characterization of alternative medicine as cultism continued into the second half of the twentieth century. Osteopathy was identified as "a cult practice of medicine" by the AMA until 1961, and "professional associations [with] doctors of osteopathy" were proscribed as "unethical" until that same year (60). For that reason, osteopaths were prevented from serving as medical officers during World War II; and although Congress authorized the appointment of osteopaths to military hospitals in 1956, it was to be a full decade before the first DO would actually be offered a position (61–62). Similarly, the AMA long held it unethical to refer patients to chiropractors, and staunchly opposed the extension of hospital privileges to DCs. As late as 1966, the Association's House of Delegates adopted a resolution designating chiropractic "an unscientific cult." Chiropractors fought back, in 1976 filing an antitrust suit against the AMA, the American Hospital Association, and several other medical organizations. A verdict would not be rendered until 1987, but it went against the defendants, the judge finding the AMA guilty of a "conspiracy against chiropractors . . . intended to contain and eliminate the entire profession of chiropractic." The AMA appealed, but the decision was upheld (63–64).

Osteopathic physicians were included in the Medicare reimbursement system when that act was passed in 1965, but chiropractors and naturopaths were denied participation. Chiropractic and naturopathic professional associations both appealed to Congress for reconsideration, but each was turned down in identical language: their "theory and practice are not based upon the body of basic knowledge related to health, disease, and health care which has been widely accepted by the scientific community" (65). Likewise, their programs of education "do not prepare the practitioner to make an adequate diagnosis and provide appropriate treatment" (65). Continuing pressure from the chiropractic community succeeded in winning inclusion of their practitioners under Medicare in 1974, but naturopaths remain outside as of this writing (66).

ELEVATION OF ALTERNATIVE MEDICINE'S STANDARDS

Much of this chapter has been given to discussion of the first century of unconventional medicine precisely because attitudes set during that period continue to shape interprofessional relations as the second century of alternative medicine draws to a close. But concomitant with this historical constancy, there have been profound changes over the course of the twentieth century, too. In 1900, alternative systems of practice were still bound to crude and speculative theoretical rationales; they still claimed panacea-like potency for their therapies; they operated schools with minimal requirements that admitted students of dubious qualifications; they were tainted, some more than others, with huckster-ism (chiropractic schools, a 1930s survey observed, "fairly reek of commercialism") (67); and they unrealistically aimed to overthrow rather than complement allopathic medicine. By midcentury, however, a vigorous bootstrap-ping effort was underway, which had already raised the level of education and ethics in all systems of practice. Theoretical foundations were being strengthened and therapeutic claims modified. Conventional medicine was being acknowledged as highly effective in its sphere, and alternative practitioners' longstanding competitive attitude toward allopathic physicians was giving way to a goal of cooperation.

For their part, mainstream physicians steadily assumed a more flexible stance too, first, as has been noted, toward osteopathic medicine. During the 1950s and early 1960s, the AMA gradually recognized that the quality of osteopathic academic training was comparable to that of allopathic. Then, in the mid-1960s, osteopaths were admitted into orthodox residency programs, even to membership in the American Medical Association. During that same decade, DOs in California and Washington were actually encouraged by those states' medical societies

to convert their degrees to MD and join the allopathic ranks. The medical establishment's sudden willingness to merge with osteopathy was, of course, assailed by some as an attempt to suppress competition by assimilating it. Ever since, alternative medical systems have been riven with angst that the culmination of their struggle for professional respectability might turn out to be absorption into the mainstream and loss of their identity and independence (68–70).

Therefore, although the trend of professional improvement in alternative medicine has taken an even sharper upward turn since the middle of this century, a gulf of distrust and misunderstanding remains between the sides. The aura of sectarianism cast by alternative systems for so long lingers in the memory of many mainstream practitioners, distorting their view of complementary medicine and inhibiting them from appreciating the remarkable transformation that has occurred. This blaming of complementary healers for the sins of their fathers, moreover, is as ironic as it is unjust, since allopaths' fathers committed all the same sins. Prior to this century, orthodox medicine was littered with naive theories, ineffective (sometimes dangerous) therapies, and inferior educational institutions. Whatever skeletons there are hidden in alternative medicine's closet are to be found in the allopathic closet as well, and one might reasonably think of the professional evolution of the major systems of complementary medicine as a repetition of the pattern of development of the allopathic profession, with a time lag of half a century or so. For the analogy to be fully accurate, however, more extensive and concrete evidence of the efficacy of complementary therapies is required. It was for the purpose of filling that need that the National Institute of Health's Office of Alternative Medicine was established in 1992.

THE REVIVAL OF ALTERNATIVE MEDICINE

In recent decades, the improvement of professional standards within alternative medicine has been paralleled by increased public interest and patronage. This improvement constitutes a striking turnaround from the decline experienced by most alternative systems during the middle years of this century. Although as recently as 1969 a federal study concluded "the number of naturopaths . . . is rapidly declining" (71), unconventional practice experienced an extraordinary revitalization in the 1970s. Not only did naturopathy, chiropractic, and other nineteenth-century systems regain popularity, but various newer programs of healing appeared on the scene as well. When the journal *Alternative Therapies in Health and Medicine* began publication in 1995, its editor was able to identify 39 distinct categories of alternative practice as topics acceptable for articles, everything from anthroposophy to vitamin treatments (72).

This alternative medicine revival was due in significant measure to rising public disaffection with mainstream medical practice. The reasons for dissatisfaction are a familiar litany: patient alienation from the impersonal and intimidating style of specialized, technological, hospital-based medicine; the dramatic increase during the twentieth century of chronic degenerative diseases, ailments that confound cure but demand caring and cooperative management; awareness of the too-frequent iatrogenic effects of prescription pharmaceuticals; the rise of consumerism and concern for patients' rights and autonomy (much like the 1830s' demands of Thomsonians for medical freedom); and the rising costs of medical care. However, it should be appreciated that those dissatisfactions had been building for a long time. The 1924 survey of Philadelphia patients cited earlier determined that the chief reasons they had sought alternative help were their beliefs that allopaths did not give thorough physical examinations and were "too busy to devote the time and attention that the obscurity of the symptoms . . . demanded," and that "the medicine ordered made the patient feel worse than before taking it" (73). An Illinois contemporary commented on a similar survey of public discontent with physicians that, "We have rendered wonderful service in the serious ailments. We have not looked properly after the little things," recognizing that such chronic "little things" were not little matters

for patients (74). That same year, 1923, an Indiana physician summed the situation up with the observation that, "irregular healers . . . would not exist if they did not fill a kind of need . . . . This indicates that the people of this country are demanding of the medical profession something more than shaking up test tubes and looking through microscopes" (75).

To the allopathic profession's credit, that "something more" has been recognized and energetically pursued by physicians in recent years. The 1970s, in particular, were the pivotal decade for a liberalization of mainstream attitudes toward illness and treatment. Family medicine as an area of specialization came into its own in the seventies, dedicated to restoring a more personal and empathic touch to physician-patient interactions. By that time also, the understanding of psychosomatic medicine was undergoing a transformation that would foster a stronger belief in the power of mind to influence body function. The notion that mind and body are fully integrated, and that emotional states affect health, had been part of medical thinking from the time of Hippocrates, and since the 1930s there had in fact been a distinct area of investigation identified as psychosomatic medicine. However, in its initial phase of evolution, psychosomatic medicine had been preoccupied with relating specific physical ailments (e.g., hypertension) to emotional stress. During the 1960s and 1970s, a more complex interpretation emerged, one that identified psychological forces as one element in the multifactorial etiology of all illnesses. The mind was now being viewed as an ever-present participant in physical functioning (76–77). By the end of the 1970s, both the biopsychosocial model of disease and the discipline of psychoneuroimmunology had been developed within allopathic medicine; the former incorporated social pressures into the psychosomatic analysis and the latter clarified neural, endocrine, and immunological pathways by which mind could influence health. During the same period, the introduction of biofeedback practices demonstrated the power of the mind to affect the body therapeutically, and not just pathologically (78). In short, mind/body medicine was becoming a respectable branch of conventional practice.

Nevertheless, the concept of the mind as healer is more fully associated with alternative medicine, constituting not just an integral part of nineteenth- and early twentieth-century alternative healing philosophy, but also emerging as a distinctive area of practice unto itself in the last third of the twentieth century. One source of this growth has been religion—a significant proportion of Americans have always believed in the power of prayer and have sought spiritual content in their medicine. Scientific medicine's determination to reduce vital phenomena to wholly material, mechanical explanations makes it seem spiritually barren to many and has fueled a revival of healing through prayer. The Human-Potential Movement, which originated in the early 1960s, has been equally important. This movement involves a search for higher and nobler states of consciousness than the base impulses central to Freudian psychology. This quest for self-actualization supposed the existence of untapped sources of awareness and psychic energy, including the energy to restore the body. During that same decade, the antimaterialist hippy counterculture sparked a fascination with the mystical religious and philosophical traditions of Asian culture, and promoted practices such as transcendental meditation. East and West have since been blended through the New Age healing philosophy that aims at reconciling scientific and spiritual ways of looking at the world and health into a unified intellectual scheme. In this attempt, acupuncture, Ayurveda, and other ancient healing traditions of the Far East—traditions that have always focused on the functional rather than organic disequilibria of the body—have been embraced as particularly powerful ways of comprehending the extraphysical components of health and wholeness. Much like the animal magnetism of the mid-nineteenth-century Mesmerists and the Innate Intelligence of turn-of-the-century chiropractors, the *qi, prana,* and human energy fields of today's holistic healers are conceptualizations of immaterial agents that sustain harmony both within the body and between the body and the cosmos (79–81).

New Age medical mysticism is representative of a final obstacle in alternative medicine's climb toward scientific respectability. Like every other alternative approach, New Age philosophy wraps itself in the banner of holism: in the current climate of healing, one cannot expect to be taken seriously unless one is holistic. The rhetorical use of the term as a label of legitimacy has resulted in a promiscuous crowding of therapies under the broad holistic umbrella. Much of allopathic medicine's remaining reluctance to give complementary medicine a serious hearing is the side-by-side intermingling of methods that are relatively easy to rationalize scientifically (herbs, massage, acupuncture) with therapeutic aromas, personal auras, and mushy empowerment philosophies: "Empathology finds and clears the underlying causes of your . . . health issues [and] facilitates your personal truth" (1997 coupon advertisement). But even the most extraterrestrial-seeming of today's holistic therapies can be appreciated historically as striving to do what alternative approaches to care have always attempted: to assist the body in its effort to heal itself.

The value of supporting nature's healing labor has never been stated more eloquently than by the renowned American journalist Finley Peter Dunne, commenting in 1901 on the differences between Christian Science and medicine. "If th' Christyan Scientists had some science," his Irish protagonist Mr. Dooley proposed, "an' th' doctors more Christianity, it wudden't make anny diff'rence which ye called in—if ye had a good nurse" (82). The nursing profession has been one of the most active and effective groups in promoting complementary medicine in our own time, and that has been true from its beginnings as a profession. "Nature alone cures," Florence Nightingale wrote in 1859 as part of her definition of the art and goal of nursing. "What nursing has to do," she maintained, "is to put the patient in the best condition for nature to act upon him" (83). This approach has served as the core principle of complementary medical philosophy from the start, since Thomsonian doctors began rescuing patients from the slough of disease by pulling them up the steps of common sense. The best medicine, as Mr. Dooley realized, has always been good nursing.

The history of alternative medicine has, under various names and approaches, been a competitive dance with the dominant orthodox system of treatment. Alternative systems have always risen when the prevailing approaches have become too abstract, too impersonal, too harsh, or too costly for full public support. Alternative systems have usually started by relying on empiricism and outcomes reports, and then often either degenerate into dogma or get absorbed into an orthodoxy-like professionalism; when this happens, they become more distant from the patient, and this makes room for newer alternative systems to arise. Throughout this process, the battle for legitimacy is played out on semantic, regulatory, political, and economic grounds, with each side claiming "nature," "science," "holism," and "healing" on its side. To the degree we can understand and learn from the recurring themes that alternative medicine brings, we will be able to better balance the empirical and rational elements of medicine for the benefit of the ill.

REFERENCES

1. Bartlett E. An inquiry into the degree of certainty in medicine. Philadelphia: Lea and Blanchard, 1848:9.
2. Gevitz N, ed. Other healers. Unorthodox medicine in America. Baltimore: Johns Hopkins University Press, 1988.
3. Gevitz N. Unorthodox medical theories. In: Bynum WF, Porter R, eds. Companion encyclopedia of the history of medicine. Vol. 1. London: Routledge, 1993:603–633.
4. Bynum WF, Porter R, eds. Medical fringe and medical orthodoxy 1750–1850. London: Croom Helm, 1987.
5. Cooter R, ed. Studies in the history of alternative medicine. New York: St. Martin's Press, 1988.
6. Fuller R. Alternative therapies. Social history. In: Reich W, ed. Encyclopedia of bioethics. 2nd ed. New York: Simon and Schuster Macmillan, 1995:126–135.
7. Berman A. The Thomsonian movement and its relation to American pharmacy and medicine. Bull Hist Med 1951;25:405–428, 519–538.
8. Kaufman M. Homeopathy in America; the rise and fall of a medical heresy. Baltimore: Johns Hopkins University Press, 1971.
9. Coulter H. Divided legacy: the conflict between homeopathy and the American Medical Association. Richmond, CA: North Atlantic Books, 1982.
10. Weiss H, Kemble H. The great American water-cure craze. A history of hydropathy in the United States. Trenton, NJ: Past Times Press, 1967.
11. Donegan J. Hydropathic highway to health. Women and water-cure in antebellum America. New York: Greenwood Press, 1986.
12. Cayleff S. Wash and be healed: the water-cure movement and women's health. Philadelphia: Temple University Press, 1987.
13. Fuller R. Mesmerism and the American cure of souls. Philadelphia: University of Pennsylvania Press, 1982.
14. Haller J. Medical rotestants. The eclectics in American medicine, 1825–1939. Carbondale, IL: Southern Illinois University Press, 1994.
15. Gevitz N. The D.O.'s. Osteopathic medicine in America. Baltimore: Johns Hopkins University Press, 1982.
16. Moore J. Chiropractic in America. The history of a medical alternative. Baltimore: Johns Hopkins University Press, 1993.
17. Kirchfeld F, Boyle W. Nature doctors. Pioneers in naturopathic medicine. Portland, OR: Medicina Biologica, 1994.
18. King D. Quackery unmasked. Boston: Clapp, 1858:332–334.
19. Rosen G. The structure of American medical practice 1875–1941. Rosenberg C, ed. Philadelphia: University of Pennsylvania Press, 1983:16.
20. Haller J. Acupuncture in nineteenth century Western medicine. N Y St J Med 1973;73:1213–1221.
21. Thomsonian Botanic Watchman 1834;1:8.
22. Thomson S. A narrative of the life and medical discoveries of the author. Boston: Author, 1835:9,45.
23. Trall R. Hand-book of hygienic practice. New York: Miller and Wood, 1864:3.
24. Lust B. Quoted in: Kirchfeld F, Boyle W. Nature doctors. Pioneers in naturopathic medicine. Portland, OR: Medicina Biologica, 1994:193.
25. Lane MA. Dr. A. T. Still. Founder of osteopathy. Waukegan, IL: Bunting, 1925:44, 182.
26. Hahnemann S. Organon of homeopathic medicine. 1st American ed, from 4th German ed. Allentown, PA: Academical Bookstore, 1836:151.
27. Thomson S. A narrative of the life and medical discoveries of the author. Boston: Author, 1835:9.
28. Numbers R. Do-it-yourself the sectarian way. In: Risse G, et al., eds. Medicine without doctors. Home health care in American history. New York: Science History Publications, 1977:49–72.
29. Whorton J. Crusaders for fitness. The history of American health reformers. Princeton, NJ: Princeton University Press, 1982.
30. Trall R. Handbook of hygienic practice. New York: Miller and Wood, 1864:4.

31. Trall R. The hydropathic encyclopedia: a system of hydropathy and hygiene. Vol. 1. New York: Fowlers and Wells, 1852:34,51.

32. Hahnemann S. The lesser writings of Samuel Hahnemann. New York: Radde, 1852:738.

33. Cathell DW. The physician himself. 4th ed. Baltimore: Cushings and Bailey, 1885:181–182, 198.

34. Holmes OW. Medical essays, 1842–1882. Boston: Houghton Mifflin, 1899:101.

35. Hooker W. Physician and patient. New York: Baker and Scribner, 1849:136.

36. Booth ER. History of osteopathy and twentieth century medical practice. Cincinnati: Caxton, 1924:179.

37. Fishbein M. The new medical follies. New York: Boni and Liveright, 1927:52.

38. Ticknor C. A popular treatise on medical philosophy; or, an exposition of quackery and imposture in medicine. New York: Gould and Newman, 1838:17.

39. Leland PW. Empiricism and its causes. Boston Med Surg J 1852;47:292.

40. Cathell DW. The physician himself and what he should add to his scientific acquirements. 4th ed. Baltimore: Cushings and Bailey, 1885:205.

41. Shryock R. Medical licensing in America, 1650–1965. Baltimore: Johns Hopkins University Press, 1967.

42. Gevitz N. The D.O.'s. Osteopathic medicine in America. Baltimore: Johns Hopkins University Press, 1982:41–2.

43. Moore J. Chiropractic in America. The history of a medical alternative. Baltimore: Johns Hopkins University Press, 1993:151–152.

44. Kirchfeld F, Boyle W. Nature doctors. Pioneers in naturopathic medicine. Portland, OR: Medicina Biologica, 1994:188.

45. Gielow V. Old dad chiro. Davenport, IA: Bawden, 1981:103–114.

46. Gevitz N. The D.O.'s. Osteopathic medicine in America. Baltimore: Johns Hopkins University Press, 1982:59.

47. Strohecker J, ed. Alternative medicine. The definitive guide. Puyallup, WA: Future Medicine Publishing, 1994:17.

48. Flint A. Medical ethics and etiquette. The code of ethics adopted by the American Medical Association. New York: Appleton, 1883:45.

49. Cathell DW. The physician himself and what he should add to his scientific acquirements. 4th ed. Baltimore: Cushings and Bailey, 1885:178, 181.

50. Kaufman M. Homeopathy in America. The rise and fall of a medical heresy. Baltimore: Johns Hopkins University Press, 1971:48–109.

51. Rothstein W. American medicine in the nineteenth century. From sects to science. Baltimore: Johns Hopkins University Press, 1972:170–174.

52. Haller J. American medicine in transition 1840–1910. Urbana, IL: University of Illinois Press, 1980:256–267.

53. Flexner A. Medical education in the United States and Canada. New York: Carnegie Foundation for the Advancement of Teaching, 1910:197, 214, 253.

54. Kaufman M. Homeopathy in America. The rise and fall of a medical heresy. Baltimore: Johns Hopkins University Press, 1969:166.

55. Reed L. The healing cults. Chicago: University of Chicago Press, 1932:19, 35–36.

56. Moore J. Chiropractic in America. The history of a medical alternative. Baltimore: Johns Hopkins University Press, 1993:113.

57. Beardsley E. Why the public consult the pseudo-medical cults. J Med Soc N J 1924;21:277.

58. Eisenberg D, Kessler R, Foster C, et al. Unconventional medicine in the United States. N Engl J Med 1993;328:246–252.

59. Reed L. The healing cults. Chicago: University of Chicago Press, 1932:3,58.

60. Judicial Council of the AMA. Osteopathy. JAMA 1961;177:774–6.

61. Blackstone E. The A.M.A. and the osteopaths: a study of the power of organized medicine. Antitrust Bull 1977;22:405–440.

62. Gevitz N. The D.O.'s. Osteopathic medicine in America. Baltimore: Johns Hopkins University Press, 1982:124.

63. Gevitz N. The chiropractors and the AMA: reflections on the history of the consultation clause. Persp Biol Med 1989;32:281–299.

64. Moore J. Chiropractic in America. The history of a medical alternative. Baltimore: Johns Hopkins University Press, 1993:131–137.

65. Cohen WJ. Independent practitioners under medicare. Washington, DC: Department of Health, Education, and Welfare, 1969:142, 197.

66. Moore J. Chiropractic in America. The history of a medical alternative. Baltimore: Johns Hopkins University Press, 1993:115.

67. Reed L. The healing cults. Chicago: University of Chicago Press, 1932:47.

68. Gevitz N. The D.O.'s. Osteopathic medicine in America. Baltimore: Johns Hopkins University Press, 1982:99–136.

69. Blackstone E. The A.M.A. and the osteopaths: a study of the power of organized medicine. Antitrust Bull 1977;22:405–440.

70. Sirica CM, ed. Osteopathic medicine: past, present,

and future. New York: Josiah Macy, Jr. Foundation, 1996.

71. Cohen WJ. Independent practitioners under Medicare. Washington, DC: Department of Health, Education, and Welfare, 1969:140.

72. Information for Authors. Alt Ther Health Med 1995;1:61.

73. Beardsley E. Why the public consult the pseudo medical cults. J Med Soc N J 1924;21:277.

74. Keller B. The laity's idea of the physician. Ill Med J 1923;44:18.

75. Arthur I. The medical profession and the people. J Indiana State Med Assoc 1923;16:369–70.

76. Ackerknecht E. The history of psychosomatic medicine. Psych Med 1982;12:17–24.

77. Lipowski Z. Psychosomatic medicine: past and present. Can J Psych 1986;31:2–13.

78. Kiecolt-Glaser J, Glaser R. Psychoneuroimmunology: past, present, and future. Health Psych 1989;8:677–82.

79. Fuller R. Alternative medicine and american religious life. New York: Oxford University Press, 1989.

80. Cooter R. Alternative medicine, alternative cosmology. In: Cooter R, ed. Studies in the history of alternative medicine. New York: St. Martin's Press, 1988.

81. Miller C. Human-potential movement. Am J Psych 1977;37:99–109.

82. Dunne FP. Mr. Dooley's opinions. New York: R. H. Russell, 1901:9.

83. Nightingale F. Notes on nursing. New York: Dover, 1969:133.

CHAPTER 2

The Physician and Complementary and Alternative Medicine

Ronald A. Chez, Wayne B. Jonas, and David Eisenberg

INTRODUCTION

The public's use of complementary and alternative medicine (CAM) is not a peripheral practice, fad, or medical side issue. Rather, it reflects a genuine public health care need that will not disappear. What then is the conventional practitioner's responsibility for offering meaningful counsel to a patient who is considering CAM? How does a practitioner make informed decisions about a particular CAM modality to determine whether it has a role in the patient's care? In this chapter we provide the basic information needed for addressing CAM with patients who may be using or asking about non-mainstream therapies. This information includes several elements:

- the extent of CAM use.
- why patients use CAM.
- clarification of CAM.
- the role of the physician in CAM.
- questioning patients about CAM use.
- obtaining and evaluating information about CAM.
- how to provide appropriate follow-up and referral when needed.
- a discussion of training, licensing, liability, and reimbursement related to CAM.

CONVENTIONAL MEDICINE

The chief goals of medicine have recently been summarized in a report by the Hastings Institute (1). Dominant emphases relate to curing disease, promoting health and preventing illness and injury, restoring functional capacity, avoiding premature death, relieving suffering, enhancing quality of life, and caring for those who cannot be cured. These goals are the same for all practitioners, regardless of their methods or beliefs.

Critics of conventional medicine argue that these goals are not being fulfilled. Instead, they are being replaced by an approach to patients that is reductionistic, cure oriented, organ specific, mechanistic, depersonalized, and subspecialized. A dogmatic attempt to address chronic disease with this approach is infringing on the aforementioned goals. Nevertheless, even severe detractors acknowledge the great value of conventional medicine regarding competent care for acute disease and trauma, the capacity to expertly apply innovations in both diagnosis and treatment, and the ability to translate basic science discoveries into clinical care.

Most physicians are aware of the finite aspects of their scope of practice. They recognize that it is impossible to be all things to all patients and keep current with every aspect of the rapid continuous advance of conventional medicine. Coupled with this knowledge is the diminishing ability of physicians to fulfill their responsibility to function as a patient advocate. Medical decision making is increasingly altered because of economic considerations in the provision of health care, which includes the actions of hospital boards and administrators, employers, third-party payers, the legal profession, and government regulations.

COMPLEMENTARY AND ALTERNATIVE MEDICINE

Extent of CAM Use

The best data on rates of usage of CAM come from two identical surveys conducted by Eisenberg and colleagues in 1990 and 1996 (2, 3). These authors extrapolated data from a 1990 U.S. telephone survey of approximately 1500 respondents. In 1990, they found that one-third of Americans (representative of all sociodemographic groups) used CAM that year. Almost all of these patients were also being cared for by traditional medical doctors. However, approximately 90% self-referred to alternative providers, and, importantly, three of four did not tell their physicians about use of the alternative care. A repeat of this survey in 1996 with more than 2000 respondents showed a dramatic increase in CAM use—to 42% of the population—and out-of-pocket CAM expenditures equaling the amount spent out-of-pocket for conventional medicine (3). The rate for women was 49%.

Other surveys have shown that approximately 50% of patients who have cancer (4) or human immunodeficiency virus (5) will use unconventional practices at some point during their illness. The medical records of these patients were incomplete, however, because they did not reflect the use of CAM therapies. Therefore, Americans are using CAM in substantial and increasing numbers. Similar and even higher figures are found in Europe (6), Australia (7), and other countries. This fact should stimulate each practicing physician to ask why his or her patients are seeking out these therapies, pay attention to the patients' answers, and decide how the practitioner should respond as a health care provider.

Why Do Patients Use CAM?

The predominant conditions for which Americans use CAM are chronic and stress-related conditions such as back problems, arthritis, headaches, digestive problems, depression, cancer, hypertension, and autoimmune syndromes—in other words, conditions for which there are no cures and for which inadequate treatment regimens sometimes produce adverse side effects.

Patients use alternative practices because these modalities are part of their social network, they are not satisfied with the process or result of conventional care, or they are attracted to CAM philosophies and health beliefs (8, 9). Patients who use CAM do not generally hold anti-science or anti-conventional medicine sentiment, nor do they represent a disproportionate number of the uneducated, poor, seriously ill, or neurotic (8–11). Included in these multiple motivations is the patient's wish to obtain faster resolution of illness. Some patients are motivated by the desires to prevent illness or injuries and maintain wellness. Most of these patients function as active participants in their own health care (9).

TYPES OF CAM MODALITIES USED

Patients who use unconventional medicine are not necessarily unconventional patients. Many interventions used by the patients in the Eisenberg studies (2, 3) straddle or are part of current conventional medical practice. This can result in confusion as to the definition of CAM. For instance, the more frequently used interventions included exercise, relaxation techniques, and massage; all of these are part of treatment programs prescribed by medical doctors. Other approaches included imagery, prayer, and spiritual healing. Medical doctors usually do not interfere with the use of these modalities.

Chiropractic manipulation was also a frequently used intervention (2, 3). Although there has been resistance by organized medicine to chiropractic, this modality has been demonstrated to be equally effective as other treatments that can be offered for acute lower back pain of nonorganic etiology. It has even been recommended as such by the United States Public Health Service (12).

The list of the more frequently used CAM modalities in the Eisenberg study also included herbal medicines and megavitamins. Herbal medicine is a difficult area for most medical doctors because most lack formal training in it, many of the medicaments are unfamiliar, and only recently has there been an authoritative source, such as the *Physicians Desk Reference* for prescription items (12a). Also, there is little required Food and Drug Administration overview and labeling of herbal products sold in the United States, although other countries (such as Germany and Australia) have established guidelines and oversight procedures. These same factors apply to the difficulty that physicians find in sanctioning the use of megadose vitamins. As a result, physicians cite generalized concerns about safety and efficacy if these products are used by their patients.

Content of CAM

CAM is defined as that subset of medical and health care practices that is not an integral part of conventional (Western) medicine. Many practices overlap with conventional medicine, and some eventually become part of it (13).

More than 350 modalities can be listed under the broad category of CAM. The United States NIH classification divided the modalities into seven major categories (Table 2.1) (14). These categories are not equivalent in terms of understanding or acceptance by conventional medicine, and there is no consensus on definitions or classification schemes.

For instance, mind-body interventions include biofeedback, meditation, relaxation techniques, support groups, guided imagery, and yoga. Biofeedback is now integrated in conventional medicine for treating urinary and fecal incontinence, swallowing disorders, and chronic pain relief, including headaches. The category of manual healing methods includes physical therapy and massage as well as chiropractic manipulations. Again, elements of these are included in conventional medicine. For the bioelectromagnetic application category, both the electroencephalogram and electrocardiogram use the body's endogenous electromagnetic elements. Diathermy, laser, and radiofrequency surgery are part of the low-frequency thermal

aspects of this category. The diet and nutrition category presently includes prescribed physician regimens of specific food elimination diets and lifestyle programs that have successfully treated patients who have cardiovascular disease.

In contrast, Western medicine has difficulty accepting and understanding the place for other alternative medical systems, such as Ayurveda, homeopathy, and traditional Chinese medicine. Similarly, the biofield approaches, such as therapeutic touch, Reiki, polarity therapy, and reflexology, all deal with life forces and subtle energy fields, concepts that are not part of the usual thought processes of Western medical doctors.

Conventional medical pharmacotherapy was founded on the use of plants as sources of medicines, but the present pharmacological manufacturing system focuses on synthetic compounds that may be costly and, in some cases, cause severe side effects. Currently, several herbs have been studied in prospective randomized controlled trials from which data have been published in peer-reviewed journals. The possibility that herbal medicines may achieve the same or better outcomes as prescription medicines, but at less cost and with fewer side effects, must be considered and examined. One difficulty is how to define the proper dosing for these products, because too frequently a disparity exists between one brand and another, caused by lack of manufacturing standardization. Phytomedicines and ethnobotany will become more prominent as a source of conventional pharmacological and biological treatment. As an example, the estrogen-like isoflavins in soy protein may have value for the perimenopausal and postmenopausal patient. In contrast, the acceptance of blood-processed products, apitherapy, and many folk medicine products remains doubtful.

Common Themes in CAM

Common themes are promulgated in the CAM literature that traverse the seven large categories shown in Table 2.1. However, as previously stated, these categories are not all equivalent, neither in acceptance nor in understanding by conventional medicine. Some familiar themes

Table 2.1. NIH Model for CAM Classification
1. Mind–body interventions
2. Alternative systems of medical practice
3. Manual healing methods
4. Pharmacological and biological treatments
5. Bioelectromagnetic applications
6. Herbal medicine
7. Diet and nutrition

focus on the enhancement of wellness and prevention of disease, whereas others emphasize self-healing and the use of recuperative powers. These themes are also espoused in conventional medicine. Other themes, such as an orientation toward mind–body–spirit relationships and the restoration of balance and subtle energy fields or life force, are difficult to comprehend for medical doctors trained in the classical sciences of physics and biochemistry. The introduction to Part I of this book provides a framework for conceptualizing the diverse themes that cut across both conventional and complementary medicines.

What can be readily applied to the everyday medical care of all patients is the distinction between disease and illness, curing and healing, and pain and suffering. Specifically, if disease is the diagnosis that derives from the patient's presenting signs, symptoms, and laboratory tests, then illness is the human experience of the disease that takes place in the context of an individual person's singular set of beliefs, fears, expectations, and meaning. If cure is an externally applied medical intervention that removes all evidence of the diagnosed disease, then healing is the internal process of recovery that takes place on a physical, emotional, mental, and spiritual level. People can heal when they believe that it is not only possible to be well, but also that they are worthy of being well (a spiritual or psychological element). Finally, because we as human beings have bodies and minds, pain as part of our existence is inevitable. Because suffering is the person's response to pain, it is not inevitable that suffering be extreme or negative, and in that sense suffering is a focus of interventions aimed at healing (15).

ADDRESSING CAM IN PRACTICE

The Role of the Physician

Patient advocacy encompasses promoting patients' well-being, protecting them from harmful practices, facilitating informed choice, honoring their values and decision making, and promoting dialogue and partnership. It also includes the purposeful identification of the physicians' own medical experience and knowledge within the limits of their training, which results in the responsibility to seek appropriate consultation and referral. The interplay of patient advocacy, the difficulty in achieving the goals of medicine, the perceived and real limits of conventional medicine, and the reality of today's practice environment serves as the motivation to 1) learn why patients are seeking and using complementary and alternative practices for their health needs; and 2) help define the significant role physicians play in these areas. We recommend that physicians follow the framework of "Protect, permit, promote, and partner" when approaching CAM in their clinical practices (16):

- Protect patients against dangerous practices.
- Permit practices that are harmless and may assist in comfort or palliation.
- Promote and use those practices that are proven safe and effective.
- Partner with patients by communicating with them about the use of specific CAM therapies and products.

Protecting Patients from CAM Risks

Given the extensive public use of CAM products and practices, the poor communication between patients and physicians about this use, and the paucity of knowledge about the safety and efficacy of most CAM treatments, a situation exists for harm from these treatments (17). Many CAM practices, such as acupuncture, homeopathy, and meditation, are inherently low-risk modalities, but if they are used by unskilled practitioners or in place of more effective treatments, adverse consequences may result. Only fully competent and licensed practitioners are qualified to help patients avoid such inappropriate use (18). Also, some alternative medicine products, such as herbal preparations, contain powerful pharmacological substances that can produce direct toxicity and herb–drug interactions (19). Contamination and poor quality control are also more likely with these products than with conventional drugs, especially if they are shipped from overseas (20).

Patients need to be especially cautious about products and practices that can produce direct adverse effects from toxicity. The conventional physician can help patients distinguish between CAM practices with little direct toxicity potential (e.g., homeopathy, acupuncture) versus those with potential for such toxicity (e.g., megavitamins and herbal supplements). In addition, physicians can work with patients to be sure they do not abandon effective care, are alert to signs of possible fraud or abuse, and are aware of unintended effects from interactions between conventional medicine practices and alternative therapies. Practices that rely on *secret* formulas, promise cures for multiple unrelated conditions, use either slick advertising for mail order products or pyramid marketing schemes, and recommend abandoning conventional medicine for their practice should be suspect (21).

PERMITTING PRACTICES THAT ARE HARMLESS AND MAY ASSIST IN COMFORT OR PALLIATION

Clinical improvement due to nonspecific factors that arise from the doctor-patient interaction, spontaneous healing, statistical regression to the mean, expectation, and placebo effects account for much of the benefit seen in medical practice (22, 23). Science is concerned with separating these factors from those thought to be attributable to specific and isolatable aspects of a therapy. Practitioners, however, are mainly concerned with how to achieve maximum benefit for individual patients with little harm (24). Many CAM systems attempt to enhance these nonspecific factors by emphasizing high-touch, personalized, self-care approaches that may be useful in symptom reduction and palliation in chronic disease. The physician can help patients optimize chances for recovery by permitting the use of beliefs and treatment approaches that

increase hope, bolster expectation, reduce symptoms, and enhance well-being if these beliefs and approaches are neither harmful nor expensive.

PROMOTING SAFE AND EFFECTIVE CAM THERAPIES

There is accumulating evidence that CAM practices have value for the way physicians treat, manage, and understand health and disease. Botanic medicine research has shown the benefit of herbal products such as *Ginkgo biloba* for improving dementia due to circulation problems and possibly Alzheimer's (25, 26); saw palmetto and other herbal preparations for treating benign prostatic hypertrophy (27); and garlic for the prevention of heart disease (28). Several randomized, placebo-controlled trials report that *Hypericum* (St. John's Wort) is effective in the treatment of depression. Additional studies have compared its effects with those of conventional antidepressants. These studies report that *Hypericum* is not only as effective as conventional antidepressants, but produces one tenth the side effects and represents one third the cost (29).

In addition, when controlled trials demonstrate that a widely used CAM therapy is not effective (such as acupuncture for smoking cessation or for the treatment of obesity), the physician can recommend against its use even though it may produce little harm (30).

As research provides credible information on the less-explored areas, expanded options for managing clinical conditions will arise. For example, studies on arthritis suggest improvements using homeopathy (31), acupuncture (32), vitamin and nutritional supplements (33), herbal products (34, 35), diet therapies (36), mind-body approaches (37), and manipulation (38). Similar collections of usually small studies exist for many other common conditions, such as heart disease, depression, asthma, and addictions. The physician can play a central role in assisting the patient to determine the value of evidence for his or her condition and situation. Searching the published medical literature and evaluating its applicability for specific problems is a service conventional physicians can provide. When no good research exists, this information can also be useful for many patients (39). Chapter 5 outlines a step-by-step and time-efficient approach for using research evidence to assist in decision making about using CAM practices.

PARTNERING WITH PATIENTS REGARDING CAM

There is a major communication gap between physicians and the public about CAM (2, 3). The physician has a responsibility to help fill this communication gap by asking patients about their CAM use and working with them to assure that it be done responsibly (40). The physician can become familiar with the basic concepts of CAM modalities, distinguishing the features and research bases of the main unconventional practices. In addition, conventional physicians can identify responsible CAM practitioners (including other physicians) who provide specific services. Learning about CAM practices will become an increasingly important aspect of both medical school education and medical practice in the future.

Questioning Patients about CAM Use

How does the physician answer when the patient asks if there is an alternative caregiver in the area to whom the physician would refer him or her, or asks about a specific alternative medicine about which he or she has been reading? For many medical doctors, this is, first, an issue of safety. It is dangerous for the public to believe that the term natural is synonymous with the terms safe, benign, or effective.

It is necessary to recognize that there are both direct and indirect adverse effects from some CAM interventions and treatments. The chapters in Part II of this book, "The Safety of CAM Products and Practices," deal with these issues in detail. It is pertinent that there is little federal supervision of most CAM products derived from plants, including herbs sold over the counter. Also, it is disconcerting that there is a paucity of authoritative licensing and certification bodies for CAM providers equivalent to those extant in conventional medicine. These oversight and supervisory structures are gradually being developed both inside and outside the CAM and conventional communities.

How then does the physician become more knowledgeable about CAM? Each individual physician will have to consider how well informed he or she wants to be about CAM—in terms of both general and specific aspects. The American Medical Association Council on Scientific Affairs and the Federation of State Medical Boards recently recommended that physicians routinely inquire about the use of CAM by their patients, educate themselves and their patients about the state of scientific knowledge regarding CAM, and educate their patients who choose CAM about the potential hazards of stopping conventional treatment (18).

Asking the patient during the intake interview whether he or she has been using or considering other kinds of treatments, medications, supplements, or seeing nonphysician therapists for relief of symptoms is a valuable source of information. If the answer is "Yes," then the physician can follow with questions similar to those presented in Table 2.2.

According to the responses, the physician may be able to inform the patient that: 1) a conventional treatment is available; 2) the patient may not need the particular CAM intervention; 3) the CAM practice is unnecessarily high in cost and low in value; or 4) the practice may be useful and can be continued. It may also become clear that the patient turned to CAM because conventional medicine was failing him or her, or that the patient in fact distrusted or was afraid of conventional medicine.

The physician has an obligation to warn, discourage, or monitor the patient when a potentially dangerous CAM intervention is being

Table 2.2. Doctor-to-Patient Questions Related to CAM Use
• How was the decision to use CAM made?
• What were the goals?
• Why was this particular intervention or treatment chosen?
• How was the particular provider selected?
• Did the intervention help?
• Did the intervention result in new problems?

considered or used. Some examples include the use of intravenous products of unknown quality or toxicity (e.g., hydrogen peroxide, herbs), colonics, and high doses of vitamins or pharmacological agents of unknown risk or value. The physician need not automatically interdict all CAM interventions on the assumption that there is a real or potential danger. Appropriate questions regarding the safety of a particular CAM treatment relate to whether it prevents or precludes needed conventional care, and if it can be continued in conjunction with conventional treatment without harm to the patient. When the patient uses interventions associated with few adverse effects, such as acupuncture, biofeedback, or homeopathy, there may be no contraindication to its continued use. If the physician acknowledges this, it may benefit the patient with little risk and help the physician gain a better understanding of the particular practice.

In all cases, the physician will want to pursue the patient dialogue in such a way that the patient will continue to seek medical care and receive appropriate conventional care. This is facilitated if the patient understands that his or her best interests are being explored with a purposeful focus on safety and efficacy. By focusing on the four goals outlined earlier in this chapter (protect, permit, promote, partner), a more integrated practice that appropriately addresses CAM with conventional medicine can be developed. These goals are organized into a series of operational questions that the physician can self-query as patients describe their use or interest in CAM practices and products (Table 2.3).

Working with Patients Who Visit CAM Practitioners

Table 2.2 outlines questions that the physician can ask of the patient, and Table 2.3 outlines questions physicians can ask of themselves when confronted with CAM practices. Because there are more visits to CAM practitioners than to conventional primary care physicians in any one year, however, the physician may frequently be faced with managing patients who visit CAM

Table 2.3. Evaluating CAM Use with Patients
• Is the CAM treatment dangerous? (Consult Part II, "The Safety of CAM Products and Practices," of this book.)
• Does the CAM therapy prevent the patient from receiving needed medical management?
• Can the CAM therapy be continued in conjunction with conventional treatment?
• Has the patient sought out CAM therapy because of distrust or a bad experience with conventional medicine?
• Is conventional medicine failing the patient in some way that might be addressed by CAM? (Consult Part III, "Overviews of CAM," and the summary charts at the end of this book.)

Adapted from Spigelbatt L. Alternative medicine: a pediatric conundrum. Contemporary Pediatrics 1997;4:51–61.

practitioners on a regular basis. How can the physician work with patients who are already visiting CAM practitioners and address the safety and management issues involved? Eisenberg has outlined a series of steps for this type of situation. In addition to the safety and screening questions previously discussed, the physician can ask the patient to begin a symptom diary and provide a set of questions for the alternative provider; for example, "What previous experience have you had with the condition?" "What will be the number of treatments and expected time table for a 'fair' trial?" and "Are you willing to communicate with my conventional physician?" (Table 2.4). After CAM therapy has been provided for a "fair" amount of time, the physician should review the results with the patient, including a symptom diary, and discuss continuation or discontinuation of the therapy and other treatment options (40). Contact with the CAM provider is encouraged early during treatment, as is thorough documentation of the process. Documentation should include advice to the patient, symptom diaries, safety issues, discussions with the CAM provider, outcomes, and conventional options tried or refused. If effective conventional care is available and is refused by the patient, termination of further management or, at the minimum, detailed documentation of the physician's recommendations may be necessary (40).

Table 2.4. Questions for the Patient to Ask the CAM Provider

- Is there evidence of efficacy and safety of the treatment?
- What is the provider's experience with the CAM treatment?
- How many treatments will be needed?
- What is a reasonable time frame for a "fair" trial of the treatment?
- What are the costs, and are they reimbursed by insurance?
- What are the toxicity and safety risks or adverse effects of the treatment?
- Will the CAM provider communicate with the patient's conventional physician?

Obtaining and Evaluating Information About CAM

Traditionally, once medical doctors complete their formal education, they continue to expand their medical knowledge base through self-study. When the physician decides how much detail about CAM he or she might want to provide, there are an increasing number of information sources available. This book and its companion, *Textbook of Complementary and Alternative Medicine,* are two sources of basic information about alternative practices, their safety, their main uses, and their organizational status. In addition, many peer-reviewed medical journals now contain clinical research articles related to CAM. There are also several peer-review journals published with a specific focus on CAM. Examples are *Complementary Therapies in Medicine, Alternative Therapies in Health and Medicine, Integrative Medicine, The Journal of Alternative and Complementary Medicine, Forschung Komplementarmedizin, The Scientific Review of Alternative Medicine, Focus on Alternative and Complementary Medicine, Advances,* and others. Another efficient way to become informed about current CAM therapies is through newsletters such as *Self Healing, Complementary Medicine for the Physician,* and *Alternative Medicine Alert.*

Herbal medicines are one of the more confusing areas for physicians. The American Botani-

cal Council is an excellent informational resource, with its publication of the translation of the German Commission E monographs, its own journal called *HerbalGram,* and therapeutic monographs describing dosage, safety, and use of individual herbs. Verro Tyler, former professor of pharmacognosy at the University of Indiana, has written several excellent books (*The Honest Herbal, Herbs of Choice*). Other books included *Healing Power of Herbs* by Michael Murray, *Out of the Earth* by Simon Mills, and *Herbal Drugs and Pharmaceuticals* by Norman Disset (editor). For information about safety, see Part II of this book, "The Safety of CAM Products and Practices"; McGuffin, Hobbs, Upton, and Goldberg's book *Botanical Safety Handbook;* or Newell, Clarkson, and Phillipson's *Herbal Medicine for the Healthcare Professional.* This last book has tables of indications, contraindications, and potential drug–herb interactions and is especially helpful for identifying possible adverse interactions of herbs with conventional medicines. Finally, the Physician's Desk Reference has recently published a PDR for herbs.

The Internet also is an important source of information. Several citation databases are dedicated to CAM. In addition, the National Library of Medicine's electronic database, MEDLINE, is currently revising its keyword headings to better capture CAM citations. Also, several medical organizations and CAM professional organizations have Web pages. The search engine, Yahoo, has more than 300 sites related to CAM and is a frequent source used by the public. Table 2.5 lists some Internet sites that the physician and health care professional may find particularly useful.

Evaluating the validity and applicability of CAM research literature is one of the primary responsibilities of the physician. Most patients cannot use evidence-based principles and research information, so they often come to the physician for this type of information. Because the physician cannot become knowledgeable and skilled in all CAM therapies, it is important that he or she become skilled in using an evidence-based evaluation approach to CAM. Quality systematic reviews and randomized controlled trials are the best source of valid in-

Table 2.5. Selected Internet Sources of CAM Information

General CAM

altmed.od.nih.gov/NCCAM (contains the CCI and links to NCCAM–supported research centers around the United States)

gn.apc.org/rccm (e-mail address for Research Council for Complementary Medicine, United Kingdom)

cpmcnet.columbia.edu/dept/rosenthal (Columbia University, New York, NY)

pitt.edu/~cbw/altm.html (University of Pittsburgh, PA)

gen.emory.edu/medweb/medweb.altmed.html (Emory University, Atlanta, GA)

chprd.sph.uth.tmc.edu/utcam (University of Texas CAM Cancer Center)

cgi.pathfinder.com/drweil (Andrew Weil's home page)

probe.nalusda.gov (United States Department of Agriculture)

healthy.net (commercial health information source)

teleport.com/~mattlmt (directory of CAM practitioners)

quackwatch.com (focuses on fraud, quackery, and CAM abuse)

General Medicine

medline.nlm.nih.gov (Medline and PubMed)

cochrane.co.uk (systematic reviews and randomized controlled trials)

biomednet.com (access to full text publications in biology and medicine)

webcom.com/mjljweb/jrnlclb/index.html (selected articles from *Annals of Internal Medicine* and *New England Journal of Medicine*)

oncolink.upenn.edu (University of Pennsylvania cancer information)

Acupuncture

acupuncture.com (United States site for acupuncture)

medicalacupuncture.org (American Academy of Medical Acupuncture)

users.aol.com/acubmas/bmas.html (British Medical Acupuncture Society)

acuall.org (U.S. National Acupuncture and Oriental Alliance)

Manipulation

amtamassage.org (American Massage Therapy Association)

osteopathy.org.uk (British Osteopathic Information Service)

amerchiro.org/index.html (American Chiropractic Association)

Homeopathy

homeopathic.com (Homeopathic Educational Services)

antenna.nl./homeoweb (a site for discussion and news)

homeopathic.org (National Center for Homeopathy, United States)

Herbal Medicine

herbalgram.org (American Botanical Council)

herbs.org (Herb Research Foundation)

pharm.usyd.edu.au (University of Sydney, Australia herbal site)

---

formation for determining safety and efficacy. The Cochrane Library, which is available online and on CD-ROM (see Table 2.5) is a rich source of this type of information for all of health care; with its CAM Field Group, it is an increasingly important source of quality CAM information. The National Center for Complementary and Alternative Medicine (NCCAM) at the National Institutes of Health (NIH) also mounts a listing of MEDLINE–derived information on its website (called the CAM Citation Index, or CCI) that is searchable by condition, CAM modality, or study type.

One result of this type of continuing medical education is acquiring knowledge of CAM treatments that may be useful for patient care. In cases when conventional medicine is not succeeding, the physician can recommend a proven treatment if it will serve the patient's needs, despite its categorization as CAM or conventional.

Obtaining Information on Licensing, Training, and Referral

The physician may have difficulty responding when asked by the patient for a referral to a CAM provider. Physician-to-physician referral is facilitated by state licensure requirements, knowledge of the center where formal medical education was acquired, and specialty board certification. The formal components of medical doctor licensure are not always required of various CAM providers. These components include the content and length of time of training, testing, and certification; a defined scope of practice; review and audit; and professional liability with regulatory protection and statutory authorization complete with codified disciplinary action (41).

All 50 states do provide licensure requirements for chiropractic, but only approximately half do so for acupuncture and massage therapy, and fewer do so for homeopathy and naturopathy. Only Connecticut and the state of Washington license all five of these provider types. Table 2.6 lists licensure status for the top CAM professions in the United States as of 1998. In England, only physicians are licensed to practice medicine, but other practitioners and patients can engage in other therapies without legal restraint. Special classifications of alternative medical practitioners also exist in Germany, France,

Australia, and other countries. In many Asian countries, full licensure and regulation of traditional practitioners occurs. In many developing countries, no regulation of such healers exists. Because the situation is constantly changing and varies from country to country and state to state, physicians should contact their own country or state licensing authorities for current information.

Many CAM organizations have requirements for membership that include some aspects of formal training, defined tutoring or mentoring internships, and testing. Although not equivalent to medical doctor licensure and board certification, these requirements represent an attempt to set standards, set scope of practice, and identify more credible and competent practitioners.

Therefore, the establishment of a CAM referral network may be more subjective than that for conventional medical referrals. In addition

Table 2.6. Licensing Status of CAM Professions by United States and Its Jurisdictions

STATE	ACUPUNCTURE	CHIROPRACTIC	HOMEOPATHY	NATUROPATHY	MASSAGE THERAPY
Alabama	—	SB	—	—	SB
Alaska	NB	SB	—	SB	—
Arizona	—	SB	SB	SB	—
Arkansas	—	SB	—	—	SB
California	1	SB	—	—	—
Colorado	NB	SB	—	—	—
Connecticut	—	SB	SB	SB	JB
Delaware	NB	SB	NB	NB	SB
District of Columbia	1	1	—	NB	SB
Florida	SB	SB	—	NB	JB
Georgia	1	SB	—	—	—
Guam	—	—	—	—	—
Hawaii	SB	SB	—	SB	JB
Idaho	—	SB	—	—	—
Illinois	—	1	—	—	—
Indiana	—	SB	—	–	—
Iowa	1	SB	—	—	SB
Kansas	—	SB	—	—	—
Kentucky	—	SB	—	—	—

continued

Table 2.6. Licensing Status of CAM Professions by United States and Its Jurisdictions

STATE	ACUPUNCTURE	CHIROPRACTIC	HOMEOPATHY	NATUROPATHY	MASSAGE THERAPY
Louisiana	1	SB	—	—	SB
Maine	JB	SB	—	JB	JB
Maryland	SB	SB	—	—	JB
Massachusetts	1	SB	—	—	—
Michigan	—	SB	—	—	—
Minnesota	—	SB	—	—	—
Mississippi	—	SB	—	—	—
Missouri	—	SB	—	—	—
Montana	1	SB	—	SB	—
Nebraska	—	SB	—	—	JB
Nevada	SB	SB	SB	SB	—
New Hampshire	NB	SB	NB	SB	JB
New Jersey	SB	SB	—	—	—
New Mexico	SB	SB	—	—	SB
New York	1	1	—	—	SB
North Carolina	SB	SB	—	—	—
North Dakota	—	SB	—	—	SB
Ohio	—	SB	—	—	JB
Oklahoma	—	SB	—	—	—
Oregon	1	SB	—	SB	SB
Pennsylvania	1	SB	—	—	—
Puerto Rico	—	SB	—	—	—
Rhode Island	NB	SB	—	—	JB
South Carolina	1	SB	—	—	JB
South Dakota	—	SB	—	—	—
Tennessee	—	SB	—	—	SB
Texas	SB	SB	—	—	JB
Utah	SB	SB	—	SB	JB
Vermont	SB	SB	—	NB#	—
Virginia	1	1	—	1	JB
Virgin Islands	—	—	—	—	—
Washington	SB	SB	—	SB	JB
West Virginia	NB	SB	—	—	JB
Wisconsin	SB	SB	—	—	—
Wyoming	—	SB	—	—	—

SB = profession regulated by its own separate board
JB = Joint Board; Board of Complementary Medicine or other
NB = profession regulated but under no board
1 = one board regulates MDs, DOs, PAs
— = Profession not reported as being regulated
= most register with Office of Professional Regulation
Adapted with permission from The Federation of State Medical Boards of the United States, Inc, 1995–1996 Exchange. Section 3: Licensing Boards Structure and Disciplinary Function.

to informal discussion with physician–colleagues, other patients may be a helpful source of information. When a referral is made, direct follow-up with the patient to assess clinical outcomes will provide additional information. As with physician referral, it is appropriate to expect a direct follow-up report from the CAM provider with details as to plan of care, defined goals of treatment, and a time line for results (42).

Reimbursement

In some countries (e.g., England and China), many CAM products and some practices are included under the national health insurance systems. In other countries (e.g., Germany), a combination of government health benefits and private insurance covers CAM benefits under conditions of special patient evaluation and follow-up.

In the United States, an increasing number of third-party payers now reimburse for some CAM interventions. This is a result of patients' desire for such services and employers responding to their employees' requests to do so as a benefit of the workplace. Thus, to be competitive in the marketplace, the third-party payer, such as a managed care company, agrees to provide a rider for some CAM modalities. Also, government health care support services are increasing their coverage of CAM, so the physician is likely to see such services available to a wider range of patients than currently exists (43).

Reimbursement can carry the imprimatur that: 1) CAM professional standards are in place; 2) there are appropriate indications for its use; 3) there is a favorable risk–benefit ratio in its application; and 4) the intervention is clinically efficacious and cost effective. Important operational issues must be established before affirming that these conditions exist. This includes establishing an authoritative panel of experts who will create criteria for: 1) appropriate referral and use; 2) cost and clinical effectiveness; 3) audit; and 4) determination of liability. Reimbursement is then based on a service done by payer-accredited providers. A provider

can be a CAM provider, but also can be a physician provider who is trained in a CAM modality (44).

Reimbursement also can result in the creation of protocols and plans of care for specific diagnoses that require shared responsibility between conventional and CAM providers. Such an integrated health plan assumes that both medical doctors and CAM providers understand each others' performance standards, share the same outcome goals for the patient, will be responsible for and responsive to monitoring and evaluating the treatments being given, and will work together in respectful and cooperative tandem. Given the level of antipathy that can exist between CAM and conventional groups, it is not certain that this cooperative venture can and will happen, although many groups are moving toward developing such integrated models of practice.

Liability and Regulatory Considerations

As the physician begins to address CAM in his or her practice, it is likely that referral to CAM practitioners and use of CAM practices and products along with conventional medical management will increasingly occur.

What risks does the practitioner take in beginning to address and use CAM alongside conventional practice? Is there an increased risk of malpractice or medical board action and scrutiny? The development of legal and regulatory issues related to integrated practice is still in its infancy, and at the same time is changing rapidly. A more personal and communicative practice generally reduces the risk of malpractice difficulties from patients in general. A limited scope of practice can also reduce the degree of risk. Full-time CAM practitioners have lower malpractice risk and insurance rates than do conventional physicians. However, in the legal system, conventional practitioners who use CAM may have less protection related to scope of practice and assumption of risk. Thus, although the improved patient communication and satisfaction that may come with an integrated practice may reduce the risk of malpractice claims from patients, liability may not be reduced if such a claim is filed.

Studdert (16) has evaluated malpractice liability issues for CAM providers. He has found that, although the number of claims and the claim rates for CAM providers are lower than for conventional providers (e.g., about one-third the rate for chiropractors than for medical doctors), the type and reasons for bringing claims against CAM providers are similar to claims against conventional physicians: misdiagnosis, failure to diagnose, continued treatment in the face of adverse effects, overly aggressive treatment, and so on (16).

Increasingly, courts have been willing to recognize school-specific standards for diagnosis and treatment where the legislature has recognized the legitimacy of the alternative practice through licensure. Patient "assumption of risk" is often cited as the rationale for adopting this position. It is reasonable to expect that for conventional physicians, conventional standards of care will be applied (including more stringent standards of "assumption of risk"), although there is little current case law to confirm this.

Disciplinary action from state medical boards and country regulatory authorities may also pose a risk for physicians who decide to make CAM services available in their own practice. Historically, use or association with CAM therapies has been a reason for professional and regulatory discipline. (The reader is referred to Chapters 1 and 3 for a discussion of historical and ethical aspects of professional discipline related to CAM.) Recently, some state medical boards have taken action against physicians who incorporate CAM practices based on standard of care and prevailing practice rules. The risk of prevailing practice as the basis for disciplinary action may decline as the awareness of wide practice variations in conventional medicine is documented, and also as states adopt laws for legal protection from such action brought solely on the basis of CAM use (so-called *access to treatment laws*). A summary of these issues and current legal precedents is available elsewhere (45).

Although the risks of malpractice and medical discipline appear relatively small, the conventional practitioner is best advised to take precautions when beginning to address CAM areas in his or her practice. Table 2.7 summarizes these steps. Ensuring that treatment or advice for patients using CAM is above standard-of-care for conventional medicine is wise. In addition, one should ensure that 1) competent conventional medicine (either from the physician or by referral) is provided; 2) potential risks (both direct and indirect) are minimized; 3) some reasonable body of competent opinion or published evidence exists for the practice; and 4) all treatments, referrals, and recommendations are thoroughly documented in patient records.

It is *not* advisable to rely on more liberal strategies, such as assumption of risk by the patient, reliance on a respected minority opinion only, use of an innovative (not experimental) approach or rationale, or an expanded informed consent form. Although such approaches are often used for defense in conventional medicine, using more conservative strategies with CAM is best (see Table 2.7), even when documented safety and efficacy data exist

---

Table 2.7. Guidelines for Reduction of Malpractice and Liability Risk

Recommended Actions

- Be sure that one's actions in case management are above the standard of care.

- Assure that competent conventional management is provided.

- Take steps to reduce risks (both direct and indirect).

- Determine if there is a reasonable body of professional opinion about the practice.

- Find published evidence indicating effectiveness of the practice.

- Document all treatments, referrals, and recommendations thoroughly.

Actions Not Recommended

- Assume that, by requesting treatment, the patient assumes full risk.

- Assume that an informed consent form— whether it is *detailed* and/or *expanded*—is protective.

- Rely only on a minority opinion.

- Assume that the approach is *innovative* rather than *experimental*.

for the treatment. Because regulatory and disciplinary bodies, such as state and federal legislatures, state medical boards, and the courts, have not provided guidelines in these areas, the true risk is unknown, and the aforementioned points should be taken only as suggestions. A detailed summary of the legal issues surrounding CAM practice in the United States is available in a recently published book by Cohen (45); these issues are summarized in a chapter in the *Textbook of Complementary and Alternative Medicine.*

FUTURE PROSPECTS FOR INTEGRATED MEDICINE

We can assume that patients will continue to use CAM, particularly for the symptomatic relief of chronic and stress-related disease. Also, patients will expect to be reimbursed for a growing number of CAM interventions. Physicians, therefore, will find themselves increasingly approached by patients who expect them to have knowledge of and be willing to work with CAM.

Many medical schools now offer elective CAM courses (45a). Also, formal CAM instruction is provided by many family practice residency programs (46) and increasingly in CME (continuing medical education) courses from universities. These educational approaches may result in an increase in physician referral to CAM providers and in the learning and use of various CAM interventions by medical doctors.

Historically, the mutual resistance of both conventional medicine and CAM to work together for the benefit of the patient has resulted in name calling and the use of pejorative adjectives. As the ethical principles of beneficence and respect for patient autonomy come to the forefront, we can hope to find that all such adjectives are replaced with the new term *integrated health care.*

REFERENCES

1. Hastings Center Report. The goals of medicine: setting new priorities. Briarcliff Manor, NY: The Hastings Center, 1996.
2. Eisenberg DM, Kessler RC, Foster C, et al. Unconventional medicine in the United States—prevalence, costs, and patterns of use. N Engl J Med 1993;328:246–252.
3. Eisenberg DM, Davis RB, Ettner S, et al. Trends in alternative medicine use in the United States. JAMA 1998;280:1569–1575.
4. McGinnis LS. Alternative therapies, 1990. Cancer 1991;67:1788–1792.
5. Anderson W, O'Connor BB, MacGregor RR, Schwartz JS, et al. Patient use and assessment of conventional and alternative therapies for HIV infection and AIDS. AIDS 1993;74:561–564.
6. Fisher P, Ward A. Complementary medicine in Europe. BMJ 1994;309:107–111.
7. MacLennan AH, Wilson DH, Taylor AW. Prevalence and cost of alternative medicine in Australia. Lancet 1996;347:569–573.
8. Furnham A, Forey J. The attitudes, behaviors and beliefs of patients of conventional vs complementary (alternative) medicine. J Clin Psychol 1994;50:458–469.
9. Astin JA. Why patients use alternative medicine. JAMA 1998;279:1548–1553.
10. Cassileth BR, Lussk EJ, Strouss TB, Bodenheimer BJ. Contemporary unorthodox treatments in cancer medicine: a study of patients, treatments, and practitioners. Ann Intern Med 1984;101:105–112.
11. Vincent C, Furnham A, Willsmore M. The perceived efficacy of complementary and orthodox medicine in complementary and general practice patients. Health Education: Theory and Practice 1995;10:395–405.
12. Bigos S, Bowyer OB, Braen G. Acute low back problems in adults: clinical practice guideline No 14. AHCPR Publication No. 95-0642. Rockville, MD: Agency for Health Care Policy and Research, 1994.
12a. PDR. The herbal Physicians Desk Reference. Philadelphia: PDR Press, 1999.
13. Panel on Definition and Description. Defining and describing complementary and alternative medicine. Altern Therap Health Med 1997;3:49–57.
14. Alternative Medicine: Expanding Medical Horizons. Washington, DC: Government Printing Office, 1993.
15. Ornish D, Brown SE, Scherwitz LW, et al. Can lifestyle changes reverse coronary heart disease? The lifestyle heart trial. [See this article's "Comments" section.] Lancet 1990;336:129–133.
16. Studdert DH, Eisenberg DH, Miller FH, et al. Medical malpractice implications of alternative medicine. JAMA 1998;280:1610–1615.
17. Ernst E. Bitter pills of nature: safety issues in complementary medicine. Pain 1995;60:237–238.
18. Report on Health Care Fraud from the Special

Committee on Health Care Fraud. Austin, TX: Federation of State Medical Boards of the United States, 1997.

19. De Smet PAGM, Keller K, Hänsel R, Chandler RF. Adverse effects of herbal drugs. Heidelberg: Springer-Verlag, 1997.

20. Bensoussan A, Myers SP. Towards a safer choice. Victoria, Australia: University of Western Sydney Macarthur, 1996.

21. Barrett S. The public needs protection from so-called "alternatives." The Internist 1994;Sept: 10–11.

22. Roberts AH, Kewman DG, Mercier L, Hovell M. The power of nonspecific effects in healing: implications for psychological and biological treatments. Clin Psychol Rev 1993;13:375–391.

23. Thomas KB. The placebo in general practice. Lancet 1994;344:1066–1067.

24. Chaput de Saintonage D, Herxheimer A. Harnessing placebo effects in health care. Lancet 1994;344:995–998.

25. Kleijnen J, Knipschild P. Gingko biloba for cerebral insufficiency. Br J Clin Pharm 1992;34: 352–358.

26. Kanowski S, Herrmann WM, Stephan K, et al. Proof of efficacy of the ginkgo biloba special extract EGb 761 in outpatients suffering from mild to moderate primary degenerative dementia of the Alzheimer type or multi-infarct dementia. Pharmacopsychiatry 1996;29:47–56.

27. Wilt TJ, et al. Saw palmetto extracts for treatment of benign prostatic hyperplasia: a systematic review. JAMA 1998;280:1604–1609.

28. Neil A, Silagy C. Garlic: its cardio-protective properties. Curr Opin Lipidol 1994;5:6–10.

29. Linde K, Ramirez G, Mulrow CD, et al. St. John's Wort for depression—an overview and meta-analysis of randomised clinical trials. [See this article's Comments section]. BMJ 1996;313:253–258.

30. ter Riet G, Kleijnen J, Knipschild P. A meta-analysis of studies into the effect of acupuncture on addiction. Br J Gen Pract 1990;40:379–382.

31. Gibson RG, Gibson S, MacNeill AD, Watson BW. Homeopathic therapy in rheumatoid arthritis: evaluation by double-blind clinical therapeutical trial. Br J Clin Pharm 1980;9:453–459.

32. Berman BM, Lao L, Greene M, et al. Efficacy of traditional Chinese acupuncture in the treatment of symptomatic knee osteoarthritis: a pilot study. Osteoarthritis Cartilage 1995;3:139–142.

33. Jonas WB, Rapoza CP, Blair WF. The effect of niacinamide on osteoarthritis: a pilot study. Inflamm Res 1996;45:330–334.

34. Tao XL, Dong Y, Zhang NZ. [A double-blind study of T2 (tablets of polyglycosides of *Tripterygium wilfodii* hook) in the treatment of rheumatoid arthritis.] [Chinese]. Chung-Hua Nei Ko Tsa Chih Chinese J Intern Med 1987;26:399–402, 444–445.

35. Altman RD. Capsaicin cream 0.025% as monotherapy for osteoarthritis: a double-blind study. Semin Arthritis Rheum 1994;23:25–33.

36. Kjeldsen-Kragh J, Mellbye OJ, Haugen M, et al. Changes in laboratory variables in rheumatoid arthritis patients during a trial of fasting and one-year vegetarian diet. Scand J Rheumatol 1995; 24:85–93.

37. Lavigne JV, Ross CK, Berry SL, et al. Evaluation of a psychological treatment package for treating pain in juvenile rheumatoid arthritis. Arthritis Care Res 1992;5:101–110.

38. Assendelft WJ, Koes BW, van der Heijden GJ, Bouter LM. The efficacy of chiropractic manipulation for back pain: blinded review of relevant randomized clinical trials. J Manipulative Physiol Ther 1992;15:487–494.

39. Jonas WB. Evaluating unconventional medical practices. J NIH Res 1993;5:64–67.

40. Eisenberg DM. Advising patients who seek alternative medical therapies. Ann Intern Med 1997; 127:61–69.

41. Fund MM. Enhancing the accountability of alternative medicine. New York: Milbank Memorial Fund, 1998.

42. Homola S. Finding a good chiropractor. Arch Fam Med 1998;7:20–23.

43. Weeks J. Alternative medicine integration and coverage. 1998; see volumes 1 & 2.

44. Weeks J. Operational issues in incorporating complementary and alternative therapies and providers in benefit plans and managed care organizations. Bethesda, MD: Agency for Health Care Policy and Research and Office of Alternative Medicine, National Institutes of Health, 1997. Available from the NCCAM Information Clearing House 1-800-644-6226.

45. Cohen MH. Complementary and alternative medicine: legal boundaries and regulatory perspectives. Baltimore: Johns Hopkins University Press, 1998.

45a. Wetzel MS, Eisenberg DM, Kaptchuk TJ. A survey of courses involving complementary and alternative medicine at United States medical schools. JAMA 1998;280:784–787.

46. Carlston M, Stuart M, Jonas W. Alternative medicine instruction in medical schools and family medicine residency programs. Fam Med 1997;29: 559–562.

CHAPTER 3

Ethics at the Interface of Conventional and Complementary Medicine

Howard Brody, Janis M. Rygwelski, and Michael D. Fetters

INTRODUCTION

Every medical and healing practice applies general laws to each individual case, and the intended outcomes are to promote the health of the patient and to avoid doing harm (1). Thus, all healing practices are moral enterprises—intended to do good and to avoid doing wrong—and most healing decisions involve a moral dimension. For centuries in Western conventional medicine, these moral and ethical issues were assumed as the almost exclusive province of physicians. However, since the 1960s, this assumption has been challenged, and there is now active research in medical ethics involving both nonphysicians (mostly philosophers, theologians, and legal scholars) and physicians. The result of this academic interest has deepened and broadened our understanding of medical ethics and has exposed some aspects of historical medical ethics as narrow and unjustifiable.

This chapter addresses some ways of conceptualizing medical ethics today to show how medical ethics applies equally well to both conventional and complementary medicine. Detail is provided for some specific issues raised by complementary medicine, both for its own practitioners and for conventional practitioners.

HISTORICAL BACKGROUND

For much of the past 100 years, medical ethics has exacerbated tension between conventional and complementary practitioners. It is important to distinguish carefully between this historical experience and what we mean by *medical ethics* and *medical morality* today. To understand this distinction, a brief discussion of power may be helpful.

Power and Ethics

The relationship between power and ethics sometimes goes unnoticed. From one perspective, ethics is about the appropriate use and misuse of power (2). In human relationships that have an imbalance of power, the exercise of power (especially when used with good intentions) tends to be relatively invisible to the person in the more powerful position. To the person with less power, the exercise of power is obvious, as is how exactly it works to his or her disadvantage. However, to the person with more power, it is relatively easy to construe that being in and exercising power is simply a manifestation of the fixed and normal order of the universe. In this scenario, the use of power escapes any critical scrutiny from within the more powerful group. And, from the viewpoint of this dominant class, any rival interpretation may be dismissed as groundless because the interpretation originates among the "wrong" people with presumably biased and incorrect viewpoints.

Sociologists have studied conventional medicine as a manifestation of this exercise of power. The medical profession may be viewed as having, in effect, struck a contract with mainstream society. Society grants conventional medicine a good deal of power and the autonomy to exercise it with little societal interference. In exchange, conventional medicine provides society with a highly valuable service—medical care in times of illness. This contract has often been very powerful (e.g., when physicians have literally risked death to deliver care during epidemics). One of the powers granted to conventional medicine by society is the privilege of defining *truth* as it pertains to a number of health-related issues. For example, when a person who has been absent from work is told to provide a note from his or her physician to certify the legitimacy of the absence, a minor and commonplace example of this delegation of power from society to the medical profession is seen. The employer views the employee's report of illness as unreliable, but the physician's certification of the same phenomenon is socially unchallenged. Although a critic may see this as an act of social dominance, physicians presume that they are merely reporting *the truth* as any rational person would see it. In this manner, physicians have gradually become less aware of the extent of their own exercise of social power than actually exists; that is, even though their intentions have been good, physicians may not realize how their use of power affects people.

The obvious, if unconscious, temptation this power creates within conventional medicine is to use the power to secure its own economic dominance over potential competitors and to justify these practices in the name of *scientific truth*, to which only regular physicians (and, of course, never their competitors) have exclusive access. Another power historically ceded to the medical profession is the privilege of developing its own internal code of ethics, without input or critical scrutiny from nonphysicians and society. With this power, medicine may declare that certain things are scientifically true. Good ethical physicians adhere to truth and avoid fraudulent practices; therefore, both truth and ethics require that regular physicians condemn certain types of practices engaged in by medicine's economic competitors.

This tendency is well illustrated by the history of the American Medical Association (AMA), founded in 1847. One of its first official actions was to write a code of ethics (1848). In the 1830s and 1840s, conventional medicine was increasingly beleaguered. Complementary schools of medicine flourished; simultaneously, the Jacksonian democracy movement forced the repeal of all state licensing laws that had favored the conventional profession. In hindsight, it is no accident that conventional physicians wanted an organization like the AMA during this time; nor is it surprising that the code of ethics enjoined conventional physicians to avoid contact with complementary practitioners and to work to undermine public confidence in those practices (see Chapter 1, "The History of Complementary and Alternative Medicine"). The AMA's "ethical" argument was that these practices were unscientific and grounded in a fraudulent view of the human body, so that no "regular" practitioner could be pure and true to his or her scientific calling if he or she recognized these practices.

A telling example of this philosophy was the relationship between conventional medicine and homeopathy during this time. Homeopathy presented two particular problems for conventional medicine. First, homeopathy was extremely popular for much of the nineteenth century, especially among better educated patients. Second, by any truly objective standard, homeopathic schools were the equal of the allopathic schools in the rigor and length of the curriculum. In New York, where homeopathy was particularly powerful, the stringent AMA code placed allopaths at a disadvantage. If conventional physicians refused to consult with the homeopaths or to attend any case in which homeopathic care was being administered, they risked a marked reduction in the size of their practices. They were also enjoined from consulting with physicians whom they might well have recognized personally as decent and well-informed practitioners. The end result was a curious schism within the state medical society, lasting from 1882 to 1900. During those years, there were two conventional medical societies in New York. One society followed the AMA code and continued to send delegates to the national AMA meetings. The other society allowed its members to consult with homeopaths and was denounced by the AMA as an illegitimate renegade group (3).

Well into the twentieth century, after the dominance of conventional medicine had been firmly established, the AMA shifted its attention to chiropractic. The code of ethics forbade consulting with or referring patients to chiropractors, and the AMA engaged in extensive lobbying to limit chiropractic scope of practice. This conflict was resolved by a rewriting of medicine's social contract: after antitrust action, the AMA was prohibited by the government from its anticompetitive activities and was in effect ordered to strike the chiropractic sections from its code of ethics (see Chapter 1, "The History of Complementary and Alternative Medicine," for more details regarding these dynamics).

This brief history lesson may suggest that medical ethics is the sworn enemy of complementary medicine and is nothing other than a power grab by conventional physicians seeking to retain all of their advantages and privileges. It is therefore extremely important to distinguish between the approach to ethics used by the AMA from 1848 into the 1960s from the current and legitimate academic study of ethics in medicine. Currently, ethics require that pronouncements are grounded in principles or concepts open to all people of reason, and any concept that attributes exclusive knowledge to practitioners of medicine is rejected. By these criteria, economic self-interest cannot be accepted as an appropriate basis for any ethical pronouncement. Moreover, although the former method of ethics took for granted the physician's power and generously bestowed a benevolent intent on any such exercise of power, current ethics work from the opposite assumption. Current theories in ethics assume that any exercise of medical power is in danger of trespassing on the patient's vital rights and interests. Therefore, ethics demand that exercise of power

be critically examined and justified—not only according to what physicians think is good for the patient, but also in terms of the patient's own free and informed choice.

For these reasons, we argue, first, that complementary medicine can hope for fair treatment from today's ethics; and second, that there is reason to hold today's ethics equally applicable to conventional and complementary healing practices.

APPROACHES TO THE ETHICS OF PRACTICE

Moral Principles

This chapter looks briefly at two ways of grounding an ethics of medicine: first, in terms of general moral principles; and second, in terms of what sort of activity or practice medicine is. The latter approach superficially resembles the old AMA code but differs by denying that physicians themselves have special or exclusive insight into the relevant questions.

The most widely used and cited modern textbook of medical ethics claims that the vast majority of ethical issues in medicine can be understood through the application of one or more of four general moral principles: autonomy, beneficence, nonmaleficence, and justice (Table 3.1) (4). These principles apply equally to many nonmedical aspects of living; therefore, their general relevance to moral issues helps increase our confidence that medical–ethical issues are being resolved wisely when these principles are applied to them.

In summary, *autonomy* requires that a person act in a manner that respects the rights of others to freely determine their own choices and destiny. *Beneficence* requires that a person tries to do good for others, especially those to whom one owes a professional duty. *Nonmaleficence*

Table 3.1. Principles of Medical Ethics
Autonomy
Beneficence
Nonmaleficence
Justice

requires that one avoids doing harm to others (a duty that applies generally, even in the absence of a professional obligation). *Justice* requires that one treats others fairly.

Difficult ethical dilemmas arise when one of these principles conflicts with another. The classic ethical problem of *paternalism* is a conflict between autonomy and beneficence: the paternalistic physician is inclined to ignore the patient's expressed choice because he or she believes that more good can be done for the patient that way. Because most modern thinkers believe paternalism in medicine is seldom justified if the patient is capable of making a rational, informed decision, autonomy is regarded as the dominant moral principle in this clash. The ethical–legal requirement of informed consent is a way of setting up respect for autonomy as a basic requirement of medical practice.

We see no problem in using these four principles as the basis for an ethic of either conventional or complementary medicine. The major requirement is that the terms *benefit* and *harm* are defined in ways that are neutral to the theory of healing being invoked. The most important consideration is what the patient regards as a benefit or harm; the next relevant consideration is what the practitioner, based on his or her own system of practice, regards as a benefit or harm. By contrast, it is wrong for conventional medicine to define a complementary practice as harmful *merely because* it is a complementary practice. However, if one particular complementary practice (or conventional practice, for that matter) leads to toxic reactions in a substantial percentage of patients, it is appropriate to regard that practice as harmful, assuming that the patients in question themselves label that outcome as harmful.

Type of Practice

The second approach to grounding medical ethics is through an understanding of the type of medical practice being used. This requires an understanding of the various goals of the healing practice and the means that the practice considers morally legitimate in pursuit of those goals (5). The goals and means detailed in Table 3.2 should be equally applicable to conventional

Table 3.2. Goals and Means of Eti Sound Medical Practice
GOALS OF MEDICAL PRACTICE
Reassuring the "worried well" who have no disease or injury
Diagnosing disease or injury
Helping the patient to understand the disease, its prognosis, and its effects on his or her life
Preventing disease or injury, if possible
Curing the disease or repairing the injury, if possible
Lessening the pain or disability caused by the disease or injury
Helping the patient to live with whatever pain or disability cannot be prevented
When all else fails, helping the patient die with dignity and peace
ETHICALLY ACCEPTABLE MEANS OF PRACTICE
The practitioner must employ technical competence in practice
The practitioner must honestly portray medical knowledge and skill to the patient and to the general public, and avoid any sort of fraud or misrepresentation
The practitioner must avoid harming the patient in any way that is out of proportion to expected benefit
The practitioner must maintain fidelity to the interests of the individual patient

and complementary practices. Based on the unfortunate historical precedents mentioned in the previous section, the critical terms to define are *competence* and *fraudulent*. Again, real ethical understanding requires that these terms be defined from the standpoint of the type of practice employed by the practitioner in question. It is fraudulent for a conventional physician untrained in homeopathy to prescribe homeopathic remedies, and it is fraudulent for an herbalist to prescribe methotrexate for cancer therapy. However, if each practitioner clearly states his or her intended approach to the patient and uses methods in which he or she has been properly trained, then no ethical duty has been breached.

If our analysis in this section is correct, then we have shown that there is no fundamental, ethical difference between the general goals and guiding principles of conventional and complementary medicine. These practices differ in their understanding of how the human body works and what methods most effectively alter bodily processes to maintain health and eliminate illness. However, both conventional and complementary practices are virtually identical in their goals and desired outcomes and in their aspirations toward a high level of professional legitimacy in how they are conducted.

ETHICS AT THE INTERFACE

This section addresses four basic issues:

1. Ethical duties conventional medicine owes to complementary medicine.
2. Ethical duties complementary medicine owes to conventional medicine.
3. Ethical duties of complementary medicine: legitimate research of its methods.
4. Other ethical duties of practitioners.

Ethical Duties Conventional Medicine Owes to Complementary Medicine

As our historical discussion shows, these duties do not arise in a vacuum. We believe that there is an unfortunate historical precedent. Conventional medicine today should seek not only to start on a fresh footing, but also to redress its questionable aspirations toward power and economic dominance.

This ethical duty begins with fidelity to the interest of the patient. Widely quoted research has shown that many patients who see conventional physicians have also used complementary healing (6). Therefore, physicians should assume, until proven otherwise, that their patients have seen a complementary practitioner. An overall appreciation of the patient's health and treatment requires an understanding of this aspect of care and sometimes cooperation between conventional physicians and complementary healers.

Both the nature of the complementary method used and the patient's reasoning in choosing to employ that method are part of the conventional physician's *holistic* approach to patient care. Some have used the term *holistic* to distinguish some complementary approaches from conventional medicine. We dissent from use of this term and insist instead that conventional medicine *should be* holistic in its approach to the patient (in which holism may be seen as identical with the so-called biopsychosocial model) (7). To us, this means that the patient should be approached as a whole person, not as a collection of organs containing a disease, and that the patient's body, mind, spirit, community, and culture are all part of the broad understanding required for successful healing. This approach is not a public relations ploy on the part of conventional medicine; it is instead required by a scientific understanding of human health and disease. To practice in a nonholistic, reductionistic manner is, simply put, unscientific. A holistic physician should account for the patient's use of any complementary remedies and what the patient thinks about his or her illness that led him or her to try these remedies.

An ethical and holistic approach to medicine is also a *relational* approach. A model of *sustained partnership* should mark the physician's approach to patient care, especially in the primary care specialties (8). We believe that physician and patient can be effective partners if the physician is open to learning about any and all remedies the patient uses and how these remedies relate to the treatments the physician recommends.

The following are recommended approaches for conventional physicians.

Duty to Warn the Patient

In a few cases, complementary practices are known to be positively harmful to patients, based on firm data; and a few complementary claims for healing are grossly exaggerated. In these cases, the conventional physician has the same duty to warn the patient as he or she would in the case of another conventional practitioner who is behaving incompetently.

Benefit of the Doubt

In the absence of firm data that a treatment is harmful, which will almost always be the case (see Chapter 4, " Evaluating Complementary and Alternative Medicine: The Balance of Rigor and Relevance"), the conventional physician should give the complementary practitioner the benefit of the doubt as long as the delivery of good medical care is not compromised. The physician should investigate sufficiently to be assured that the complementary practitioner is competent and that the healing employed is efficacious for the healer's intended purposes, or is at least harmless to the patient.

UNDERSTANDING COMPLEMENTARY MEDICINE

Ideally, the physician would become sufficiently versed about complementary practices so that he or she can discuss them with the patient and become familiar with local complementary practitioners and their degrees of skill. Realistically, however, this scenario is unlikely. In the absence of detailed knowledge, the physician may inform the patient that some complementary therapies seem to work, at least for some patients; that conventional medicine does not understand fully the means by which these remedies work; that the physician appreciates the patient discussing this with the physician and hopes he or she will continue this discussion in future visits; and that the physician welcomes this opportunity to learn more about specific complementary practices. Agreeing to search the medical literature to examine the evidence for CAM is useful (see Chapter 5, "How to Practice Evidence-Based Complementary and Alternative Medicine"). We believe this type of exchange reinforces the ideal partnership between physician and patient without going beyond the physician's actual knowledge base.

CONSULTING WITH COMPLEMENTARY PRACTITIONERS

The complexity of the patient's case may require the conventional physician to consult with the complementary practitioner to effectively coordinate the patient's care. Some models for this approach exist in the United States Indian Health Service, which has encouraged conventional physicians and native healers to practice cooperatively.

Once the conventional physician becomes aware of local, skilled complementary practitioners and of the efficacy of their treatments for certain classes of patients, and once he or she has examined the medical literature for evidence of safety and effectiveness, he or she may recommend these approaches to patients who demonstrate openness to such recommendations, precisely as he or she would recommend the use of other medical specialists and allied health services.

However, because of the multitude of complementary approaches available and the wide variability in state credentialing or licensure of complementary practitioners, this may be a more daunting task than it appears. Although the state may not recognize a complementary modality, local practitioners frequently belong to organizations or possess certification that assures a prescribed level of training.

In the absence of official licensure or prescribed legal standards, conventional practitioners must select complementary "colleagues" partially based on local reputation and community acceptance, partially based on knowledge of their training, and partially based on trust and goodwill.

Once a complementary medical practice has been validated by adequate scientific evidence, conventional practitioners should either provide the treatment themselves if possible, or provide the patients with access to that treatment through referral or other channels (see Chapter 2, "The Physician and Complementary and Alternative Medicine").

Ethical Duties Complementary Medicine Owes to Conventional Medicine

If conventional and complementary practitioners are to pay equal ethical respect to each other, they must recognize ethical obligations in both directions. It might seem to complementary practitioners that, because conventional medicine remains socially more powerful and wealthy, the principal ethical duties should lie on that side. However, we argue for reciprocal obligations.

REFERRALS

Proper care for patients requires that complementary practitioners refer patients to the conventional system when conventional medicine offers effective treatment for the particular disease from which the patient suffers (e.g., bacterial pneumonia). These referrals may include a promise to continue to provide supportive or supplemental complementary healing in addition to conventional medical treatment. Except in cases in which a direct conflict exists between complementary and conventional therapies, neither side should require that the patient declare an exclusive allegiance to one school of treatment as a precondition of care.

PATIENT EDUCATION

Some complementary systems rely on different definitions or measures of "benefit" from those employed by conventional medicine, and thus the patient should be educated as to these tenets of the complementary school of healing. This will allow the patient to make an informed choice of treatment modalities (9).

TOLERANCE

We contend that a complementary practitioner should not deny the potential benefit of a medicine just because it is prepared in a pharmacological laboratory using synthetic compounds, as long as the patient would deem the response to the medication as positive and desirable. Because there may never be a full reconciliation between complementary and conventional paradigms, the patient's view of what is a harmful or beneficial reaction can serve as a framework for judgment.

SPIRITUAL CONSIDERATIONS

Several complementary systems especially stress the spiritual aspects of healing; this dimension has been largely ignored by conventional medicine. To the extent that conventional medicine now accepts a scientific obligation to seek more holistic approaches to the care of the patient, complementary medicine can help conventional to better understand the importance of the spiritual dimension. Moreover, complementary healing traditions may be particularly adept at avoiding the mind–body dualism that conventional medicine tends to propagate. Conventional medicine stands to benefit from this expertise developed in many of the complementary traditions.

Ethical Duties of Complementary Medicine: Legitimate Research of Its Methods

A profession that seeks the good of others and of society maintains high ethical standards when it is maximally accountable. One of the more exemplary features of conventional medicine has been its reliance on scientific research; it has been willing to discard remedies which, however well grounded in biological theory they may at first have appeared, have been shown by empirical trial to lack efficacy. However, some complementary schools of medicine employed sophisticated research techniques even before conventional medicine did; for example, homeopathy introduced blinding into its routine research design almost a century before conventional investigators did so (see Chapter 4, "Evaluating Complementary and Alternative Medicine: The Balance of Rigor and Relevance") (10).

It may seem that complementary medicine has little if any obligation in this direction, because it lacks the vast resources society has granted to conventional medicine for purposes of conducting research. However, the government and private foundations have shown interest in funding studies of complementary practices, and so the complementary medical community must begin to address its own research priorities and methods. There is a wide variation among complementary practices in the amount and type of research conducted to date.

We may distinguish healing practices based on faith and evidence. Some healing relies on faith, which, by definition, is only partly grounded in empirical evidence, and requires that one go beyond whatever can be proven or demonstrated rationally. It would be self-contradictory for advocates of faith-based healing to offer, or to demand, empirical proof of the efficacy of the healing practice. However, most complementary practices appear grounded in empirical systems of understanding the human body or the mind–body complex, regardless of how different these systems may be from the science of conventional medicine. In this case, it is not logically consistent for the complementary practice to deny the possibility of empirical proof or disproof of its claims. Moreover, practitioners who see practical possibilities for empirical investigations into the efficacy and mechanisms of their treatments but who do not avail themselves of these opportunities are lacking in accountability and thus occupy an ethically suspect position.

These comments must be understood within the context of what it means to conduct valid research on complementary practices. We reject the perspective that one can deny the value of complementary medicine simply because research conducted by the standards of conventional science fails to provide a basis for the complementary practice. It is not sufficient, in our view, for conventional medical scientists to conduct conventional-type research upon complementary practices, and then reject those practices because no conventional basis can be found for them without at least some critical scrutiny of whether the conventional research methods are truly appropriate for evaluating both the complementary approach and the setting in which it is practiced. The critical issue is about the types of research studies: can they be designed so that they are respectful of complementary practices, yet unbiased against those practices by the very nature of the research design? If so, and if resources exist for conducting such studies, then complementary practitioners *as a group* are ethically deficient if they do not take advantage of the research opportunities and report the results openly. Not every practitioner can become a scientific investigator; professional or group responsibilities must be distinguished carefully from individual responsibilities.

Despite a century of heavy reliance on the scientific method, conventional medicine includes several diagnostic and therapeutic practices that are of undocumented efficacy. Some of these practices are, in fact, efficacious; and

some practices simply do not work, despite both physicians and patients believing in them. To us, it is a sign of the ethical vitality of conventional medicine that its practitioners *care which treatments are proved or unproved,* and are willing to alter their habitual practices based on carefully conducted research showing the efficacy of a treatment. If complementary medicine seeks a secure place within society as a legitimate and ethically sound practice, then its practitioners should emulate this approach. Admittedly, the present willingness of some of the public to believe in complementary treatments (even those without scientific evidence) leaves practitioners with the power to ignore any proof-of-efficacy issues and still succeed economically and perhaps politically. But economic success, as conventional medicine knows, is not the same as the ethical high road.

Other Ethical Duties of Practitioners

Willingness to conduct properly designed research into its methods is only one of many obligations all medical practitioners owe to their patients. The scope of this chapter cannot accommodate a review of all ethical duties (e.g., informed consent) that apply equally to complementary and to conventional practitioners. However, a few issues merit specific comment.

It has been widely and generally stated that physicians are supposed to place fidelity to the patient's benefit above any interests of their own. This statement is good public relations, and physicians have made exceptional sacrifices to serve patients in need. But as a matter of day-to-day practice, physicians do not and should not act this way. According to this stringent ethical code, physicians should not take days off or vacations and should happily face bankruptcy rather than withhold services from any who cannot pay.

A much more realistic statement of medical ethics is that practitioners are constantly facing conflicts between their altruistic service goals and legitimate self-interest, and they must constantly work to find a reasonable balance. To deny the need for balance and to insist that practitioners should serve patients without regard for their own interest may have deleterious consequences. By setting an impossibly high standard, ethics become purely an idealistic exercise without practical value, because virtually all practitioners fail to live up to this standard.

All practitioners have some legitimate self-interests. Among complementary practitioners these include establishing individual economic well-being and promoting legitimacy and support for their type of practice. One can often promote these ends while simultaneously providing benefits and avoiding harm to individual patients. If some conflict exists, however, then patient benefit and professional accountability should take priority over self-interest.

The following case study provides an illustration of inappropriate balancing.

CASE EXAMPLE

A patient who had developed cancer sued both his family physician and two complementary practitioners. The family physician had initially treated him for worrisome symptoms and had advised him to return soon for further evaluation. The patient instead went to the two other practitioners who did not advise returning to the family physician. As a result, the cancer went undiagnosed for many months, probably leading to a worse prognosis.

In depositions, the deans of two schools of complementary medicine where the practitioners had trained testified that there was no standard of practice in that particular field of complementary medicine. By definition, malpractice cannot be found unless the standard of practice is violated, so this testimony stated that no complementary practitioner in that school could ever be successfully sued for malpractice. The result was that the entire burden of the lawsuit was shifted to the family physician.

COMMENTS ON CASE

The course pursued by these complementary practitioners may have been an excellent legal ploy. By denying the basis for any tort action in law, the testimony of these leaders of the field neatly shifted the total burden to the physician (and to his "deep pockets" insurance company). In terms of economic self-interest, it was a brilliant strategy.

However, the ethics of this strategy are questionable in terms of public accountability. The two deans were saying, in effect, that they had never had grounds to flunk a student; presumably, anyone who enrolled and paid fees was guaranteed graduation and a diploma. The deans were saying to the public that membership in their particular school of complementary medicine did not entail any accountability, nor did it guarantee any standards of basic professional competence. "Let the buyer beware" would be the only prudent course a patient could adopt upon consulting anyone who prac-

ticed within that system or studied at that school. Of course, we presume that the deans did not intend to say these things and would assuredly not have said any of those things were they instead addressing, for example, the local Rotary Club luncheon. But the fact that they would say one thing about their discipline in the Rotary Club and something diametrically opposed in a court of law suggests that they were allowing economic interests to override any ethical concerns about public accountability.

The final negative consequence of this type of case is that it discourages conventional physicians from trusting in the goodwill of, or offering to collaborate with, complementary practitioners. Moreover, given the lack of education among conventional physicians about the various types of complementary medicine, these actions by one group of practitioners are likely to tar the entire complementary movement.

Ethical professionals naturally wish to receive credit when their treatments succeed, but that also implies that they should accept some measure of potential blame when their treatment fails. They wish to be paid reasonable fees for their healing practices, which means they should publicly promulgate and adhere to standards of practice. To take accountability for only the positive outcomes of their practice and to refuse any accountability for the negative outcomes is an unprofessional approach.

CONCLUSION

The cooperation between conventional and complementary systems of health care is in its infancy, and the current stage is critical. If patient autonomy is indeed an important ethical value, then the patient must assume more responsibility. Conventional medicine must yield some responsibility along with some of its exclusive claims to power. Conventional physicians may feel threatened by giving up some of their historical power and esteem, but they would benefit by a new social climate that does not make them the scapegoats for any negative health outcome. Patients must recognize that they cannot expect conventional physicians to be equally well versed in all other healing systems, so that if patients decide to use a particular method outside the physician's expertise, the physician cannot be held accountable for its failure or harm.

An ideal health care system is one in which power is shared equally among the patient, the conventional physician, and the complementary healer, with the patient piloting the ship. Currently we are far from that system, and approaching it will be a challenging transition. Among other factors, this transition requires a change in thinking about health outcomes instead of focusing strictly on disease and diagnosis. A practice that focuses only on curing disease shifts power inevitably toward the practitioner, whereas a practice aimed at optimizing health tends to stress shared responsibility and the power of the individual. Moreover, the treatment's effectiveness is much more important to a patient than the healing paradigm that explains it. Whether the benefit is a placebo effect

is of little concern to the patient who feels better. Conventional and complementary medicine coexist best when both recognize that a placebo response is as favorable and important as a specific therapeutic response because the ultimate goal is the health and well-being of the patient (11). Placebo effects may have been stigmatized in the past because they were associated with deception (i.e., "dummy" pills). Today, scientifically informed practitioners of both conventional and complementary medicine can agree that all treatments, in addition to their powers to alter the body directly, exert psychological and spiritual effects that may themselves add to healing.

In the late 1970s, when textbooks of medical ethics in the modern era first began to be published, it was typical for each text to be liberally illustrated with case examples. Some monographs on medical ethics consisted entirely of cases and commentaries. By highlighting real dilemmas and indicating some of the ethically problematic features of actual practice, this case focus was helpful for the developing field of medical ethics. Unfortunately, these case studies were only rarely accompanied by any true epidemiology of ethics, in which one sought to find out exactly how common or how rare specific sorts of cases and dilemmas were in practice overall.

Ethics of complementary medicine today is in much the same state as the ethics of conventional medicine in the 1970s. Collections of case studies, with quantitative assessments of the most common, most vexing, and most clinically relevant ethical problems for complementary healers, would help focus attention on the matters of greatest concern to the front-line practitioners and help guide future research and education.

Some conventional physicians in the 1970s attacked or ignored this new field of ethical inquiry because it was a threat to their historical prerogatives or because they felt that nonphysicians could say nothing useful to them about their practices. But many other physicians embraced this line of inquiry as a way of improving the quality of practice and making practice more emotionally satisfying. We anticipate both types of reactions among today's complementary practitioners who have even more reason to be skeptical of anything emanating from conventional medicine. We hope that the latter reaction will ultimately dominate.

References

1. Pellegrino ED, Thomasma DC. A philosophical basis of medical practice. New York: Oxford University Press, 1981.
2. Brody H. The healer's power. New Haven: Yale University Press, 1992.
3. Starr P. The social transformation of American medicine. New York: Basic Books, 1982.
4. Beauchamp TL, Childress JF. Principles of biomedical ethics, 4th ed. New York: Oxford University Press, 1994.
5. Miller FG, Brody H. Professional integrity and physician-assisted death. Hastings Center Report 1995;25(3):8–17.
6. Eisenberg DM, Kessler RC, Foster C, et al. Unconventional medicine in the United States: prevalence, costs, and patterns of use. N Engl J Med 1993;328:246–252.
7. Engel GL. The need for a new medical model: a challenge for biomedicine. Science 1977;196:129–136.
8. Leopold N, Cooper J, Clancy C. Sustained partnership in primary care. J Fam Pract 1996;42:129–137.
9. Clouser KD, Hufford DJ, O'Connor BB. Informed consent and alternative medicine. Altern Ther 1996;2:76–78.
10. Kaptchuk TJ. When does unbiased become biased? The dilemma of homeopathic provings and modern research methods. Br Homeop J 1996;85:237–247.
11. Lynoe N. Ethical and professional aspects of the practice of alternative medicine. Scand J Soc Med 1992;4:217–225.

CHAPTER 4

Evaluating Complementary and Alternative Medicine: The Balance of Rigor and Relevance

Klaus Linde and Wayne B. Jonas

INTRODUCTION

THE SCIENTIFIC APPROACH TO MEDICINE

Applying scientific methods to medicine is a relatively recent phenomenon. Technologies for examining basic life processes, such as cellular functioning, genetic regulation of life, and mechanisms of infectious agents and environmental stressors to disease, have developed only in the last 100 years. The randomized controlled clinical trial is only 50 years old and has been an established standard for accepting new drugs for only about half that time. Statistical principles and approaches for analyzing large data sets have also only recently evolved. The use of scientific methods has taken much of the guesswork and unverifiable theory out of medicine by providing more precision and control over the body and the public's health than ever before. The continued development and refinement of science and technology promise even greater benefits to medicine in the future.

Despite the rather recent development of science-based approaches to biology and medicine, a wide array of research methods now exists for acquiring information useful for treating disease and illness. We discuss methods of investigation frequently used in medical research and the general type of information that these approaches provide. Figure 4.1 illustrates how these methods of investigation are put together into strategies of medical research.

- **Qualitative research,** such as detailed case studies and patient interviews, describe diagnostic and treatment approaches and investigate patient preferences and the relevance of those approaches. Qualitative approaches have been extensively developed in the nursing profession and are becoming increasingly common in primary care.
- **Laboratory and basic science approaches** investigate the basic mechanisms and biological plausibility of practices. In vitro (e.g., cell culture, intracellular with probe technology), in vivo (e.g., testing in normal, disease prone or genetically altered animals), and mixed approaches are now extensively used.
- **Observational studies,** such as practice audit, outcomes research, and other types of observational research, describe associations between interventions and outcomes. Practice audit involves monitoring outcomes on all or a selected sample of patients who receive treatment with evaluation before and after an intervention to measure effects. These studies may not have a comparison group; or, comparison groups may be developed by sampling patients not treated with the interven-

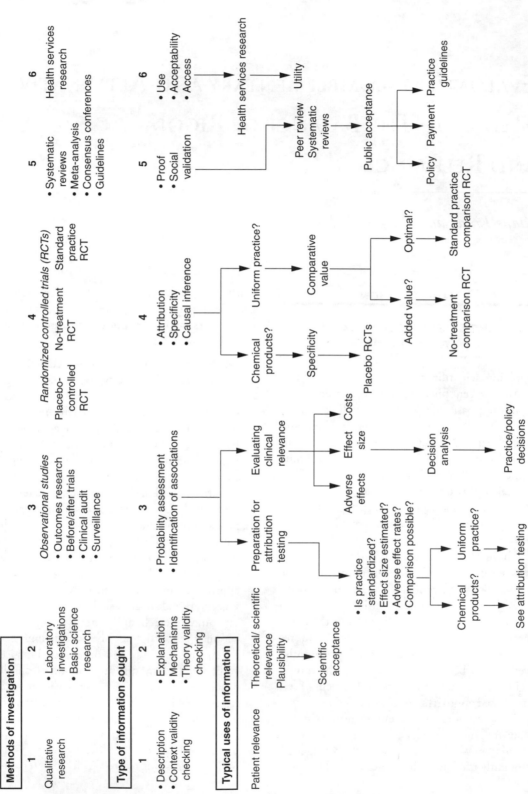

Methods of investigation

1	2	3	4	5	6
Qualitative research	• Laboratory investigations • Basic science research	*Observational studies* • Outcomes research • Before/after trials • Clinical audit • Surveillance	*Randomized controlled trials (RCTs)* Placebo-controlled RCT No-treatment RCT Standard practice RCT	• Systematic reviews • Meta-analysis • Consensus conferences • Guidelines	Health services research

Type of information sought

1	2	3	4	5	6
• Description • Context validity checking	• Explanation • Mechanisms • Theory validity checking	• Probability assessment • Identification of associations	• Attribution • Specificity • Causal inference	• Proof • Social validation	• Use • Acceptability • Access

Typical uses of information

FIGURE 4.1. Research strategy chart.

tion from other practices or in the same practice previous to the intervention.

- **Randomized controlled trials (RCTs)** which attempt to isolate or compare the specific contribution of different interventions on outcomes. These studies usually involve assigning patients to one treatment group or another using a method that assures the groups are comparable on all factors that might influence outcomes, except for the treatment. Various methods, such as randomly selected numbers or computer-generated assignment, are used. The treatment may be evaluated without knowledge of this assignment; these trials are best done by concealing knowledge of which patients will get which treatment at the time of assignment.
- **Meta-analysis, systematic reviews, and expert review and evaluation** assess the accuracy of the previously mentioned methods. Methods for expert review and summary of research have evolved over the last several years. Systematic, protocol-driven methods, such as meta-analysis, are used increasingly to try and prove that the effects found in clinical research are accurate and applicable across populations.
- **Health services research** examines the actual use and impact of interventions in context of social factors, such as access, feasibility, cost, practitioner competence, patient compliance, and so on. This type of research often involves surveys or sampling from groups already receiving an intervention; the research looks at the quality and costs of the intervention, as well as other factors. Random sampling may or may not be used.

Although certain groups may preferentially seek out one or more of these methods and the type of information they provide (e.g., basic scientists may have more interest in laboratory research results), information from all of these methods may be needed for making clinical decisions.

Tension often exists between research that tries to isolate specific mechanisms and effects (e.g., laboratory, RCTs, meta-analyses) and research that tries to identify the pragmatic use and patient-specific relevance of a practice in the real world (e.g., qualitative, observational, health services). Because addressing more than one question in a single research project is rare, designing research strategies that attempt to address both specific and pragmatic questions simultaneously is often difficult. To address both specificity and pragmatism, strategies for applying and interpreting multiple research methods are needed. Without such strategies, research methods and their interpretation are inconsistently applied in both conventional and complementary medicine. A consistent set of decision rules for the strategic application of research methods in medicine is a needed step in the continued development of science-based medicine (1). Figure 4.1 illustrates a framework for developing such strategies.

Evaluating and Researching CAM Treatments

Complementary and alternative medicine is no different from conventional medicine when it comes to the application of research methods (2). In addition, the interaction of conventional and unconventional medicine has often resulted in improvements in the scientific method. Fifty years ago, for example, current methods of blinding and randomization became accepted parts of orthodox medical research after they were first developed and applied to unorthodox practices, such as mesmerism and psychic healing, in an attempt to disprove them (3). Thus, research in CAM may help us develop the decision rules for a consistent strategic approach to the application and interpretation of science in medicine. We illustrate the application of research methods to the CAM modalities of herbalism (phytotherapy), acupuncture, homeopathy, and complex naturopathic interventions, and show some of the strategies that have emerged. We then outline how these research strategies may help us develop decision rules for the assessment of chronic disease in both conventional medicine and CAM.

EFFECTIVE TREATMENT

Is the treatment effective? This is the most crucial question for all therapies, regardless of whether they are considered conventional or complementary. A therapeutic intervention is effective if it beneficially influences the course of a patient's disease. The concept of effectiveness includes a causal element (i.e., *Is it the treatment that makes the difference?*) and a quantitative element (i.e., *What is the degree of change?*). For determining whether a therapy is effective in a single patient, one would essentially have to compare the course of the disease both with and without the treatment in that patient. This is rarely possible, and in most conditions the untreated course is not predictable.

The next most straightforward way to evaluate effectiveness is in controlled trials with groups of approximately comparable patients, where one group receives the treatment and the other group receives no treatment. A placebo-controlled condition should be included if the research is more narrowly focused than on the question, *Is the treatment effective?* For example, the research may aim to find the proportion of the *specific effects* attributable to a particular feature of the intervention under scrutiny (e.g., needling a specific acupuncture point in a specific way) in comparison to the *nonspecific effects* from the act of treating in general (e.g., the act of needling in general). This type of research gives information about the treatment's effectiveness over placebo, rather than effectiveness in general. This information may or may not be important for the individual patient, depending on the risks, costs, feasibility, and other factors involved in the treatment. However, this information does not answer the question regarding the treatment's effectiveness; in actual practice, a patient is not given the option of placebo treatment or no treatment based on a random selection process.

Frequently, the clinician and patient want to know if the therapy they choose is the most effective treatment out of several treatment options. This is an attempt to find an answer to another question, *Is this the most effective treatment?* Determining the answer to this question requires direct comparison of two active treatments to evaluate their relative merits (*comparative effectiveness*). In any of these tests, ensuring that the groups are comparable before treatment requires, whenever possible, randomization. The outcomes evaluated should be relevant primarily for the patient, but these or other outcomes may also be needed either for the provider or for public policy decisions. The methodology of the study should minimize the influence of chance and systematic error, but this needs to be balanced as much as possible with how the treatment is actually delivered in the health care system. Table 4.1 illustrates these questions and their relationship to some of the research methods from Figure 4.1.

Evidence from research (i.e., evidence showing scientifically that a treatment works on groups of individuals who have a condition similar to the one that the physician is treating) is only one type of information needed for decision making in daily practice. These are some other factors:

- **A clinician's personal experience.** The physician has seen the therapy benefit similar patients.
- **Plausibility.** It makes sense that the therapy should benefit the patient.
- **Patient acceptability.** The therapy will be acceptable for patients and is most likely to serve their objectives.
- **Economic and social reasons.** The therapy costs less and is wanted by payers and policymakers.

Table 4.1. Clinical Questions and Research Designs	
1. Is the treatment effective for this patient?	Therapeutic trial with the patient
2. Is the treatment effective on average for patients with conditions like this?	No-treatment comparison controlled trial
3. Is an aspect of the treatment effective on average for patients with conditions like this?	Sham (placebo)–controlled trial
4. Is this a more effective treatment on average for patients with conditions like this than another treatment?	Two-treatment comparison controlled trial
5. Is the effect biologically demonstrated?	Laboratory experimentation

In conclusion, both the question *"Is it effective?"* and the principal approach to answer that question are the same for all therapies. However, the optimal strategy for applying these approaches when evaluating a therapy may be different for different types of interventions, as illustrated with the following CAM examples.

EVALUATION OF SPECIFIC CAM PRACTICES

Phytotherapy

Phytomedicine is the use of plants and their preparations for preventative or therapeutic purposes. Phytomedicine is a central part of traditional medicine in almost all cultures, and many drugs used today in Western medicine have been directly or indirectly derived from active plant components.

What is unconventional about phytomedicine? First, knowledge about using a specific plant or plant extract for a defined ailment is almost always based on empirical experience instead of systematic scientific research. As a consequence, a plant is often in widespread use *before* it becomes an object of scientific investigation. In contrast to the development of conventional drugs—defining the substance, screening and toxicity tests in vitro and in animals, pilot trials in small patient groups, larger randomized trials, and postmarketing surveillance—the development of phytomedicine does not proceed in the same order.

Second, plant extracts always contain a variety of bioactive substances in relatively small concentrations. This complex composition makes the identification of a mechanism of action difficult. The relatively low concentrations of single components further decrease the *a priori* credibility of effectiveness (at least among scientists). Given this situation, the strategy to evaluate a widely used plant preparation cannot be exactly the same as for a newly developed drug.

The primary questions are safety and effectiveness in actual use. In addition, there is a problem common for phytomedicine—the comparability of plant preparations. *Echinacea*, a plant originally used by North American Indians and now in widespread use for the prevention and treatment of upper respiratory tract infections, is an example of this comparability problem. Three different species of *Echinacea* are in medicinal use (*E. purpurea, E. angustifolia, E. pallida*); sometimes only the roots are used, sometimes only the stems and leaves are used, and sometimes both are used. Some preparations contain pressed juice from fresh plants, whereas other preparations contain alcoholic extracts from dried plants. Depending on these variables, the composition and the concentrations of components can vary widely. Even within one product, the concentrations of components may vary according to the origin or quality of the plant material, the timing of collection, and other related factors. In some widely used plant preparations, such as St. John's Wort (*Hypericum perforatum*), garlic, ginkgo, horse chestnut, or hawthorn, the problems, although in principle the same, are less pronounced. This is because high-quality preparations of these plants are standardized in their content of a characteristic component, which in most cases—but not always—is related to the clinical effects.

An efficient strategy for evaluating herbal preparations must integrate research on effectiveness and safety with a certain amount of basic research. This research must determine a minimum of comparability in the content of active or marker ingredients. Such a strategy is expensive, and most manufacturers of herbal preparations have neither the resources nor the expertise for such a program. Because plant extracts tend to have relatively moderate effects, the risk of getting nonsignificant results in a clinical trial is relatively high; also, it may not be possible to recruit the large numbers of subjects needed for a trial to show statistical significance. Furthermore, patents of plant extract processes do not secure exclusive market advantage on the product, so companies that produce herbal preparations have limited interest in investing large amounts of money into research. In addition, if certain herbal products come into direct competition with highly profitable prescription drugs, research may develop in an attempt to discredit such herbal research if the market share of the prescription drug is threatened.

CURRENT RESEARCH

Example 1: St. John's Wort

Several hundred randomized clinical trials of herbal preparations are available. Most clinical trials of herbal preparations are placebo-controlled. No plant preparation has reached the status of a standard treatment on a worldwide level. A possible candidate to achieve this status is St. John's Wort (*Hypericum*), which has been tested in approximately 40 randomized trials (4–7). There is evidence that *Hypericum* extracts are more effective than placebo and are as effective as standard antidepressants in treating mild and moderately severe depression (4, 5). However, the existing trials suffer from weaknesses in the characterization of patients, and the doses of standard antidepressants used in comparative trials have been low. Also, it is not clear to what extent the results obtained with one specific extract can be extrapolated to another. Good-quality *Hypericum* preparations are standardized in their content of hypericins. Hypericins, however, are only one of the possibly active component groups of *Hypericum* extract; the existing evidence suggests that a number of components synergistically influence various metabolic pathways involved in depression (8).

Future research regarding this herb has to fill the gaps left by existing clinical trials, such as effectiveness in more severe depression, long-term effectiveness, and safety. Also, pharmaceutical and pharmacological research on product comparability and mechanisms of action are needed to complement the clinical data. Given the huge public interest and the financial interest by the pharmaceutical industry, it seems possible that sufficient resources will be available to realize such research.

Example 2: Ginkgo biloba

Another promising group of plant preparations is *Ginkgo biloba* extracts. Approximately 40 controlled trials done on dementia patients have established that these extracts effectively enhance cerebral functioning and diminish a number of symptoms of cerebral insufficiency in the elderly (9–11). These trials measured only cognitive functioning rather than activities of daily living, which today are considered the most important outcomes. A number of further trials suggest that *Ginkgo* is also effective in treating certain aspects of other conditions, including cardiovascular and peripheral arterial disease (9, 12–14). Again, several constituents seem to be involved in the clinical effects of *Ginkgo*, but defined pharmacological effects can often be attributed to single substance groups; for example, the inactivation of toxic oxygen radicals is mainly caused by the action of *Ginkgo* flavanoids.

The research conducted on *Hypericum*, *Ginkgo*, and other relatively well-investigated plant preparations, such as garlic (15–19); evening primrose oil (20–22); ginseng (23); *Echinacea* (24), mistletoe (25, 26); horse chestnut (27), Kava (28); *Valeriana* (29); hawthorne (30), saw palmetto (31); or feverfew (32), should not obscure the fact that most medically used plant preparations have not been evaluated in rigorous clinical trials. Although it seems realistic that some plant preparations will be systematically investigated in-depth over the next several years, some efficient, simplified strategies must be established to deal with the majority that will not.

These strategies are necessary because, although most herbal preparations have relatively few side effects if taken orally and if instructions on dosage and duration of use are followed, these preparations are not free of risks, and cases of severe adverse effects have been reported (see Chapter 6) (33, 34). It seems that standards specific to phytotherapy need to address product quality, safety monitoring, and some reasonable measure of benefit. The evaluation of efficacy with expensive and time-consuming randomized trials is difficult in phytomedicine because of the moderate effects of these substances and their use mainly for chronic, non–life-threatening diseases with subjective endpoints.

Acupuncture

Most people see the logic in asking, *Is garlic effective for lowering blood pressure?* and not, *Is phytomedicine effective for lowering blood pres-*

sure? However, the logic of asking about specific treatments rather than whole systems of therapy is frequently forgotten in the case of acupuncture. *Is acupuncture effective for chronic pain?* or *Is acupuncture effective for asthma?* are questions typically asked by those unfamiliar with acupuncture rather than questions as to whether a specific type of acupuncture treatment is effective. For example, if a group of asthma patients who meet defined inclusion criteria is randomized to receive acupuncture at certain points, at a certain depth, with or without achievement of *de-chi* (a specific needling sensation), with or without electrical stimulation, and so forth, and if this group does better than the group receiving placebo (superficial needling or at different acupuncture points), does that mean that acupuncture works for treating asthma? Conversely, if such studies do not provide consistent evidence for an effect over placebo, does that mean that acupuncture is only placebo?

The first major problem in evaluation is that acupuncture is not a uniform treatment as is the application of a 1-mg aspirin tablet. Acupuncture, like physical therapy or surgery, is applied in very different ways. If a treatment strategy in a trial is interpreted as *the acupuncture treatment of asthma,* it must be *representative*, at least for a defined group of providers and a defined group of patients. In a systematic review of 15 randomized trials of "acupuncture for asthma," variable results and very different treatment strategies were found (35). Only two trials by the same author used the same acupuncture points. This makes one wonder if acupuncture treatment (like psychotherapy or surgery) is practitioner-dependent, which makes it difficult to determine the consistency of both acupuncture theory and practice.

However, one should not rush to conclusions based on a small sample of trials with a variety of study models in heterogeneous patient samples. What can be concluded from the available asthma trials? Surely, that not all acupuncture works in all asthma patients in each study model. But are some acupuncture strategies effective, and others not? Do we need 10 further studies with 10 further treatment strategies with uncertain generalizability? Should acupuncture be reimbursed? Acupuncturists should be en-

couraged to do research on what they are doing in actual practice and why they do it. They should monitor the outcomes of their patients carefully and check if there are major discrepancies and differences in findings. This type of research will not convince skeptics or answer the question, *Does acupuncture have specific effects?* It can, however, help develop guidelines and establish clinically relevant hypotheses that can then be tested in a randomized clinical trial to determine the probability of an effect with a certain treatment approach.

In some of the available asthma trials, lung function, symptoms, and medication use did not change during the study. However, a simple prospective observational study would give us similar information and would not require a controlled trial. The idea behind this is that if you have no change at all (i.e., a nonprogressive condition), you do not need an RCT. A prospective case series with no differences between before treatment and after treatment is sufficient. If the results of an observational study and a randomized trial are conflicting (e.g., a clear improvement in the observational study versus no change, even within groups in the randomized trial), this information is important, but its interpretation is difficult. For example, are the discrepancies due to bias? Or did the experimental design interfere with the context or delivery of the normal acupuncture procedure?

ACUPUNCTURE AND PLACEBO

A second major problem with acupuncture research is the subject of placebo. Most randomized acupuncture trials include some form of placebo control (see references 36 through 43 for systematic reviews of acupuncture treatment for various conditions). Acupuncture is a complex intervention. Randomized trials of conventional complex interventions are rarely placebo-controlled; for example, the idea of comparing physical therapy and placebo-physical therapy seems at least questionable, and comparing coronary care units to placebo coronary care units is absurd. However, one reason for the extensive use of placebo controls in clinical trials of acupuncture is the relatively low plausibility (in the

West) that needling specific points in a specific way should have specific effects over needling in general. Many studies are initiated and designed to disprove this general placebo hypothesis. It is definitively important to determine whether where and how the acupuncturist inserts a needle makes any difference. However, this question should be investigated in simple models when independent replication is possible. The cause and the influence of a treatment on this cause (i.e., chronic diseases) are accessible only in long-term studies. In these circumstances, placebo-controlled studies are rarely feasible or useful. An example of such a simple model is the stimulation of acupuncture point P6 (located centrally about 5 cm above the wrist) for relieving nausea and vomiting. This is discussed further in the next section.

Another more important argument for placebo control is that it allows the blinding—at least in theory—of both patients and evaluators. Because acupuncture is mainly used for treating non–life-threatening diseases with subjective outcomes, unblinded clinical comparisons are prone to bias.

Finding an adequate placebo control for acupuncture is difficult. Typical placebo procedures include stimulating nonacupuncture points, stimulating points thought not to be indicated in the condition being investigated, superficial needling, using devices for electrical or laser stimulation that can be switched off. Although placebo treatments that involve deep needling are unlikely to be inert and might increase the risk of false-negative results, treatments that do not involve needling are likely to be distinguishable. Patients know if they got "true" or "sham" treatment. It remains unclear whether the introduction of placebo controls and blinding enhances or confuses the conclusions of acupuncture trials. This situation makes it difficult to discern whether this feature of the treatment is effective on average for these types of patients (see Table 4.1, question 3). Which proportion of the effects result from which specific component of the treatment is secondary to most patient care. The question that matters most is whether acupuncture benefits the patients (see Table 4.1, question 2). With that goal in mind, careful, multidimensional measurement of out-

comes and inclusion of independent—and, if possible, blinded—evaluators and rigorous monitoring might be better ways to minimize bias than the introduction of questionable placebo-controlled conditions.

BALANCING RESEARCH EVIDENCE AND CLINICAL RELEVANCE

The dynamics between *evidence* and *relevance* is nicely illustrated with two examples. The first is the study of the stimulation at acupuncture point P6 for relieving postoperative or chemotherapy-associated nausea and vomiting. This use was one of the few indications for acupuncture recommended by a panel at a National Institutes of Health Consensus Conference on Acupuncture in 1997. More than 30 trials have investigated this study model, and the overwhelming majority had positive results (40). This model has relatively little relevance for the daily practice of acupuncturists, but it is perfect for researchers looking for specific effects. Blinding is thought to increase validity, but whether this is truly achieved is unclear. This model is based on a simple intervention that can be standardized (almost like a drug treatment) and involves a condition in which outcomes are straightforward and follow-up times are short. Thus, acupuncture point P6 is the most studied area in acupuncture, not because it is the most important potential indication for acupuncture, but because it is simple to study. Thus, evidence of nausea and vomiting and its treatment approach is easily gathered. However, as previously stated, the findings are not very useful for the average acupuncture practitioner, and the indication is not the main one of interest for the public. Acupuncture is more frequently used to treat conditions such as chronic pain or drug addiction, for which placebo-controlled evidence is much less convincing (37, 38), primarily because it is difficult to develop rigorous trials in such complex situations.

In smoking cessation, there is quite clear evidence that acupuncture acts only as a placebo effect (41, 42). However, smoking cessation is of particular interest regarding the placebo problem previously discussed. Although there was no difference in smoking cessation rates between acupuncture and placebo-acupuncture, there was also no difference between acupuncture and conventional, effective smoking cessation treatments (42). If these results are valid, however, this would mean that acupuncture, despite being a placebo, would be equally effective as specifically effective, conventional interventions. These two examples show the complexity and inefficiency of trying to answer both questions of effectiveness and specificity (see Table 4.1, question 3 and question 4) of complex treatment approaches with the same research strategy. In addition, it may not be reasonable to try to answer all these questions for all conditions. Again, do patients and many clinicians care if they stopped smoking because of a *placebo* effect or a *specific* effect with a safe and inexpensive procedure? For scientific and reimbursement purposes, however, these may be important questions.

ACCEPTANCE OF TREATMENTS WITHOUT SCIENTIFIC PROOF

Acupuncture is also a good example of how a therapy becomes increasingly accepted despite lack of convincing evidence from randomized trials, which is a phenomenon that also frequently occurs in conventional medicine (44). Recently, a National Institutes of Health (NIH) consensus panel concluded that acupuncture is effective for treating some conditions and should be integrated into standard medical practice. Yet only two relatively minor conditions (postoperative and chemotherapy-associated nausea and vomiting, and acute, postoperative dental extraction pain) out of a dozen conditions evaluated were proven effective by acupuncture treatment. Nevertheless, insight into mechanisms of action, positive experiences by patients and by a growing number of providers and physicians, and interest from consumers and insurance companies are contributing to the acceptance and use of acupuncture even in the absence of proof for most conditions for which it is used. Thus, the simplicity and safety of acupuncture made the NIH panel willing to recommend that this treatment be accepted with less evidence than would other, higher-risk interventions. It seems reasonable, then, for

initial risk stratification to be a strategic element in evaluating CAM before setting the type and level of evidence required for acceptance. The application of risk strategies in evidence-based CAM is illustrated in Chapter 5.

More and better randomized clinical trials of acupuncture are clearly desirable. However, an effective strategy requires a number of preconditions for such trials:

1. The investigated treatment strategy should represent an actual practice of at least a defined group of acupuncturists. Representativeness should be shown empirically by observational studies. An alternative is to use a treatment approach recommended officially by a professional society.
2. Before starting the randomized trial, pilot studies are mandatory.
3. The exclusive use of placebo-controlled conditions for the purpose of determining what techniques are adopted in practice should be avoided.
4. Standard therapies of proven effectiveness should be used for direct comparison to acupuncture if acupuncture offers a potential advantage (e.g., lower cost or side effects) over the standard therapy.

In addition, acupuncture societies and their members should be encouraged to perform clinical audit and outcome studies to monitor their performance. There is a growing awareness of the need for evaluation as a precondition for more extensive, broadly based, high-quality research, like rats. In addition, audit and outcome studies might identify areas of both strength and weakness in acupuncture practices to better guide both practice and research.

Homeopathy

Research questions in acupuncture are usually narrowed to whether acupuncture is effective in treating certain conditions, but usually not narrowed so much as to ask whether a specific type of acupuncture is effective, as in phytotherapy. In the case of homeopathy, however, the questions usually asked by those unfamiliar with the practice are even more general than for acupuncture. In homeopathy, the most frequently asked question is: *Isn't ALL of homeopathy due to placebo effects?*

Homeopathy is one of the most widespread and most controversial of CAM systems. The fundamental principle of homeopathy is the *simile* principle, which states that patients who have particular signs and symptoms can be cured if given a drug that produces the same signs and symptoms in a healthy individual. The *simile* principle is not accepted by conventional medicine, but the main reason for the often vigorous rejection of homeopathy is its second tenet: the idea that remedies retain biological activity if they are repeatedly diluted and agitated or shaken between dilution steps. These dilutions are said to produce effects even when diluted beyond Avogadro's number, for which no original molecules of the starting substance remain.

Many scientists think that homeopathy violates natural laws (45), and thus any effect *must* be a placebo effect (46, 47). Apart from some speculative hypotheses, there is no good theory for a possible mechanism of action. Academic institutions are reluctant to do any research on homeopathy. For example, the German Society for Pharmacology and Toxicology in 1993 considered such research a waste of time and money (48), and discussion of homeopathy in journals continues to revolve around the value of researching this therapy at all (49). At the same time, practicing homeopaths are convinced that they offer a highly effective therapy, and many consider rigorous clinical research inadequate, unethical, and unnecessary.

This climate has not been supportive for developing an effective and competent research infrastructure. Nevertheless, individuals and small groups have done a considerable number of clinical trials. Recent systematic reviews have identified approximately 190 controlled clinical trials, 120 of which were randomized (50, 51). Overall, the available evidence clearly suggests that homeopathy can have an effect over placebo. However, there is a lack of independent replication of study models (as is done with P6 acupuncture) that convincingly proves the effectiveness of a single homeopathic strategy in a defined condition.

BALANCING SCIENTIFIC PLAUSIBILITY AND CLINICAL RELEVANCE

Given the implausibility of homeopathy, it is not surprising that clinical research focuses almost exclusively on the placebo question. But "placebo" in clinical trials of homeopathy has a more fundamental meaning than in conventional medicine. If, for example, *d*-sotalol (an anti-arrhythmic) is tested in a placebo-controlled trial, no one has any doubt that it has— regardless of its clinical usefulness—strong biological effects. However, homeopathic remedies—particularly when delivered in high dilutions—are assumed, *a priori*, to be completely inactive. If a clinical trial showed that significantly more side effects occurred in the homeopathic group compared with placebo, this might be interpreted as evidence for biological activity (in fact, such a trial exists [52]). Clinical trials in homeopathy are not really true clinical trials (attempting to answer questions 1–4 in Table 4.1); they often try to also answer what would normally be considered a basic science question that might only be answered in the laboratory (see Table 4.1, question 5). Mixing these questions in a single trial or series of trials usually produces ambiguous answers for both questions and is not a reasonable strategy.

Not only do such studies not answer the placebo question, most current studies in homeopathy do not represent actual practice and so are largely irrelevant for everyday homeopathic practice. The two most frequently investigated study models—administration of *Galphimia glauca* for treatment of hay fever (53) and administration of a complex of opium, *Raphanus*, arnica, or China for postoperative ileus (51)— illustrate this point. The remedy *Galphimia* is rarely used by homeopaths to treat hay fever, and postoperative ileus is hardly ever addressed in homeopathic daily practice.

These models are studied because they are easy to study. As in the case of acupuncture, the best scientific evidence for homeopathic medicine's effectiveness exists in areas that are simple to investigate but not necessarily useful for guiding treatment decisions. Thus, the pressure to answer the broad question of placebo effect with rigor results in neglect of research that would be the most relevant for clinical practice.

In recent years, the quality of research in homeopathy has improved considerably; a number of excellent studies are available that, in principle, seem more representative and relevant for actual practice (54–56). Many homeopaths practice a form of homeopathy (classical homeopathy) in which patients who have the same conventional diagnosis (e.g., migraine) receive different homeopathic remedies that fit their individual subjective symptom picture. Also, classical homeopathy involves extensive case-taking and poses considerable problems for clinical trial methodology. In recent studies of classical homeopathy, all included patients went through this case-taking procedure and then were prescribed their individual remedies. Only after that were these patients randomized to receive the true treatment or placebo by a third party. This method allows classical homeopathy to be studied more closely. However, it also brings up new problems. As with acupuncture, the intervention is no longer well defined (i.e., the remedy process is quite individualized), so possible placebo effects induced by the intense homeopathic case-taking might lead to underestimating the complete intervention's clinical effectiveness (56). Furthermore, such a design is associated with a number of logistic and ethical problems in long-term trials with patients who have chronic disease. Again, in such situations, direct comparisons of homeopathic treatment approaches to standard therapies of proven effectiveness appear more useful than do placebo-controlled trials.

Unless a breakthrough in basic research provides a plausible and reproducible mechanism for the action of high dilutions, scientific controversy about homeopathy will probably not be solved if the questions asked remain limited and dogmatic rather than pragmatic (see Table 4.1, question 4). Because the use of homeopathy continues to grow, the inability of science to provide answers to the questions posed by society is a cause for concern. Therefore, a variety of research methods must be applied to get a better understanding of what is going on in homeopathic practice: that is, determining whether its observed effects are caused by placebo or by a process outside of the current biological paradigm. As with acupuncture, research in homeopathy needs a broader base and more systematic strategy. Homeopaths must learn to evaluate their performance and use clinical research as a tool for improvement. Data collected in everyday practice might then contribute to planning randomized studies that evaluate the usefulness of homeopathy beyond the placebo question.

Complex Naturopathic Interventions

The prevalence of chronic diseases is increasing, especially in Western countries. The management of chronic diseases is considered a cornerstone of complementary medicine. A number of treatment centers offer complex life-style and naturopathic programs for the management of a variety of chronic conditions. These programs are rarely restricted to one complementary therapy; they consist of a mixture of different treatment modalities compiled according to both the complaints of the individual patient and the skills or experiences of the providers. Besides acupuncture, treatments such as aromatherapy, or herbs, counseling, behavioral therapies, and nutritional and life-style changes are central components of such programs.

With a few exceptions (57, 58), there are no randomized clinical trials of such complex naturopathic systems. Doing good research on such programs is difficult for a variety of reasons, including lack of funding for such research and difficulty in both recruiting patients and obtaining sufficiently long observational periods. In addition, generalizability of any findings is unlikely unless the program is well standardized and transferable to other facilities. Studies on isolated components are of little value for determining the whole program's effectiveness. A more promising strategy in such a situation might be to perform long-term outcome studies and clinical evaluation of centers providing such programs. The results of such nonexperimental observation will not allow the same scientific conclusions as would a randomized trial. However, it is unlikely that randomized trials will ever be done for many of these programs. Observational studies are feasible in many instances and could even be a precondition for reimbursement. Such studies might provide sufficient information to enable patients, health care providers, and policymakers to make rational, data-based choices.

DEVELOPING DECISION RULES FOR A STRATEGIC SCIENCE IN CAM

Balancing Relevance, Rigor, and Realism in Practice

As the four examples previously described have shown, evaluating the effectiveness of CAM practices is an extremely complex issue. A handful of rigorous, large-scale randomized trials will not solve the problem. The huge resources needed for systematic and extensive research will not be available in the next few years, even for the most prevalent interventions. At the same time, CAM use will likely increase. Given such a situation, the choice of an adequate research methodology should not be fixed *a priori,* but should reflect a balance among relevance, scientific rigor, and feasibility. Finally, we must keep in mind that there are several different public groups that the results of such research must serve, including patients, practitioners, the scientific community, and policymakers. Usually, these groups are each interested in different types of information that require different types of research methods. Considering how these groups plan to use the resulting information can also help guide the design of research on CAM.

When considering complementary treatments, the conventional physician will ask, *How should I advise or warn my patient about a given treatment? Should I consider using or recommending it myself?* These questions can be answered relatively easily by checking the evidence in the medical literature and by using available readers' guidelines (see, for example, Chapter 5, "How to Practice Evidence-Based Complementary and Alternative Medicine"). In the case of a clearly defined and characterized single intervention for a specific condition, such as giving *Hypericum* to a patient who has depression, a "conventional" framework can be used. However, getting a rational answer becomes much more difficult if the questions deal with complex therapeutic systems, such as acupuncture, naturopathy, traditional Chinese medicine, or homeopathy. The physician has to consider that the research evidence in most cases will be scarce, and even good research may not be relevant for making clinical decisions. In addition, issues like plausibility; the specific circumstances of the patient; the cost, feasibility, and risk of the treatment; severity of the condition; and the physician's own experiences and confidence in the particular provider must all be considered. In Chapter 5, the steps in developing an evidence-based approach to CAM are outlined.

Choosing Research Strategies in CAM

Basic decisions about choosing research methods and the interpretation of existing research may be approached in flowchart fashion from the framework of the types of research and use of research information previously described (see Figure 4.1). The decision to pursue a particular approach depends on a number of factors, including the following:

- Simplicity or complexity of the therapy being investigated
- Type of information sought
- Purpose or planned use for the information found
- Methods of investigation available and whether feasible, ethically acceptable, and affordable

By determining the main use for which information from a research project is to be put, the appropriate corresponding method can be determined (see Figure 4.1). For complex practices that are not well described, observational data and outcomes research or pilot trials may be the best initial approach (e.g., naturopathy). For well-described CAM practices, outcomes data coupled with decision analysis may provide the best strategic approach (e.g., defined acupuncture techniques). This may or may not be followed by selective application of randomized controlled trials, depending on the need for and ability to obtain information about specific effects. For CAM products whose constituents are unknown (e.g., complex herbal combinations), consultation with expert practitioners, followed by basic laboratory characterization of the products, may be needed before clinical research is undertaken. For well-characterized CAM products (e.g., standardized plant extracts), randomized controlled trials are appropriate and feasible provided their likely cost-risk-benefit ratios and potential public health impact warrant such an investment. The results of placebo studies may be more useful for making policy decisions (e.g., public benefit plans) than for individual decision making. The United States National Institutes of Health study of the efficacy of the herb St. John's Wort for depression using a large, three-armed, multi-centered, placebo-controlled trial is an example of this latter approach.

For a physician who is considering referring a patient for a CAM intervention such as acupuncture, it might be more valuable to know which patients are seen in the acupuncture practice, how they are treated, whether they are satisfied with treatment, and what their outcomes are rather than to rely on the results of small-scale, placebo-controlled randomized trials done in another continent with practitioners and populations quite different from those in the patient's community. Unfortunately, the methods of simple observational studies have not been used by biostatisticians and clinical epidemiologists who are under the dominance of industry-sponsored randomized trials for more easily tested and profitable products. Thus, the methodologies of observational studies may need to be developed further in ways applicable to CAM. Data collection and monitoring in observational studies must be performed at least as carefully as in experimental studies. The interpretation of such data must also be done carefully. Efficient systems of quality assurance should at least allow us to identify areas of particular risk and clinically significant benefits. Straightforward regulations requiring a certain level of quality would increase the probability that a treatment provided has at least limited risk.

Finally, for empirical observations that do not fit into our current assumptions about the nature of reality (e.g., psychic healing, homeopathy) but are of high public use, a carefully thought-out strategy with a basic science component is needed. Given the high public interest in some of these areas, it seems irresponsible for science to ignore studying these phenomena.

CAM AND THE EVOLUTION OF SCIENTIFIC MEDICINE

It is likely that only a small proportion of most therapies, whether conventional or complementary, will ever be established as fully evidence-based (i.e., answering all five questions in Table 4.1). Thus, practical methods for collecting information relevant for patient and practitioner decisions should be developed and implemented. In addition, a more careful examination of what role science should play in providing information for the management of chronic disease and investigating anomalous findings is needed. Because only incremental, answerable questions can be addressed with science, the public must understand that research can never answer all questions of public interest. Skepticism among conventional physicians about unorthodox practices is often higher than for conventional practices, so a demand for data is often required before CAM practices are accepted. The continuing interface between orthodox and unorthodox medicine today provides the opportunity for new research strategies and methodologies to arise. By purposefully maintaining a creative tension between the established and the frontier, we can advance scientific methods and more clearly define the boundaries and purpose of the scientific process for medicine.

REFERENCES

1. Eddy DM. Should we change the rules for evaluating medical technologies? In: Gelijns AC, ed. Modern methods of clinical investigation. Washington, DC: National Academy Press, 1990:117–134.
2. Levin JS, Glass TA, Kushi LH, et al. Quantitative methods in research on complementary and alternative medicine. A methodological manifesto. Med Care 1997;35:1079–1094.
3. Kaptchuk TJ. Intentional ignorance: a history of blind assessment in medicine. Bull Hist Med 1998;72(3):389–433.
4. Ernst E. St. John's Wort, an anti-depressant? A

systematic, criteria-based review. Phytomedicine 1995;2(1):67–71.

5. Linde K, Ramirez G, Mulrow CD, et al. St John's wort for depression—an overview and meta-analysis of randomised clinical trials. BMJ 1996;313: 253–258.

6. Harrer G, Schulz V. Clinical investigations of the antidepressant effectiveness of hypericum. J Geriatr Psychiatry Neurol 1994;7(suppl 1):S6–S8.

7. Volz HP. Controlled clinical trials of hypericum extracts in depressed patients—an overview. Pharmacopsychiatry 1997;30(suppl):72–76.

8. Müller WE, Rolli M, Schäfer C, Hafner U. Effects of hypericum extract (LI160) in biochemical models of antidepressant activiy. Pharmacopsychiatry 1997;30(suppl):102–107.

9. Weib G, Kallischnigg G. Gingko-biloba-Extrakt (EGb 761)—Meta-Analyse von Studien zum Nachweis der therapeutischen Wirksamkeit bei Hirnleistungsstörungen bzw. Peripherer arterieller Verschlubkrankheit. Muench Med Wschr 1991; 10:138–142.

10. Kleijnen J, Knipschild P. Gingko biloba for cerebral insufficiency. Br J Clin Pharmacol 1992;34: 352–358.

11. Hopfenmüller W. Nachweis der therapeutischen Wirksamkeit eines Ginkgo biloba- Spezialextraktes-Meta-Analyse von 11 klinischen Studien mit Patienten mit Hirnleistungsstörungen im Alter. Arzneim-Forsch/Drug Res 1994;44(2):1005–1013.

12. Letzel H, Schoop W. Gingko-biloba-Extrakt EGb 761 und Pentoxifyllin bei Claudicatio intermittens. Sekundäranalyse zur klinischen Wirksamkeit. VASA 1992; 21:403–410.

13. Schneider B. Ginkgo-biloba-Extrakt bei peripheren arteriellen Verschluβkrankheiten. Meta- Analyse von kontrollierten klinischen Studien. Arzneimittelforschung 1992;42:428–436.

14. Dalet R. Rökan bei Kopfschmerzen und Migräne. In: Diehm C, Müller D, eds. Rökan:Ginkgo biloba EGb 761. Vol 2. Berlin: Springer, 1992:321–326.

15. Kleijnen J, Knipschild P, ter Riet G. Garlic, onions and cardiovascular risk factors. A review of the evidence from human experiments with emphasis on commercially available preparations. Br J Clin Pharmacol 1989;28:535–544.

16. Warshafsky S, Kamer RS, Sivak SL. Effect of garlic on total serum cholesterol. Ann Intern Med 1993;119:599–605.

17. Silagy C, Neil A. Garlic as a lipid lowering agent—a meta-analysis. J R Coll Physicians Lond 1994; 28:39–45.

18. Neil HAW, Silay CA, Lancaster T, et al. Garlic powder in the treatment of moderate hyperlipidae-

mia: a controlled trial and meta-analysis. J R Coll Physicians Lond 1996;30:329–334.

19. Kleijnen J. Controlled clinical trials in humans on the effects of garlic supplements. In: Kleijnen J, ed. Food supplements and their efficacy. Maastricht, The Netherlands: Rijksuniversiteit Limburg, 1991: 73–82.

20. Morse PF, Horrobin DF, Manku MS, et al. Metaanalysis of placebo-controlled studies of the efficacy of Epogam in the treatment of atopic eczema. Relationship between plasma essential fatty acid changes and responses. Br J Dermatol 1989;121:75–90.

21. Kleijnen J, ter Riet G, Knipschild P. Evening primrose oil. In: Kleijnen J, ed. Food supplements and their efficacy. Maastricht, The Netherlands: Rijksuniveriteit Limburg, 1991:51–61.

22. Budeiri D, Li Wan Po A, Dornan JC. Is evening primrose oil of value in the treatment of premenstrual syndrome? Control Clin Trials 1996;17: 60–68.

23. Knipschild P. Ginseng: Pep of nep? Een overzicht van experimenten by ouderen met stoornissen van de vitaliteit. Pharmaceutisch Wekblad 1988:123: 4–11.

24. Melchart D, Linde K, Worku F, et al. Immunomodulation with Echinacea—a systematic review of controlled clinical trials. Phytomedicine 1994;1: 245–254.

25. Kiene H. Klinische Studien zur Misteltherapie der Krebserkrankung. Eine kritische Würdigung. Herdecke: Dissertation, 1989.

26. Kleijnen J, Knipschild P. Mistletoe treatment for cancer. A review of controlled trials in humans. Phytomedicine 1994;1:255–260.

27. Diehm C. The role of oedema protective drugs in the treatment of chronic venous insufficiency: a review of evidence based on placebo-controlled clinical trials with regard to efficacy and tolerance. Phlebology 1996;11:23–29.

28. Volz HP. Kava-Kava und Kavain. Münch Med Wschr 1997;139:42–46.

29. Loew D. Phytotherapy in heart failure. Phytomedicine 1997;4:267–271.

30. Schulz V, Hübner WD, Ploch M. Klinische Studien mit Psycho-Phytopharmaka. Ztschr Phytotherapie 1997;18:141–154.

31. Wilt TJ, Ishani A, Stark G, et al. Saw palmetto extracts for treatment of benign prostatic hyperplasia. JAMA 1998;280:1604–1609.

32. Murphy JJ, Heptinstall S, Mitchell JRA. Randomised double-blind placebo-controlled trial of feverfew in migraine prevention. Lancet 1988;2: 189–192.

33. Ernst E, de Smet PAGM. Risks associated with complementary therapies. In: Dukes MNG, ed.

Meyer's side effects of drugs. 13th ed. Amsterdam, The Netherlands: Elsevier, 1996:1427–1454.

34. de Smet PAGM. Health risks of herbal remedies. Drug Safety 1995;13:81–93.

35. Linde K, Worku F, Stör W, et al. Randomized clinical trials of acupuncture for asthma—a systematic review. Forsch Komplementärmed 1996;3: 148–155.

36. Patel MS, Gutzwiller F, Paccaud F, Marazzi A. A meta-analysis of acupuncture for chronic pain. Int J Epidemiol 1989;18:900–906.

37. ter Riet G, Kleijnen J, Knipschild P. Acupuncture and chronic pain: a criteria-based meta-analysis. J Clin Epidemiol 1990;43(11):1191–1199.

38. ter Riet G, Kleijnen J, Knipschild P. A meta-analysis of studies into the effect of acupuncture in addiction. Br J Gen Pract 1990;40:379–382.

39. Kleijnen J, ter Riet G, Knipschild P. Acupuncture and asthma: a review of controlled trials. Thorax 1991;46:799–802.

40. Vickers AJ. Can acupuncture have specific effects on health? A systematic review of acupuncture antiemesis trials. J R Soc Medicine Lond 1996;89: 303–311.

41. White AR, Resch KL, Ernst E. Smoking cessation with acupuncture? A 'best evidence synthesis.' Forschende Komplementärmedizin 1997;4:102– 105.

42. White AR, Rampes H. Acupuncture in smoking cessation. In: Lancaster T, Silagy C, eds. Tobaccos addiction module of The Cochrane Database of Systematic Reviews. Available in The Cochrane Library. The Cochrane Collaboration. Oxford, England: Update Software, 1998.

43. Ernst E, White AR. Acupuncture as an adjuvant therapy in stroke rehabilitation? Wien Med Wschr 1996;146:556–558.

44. Eddy DM. Should we change the rules for evaluating medical technologies? In: Gelijns AC, ed. Modern methods of clinical investigation. Washington, DC: National Academy Press, 1990:117–134.

45. Sampson A. Homeopathy does not work. Altern Therap 1995;1:48–52.

46. O'Keefe D. Is homoeopathy a placebo response? Lancet 1986;29:1106–1107.

47. Götzsche P. Trials of homoeopathy. Lancet 1993;341:1533.

48. Deutsche Gesellschaft für Pharmakologie und Toxikologie. Forschungsgelder für naturwissenschaftliche Methoden. Münch Med Wschr 1993;135, 6:14–15.

49. Reilly's challenge. Lancet 1994;344:1585.

50. Boissel JP, Cucherat M, Haugh M, Gauthier E. Critical literature review on the effectiveness of homoeopathy: overview of data from homoeopathic medicine trials. In: Homeopatic Medicine Research Group. Report to the Commission of the European Communities. Brussels, Belgium: 1996: 195–210.

51. Linde K, Clausius N, Ramirez G, et al. Are all effects of homeopathy placebo effects? A meta-analysis of randomized placebo-controlled trials. Lancet 1997;350:834–843.

52. Attena F, Toscano G, Agozzino E, del Giudice N. A randomized trial in the prevention of influenzalike syndromes by homoeopathic treatment. Rev Epidem et Santé Publ 1995;43:380–382.

53. Wiesenauer M, Lüdtke R. A meta-analysis of the homeopathic treatment of pollinosis with Galphimia glauca. Forsch Komplementärmed 1996;3: 230–236.

54. Jacobs J, Jimenez LM, Gloyd SS, et al. Treatment of acute childhood diarrhea with homoeopathic medicine: a randomized clinical trial in Nicaragua. Pediatrics 1994;93:719–725.

55. de Lange de Klerk ES, Blommers J, Kuik DJ, et al. Effects of homoeopathic medcines on daily burden of symptoms in children with recurrent upper respiratory tract infections. BMJ 1994;309:1329– 1332.

56. Walach H, Haeusler W, Lowes T, et al. Classical homeopathic treatment of chronic headaches. Cephalalgia 1997;17:119–126.

57. Ornish D, Brown SE, Scherwitz LW, et al. Can lifestyle changes reverse coronary heart disease? The lifestyle heart trial. Lancet 1990;336:129–133.

58. Kjeldsen-Kragh J, Haugen M, Borchgrevink CF, et al. Controlled trial of fasting and one-year vegetarian diet in rheumatoid arthritis. Lancet 1991; 338:899–902.

CHAPTER 5

How to Practice Evidenced-Based Complementary and Alternative Medicine

Wayne B. Jonas, Klaus Linde, and Harald Walach

INTRODUCTION

Previous chapters in this section have described the history of complementary and alternative medicine (CAM), an approach to discussing CAM with patients in the modern medical environment, and its implications for medical ethics and science. The topics dealt with in CAM will continue to be increasingly important for the health care system and for physicians in general. The establishment of the Office of Alternative Medicine at the U.S. National Institutes of Health in 1992 (now the National Center for Complementary and Alternative Medicine), although not the beginning of interest about CAM in this country, in many ways symbolizes the likely permanence of these topics. The fact that the first official entity established to address CAM in the West is located in a research organization, rather than a practice, licensing, or economic organization, demonstrates the coming-of-age of science in relation to medicine.

THE ADVENT OF EVIDENCE-BASED MEDICINE (EBM)

The idea that science can provide important information for making medical decisions has only recently started to become a reality. As early as 100 years ago, there were practically no scientific tools to provide medical information. It is interesting that the first double-blind experiment in the history of medicine was done by homeopaths in Nuremberg, Germany, in 1835. To end a public debate about the correctness of homeopathic allegations, an experiment was conducted in which volunteers were divided in two groups. The public surgeon of Nuremberg had a homeopathic pharmacist prepare Natrum muriaticum C30 and dispense it in labeled vials together with sham vials containing only water. The volunteers were to take the substances and report later on the observed effects. Although the results of the experiment were inconclusive, it was the first double-blind study in medical history (1).

Clinical trials are also a recent event. The first true experiment on humans, a randomized controlled trial, occurred only 50 years ago. The scientific basis for approving drugs for medical use through the U.S. Food and Drug Administration (FDA) is only approximately 20 years old. Only in the past 10 years has a serious emphasis on EBM—the use of up-to-date published research evidence to guide decisions in patient care—occurred. The official debut of EBM in the United States occurred in 1992 (the same year the Office of Alternative Medicine was established) with a series of articles published in the *Journal of the American Medical Association* (2).

In conventional medicine, the need for an evidence-based approach to medical decision making has been evident for a long time. A similar need for CAM is equally evident (although not always acknowledged). The introduction, diffusion, adoption, and abandonment of procedures in medical practice are predominantly influenced by social prestige, power, or potential profit rather than by evidence of public benefit (3–5).

Clinical experience is notoriously flawed for accurately judging the probability of risk and benefit. Global judgments by experts using informal methods are no better, often reflecting lack of rigor (6) and shifting recommendations based on specialty interests (7). The subjective and unreliable nature of clinical decision making and expert opinion is demonstrated by the wide variation of standard procedures in practice, even within relatively small geographic areas (8). The variation can be up to 20-fold across wide geographic areas (9, 10). Part of this variation is caused by legitimate differences in data that come from research conducted on different populations and relate to different specialties (11). Another part of this variation is caused by errors and inconsistencies in clinical judgment, even within the same specialty (12).

VARIATIONS IN CAM PRACTICE

Complementary medicine has similar, and probably even more extreme, problems with clinical variation. In a systematic review of 15 randomized trials of acupuncture treatment of asthma, for example, very different treatment strategies were found (13). Only two trials by the same author used the same acupuncture points (14). The type of acupuncture treatment (like many CAM and conventional procedures) largely depends on the practitioner, and perhaps also on the patient.

Likewise, in a meta-analysis of clinical trials of homeopathy, the authors were unable to find three trials by different authors that used the same treatment approach for the same clinical condition (15). This is partly caused by the greater individualization of CAM therapies, which confounds the problem of accurately estimating the clinical effects. Continuous collection of local patient characteristics and outcome data for CAM practices may help make more precise estimates of potential benefits and harms as they relate to individual decision-making. Such data, although helpful in estimating the

likelihood of benefit, cannot determine whether such effects are specific to the therapy. This information can come only through randomized controlled trials.

MANAGING THE EXPLOSION OF MEDICAL INFORMATION

From the perspective of EBM, CAM is but another topical addition to the current explosion of biomedical information. Clearly, no one can master all this information, so the need for evidence-based problem-solving skills is essential. The recurring call for both more generalist medical education and the development of problem-oriented medical training reflects efforts to provide such skills to medical students (16). The complete practice of EBM, however, would require information from all six knowledge domains discussed in Chapter 4:

1. Patient preferences and meaning.
2. Mechanisms of action.
3. Safety and efficacy.
4. Treatment effect probabilities in the open clinical setting from observational and outcomes research.
5. Precise estimates of effects through systematic summaries and calculations of confidence intervals when possible.
6. Demonstration of utility and benefit under normal health service conditions examining the impact of access, feasibility, and costs.

In addition, a practitioner would need to be able to assess the relevance of all this information to the particular clinical case at hand, with all its unique nuances and circumstances. Rarely will any intervention have such a breadth and depth of information available, and few, if any, practitioners or even groups of experts could obtain and analyze all such information.

Knowledge Domains: What Is Needed for Clinical Practice?

Fortunately, most clinical decisions can be made with information from two of the six domains listed above, through randomized controlled trials and outcomes research. This presumes that the practitioner is well trained clinically and has the communication and interpersonal skills needed to assess and incorporate patient preferences and relevance into the decision-making process. This three-legged stool—clinical expertise, patient relevance, and research evidence—is the foundation for evidence-based clinical decisions (17, 18).

The level of EBM skill used is currently up to the practitioner. It can vary from using pre-evaluated literature to quick summary sheets to week-long continuing medical education courses on how to practice EBM. With concerted effort, it is possible for physicians in general practice to base the vast majority of clinical decisions in conventional medicine on good evidence (19). Once the habit of EBM is established, the practitioner can incorporate CAM

topics into this process. Table 5.1 lists some *bare-bones users guidelines* developed by Haynes and colleagues for appraising the validity of the most common types of clinical studies (20).

The physician may be approached by (or discover on questioning) patients already using CAM. Or patients may request information about CAM practices being considered. Patients come to physicians to get their opinion about a therapy because of their clinical expertise, or to ask whether there is any research evidence supporting the practice. The physician can fulfill this professional role if he or she evaluates the medical literature for the relevance of the therapy to the patient's situation. As discussed in Chapter 2 of this book, the first step is to determine why the patient is seeking alternative therapy and whether conventional medicine has been inadequate in some way or simply not

Table 5.1. Minimum Guidelines for Assessment of Study Validity

PURPOSE OF STUDY	GUIDELINES			
Therapy	Was there concealed random allocation to comparison groups?	Were outcome measures of known or probable clinical importance?	Were there few patients lost to follow-up compared with the number of bad outcomes (<20%)?	
Diagnosis	Were the patients those to whom you would want to apply the test in practice (ambiguous cases)?	Was an objective or reproducible diagnostic standard applied to all participants?	Was a blinded assessment of the test and diagnostic standards ("gold standard") done?	
Prognosis	Was the group being assessed (the inception cohort) gathered early in the course of the disorder and initially free of the outcome of interest?	Was there an objective or reproducible assessment of clinically important outcomes?	Were there few lost to follow-up compared with the number of bad outcomes (<20%)?	
Etiology	Was there a clearly defined comparison group, or those at risk for or having the outcome of interest?	Was there blinding of observers to the status of the exposure to the outcome of interest?		
Reviews	Were there explicit criteria for selecting articles and rating their validity?	Was there a comprehensive search for all relevant articles? Were negative and unpublished articles found?		
Observational and outcomes studies	Were there outcome measures of known or probable clinical importance?	Were there few lost to follow-up compared with the number of bad outcomes (<20%)?	Was the probability of benefit reported worth the inconvenience, risk of side effects, and costs of the treatment?	Were confidence intervals reported, and were they narrow?

Adapted from Haynes RB, Sackett DL, Gray JA, Cook DL, Guyatt GH. Transferring evidence from research into practice: 2. Getting the evidence straight. *ACP J Club* 1997;126:A14–A16.

been adequately applied. If proven conventional therapy has not been adequately applied, then this is explained to the patient and rectified. If the patient has a strong preference for CAM or if conventional medicine does not offer adequate therapy, the physician can seek out evidence for alternatives.

Finding Good Information

With computerized access, a ready source of credible information is possible. Information on CAM for assisting with evidence-based decisions for patient care is becoming increasingly available. A number of groups are working to collate and produce CAM-specific databases; for example, the National Library of Medicine and the National Center for Complementary and Alternative Medicine (National Institutes of Health) in the United States, the Research Council for Complementary Medicine in England, the BMBF Coordinating Group in Germany, the international Cochrane Collaboration, and some universities and private organizations. Practitioners can anticipate that,

within the next few years, a number of comprehensive and easily accessible sources of quality CAM literature will become available. Some on-line sources of high-quality information that are indispensable for obtaining up-to-date information are listed in Table 5.2 as well as in Table 2.5 in Chapter 2.

SEARCHING THE LITERATURE

If a physician uses the approach outlined in Chapter 3 (see Table 3.3) and determines that an alternative therapy is already being used by the patient or may be useful to the patient, the physician can search for data on the effects of CAM for that condition. Three types of information should be sought on the CAM therapy:

1. Meta-analyses, or systematic reviews.
2. Randomized controlled trials.
3. Observational or prospective outcomes data.

Table 5.3 lists the most common search categories that capture this type of data from standard MEDLINE-type databases. If relevant citations are not found using the main terms, one can try the other terms listed under the main

Table 5.2. Some On-line Sources of Quality Medical Information

NAME	INTERNET ADDRESS	SOURCE
Sources of Primary Literature		
MEDLINE	www.medline.nlm.nih.gov or www.ncbi.nlm.nih.gov/PubMed	National Library of Medicine PubMed (free Internet access to MEDLINE)
CAM Citation Index (includes the Cochrane Database of CAM–controlled trials; see Appendix 4)	www.altmed.od.nih.gov/nccam/ resources/cam-ci	Office of Alternative Medicine, NIH (now the National Center for Alternative & Complementary Medicine)
CISCOM	www.gn.apc.org/rccm/ ciscom.html	Research Council for Complementary Medicine, U.K.
Sources of Secondary Literature		
The Cochrane Library	www.nihs.go.jp/acc/cochrane/ revabst/ccabout.htm	Cochrane Library's field group in CAM (CD-ROM available also)
Best Evidence Selection	www.webcom.com/mjljweb/ jrnlclb/index.htm	ACP Journal Club and Evidence-Based Medicine (CD-ROM available also)
Agency for Health Care Policy and Research (AHCPR)	www.ahcpr.gov	Evidence-Based Practice Guidelines Database
Focus on Alternative and Complementary Therapies (FACT)	www.exeter.ac.uk/FACT/	Quarterly Journal Club for CAM

Table 5.3. Citation Categories and Terms for Searching Databases for Clinical Evidence

CATEGORY	TERMS
Systematic Reviews or Meta-Analyses	Systematic review Meta-analysis Clinical practice guideline Consensus conference statement
Randomized Controlled Trials (RCTs)	Randomized controlled trials Multi-site, large-scale RCT (N > 100) Large-scale RCT (N > 100) Small-scale RCT (N < 100)
Observational Studies and Clinical Studies (Non-RCTs)	Intervention outcome study (nonrandomized) Clinical study, pre- and postuncontrolled, epidemiological study Noncontrolled prospective study Practice audit Postmarketing surveys Clinical trial, noncontrolled *Other possibilities* Controlled observational study Controlled cohort study Case-controlled study Retrospective comparative (controlled) study

terms in Table 5.3 to see if they yield studies in that category. Other types of data (e.g., from controlled studies, cross-sectional, or retrospective epidemiological studies; cost and health service information; laboratory research and editorials; letters; and so forth) are generally less useful for evidence-based decision making. Limiting the literature search to the evidence domains of *attribution* and *association* (which a search in the three aforementioned categories of data will do) focuses on the areas most relevant for making decisions in practice.

When No Research Information Is Found

If the search yields no information from relatively comprehensive database sources, one can reasonably assume that there is scant or no good clinical evidence for the CAM therapy with that condition. Knowing that no good information exists is useful, and patients are often grateful for this effort. The physician then knows with reasonable confidence that any decisions to use or discourage the CAM therapy are not evidence based and must rely on the physician's own clinical judgment or other information.

Not having access to information about CAM practices and products can represent a risk to quality patient care, because patients will often use the product or practice without their physician's knowledge or without reliable information. A physician's skill and ability to search for and evaluate reliable quality data can assist both physician and patient in making the decision to stop or go forward with a treatment. Providing information about research on CAM practices and combining it with good clinical judgment are two of the main services patients seek from physicians.

When Research Information is Found

If a practitioner uses the proper search terms and information sources and finds clinical data documenting the effects or efficacy of a CAM practice for the condition of interest, a more evidence-based decision can be made. This information can then be communicated to the patient in the clinical setting. Patients are grateful for this effort, because they often seek out a CAM practice after receiving information derived from sources that may not be reliable, such as articles in magazines, newsletters, the Internet, radio shows involving advocates of a practice, or the urging of friends and family to try an alternative therapy.

What Is the Risk and Cost of the CAM Therapy?

When reasonable clinical data about a CAM practice are found in meta-analyses and systematic reviews, randomized controlled trials, or observational studies, the physician can then decide on its validity and relevance to the patient at hand. The amount and type of evidence required to use or reject the use of each CAM therapy depend on a number of factors. However, there are two key screening issues to be considered before evaluating the evidence: the degree of direct risk or toxicity, and the cost of the therapy (14). Many CAM practice involve over-the-counter (OTC) supplements—medications or self-care techniques that are reasonably safe and inexpensive when properly monitored. The physician should distinguish between CAM practices that are low in both risk and cost and those that are higher in risk and cost. Practices that are low in risk and often low in cost for most patients include:

- OTC homeopathic medications.
- Properly delivered acupuncture and manipulation.
- Mind–body techniques, such as meditation, relaxation, and biofeedback.
- Vitamin and mineral supplementation that is below known toxic ranges and is without potential vitamin/drug interactions.

The financial status of the patient and reimbursement status of the practice should be considered with the patient. When a practice is low risk and low cost, the physician and patient want to know the probability of benefit from its use. This information can be obtained from either randomized trials or good observational and outcomes studies that are not randomized.

Deciding on the Use of Outcomes Data or Randomized Trials in Practice

Although data from observational and outcomes research may provide sufficient evidence for clinical decisions on low-risk, low-cost practices, data from randomized controlled trials are required for practices that have significant potential risk or cost. This includes practices such as:

- Herbal therapies.
- High-dose vitamins and minerals.
- Blood-derived vaccine products.
- Instrumentation such as colonics.
- Intravenous administration of substances such as hydrogen peroxide and ozone.
- Repeated visits or long distance travel for treatments.

These types of practices require specific risk–benefit comparison to either no treatment, placebo, or a standard conventional treatment. In addition, some products and practices are extremely expensive, require the patient to travel to obtain services, and are not reimbursable. Even if a therapy is relatively harmless, the high cost and inconvenience of such therapies make the use of noncontrolled information inadequate for decision making. Depending upon the category of risk and cost of the potential practice, the physician can then obtain and examine the abstracts or research articles found (often also online). For high-risk, high-cost interventions, the physician should rely on randomized controlled trials only.

In summary outcomes research, randomized controlled trials, and meta-analyses of controlled trials can provide information about the probability of benefit from a practice. Outcomes data alone can often provide evidence for clinical decisions if the practice is safe and low-cost (21). For example, if outcomes studies show that a nontoxic and low-cost OTC homeopathic remedy has a 75% probability of improving allergic rhinitis (22), this information can assist the physician and patient in deciding on whether to try it. If, however, the CAM practice is high risk or high cost (e.g., intravenous H_2O_2 for allergic rhinitis), a stricter level of evidence on benefits and risks from randomized controlled trials is required (23).

Assessing Study Quality: Is the Information Any Good?

Once data are found, the physician should apply the minimum available assessment guidelines (see Table 5.1) for evaluating the research.

Three criteria can be checked quickly:

1. Blind and random allocation of subjects to comparison groups (in controlled clinical trials).
2. Clinical relevance and reliability of the outcome measures.
3. The number of subjects entered in and then analyzed at the end of the study.

How to apply these criteria to any study set is described in more detail below.

TREATMENT ALLOCATION

When assessing a treatment trial, the physician should examine whether there was adequate concealment of allocation from one treatment group to another, even if the treatment itself is not blindable. If the investigators did not know which subjects were going to be assigned to treatment groups, or if a random numbers table was used to make subject assignments, the trial's validity is more likely.

RELEVANT AND RELIABLE OUTCOMES

Second, were the outcomes important? Objective outcomes should have been used whenever possible, but not at the expense of more patient-relevant measures. *Surrogate* outcomes–those easy to measure and used as a marker for a disease or illness–should be suspect unless they are known to be tightly linked to the relevant clinical outcomes. When the outcome involves a subjective condition (e.g., pain), the investigators should have checked for reliability of measurement. This means that the outcome was measured several times (either in this trial or previous tests) and consistently came up with the same results.

WHAT WAS ANALYZED?

Finally, was the number of patients analyzed comparable with the number who entered into the study at the beginning—that is, what was the dropout rate? Dropout rates of more than 20% in most studies should make the value of the trial information suspect. Ideally, the analysis should be done on all individuals who entered into the trial from the beginning of the study. This is called an *intention-to-treat* analysis. Some assessment of the number of outcomes measured should also be made. The practitioner should ascertain whether the outcomes reported in the study were the original focus of the study (part of the main hypothesis), or whether there were multiple outcome measures assessed, and only those that were statistically significant were reported. If the latter is true, the value of information from the trial should again be suspect.

OBSERVATIONAL STUDIES

These same minimum study quality criteria apply to observational studies, except that concealed random allocation to treatment and comparison groups (see Guideline 1, Table 5.1) does not apply. In observational or outcomes studies, the physician should also carefully examine the magnitude of benefit. Two questions should be asked:

1. Was the probability of benefit reported worth the inconvenience, risk of adverse effects, and costs of the treatment?
2. Were confidence intervals reported, and were they narrow or broad?

Confidence intervals are the range of minimum-to-maximum benefit expected in 95% of similar studies. If the confidence intervals are narrow, the physician can be more confident that the likelihood of benefit found with the patient will be close to that reported. If confidence intervals are broad, one can expect that the likelihood of benefit from the treatment will be unpredictable.

If the answers to these quality questions show that there are marked quality flaws in the studies retrieved, the physician can conclude that the evidence for the practice is insufficient and should not be used as a basis for clinical decisions.

WHAT POPULATION WAS STUDIED?

If quality evidence *is* found, the next most important step is to ask whether the population studied is reasonably similar to the patient at hand. Research involves attempting to bring together homogeneous groups of patients to control for, as far as possible, extraneous and confounding variables that might influence the outcomes. These study groups are created through a series of inclusion and exclusion criteria that may result in the study findings being applicable to only a very narrow range of patients. The challenge for the physician is to identify whether the patient group reported in the study is similar enough to warrant its application to his or her patient. Although this matching is somewhat subjective, practitioners can compare at least five areas of how a study has been conducted to help judge this match. These areas are:

1. Age of the study population.
2. Gender of the study population.
3. A setting similar to the patient's own (e.g., primary, secondary, or tertiary care center).
4. A culture similar to the patient's own (e.g., Western, Eastern, developing, industrialized).
5. A population in which the accepted diagnostic criteria for the condition are similar to that used in that population's system of medicine (e.g., do patients in a United States study meet the accepted criteria for diagnosis of diseases such as osteoarthritis or congestive heart failure?).

Other factors, of course, such as the severity of the illness and the magnitude of the patient's desire for treatment, must also be considered in the decision. If the characteristics of the population studied are not close to that of the patient, then it is unlikely that even valid data can be reasonably applied, because insufficient evidence exists for the use of that CAM therapy in that patient population. However, if the match is close, then the data provide an appropriate body of evidence for moving forward with a therapeutic trial.

Efficiency of EBM

One of the concerns many physicians have about practicing EBM is the time it takes to search and evaluate the literature, apply the quality criteria, and decide whether the data apply to the patient. Skills for efficient use of the current medical literature—rapid access, accurate screening, skilled quality assessment, and

application—are usually not taught in medical school or residency. With practice, however, the clinician can rapidly screen and assess the literature for the likelihood that an evidence-based decision can be made. It is possible to make the majority of clinical decisions using an evidence-based process (19). Obviously, a separate complete literature search and evaluation procedure is not needed for every patient who comes into the office. Only in circumstances in which an alternative practice is already being used or in which an alternative practice is sought for the first time would such a procedure be needed. Once this procedure is done for the first few patients, this information can often be used for subsequent patients who have similar problems and are using similar CAM practices. If the study assessment criteria mentioned previously and summarized in Figure 5.1 are not met anywhere along the decision path, then the patient should be informed that there is insufficient quality research to make an evidence-based decision about the practice. If, however, the physician finds adequate evidence, a therapeutic trial with proper monitoring may be warranted. The reader is referred to Chapter 2, Table 2.4, for guidelines on how to follow patients using CAM practices. Assurance of adequate training of the practitioner and quality of the products involved must be considered. The reader is referred to Chapter 2 and to the descriptions of the main CAM systems in Part III of this book.

Balancing Belief, Plausibility, and Evidence in Medical Decisions

Although EBM is necessary to make sound decisions, the practitioner must be aware of several items requiring caution.

Randomized controlled clinical trials (RCTs) assume an important presupposition: namely, that the participants do not have any strong preference for one of the treatments offered. This presupposition generally is met when the RCT is an evaluation of a new conventional drug. In this case, the drug and its effects are usually unknown, and there are no strong inclinations among practitioners or patients. In addition, an RCT is the only way a drug can be marketed.

In CAM treatments, however, there are usually strong preferences, either by the patient, the doctor, or both, and the treatments are already on the market and in use. If the *a priori* probability is high for a patient (e.g., he or she has a strong belief in and preference for the treatment), then this patient is probably different from typical patients in clinical trials. Furthermore, some forms of CAM—mainly, traditional healing systems like acupuncture, homeopathy, and folk medicine—rely on a long history of uncontrolled experience, which lends high credibility to its application in the eyes of those practitioners. If this high prior probability on the side of the practitioner is met with a high prior probability for the patient—that is, when a believing patient meets with a charismatic doctor who is convinced of what he or she practices—then strong nonspecific effects may occur. This effect may not have been seen in RCTs and meta-analyses. Many of the effects of CAM may be nonspecific or placebo. Nevertheless, from the clinical (not scientific) perspective, if there is a high prior probability on the side of the patient and practitioner, a CAM practice may trigger self-healing responses even in the face of missing or negative evidence.

EBM is currently the best way to make decisions about general effectiveness and the specific efficacy of CAM and conventional medicine alike. However, in day-to-day medical practice, it may be unclear to what extent this evidence applies to individual patients and to what extent nonspecific effects are responsible for healing.

Most patients and physicians agree that within the boundaries of ethical practice, as outlined in Chapter 3, the power of these effects should be harnessed as much as possible for the welfare of the patient. In this sense, the prior belief system of patient and practitioner may often turn out to be paramount and can lead to the effectiveness of otherwise ineffective treatments (24).

Given this situation, how should the goal of scientifically identifying therapeutic options be balanced against the clinical need to maximize optimal healing responses? The authors suggest

that the physician explicitly consider plausibility and belief in the therapy of both patient and practitioner.

In conventional medicine, plausibility is usually implicitly accepted by both patient and physician, but this is not the case for CAM. Belief in therapeutic agents, even those with specific effects, has long been known to affect outcome; high belief and expectation enhance positive outcomes, and low belief and expectation interfere with positive outcomes (25–28).

A physician may believe that a CAM practice has incredibly low plausibility (e.g., faith healing, homeopathy). If a practice is far outside the belief systems of both the physician and patient, permitting such a practice is ethically unacceptable. However, the patient may have a strong belief in the therapy and find it completely acceptable. This *prior probability* of belief by the physician and patient should be considered in the decision to use or allow the practice to go forward. If both the physician and the patient can reasonably believe in the plausibility or potential benefit of the practice, and a physician has found good evidence to support such a belief, then a therapeutic trial is warranted. If, however, the patient has only marginal belief and the plausibility for the practitioner is extremely low, then, even in the face of clinical evidence, discouragement from the practice or referral elsewhere for treatment is appropriate. In some circumstances, the patient may have a strong belief in the practice, whereas the physician may find it extremely unbelievable. In those situations, the physician must work with the patient to decide the best action, and referral elsewhere may be the best option. In conventional medicine, the disparity between plausibility and belief is rarely addressed because it is assumed that both the patient and physician believe in the plausibility of the practices in which they engage. Such assumptions should be explored to make sure that they are true for CAM practices.

Is the Diagnostic System Working?

In some cases, a conventional Western diagnosis may not be useful for the treatment and management of a patient. This occurs most often for chronic conditions with vague or unknown etiologies characterized by subjective symptoms and lack of general well-being. Examples include chronic fatigue syndrome, fibromyalgia, chronic idiopathic urticaria, and functional and psychosomatic problems. If the conventional diagnosis does not help for improving the patient's condition, the clinician may want to consider complete evaluation with a complementary and/or alternative system. Because these systems use different diagnostic classifications and approaches (e.g., deficient kidney *chi* in Traditional Chinese medicine, *pitta* imbalance in Ayurvedic medicine, or the sepia syndrome in homeopathy), obtaining an assessment by one of these alternative systems may prove useful. The reverse situation may also occur. A patient may undergo diagnosis and treatment based on a CAM system with little effect when the condition could be managed simply and effectively with a conventional medicine approach. The physician should be alert to both possibilities.

Because CAM systems are generally not studied scientifically using their own diagnostic classifications, it is rare to find research evidence using such classifications. In such cases, a professional consultation may be needed, and the guidelines outlined in Chapter 2 should be followed. A competent complementary practitioner should be able to inform both the physician and patient whether the diagnostic category of the alternative system is clear and is likely to be useful.

For example, a patient with chronic idiopathic urticaria and fatigue was not helped after evaluation and treatment from an allergist, psychiatrist, nutritionist, dermatologist, and general practitioner. Conventional diagnostic workups were negative and therapeutic trials with antihistamines, antidepressants, steroids, and other treatments were ineffective or produced unacceptable side effects. The patient was sent for a complete homeopathic evaluation, which showed a clear homeopathic diagnostic category. Homeopathic treatment was initiated and resulted in rapid and permanent resolution of both problems.

Sometimes, however, vague symptoms are simply vague symptoms, and both conventional and alternative systems cannot make sense of them. In cases when the alternative diagnostic classification is not clear, a therapeutic trial is not warranted, and the physician should consult guidelines previously mentioned (Chapter 2).

SUMMARY OF STEPS

Figure 5.1 summarizes the approach to evidence-based CAM. The steps (or criteria) are:

Step 1 Is the patient already using or wanting to use a CAM approach, or is an alternative sought (see Chapter 2, Tables 2.2 and 2.3)?

Step 2 Is the practice inexpensive and unlikely to produce direct (toxic) adverse effects?

Step 3 Is there evidence for this practice from randomized controlled trials or observational and outcomes studies?

Step 4 Does the quality of the studies meet the minimum quality criteria (see Table 5.1)?

Step 5 Is the population in these studies similar to the patient at hand?

Step 6 Is the belief and rationale for the therapy acceptable to both patient and physician?

Step 7 If yes to all the above, consider a therapeutic trial provided:
A A quality product or procedure by a competent practitioner can be obtained (see Chapter 2, Tables 2.4 and 2.6), and
B The patient can be monitored while undergoing the treatment (see Chapter 2, Table 2.4).

Step 8 Also consider if a new diagnostic assessment by a CAM system is in order.

By following these steps, the physician can increase the likelihood that decisions about

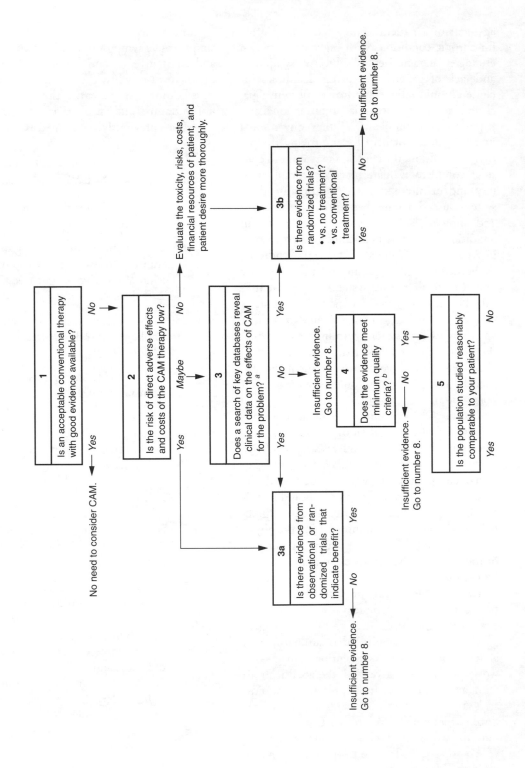

1

Is an acceptable conventional therapy with good evidence available?

Yes — No need to consider CAM.

No →

2

Is the risk of direct adverse effects and costs of the CAM therapy low?

Yes / Maybe / No

No → Evaluate the toxicity, risks, costs, financial resources of patient, and patient desire more thoroughly.

3

Does a search of key databases reveal clinical data on the effects of CAM for the problem? [a]

Yes / No

No → Insufficient evidence. Go to number 8.

Yes →

3a

Is there evidence from observational or ran-domized trials that indicate benefit?

No — Insufficient evidence. Go to number 8.

Yes

3b

Is there evidence from randomized trials?
• vs. no treatment?
• vs. conventional treatment?

Yes / No

No → Insufficient evidence. Go to number 8.

4

Does the evidence meet minimum quality criteria? [b]

No — Insufficient evidence. Go to number 8.

Yes

5

Is the population studied reasonably comparable to your patient?

Yes / No

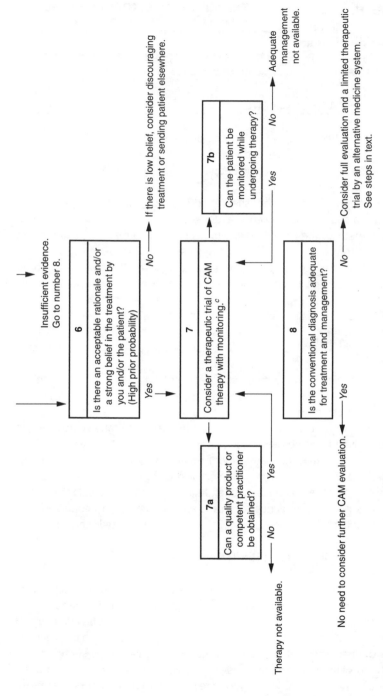

FIGURE 5.1. Decision tree for evidence-based complementary and alternative medicine.

[a] See Appendix B and Table 5.3.
[b] See Table 5.1 for quality criteria.
[c] See Chapter 2 for management guidelines.

CAM practice are based on research evidence; or, if there is no research evidence, the practitioner can be clear that clinical decisions are based on other criteria (e.g., opinion, clinical judgment).

EXAMPLES OF EVIDENCE-BASED APPROACHES TO CAM

The following case examples help illustrate the use of an evidenced-base approach.

CASE 1: ALLERGIES

A 23-year-old woman comes to her practitioner for the treatment of seasonal allergies. She is in good health and has normally taken standard antihistamines and decongestants for her condition. However, these agents make her sleepy, so when she came across a homeopathic allergy remedy in the drug store, she tried it for several days. It seemed to help.

Step 1. Now she would like your opinion on whether she should continue with this preparation.

Steps 2 and 7A. The product is a combination of very low doses of plant extracts and is said to be manufactured according to the standards of the United States Homeopathic Pharmacopoeia–a product for which the Food and Drug Administration does provide some regulation and oversight.

Step 3. A search of the available databases comes up with two meta-analyses of randomized controlled trials and several other randomized controlled trials on the treatment of allergies with homeopathic preparations (15, 17).

The effect size for these studies shows that approximately 75% of patients will experience clinically significant relief, but the preparations in the studies are not exactly the same as the ones in the product she has found. No significant adverse effects have been reported from these dilutions, nor are any expected given the extremely low dose.

Step 4. A review of two controlled trials with the minimum quality criteria mentioned earlier in the chapter shows that these studies meet these standards.

Step 5. The populations in the studies are varied enough to be similar to this patient's situation.

Step 7B. The patient is very happy to have the physician monitor the treatment and switch back to conventional treatment if the alternative practice proves inadequate.

Step 6. However, the physician believes that the plausibility of homeopathy's effect is very unlikely.

Thus, all of the steps in establishing the evidence criteria are fulfilled except for step 6 (plausibility), with some disparity of belief between the patient and practitioner. In addition, the product is not exactly the same as that studied, so there is no direct evidence for this exact product on this condition. The physician must then decide with the patient the proper course of action (referral, limited therapeutic trial with reevaluation, etc.).

CASE 2: DEPRESSION

A 45-year-old woman suffering from depression in combination with a dependent-depressive personality disorder seeks help, primarily psychotherapy. History reveals a series of losses in her past: her grandmother, who was very kind and important to her, had died when she was 5. Her father, whom she admired and who doted on her, died when she was 12. From the time her father died, she had taken on considerable responsibility for herself and her younger sister. When she was in her teenage years, she started dating a young man from her neighborhood with whom she fell in love. Because he was a Protestant and she was a Catholic, a relationship seemed impossible, given the strong religious background of both families. After several years, the young man was diagnosed with leukemia and soon died. This was the same disease the patient's father had died of. Shortly afterward, she married a close friend of her deceased boyfriend who courted her but whom she did not really love. Recently, a son of a good friend of hers had committed suicide, which started the patient's suicidal impulses and brought her to therapy. From reading popular books she had taken a fancy for homeopathy and inquired whether her problems could benefit from taking homeopathic remedies.

Step 1. Under no circumstances is the patient willing to take any conventional psychotropic medication or consider seeing a psychiatrist. Verbal psychotherapy in a general psychodynamic framework with behavioral elements is initiated, but the patient persistently requests homeopathic treatment.

Step 2. The risk of adverse effects is low if the treatment is embedded in a general psychotherapeutic environment in which the patient is not alone with her experiences. If such a patient is left unmonitored with only CAM intervention, this approach would be very risky. Direct risk of adverse effects in this situation is low and costs are negligible, but refusal of potentially effective conventional treatment by the patient is of concern.

Step 3. There is no evidence from clinical trials or observational studies about the effectiveness of homeopathy in depression. One could consider the herb Hypericum (St. John's wort), a phytotherapeutic alternative that has been studied and seems to be effective as a mild antidepressive, but this is also refused by the patient. It is also doubtful whether Hypericum alone is sufficient because it is used only for mild depression. The patient has been reading case histories in the homeopathic literature about positive effects of homeopathic treatment in depression. She thinks that her case would be clear to a homeopath because of depression and sadness after multiple losses, which she thinks is a key homeopathic diagnostic symptom.

Step 4. The evidence for a homeopathic intervention is weak. There are no trials and no formal observational studies, only single observations and case reports that are very likely due to placebo and nonspecific effects—something to which depression often responds.

Step 5. It is difficult to say whether the people reported on in the case studies the patient reads are comparable with the patient here. Usually, there is not enough information in the case studies to make a determination.

Step 6. The evidence certainly is not enough for relying solely on a homeopathic intervention. Given the patient's refusal of other therapies and her high belief in the system, nonspecific effects might be enhanced if a confident practitioner is found and careful follow-up with psychotherapy is maintained.

Step 7. There is no way of starting a therapeutic trial unless a responsible homeopathic practitioner is found, is willing to work with the physician (see Chapter 2), and uses standard homeopathic products overseen by the FDA. The physician also might consider this patient noncompliant and refuse further therapy. However, given the patient's propensity for alternative medicine, this may place the patient at increased risk (albeit of her own choosing).

Step 8. The diagnosis is clear. If the patient is refusing psychotropic medication (which she does), psychotherapy is the only alternative left. If the circumstances in step 7 for referral and follow-up exist, it is possible that additional benefit from adding a therapeutic trial of homeopathy may occur.

Follow-up: A homeopathic treatment is initiated in parallel to continuous psychotherapy. Over the course of 1 year, this brought out a variety of destructive impulses, sadness and mourning—feelings she had not allowed herself before. In the course of this treatment, the homeopathic practitioner says that a decisive homeopathic symptom surfaces. The patient relates the single fear she is most ashamed of—losing her financial and economic security and becoming poor. However, this fear is irrational (the family is quite rich) and is correlated as a key symptom to the homeopathic remedy Aurum, made from gold. Homeopathic treatment is initiated and gradually the patient loses her self-hate and self-destructive impulses. Psychotherapy seems to progress better. When therapy was terminated, the patient said that her major gain was that she could never think of harming herself any more.

It is not clear in this case whether homeopathy in itself was helpful. Subjectively it was, but it is doubtful whether the effect would have been visible without ongoing psychotherapy. Certainly, the evidence for a homeopathic treatment alone was weak and the decision to proceed was not determined by convincing evidence. If the prior probability (step 6) had been low either on the side of the patient or on the side of the therapist, proceeding with CAM therapy could not be recommended. Had the prior probability been low on the side of the patient, homeopathy or any alternative treatment could have sustained a false hope, diverting the patient from the need to seek definitive treatment. If the prior probability had been low on the side of the therapist, it is doubtful whether he or she could have integrated both perspectives, which again could interfere with an effective therapeutic process.

CASE 3: SMOKING CESSATION

A 32-year-old woman who has smoked a pack of cigarettes a day for 15 years saw an advertisement for a smoking cessation clinic that used acupuncture. She comes to her physician's office seeking advice about this program, which claims to have great results. When she visited the smoking cessation clinic, there was a single practitioner with an acupuncture degree from a Midwestern institution. The practitioner claimed that lots of research proved that acupuncture is highly effective in helping people stop smoking. The practitioner gave the patient some research articles—a randomized controlled trial written up in an Italian cardiology journal claiming 60% effectiveness, and a French article showing that acupuncture was effective in helping to stop smoking (29). He said that in his clinical experience, 80% of people that he treated were able to stop smoking.

The treatment consists of ear acupuncture 3 times a week for 2 months, followed by a single monthly treatment for 1 year. Also, a small "acu-ball" is taped to points on the patient's ear for several hours daily. The cost is $35 per visit (plus $5 for the "acu-ball"). The practitioner requests 2 months' payment at the start, yet gives a discount if it is all paid upfront ($240 at the first session for eight sessions). He said this prepayment helps patients become motivated to complete the first eight treatments. The patient would like to try this treatment because she really wants to stop smoking and has failed at previous attempts. She has tried smoking cessation classes and nicotine gum, but her nonsmoking status lasts only a few days or weeks. She is enthusiastic about the acupuncture and feels it may help her. However, before spending the money, she wanted to know if her physician thought it was a good idea.

Step 1. The patient really wants to try acupuncture. She has tried smoking cessation classes and nicotine gum and patches without success. She wants to have a baby and stop smoking before she becomes pregnant.

Step 2. If properly delivered with disposable needles, ear acupuncture is unlikely to produce serious side effects. The cost and time commitment is considerable, but so is continuing to smoke.

Step 3. Her physician offers to search the literature. He logs onto the Internet and goes to the Cochrane Database of Clinical Trials in Complementary Medicine (available free on the Web page of the NIH National Center for Complementary and Alternative Medicine). Using the key words "smoking" and "acupuncture," he finds 27 controlled trials and 1 systematic review (30).

Step 4. The systematic review (published in 1990) is a criteria-based quality review of 15 trials. The review reports that the vast majority of these trials were small, of poor quality, and reported negative results. The French study provided by the acupuncturist was also on-line and, although it reports positive effects from acupuncture, it received a very poor score in the systematic review. A more recent study (1997) evaluated smoking cessation rates in groups given acupuncture, nicotine gum, both, or neither. About 6% remained off tobacco at 4 years, with no difference between any treatment (31).

Steps 5 through 9 are unnecessary because the current best evidence indicates that acupuncture is no more effective than placebo or nicotine gum for smoking cessation. The patient should be informed that using the acupuncturist for this purpose may be a waste of time and money. Once the patient's initial enthusiasm for the acupuncture treatments has subsided, a relapse to smoking is highly probable. Provided the acupuncture is delivered in a proper manner with sterile needles, the patient's main risk is the cost and time of the treatments as well as potential resignation from future attempts at smoking cessation should she return to smoking. This might prevent her from enrolling in a comprehensive smoking cessation program, which may increase her chances of success in smoking cessation. Thus, an additional risk of acupuncture in this case is substituting ineffective therapy for possible effective therapy.

REFERENCES

1. Stolberg M. Die Homoeopathie auf dem Pruefstein. Der erste Doppelblindversuch der Medizingeschichte im Jahr 1835. Muenchner Medizinische Wochenschrift 1996;138:364–366.
2. Evidence-Based Medicine Working Group. Evidenced-based medicine: a new approach to teaching the practice of medicine. JAMA 1992;268:2420–2425.
3. DiGiacomo S. Biomedicine as a cultural system: an anthropologist in the kingdom of the sick. Encounters with Biomedicine 1987:315–346.
4. Collins HM. In: Collins HM, ed. Sociology of scientific knowledge: a source book. Bath, England: Bath University Press, 1982.
5. McKinlay JB. From "promising report" to "standard procedure": seven stages in the career of a medical innovation. Health and Society 1981;59:374–411.
6. Berg AO. Clinical practice policies: believe only some of what you read. Fam Pract 1996;3:58–70.
7. Slawson DC, Shaughnessy AF, Bennett JH. Becoming a medical information master: feeling good about not knowing everything. J Fam Pract 1994;38:505–513.
8. Wennberg J. Dealing with medical practice variations: a proposal for action. Health Aff (Millwood) 1984;3:6–32.
9. Chassin MR, Brook RH, Park RE, et al. Variations in the use of medical and surgical services by the Medicare population. N Engl J Med 1986; 314:285–290.
10. Eddy DM. Clinical decision making: from theory to practice. A collection of essays from JAMA. Boston: Jones & Bartlett Publishers, 1996.
11. Ellenberg JH, Nelson KB. Sample selection and the natural history of disease. Studies of febrile seizures. JAMA 1980;243:1337–1340.
12. Feinstein AR. Clinical judgment revisited: the distraction of quantitative models. Ann Intern Med 1994;120:799–805.
13. Linde K, Worku F, Stör W, et al. Randomized clinical trials of acupuncture for asthma—a systematic review. Forsch Komplementärmed 1996;3:148–155.
14. Jonas WB. Alternative medicine. J Fam Pract 1997;45:34–37.
15. Linde K, Clausius N, Ramirez G, et al. Are the clinical effects of homeopathy all placebo effects? A meta-analysis of randomized, placebo controlled trials. Lancet 1997;350:834–843.
16. Physicians for the 21st century: the GPEP Report. Washington, DC: Association of American Medical Colleges, 1984 and 1994.
17. Haynes RB, Sackett DL, Gray JM, et al. Transferring evidence from research into practice: 1. The role of clinical care research evidence in clinical decisions. ACP J Club 1996;125:A14–16.
18. Sackett DL, Richardson WS, Rosenberg W, Haynes RB. Evidence-based medicine: how to practice and teach EBM. New York: Churchill Livingstone, 1997.
19. Gill P, Dowell AC, Neal RD, et al. Evidence-based general practice: a retrospective study of interventions in one training practice. BMJ 1996; 312:819–821.
20. Haynes RB, Sackett DL, Gray JA, et al. Transferring evidence from research into practice: 2. Getting the evidence straight. ACP J Club 1997;126:A14–16.
21. Schneider CJ, Jonas WB. Are alternative treatments effective? Issues and methods involved in measuring effectiveness of alternative treatments. Subtle Energies 1995;5:69–92.
22. Wiesenauer M, Ludtke R. A meta-analysis of the homeopathic treatment of pollinosis with galphimia glauca. Forschende Komplenemtarmedizin 1996;3:230–234.
23. Jonas WB. Clinical trials for chronic disease: randomized, controlled clinical trials are essential. J NIH Res 1997;9:33–39.
24. Frank JD. Non-specific aspects of treatment: the view of a psychotherapist. In: Shepherd M, Sartorius N, eds. Non-specific aspects of treatment. Bern: Huber, 1989:95–114.
25. Beecher HK. The powerful placebo. JAMA 1955;159:1602–1606.
26. Benson H, Epstein MD. The placebo effect: a neglected asset in the care of patients. JAMA 1975;232:1225–1227.
27. Moerman DE. General medical effectiveness and human biology: placebo effects in the treatment of ulcer disease. Med Anthropol Q 1983;14(3):13–16.
28. Roberts AH, Kewman DG, Mercier L, Hovell M. The power of nonspecific effects in healing: implications for psychological and biological treatments. Clin Psychol Rev 1993;13:375–391.
29. Circo A, Tosto A, Raciti S, et al. First results of an anti-smoke outpatient unit: comparison among three methods. Riv Cardiol Prev Riabil 1985; 3:147–151.
30. ter Riet G, Kleijnen J, Knipschild P. A meta-analysis of studies into the effect of acupuncture on addiction. Br J Gen Pract 1990;40:379–382.
31. Clavel CF, Paoletti C, Benhamou S. Smoking cessation rates 4 years after treatment by nicotine gum and acupuncture. Prev Med 1997;26:25–28.

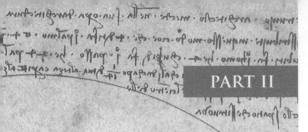

PART II

THE SAFETY OF COMPLEMENTARY
AND ALTERNATIVE MEDICINE
PRODUCTS AND PRACTICES

INTRODUCTION: EVALUATING THE SAFETY OF COMPLEMENTARY AND ALTERNATIVE PRODUCTS AND PRACTICES

Wayne B. Jonas and Edzard Ernst

COMPLEMENTARY AND ALTERNATIVE MEDICAL (CAM) PRACTICES ARE INCREASING IN POPULARITY. IN THE UNITED STATES IT IS ESTIMATED THAT AT LEAST ONE-THIRD OF THE POPULATION USES THESE PRACTICES ON A REGULAR BASIS, CONSTITUTING 425 MILLION VISITS AND SPENDING ALMOST $14 BILLION ON THESE PRODUCTS AND PRACTICES ANNUALLY; MOST OF THESE COSTS ($10 BILLION) ARE OUT-OF-POCKET EXPENSES (1). IN EUROPE, THE PROPORTION IS EVEN HIGHER, WITH 40 TO 70% OF THE POPULATION USING CAM IN SOME CASES (2). THE WORLD HEALTH ORGANIZATION (WHO) ESTIMATES THAT 80% OF THE DEVELOPING WORLD'S POPULATION DEPENDS ON TRADITIONAL PRACTICES (MOSTLY HERBAL PREPARATIONS) FOR THEIR HEALTH CARE MANAGEMENT (3). IN 1996, A STUDY IN *THE LANCET* EXTRAPOLATED ON THE BASIS OF ABOUT 3000 PERSONAL INTERVIEWS WITH SOUTH AUSTRALIAN PERSONS AGED 15 YEARS OR OLDER THAT THE AUSTRALIAN POPULATION HAD SPENT $AU621 MILLION FOR ALTERNATIVE MEDICINES AND $AU309 MIL-

LION FOR ALTERNATIVE THERAPISTS, COMPARED TO $AU360 MILLION OF PATIENT CONTRIBUTIONS FOR THE CONVENTIONAL DRUGS THAT HAD BEEN PURCHASED IN 1992–1993 (4).

As use of these practices rises, concern over safety becomes increasingly important. Toxic products can be used in a relatively safe manner if they are delivered by a well-trained practitioner with supporting medical infrastructure and close monitoring. However, many practices used in CAM involve self-care or delivery by practitioners whose training may be unknown, unmonitored, or inadequate (5, 6, 7). Because there is an increasing potential for public harm with misuse of these practices, closer scrutiny of potential adverse effects from CAM practices is needed.

On the supply side, the growth of the market for complementary medicines is promoted by active marketing, which regularly emphasizes the natural origin and harmlessness of these medicines (8–11). On the demand side (i.e., the market), the volume is increased by various factors, which vary from user to user and from product to product (12, 13). Some consumers use alternative medicines because of the health-promoting action ascribed to these products (8, 14), whereas others take them because conventional medicine does not offer an adequate prospect of being cured (15–17). The preference for alternative medicines may be partly explained by the consumer wanting to exert control over his or her own health status; also, the consumer may be attracted to the patient-oriented approach of the alternative practitioner (17–20). In addition, advice of family or friends can be a primary or additional motive to start the use of alternative products (21, 22). Finally, many conventional health care providers are increasingly tolerant of rather than rejecting toward alternative therapies (23–25).

BROAD SCOPE

Because of the broad scope of CAM, it is difficult to define what preparations should be dis-

cussed and what should be excluded in this review. The same product may be an officially licensed medicine in one country and a dietary supplement in the next, and it is also possible that the same substance is available as an approved medicine and as a health food preparation in the same country. Furthermore, current markets of dietary supplements and health food products not only comprise medicinal preparations, but also products used for other purposes, such as aphrodisiacs (26), mind-altering recreational herbs, and preparations for the enhancement of athletic performance (27–29). Although these types of products may be outside the domain of complementary medicines in a strict sense, we have included them here because they are often available through similar outlets as complementary medicines and are often perceived by the public as similar products. Also, we felt that the informational value of this chapter would benefit from a broad scope rather than a conceptually strict definition.

THE RELATIVE NATURE OF "SAFETY"

Safety is defined by Webster's Dictionary as "freedom from whatever exposes one to danger or from liability to cause danger or harm; safeness; hence the quality of making safe or secure or of giving confidence, justifying trust, insuring against harm or loss, etc." It derives from the Sanskrit word *sarva,* which is akin to the word *salus,* meaning "of sound condition, well preserved, unharmed, whole." The word *safety* is thus intimately related to the concepts of health and wholeness, or completeness, and refers more specifically to conditions that threaten wholeness or health.

The medical application of the term *safety* is relative. This is illustrated by the fact that the United States Food and Drug Administration (FDA), which is charged with ensuring safety of products and devices, has no specific definition of the term. Safety is relative to several factors, including:

1. Toxicity of the product or device being used.
2. Potential benefits incurred from use.
3. Context of use—e.g., self-care or under the

care of a competently trained professional with knowledge, skills, and abilities to ensure proper use.

4. Appropriate monitoring, marketing, and advertising to ensure that its use is accessed properly.

5. Values that underlie judgment of its proper use—for example, the desired and expected outcomes interpreted by judgments that determine whether its effects are adverse or beneficial.

To speak of safety, one must address the risk-to-benefit ratio derived from engaging in these practices or administering products with therapeutic intent. The risk-benefit ratio becomes the index by which safety is judged. For most products or practices, only the direct assessment of the risk-benefit ratio can provide reliable information with which to make evidence-based judgments about safety.

THE RELATIVE SAFETY OF "NATURAL"

CAM products are often assumed to be safer than conventional medicine and drug therapy, providing a frequent reason individuals turn to CAM (30). The term *natural medicine,* used frequently in Germany and elsewhere, attracts people to CAM practices who may be afraid of the side effects of conventional therapies. People may assume that therapies labeled *natural* are inherently safer, which is not always true.

Some CAM practices appear to be generally of low risk. Examples include meditation, mind-body techniques (e.g., visualization), psychic or spiritual healing, and whole systems of practice, such as homeopathy and acupuncture. Other complementary therapies clearly present direct risks. Examples are herbal remedies; intravenous hydrogen peroxide or high-dose megavitamin and mineral infusions; and procedures such as colonics or high-velocity spinal manipulation. Yet, given the risk-benefit definition of safety, one cannot assume any therapy, which on the surface appears mostly harmless, is safe.

Homeopathy provides an example of the need to match appropriate criteria to specific CAM therapies. Homeopathy, which uses highly dilute substances, appears to be inherently safe. Homeopathic remedies often begin with highly toxic substances. But, through a process of serial dilution, these substances end up having little or none of the toxic component remaining in the final preparation. However, specific precautions are still required. For example, not all homeopathy preparations (or those labeled as homeopathic) are extremely dilute. Some "low-potency" preparations or those mixed with herbal products may contain potentially dangerous substances (31).

One may also assume that prayer has no direct toxic effect. However, adverse effects from "psychic" phenomena have been documented (32). Whether one understands the mechanisms (e.g., psychogenic, cultural, autonomic), can we reasonably assume that these practices have no adverse effects?

Therapies with known toxic effects (e.g., herbal preparations) may actually prove to be inherently safer (given their relative benefits) than comparable conventional therapies. An example is the use of hypericum, or St. John's Wort, for the treatment of mild to moderate depression. The efficacy of this herb for this indication has been demonstrated in clinical trials and has very few adverse effects. In direct comparison with conventional antidepressant agents, hypericum has fewer side effects with comparable efficacy (33). This finding illustrates that a therapy with higher potential direct toxic effects than homeopathy or prayer may be inherently more desirable—that is, "safer"—given the indications and comparative value to a conventional therapy because of a reduced risk-benefit ratio. Therefore, decisions about safety requires evaluation using various criteria, both for systems as a whole (e.g., homeopathy, prayer, herbalism) and for specific products within systems during application for specific indications.

To be considered sufficiently safe for application, certain therapeutic systems (e.g., acupuncture and homeopathy) may require only toxicity screening and appropriate training for their use as a whole system. In this case, specific product safety testing for each indication is unrealistic. Other inventions (e.g., herbalism or megavitamin therapy) require screening of both the entire system for general safety characteristics and specific testing of standardized products for specific indications before marketing. Examples of these approaches are the WHO *Guidelines for Safe Acupuncture Treatment* (3) and ongoing work in several countries developing both safe and practical regulation of botanical products (34–36). (See Chapter 5 for guidelines on how to use potential risk in making evidence-based decisions about CAM.)

COMPONENTS OF SAFETY

Adverse effects from CAM practices can be classified into three broad categories:

- **Direct adverse effects** are either short-term, in which they are often called *toxic effects*, or long-term, in which they are called *side effects.*
- **Indirect adverse effects** are those events that occur because of incompetent delivery of the therapy or diagnostic procedure.
- **Definitional adverse effects.** Many CAM systems use different diagnostic categories, patient preferences, explanatory models, and outcome values than those commonly accepted in the West. Failure to provide clarity in these definitional and descriptive areas can lead to misunderstanding of application or attempted application of the practice, which can also produce adverse effects.

Mislabeling

Mislabeling occurs when a product or device does not contain the items it purports to contain or does not perform the actions its claims to perform. In products such as herbal preparations, mislabeling may involve the application of a specific herbal name and yet the product may not contain that herb. For example, confusion and mislabeling of various ginseng species has lead to inaccurate claims of toxicity. Herbal products sometimes are labeled as containing a single herb, but actually contain products from a variety of plants (37). Some homeopathic products are labeled homeopathic because they include highly dilute preparations combined

with plant products, or even pharmacological doses of conventional drugs. Likewise, acupuncture needles may not be prepared with appropriate manufacturing and sterility standards and yet be labeled sterile. Mislabeling may occur because good manufacturing processes are not incorporated in the manufacture of the product. In fraudulent cases, mislabeling may occur deliberately. Although fraudulent mislabeling of products occurs, its frequency is unknown and probably represents a minority of products compared to those who mislabel because of inadequate manufacturing and standardization procedures.

A significant subset of mislabeling is underlabeling. Underlabeling occurs when potentially toxic or active ingredients are not listed on the product's contents label. For example, some Traditional Chinese and Ayurvedic herbal preparations may contain toxic doses of mercury, lead, arsenic, and other heavy metals (38). In some cases, these substances are in the product because practitioners in the CAM system believes they provide important therapeutic effects. These substances are clearly toxic and have long-term damaging effects, especially if ingested by children, but may not appear on the label. Nor can the predictions about their concentration be estimated from the name of the plant product or herbal mixture. The recent Dietary Supplement Health and Education Act passed by the U.S. government may have aggravated this problem by allowing some products that are frequently used as therapeutic agents to be classified as foods. This classification results in less labeling of the content and description of appropriate usage. Underlabeling can be a serious type of mislabeling.

Misrepresentation

Misrepresentation involves claiming effectiveness for ineffective interventions or diagnostic procedures. Even in relatively benign conditions, misrepresentation can cause adverse effects because of the risk of wasting time and money, the increased use of diagnostic techniques (including repeated history-taking and physical exams), and the generation of false expectations about the outcome. In addition, misrepresentation of ineffective therapies causes harm if effective therapies are not used for the alleviation of the condition.

There are two key decisions needed to evaluate misrepresentation. The first is whether an intervention is needed at all. Many conditions have a benign natural course or recover spontaneously and require no intervention. In these cases, any intervention carries potential risks. For example, close to 80% of individuals who visit a general practice in which a specific diagnosis is not reached will have his or her problem resolve or improve with no therapy (39). In this case, any intervention with potential side effects, inconvenience, cost, or one that produces anxiety or other psychological factors is inappropriate. Thus, prognostic need is an important part of evaluating misrepresentation. Increased self-care with natural medicines and the assumption of comprehensive medical care by practitioners without extensive experience and training in the management of serious disease can lead to unfavorable, avoidable, and, therefore, adverse outcomes. Examples of these outcomes have been published, such as an attempted treatment of diabetes mellitus using ineffective herbal preparations (5–7). Other examples include the treatment of cancers in the early stages using biological or homeopathic preparations and the reliance on prayer and mental healing while serious conditions progress (40). The prevalence of such events from a public health perspective is unknown.

The first aspect of misrepresentation can only occur if there is truly an effective conventional therapy available for the condition. In many incidences, there may not be an effective therapy. For example, acupuncture or homeopathic treatment may alleviate pain and improve function in patients with pancreatic cancer because of nonspecific effects. Because the side effects of these therapies are less than those produced by chemotherapeutics used in conventional medicine for the treatment of pancreatic cancer, and because conventional treatment does not change the prognosis of this disease, the use of these two alternative modalities in the treatment of pancreatic cancer could not be considered as causing harm or misrepresentation in this sense.

Comparative Trials

Direct comparative trials of CAM therapies compared with proven conventional therapies has increased. There are now a number of examples comparing acupuncture, homeopathy, and herbal preparations, as well as spinal manipulation and Traditional Chinese Medicine with and without the incorporation of conventional medicine in randomized controlled trials. These trials often, but not always, demonstrate similar benefit with equal or reduced adverse effects from complementary therapies, although costs are rarely measured.

Examples of such direct comparison is the hypericum versus imipramine trial described previously (41), the comparison of classical homeopathy versus salicylates in the treatment of rheumatoid arthritis published by Gibson et al. (42), and the controlled trial comparing antacids, cimetidine, deglycyrrhizinated licorice, and gefarnate in the treatment of chronic duodenal ulceration (43). Hammerschlag has summarized the direct comparative trials of acupuncture versus conventional medicine in a variety of conditions. In most trials in which the benefit of conventional treatments is similar to acupuncture, adverse effects were usually equal or less (44). More trials of this type are needed in complementary medicine.

Misapplication

Misapplication of effective therapies can also result in harm. Misapplication usually occurs because of inadequate training, in knowledge, skills, or experience or from incompetence or practitioner impairment. Conventional medication has well-established training, certification, licensing, and monitoring procedures to ensure that the knowledge, skills, and qualifications of a practitioner are adequate. Even with these safeguards, misapplication occurs. If CAM practitioners engage in the entire scope of a medical practice, then their knowledge, skills, and experience in these areas must be at least comparable to those involved in conventional primary care, or their practice should be specifically restricted and defined. Appropriate referral to and from medically qualified practitioners requires knowledge by those practitioners of which conditions are best managed and under what circumstances. As the number, type, and background of complementary practitioners increases and as the identification of more effective and ineffective CAM therapies occurs, it is likely that a generalist medical coordinator with knowledge about both CAM and conventional medicine will be needed to prevent misapplication.

Misapplication can occur if practitioners fail to properly refer to or apply effective practices. Schools of acupuncture for physicians consist of about 200 to 400 hours of training in acupuncture, which is often considered inadequate in countries where extensive use and training of traditional acupuncturists has occurred for centuries. In addition, non-MD acupuncturists may have inadequate medical training. The WHO is attempting to address these problems by creating categories of acupuncturists with various training standards and scopes of practice. Thus, minimum hours and standards for the training of qualified medical doctors in acupuncture is defined, as are minimal training and experience in anatomy, physiology, pathophysiology, prognosis, and scope of practice for acupuncturists in Western diagnosis and medicine. Without such standards for all those who may engage in, refer to, or recommend complementary practices, misapplication is likely to continue unchecked. In the United States, there are at least three certifying bodies in acupuncture and Oriental medicine, each having different requirements for certification and scopes of practice. States seeking to provide appropriate laws for licensing and regulating acupuncturists may use criteria from different organizations or from none of these organizations in their certification process. A similar situation exists with homeopathic practitioners, having various certification and licensing and training requirements for MDs, NDs, DCs, and even lay practitioners. Whereas all 50 states recognize, license, and regulate chiropractors, only about 24 states have statutory regulations dealing with acupuncture, 12 with naturopathy, and 4 with homeopathy, one of which dates back to 1906. The situation in the United Kingdom is even more chaotic, where the practice of medicine does not require any certification or licensing. (See Chapter 2 for a list of current licensing laws for various practices by state.)

Misdiagnosis

Finally, harm can occur because of incorrect, inaccurate, or inappropriate diagnosis and patient classification, resulting in the application of effective therapies for the incorrect condition. Harm can also occur from failure to detect conditions that can be corrected. Harm from inappropriate diagnosis and patient classification is different from suboptimal application of effective therapies. The former involves clinical disagreement and diagnostic accuracy, or failure to detect and apply the therapy to the main cause of a condition. The practitioner should especially be alert for CAM systems that create their own diagnostic class for which their therapy is then applied. Iridology claims to diagnose specific conditions from patterns in the eye. This results in unnecessary treatments not proven to effect that particular condition (45). Many other similar diagnostic methods are available that in principle set up situations for the same risk. Electrodermal diagnostic methods, for example, claim to be able to detect functional changes in acupuncture meridians and subsequently the corresponding organ locations. These measurements then become an "electromagnetic" diagnosis of disease. These "diseases" created with such instruments are then "treated" using a variety of means. Without proof that such a "diagnosis" is important, these treatments are claimed to be "preventive," and patients may go through multiple "measurements" and "treatments." This can cause harm by creating anxiety, excessive and unnecessary testing, treatments, and expenditures of time and energy, all of which have unknown benefit. Similar CAM diagnostic systems, including combinations of endocrinological and blood measurements from normal serum, radiathesia, intuitive diagnosis, auricular diagnosis, and the use of pleomorphism, all carry the same risk of misinformed application and misdiagnosis.

Orthodox medicine has its share of similar questionable screening and diagnostic methods, including tests such as PSA for all men, mammography for younger women, occult stool blood tests, fetal monitoring in normal pregnancies, and so on. In many of these tests, their reliability and correlation with significant outcomes are questionable, yet their application leads to interventions, all of which carry risks. An overdependence on medically "correct" (e.g., objective, proven, most common, most easily verified, most high-tech) outcomes in place of attending to subjective, quality of life, and individually valued outcomes is probably a major reason why the people turn to CAM practitioners (30). These are definitional and value issues that if not addressed can lead to adverse effects from treatment.

DEFINITIONAL ISSUES

Many CAM practices are derived from the medical systems of non-Western cultures, or carry basic epistemological assumptions about the nature of man and reality that are quite different from conventional science and medicine. These issues must be considered to prevent misunderstanding that may arise regarding different values underlying these practices. Definitional issues can impact safety judgments in several areas, including decisions on the most preferred product; diagnostic and patient classifications; type of outcomes valued by the complementary medical system; the personal value placed by individuals on outcomes; and the explanatory model that drives the forgoing. (A full discussion of definitional issues and how they impact on safety in CAM is beyond the scope of this chapter, but they are discussed in each chapter in Part III of this book for particular CAM systems.)

INDIRECT RISKS

Contrary to popular belief, complementary therapies can be associated with serious health risks. In addition to the risks just described, there is the indirect risk that a complementary treatment with unproven therapeutic potential delays or replaces a more effective form of conventional therapy. This can occur if an alternative practitioner is overly optimistic about his or her diagnostic or therapeutic abilities or when a naive patient or headstrong parent of a sick child puts too much trust in the healing powers of nature. There are various case reports, both in the medical and judicial literature, to indicate that this is not just a theoretical concern (48–54). For example, life-threatening and fatal ketoacidotic coma has been observed in patients with insulin-dependent diabetes following reduction or withdrawal of insulin treatment in favor of an ineffective alternative approach (55–57). Of particular concern may be the phenomenon that non-Western patients can seek refuge in a traditional therapy of their homeland. According to Belgian researchers, for example, serious problems have arisen in Moroccan migrants with asthma or diabetes, who returned to their homeland for a holiday, where they swapped their Western medicines for local herbs (58, 59).

Scientific information about the extent of the indirect health risks of complementary medicine is still difficult to find. In a questionnaire study among Dutch family doctors about their personal experiences with negligent behavior by alternative practitioners in 1986, 120 respondents reported 10 cases of complications: 6 of the patients had received complementary treatment instead of conventional therapy, whereas the other 4 had discontinued conventional drug therapy on the advice of an alternative practitioner (60). In a systematic Swedish survey among 242 hospitals over the period 1984–1988, 233 hospitals reported a total of 123 detailed cases. In 6 cases the patient had died and another 23 patients had needed intensive care to save their lives (61). Unfortunately, without a reliable denominator, it is impossible to assess the incidence of the reported cases. Moreover, one should measure doctor's delay not only among alternative practitioners, but also among conventional physicians to allow a fair comparison between both types of health care providers. More and better research in this area is warranted.

Another indirect risk of complementary medicines is that the effectiveness of a conventional medicine may be compromised by concurrent use of an alternative product. This point is well illustrated by two fairly recent reports on adverse interactions between traditional Indian medicines and conventional medicines:

- The oleoresinous product gugulipid (derived from an ancient Indian medicinal plant, *Commiphora mukul*) was found to reduce the bioavailability of certain synthetic agents (e.g., diazepam, propranolol) by one-third (62). For conventional drugs with a narrow therapeutic window or steep dose-response curve, a decrease of this magnitude is relevant.
- Co-administration of phenytoin with an Ayurvedic syrup called Shankhapushpi (prepared from *Centella asiatica*, *Convolvulus pluricaulis*, *Nardostachys jatamansi*, *Nepeta elliptica*, *Nepeta hindostana*, and *Onosma bracteatum*) was reported to result in reduced plasma levels of phenytoin and in loss of seizure control (63). Additional studies on the risk of such interactions between traditional medicines and conventional pharmaceuticals are needed.

ADVERSE EFFECTS: TYPES A, B, C, AND D REACTIONS

Limited experience with complementary medicine can help to identify adverse effects that can develop rapidly after the start of therapy in a high proportion of users. In the clinical pharmacological literature, such acute effects are known as *type A reactions* (64). A classic example is the induction of anticholinergic symptoms, such as palpitations, dryness of the mouth, and dilation of the pupils, by herbal medicines rich in belladonna alkaloids. As Table 1 illustrates (65), type A reactions are pharmacologically predictable and dose-dependent, which implies that they can be anticipated and that they could be prevented by dose reduction. Traditional experience can bring these dose-dependencies to light and it can also help to detect ways of processing to reduce the likelihood of acute problems.

However, not all adverse reactions occur immediately after a therapy has been initiated. The importance of delayed reactions has been underlined by a recent retrospective study covering clinical safety trials with 27 different pharmaceuticals. Nine of these 27 drug compounds were associated with serious drug-related adverse events that first occurred during the second half of a 12-month testing period. For three of the compounds, these late discoveries were so serious that they eventually affected the final dose selected, the product labeling, or the target population (66). When reactions develop during chronic therapy in a pharmacologically predictable way, they are called *type C reactions* (64). An herbal example is muscular weakness due to hypokalemia in long-term users of herbal anthranoid laxatives (67). Type C reactions can be anticipated, but only after they have been identified, and such an identification may be more difficult than with type A reactions.

Table 1. Effects of Atropine in Relation to Dosage	
DOSE	**EFFECTS**
0.5 mg	Slight cardiac slowing; some dryness of mouth; inhibition of sweating
1.0 mg	Dryness of mouth; thirst; acceleration of heart rate, sometimes preceded by slowing; mild dilation of pupils
2.0 mg	Rapid heart rate; palpitation; marked dryness of the mouth; dilated pupils; some blurring of near vision
5.0 mg	All the above symptoms marked; speech disturbed; difficulty in swallowing; restlessness and fatigue; headache; dry, hot skin; difficulty in micturition; reduced intestinal peristalsis
10.0 mg and greater	Above symptoms more marked; pulse rapid and weak; iris practically obliterated; vision very blurred; skin flushed, hot, dry, and scarlet; ataxia, restlessness, and excitement; hallucinations and delirium; coma

It is also difficult for alternative practitioners and their clients to recognize *type B reactions*. These reactions are not associated with the principal pharmacological properties of a product and they do not improve when the dose is reduced—the product has to be withdrawn completely. Type B reactions are often immunologically mediated but some have a non-immunological basis (e.g., genetic cause). Although type B reactions occur in only a minority of the users, they can be so severe that withdrawal of the responsible agent from general use is warranted (64, 68). Examples of type B reactions to complementary products are the hepatotoxic reactions that have been attributed in recent years to the wall germander (*Teucrium chamaedrys*) (69), skullcap (*Scutellaria* or *Teucrium* sp.) (70, 71), and chaparral (*Larrea tridentata*) (72, 73). In chaparral, the hepatotoxic potential only became apparent after an estimated 500 million capsules had been used without concern over a 20-year period (74). At present, 5% of presumed viral hepatitis cases are not confirmed on serological testing. To what extent complementary medicines play a role in such cases is currently unknown. Doctors should definitely keep this possibility in mind, however, when they examine patients with unexplained hepatic disease (75).

Finally, *type D reactions* may be readily overlooked. This category consists of certain delayed effects, such as teratogenicity and carcinogenicity (64). It has been shown, for example, that the amines of certain Nigerian medicinal plants can be converted to *N*-nitroso carcinogens under simulated gastric conditions (76). A clinical example is the presence of aristolochic acids in various medicinal species in the genus of *Aristolochia*. These acids are potent rodent carcinogens (77), and human cases of *Aristolochia*-associated malignancy have recently been described (78, 79). The use of complementary medicines during pregnancy and lactation is also of concern. When a herb has oxytocic properties (the capacity to cause contraction of the uterus), the risks of its unrestricted use during pregnancy will be readily discovered. However, when a sick baby is born, who will attribute the disease to maternal consumption of a complementary product many months before the baby's delivery? Herbal remedies containing pyrrolizidine alkaloids may have been used since prehistoric times, but the first case report about neonatal hepatotoxicity following the use of such a remedy during pregnancy did not appear until the late 1980s. There is a need for more and better information about the embryotoxic and fetotoxic risks of complementary medicines, not in the least because the use of herbal medicines during pregnancy is sometimes encouraged by uncritical publications (80).

LIMITATIONS OF TRADITIONAL EXPERIENCE

Alternative practitioners and their customers are likely to detect some types of adverse reactions to herbal medicines less readily than other types (e.g., type A). Recognition can be particularly difficult when the signs and symptoms are not unusual in the population and could thus also be ascribed to various causes. In other words, although long-standing experience may tell much about striking and predictable acute toxicity, it is a less reliable tool for the detection of reactions that occur uncommonly, develop very gradually, need a prolonged latency period, or that are inconspicuous (80). This phenomenon of unobtrusive problems remaining undetected can be denoted as the *Aje-Mutin trap*. *Aje-imutin* is the native name used by the Nigerian Yoruba people for an African relative of the ink-cap mushroom. The literal translation of the term is "eat-without-drinking-alcohol" (81), which shows that the Yoruba have learned that ingestion of *Coprinus* mushrooms can induce a disulfiram-like sensitivity to alcohol. Yet the same Yoruba employ herbal enemas to treat diarrhea and dysentery, apparently without realizing that this can exacerbate the dehydration produced by the diarrhea, thereby reducing (instead of increasing) the patient's chance of recovery (82). Another example in Africa of inconspicuous traditional toxicity is the risk that eye medicines damage the eye by a direct action of toxic substances introduced into the conjunctival sac, by the introduction of microorganisms leading to infection, by physical trauma resulting from the application, or indirectly by delaying the patient's presentation to a clinic for therapy. Epidemiological research has shown that 25% of the corneal ulcers and childhood blindness in rural Africa is associated with the instillation of traditional eye medicines (83–85).

The risk that rare adverse reactions to complementary medicines remain unnoticed can also be illustrated by the statistical "rule of three," which dictates that the number of studied subjects must be three times as high as the frequency of an adverse reaction to have a 95% chance that the reaction will actually occur in the studied population. When an adverse reaction to a medicine occurs with a clinically relevant frequency of 1 in 1000, a practitioner treating 1000 patients with this medicine still has a 37% chance that he or she will not observe the reaction at all. To be 95% certain that the practitioner will see the reaction, he or she would have to treat at least 3000 patients (Table 2). The practitioner may need to see more than one reaction, however, before he or she can make a mental connection with the medicine. To have a 95% chance that the clinician observes the reaction three times, he or she would have to treat 6500 patients—that is, one patient every working day for almost 25 years (55). These calculations make clear that personal experience is not a reliable basis for the exclusion of uncommon reactions to complementary medicines.

Nontraditional Hazards

There is another reason why safety claims cannot always be based on long-standing traditional experience: not all complementary medicines have firm roots in traditional practices, and this issue seems underestimated. When traditional source plants are extracted in a nontraditional way (e.g., by resorting to a nonpolar solvent such as hexane), one can question whether this nontraditional extract is as safe as the traditional one. Until recently, the ostrich fern (*Matteuccia struthiopteris*) was generally considered to be a nontoxic, edible plant with a history of use as a spring vegetable that dates to the 1700s. However, recent observations of serious gastrointestinal toxicity following the consumption of lightly sauteed or blanched ostrich fern shoots suggest that this vegetable is safe only when it is thoroughly cooked before use (86). A similar example is the recent outbreak of bronchiolitis obliterans in Taiwan, which was associated with the ingestion of *Sauropus androgynus*. This herb is normally cooked before being eaten as a vegetable, but in this case the numerous victims had all consumed uncooked leaf juice as an unproven method of weight control (87).

It is also possible that an ingredient may have no medicinal tradition at all, and its route of administration or dose level may be quite different from that used in a traditional setting. The question could be raised, for example, to what extent the excellent oral safety record of certain traditional herbs is applicable to herbal cigarettes, available in Western health food stores. Certain respiratory risks attributed to tobacco smoking may extend to the smoking of nontobacco herbal products, particularly marijuana (88–93).

Table 2. Number of Persons who Need to be Exposed to a Drug to Have a 95% Chance of Detecting an Adverse Drug Reaction Occurring with a Particular Frequency at Least Once, Twice, or Three Times

FREQUENCY OF ADVERSE DRUG REACTION (ADR)	NUMBER OF ADR CASES		
	1	2	3
1 out of 100	300	480	650
1 out of 200	600	960	1300
1 out of 1000	3000	4800	6500
1 out of 2000	6000	9600	13,000
1 out of 10,000	30,000	48,000	65,000

Taken from Verrept H et al., 1994.

PRODUCT-RELATED DETERMINANTS OF ADVERSE EFFECTS

Principal determinants of the toxic potential of complementary medicines are their composition and way of use. Various examples of potentially hazardous ingredients of complementary medicines are reviewed in detail later in this section. Unfortunately, checking out a product label is not always sufficient to exclude harmfulness. In many cases the adverse effects are associated with a hidden constituent or with a higher strength than that mentioned on the product label. For example, selenium toxicity has been repeatedly caused by health food tablets, which contained many times more selenium than was stated on their label (94–96). In other words, the current adverse effects to complementary medicines can be caused by a lack of stringent quality assurance rather than to the toxicological spectrum of their declared ingredients.

TOOLS FOR SAFETY ASSESSMENT IN COMPLEMENTARY MEDICINE

Clinical Accuracy

Modern science has derived a number of methods for attempting to assess safety of conventional medical practices. Despite this safety net, it is not infrequent to find significant risks being uncovered after years of use (e.g., UV light treatments, anti-arrythmics, calcium channel blockers, prostate cancer surgery). For practical purposes, the methods needed to detect adverse events are the same for both indirect and long-term direct effects. Direct, short-term toxicological effects are much easier (depending upon severity) but in some cases can be exaggerated or underdetected without proper investigative design. First, there is often wide clinical disagreement about whether a particular adverse effect was caused by a therapy. Even pharmacologists, for example, disagree 36% of the time as to whether a particular adverse effect was caused by a drug. The rate of disagreement goes up the more serious the attribution, with a 50% disagreement on whether an admission to the hospital was due to an adverse drug reaction and a 71% disagreement on whether a death was due to an adverse drug reaction (97).

Methods of Measurement

Many methods of surveying for adverse effects —broad checklists, patient interviews, or questionnaires—often do not yield relevant associations. For example, symptoms attributable to adverse drug reactions using symptom checklists results in 81% of individuals checking "Yes," with a mean of two symptoms per individual and 7% reporting six or more symptoms (98). Most symptoms collected this way will be false positive. The true rate of adverse events, even in extensively used therapies, may not be detected without rigorously designed, hypothesis driven, prospective trials with randomization and a control group.

Rare Events and Public Health Impact

Because adverse events occur rarely for many complementary medical practices (34), relatively large numbers (i.e., 3×1 over the inverse ratio of events) and special designs are needed to be 95% confident that even one adverse event would be detected. Adverse drug reporting can significantly underestimate these effects because only 5 to 10% of such events are ever reported. However, non-random cohort or case-control evaluations of adverse events often overinflate estimates of events with odd ratios of even two or three subsequently being found to be false (99). Because of their widespread use, complementary and alternative interventions may have significant public health implications. Accurately assessing the adverse effects of a single CAM therapy would require postmarketing surveillance of upwards of 3000 individuals. In addition, the rate of rare idiosyncratic and allergic reactions needs similar, large-scale postmarketing assessment (100).

Types of Evidence in Adverse Effects Assessment

Table 3 lists various types of evidence often used for reporting on safety in medicine, its usefulness, and its major limitations. First, preclinical evidence can often give indications of areas where there is potential toxicity and guide hypothesis testing and mechanism studies. Such information may identify compounds of potentially high risk in humans that cannot be automatically inferred to be harmful in the context

Table 3. Tools for Assessment of Adverse Effects

METHODS	USED FOR	NOT USED FOR
• Laboratory	• Dose-toxicity range • Screening for teratogenicity and carcinogenicity	• Frequency and degree of effects in humans under normal use
• Historical evidence	• General indications about acute toxicity	• Subtle, delayed, or infrequent adverse effects
• Case reports; Practice experience	• Detection and description of adverse effects	• Frequency or cause of the adverse effect
• Adverse effects registries	• Trends in use or unexpected effects	• Frequency or cause of the adverse effect
• Poison control centers	• Adverse effects from misuse	• Frequency or cause of the adverse effect
• Phase I & II trials	• Detection and verification of common short term adverse effects	• Delayed, infrequent effects and confirming the cause of the effects
• Phase III trials	• Relative frequency and causation of effects	• Detecting delayed, infrequent, and many unanticipated effects
• Postmarketing surveilliance	• Detection of delayed, infrequent, or unanticipated effects	• Confirming cause of the effects

of their clinical use. For example, phenobarbital increases the rate of hepatocellular carcinoma in rats, but when prepared as a homeopathic dilution can result in decreased rates of such cancers (101).

Historical evidence is often used to indicate that natural products are self-evidently safe. It is useful for giving general indications about acute toxicity, but cannot be used to indicate potential chronic effects or indirect risks. Therefore, this type of evidence is not useful for making firm conclusions about the value of these products for chronic disease in practice (102).

Case reports in the literature are the most frequent method of illustrating and emphasizing potential toxicity from complementary treatments. Such reports on adverse effects have the same limitations as anecdotal reports of beneficial effects. Case reports allow for descriptions of possible adverse associations but cannot be used to make judgments about frequency or cause. These reports tell us that adverse events can occur, not that they must occur nor how frequently. As with anecdotal reports about benefit, they are likely to lead to an overinterpretation of the significance of such events. Lists of adverse reports have been collected for a number of practices (especially herbal practices, acu-

puncture, and megavitamin therapy) (40, 103). Most authors agree that many of the more established complementary, alternative, and traditional medical interventions do not produce many serious adverse reactions when used in the traditional and/or indicated manner. Postmarketing surveillance can provide information about prevalence, incidence, and associations related to these events. As discussed previously, however, postmarketing surveillance may require large numbers (at least 3000) to identify with any confidence the true adverse event rate. Surveys risk inflating adverse event rates because specifically searching for events among a population can lead to search intensity bias, even in case-control studies (98). All studies must be conducted using objective outcome measures in a way that provides equal opportunity for finding and extracting information from exposed and unexposed groups. Failure to use blind evaluations can lead to diagnostic suspicion bias (finding what you are looking for) which also can inflate and exaggerate the rate of these events (104).

Adverse effects-reporting registries, such as MedWatch used by the FDA in the United States, can provide an indication of the popularity of new therapies or about changes in opinion on the value of new therapies in practice. In addition, they can be used to identify new, unexpected problems, such as a sudden increase in reactions from treatment exposures. These registries, however, are notoriously subject to falsification and under-reporting. Without rigorous verification methods built in, they cannot be relied upon for accurate prevalence data.

Information on adverse reactions also comes from poison control centers. These data are valuable for the likelihood of adverse reactions that occur from misuse and abuse of therapies (e.g., overdosing, suicide attempts, fraudulent practices, accidents) (105). These sources of data cannot provide information about safety under conditions of appropriate therapeutic use, nor is the accuracy of such information high given the high rates of disagreement about true adverse drug effects previously discussed.

Phase I and Phase II controlled trials can begin to indicate adverse effects accurately. However, the frequent use of open-ended checklists of adverse effects increases the risk of missing the real effects secondary to the multiple outcome assessments. In addition, the small size of these trials and their usual short-term duration reduce the chance of detecting effects that are not frequent or that may be delayed.

Phase III, or true efficacy, trials allow us to make conclusions about cause and are likely to be accurate if properly conducted. However, unless the adverse effects themselves are hypothesis generated, real adverse effects may be obscured by the likelihood of obtaining false-positive associations from multiple outcome measures. In addition, many complementary and alternative practices may find adequate sham controls problematic. For example, sham acupuncture usually shows increased effects over no acupuncture but less effects than "real" acupuncture, indicating that both specific and non-specific effects occur (43). Likewise, delivery of sham acupuncture cannot be done blind in a way that allows a complete approximation of how the therapy is delivered in clinical practice. Such trials may necessitate a pragmatic orientation that can never positively identify adverse effects from the specific therapy. If such effects are low to begin with, identifying these effects unequivocally may be impractical and unneces-

sary. The most valuable type of evidence would be hypothesis-generated toxicity studies done in randomized placebo-controlled fashion. This has the highest likelihood of revealing accurate adverse effects. However, because of its complexity, it is rarely done. Even hypothesized-generated, RCT toxicity studies, however, will not eliminate outcome substitution bias. This occurs when the more easily measured objective outcomes become the focus of the study, although less easily measured subjective outcomes are the most relevant for the patients involved. This is like the man looking for his lost car keys under a lamp where there is more light, though he lost them in the dark somewhere else.

Finally, none of these types of evidence adequately addresses the issue of model validity and the complexities that arise in attempting to assess optimal therapy (treatment of choice). This information comes best from direct randomized comparative trials that directly compare therapies and trials incorporating patient preferences into the investigation.

THE SAFETY OF SELECTED COMPLEMENTARY PRACTICES

This section of the book gives summary information from the published literature on adverse affects from manipulation, acupuncture, herbals, vitamins, mineral and other nutritional supplements, and homeopathy. The practitioner can use these chapters to review and refer to specific products and practices in CAM. One difficulty is that little is known about the prevalence of many of these events. The best sources of information on prevalence and adverse effect rates are from postmarketing surveillance studies, poison control centers, and randomized controlled trials.

Poison Control Centers

Perharic (105) and others have surveyed the toxicological problems resulting from traditional remedies and food supplements reported to a poison control center. Of the 5536 contacts, 657 (12%) had symptoms indicative of adverse effects from the ingestion. Most of these were children under 5 years of age who had ingested vitamins in overdose. Forty-two of these had some probability of being linked to the ingestion and two had high-probability. The rates of adverse effects calculated for vitamins were 343 in 4000 (8%), for food supplements 17 in 141 (12%), and for herbal products 245 in 968 (25%) (Table 4)(105). This information gives a sense of the rate of serious adverse events in situations of abuse but does not provide information about adverse effects rates under competent use.

Randomized Controlled Trials

Adverse effects reported in randomized controlled trials of alternative and complementary medicine as published in the conventional peer-reviewed literature would be the best type of evidence for identifying the true rate of hypothesis-driven, attributable adverse effects from the use of such interventions under normal conditions. This is because inflated effects would not likely be found from blinded trials that were using randomized assignment to therapy and that were specifically reporting on adverse effects and published in non-advocacy journals.

To access this information, we downloaded all of the citations from the National Library of Medicine (MEDLARS system) that dealt with alternative and complementary medicine, from

Table 4. Adverse Effects from Misuse Reported to Poison Control Centers

PRODUCT	NUMBER REPORTED	RATE (PERCENT)
• Total reports	• 5536	• 100
• Symptoms	• 657	• 12
• Probable link to ingestion	• 41	• <1
• Vitamins	• 342 of 4019	• 8
• Other food supplements	• 17 of 141	• 12
• Herbal products	• 245 of 968	• 25

Taken from Perharic L, Shaw D, Colbridge M, et al. Toxicological problems resulting from exposure to traditional remedies and food supplements. Drug Safety 1994;11(4):264–294.

double-blind, randomized control trials that specifically looked for and reported on adverse effects. Studies that involved extracted or purified plant toxins (e.g., podophyllotoxin) that were being used in combination with or as chemotherapeutic agents for cancer or were commonly used in conventional medicine (e.g., TENS therapy, direct electrical muscle stimulation, conventional chemotherapeutic agents [vincristine]) were excluded.

A total of 121 studies were found. Of these, 27 were found to meet the inclusion criteria and were evaluated for the type of therapy, the duration of the trial, the diagnosis and indication, the number in the trial, and the rate of adverse effects as compared with the control group (either conventional therapy or placebo). For alternative therapies compared to conventional therapies, we assessed whether the rate of adverse effects was lower, higher, or equal, and for the placebo trials whether the therapeutic efficacy of the trial was positive. Twenty-two of the studies involved plant or herbal preparations, two used megadose vitamins, two involved Traditional Chinese Medicine, and one involved electromagnetic pulsed fields. Mean duration of the trials was 10.3 weeks with a range of 1 to 52 weeks (sd = 11.4 weeks). Type of condition ranged from cholesterol reduction and hay fever to nephrotic syndrome and advanced cancer. The average number of subjects enrolled in the trials was 89 with a range of 15 to 263 (sd = 73.1) (Table 5).

The total number of adverse effects in those studies that reported on patient numbers was 17 of 565 patients, or a rate of 3%. Nine studies compared the complementary therapy with a conventional therapy in a direct randomized fashion. Of these, six reported decreased side effects from a complementary therapy. All six reported that the complementary therapy was equally efficacious as the conventional therapy for the condition. One study reported increased side effects from the complementary therapy. This involved patients treated with the herb *Serona repens* for benign prostatic hypertrophy. The two remaining direct, comparative trials reported equal rates of adverse effects in both complementary and conventional therapy (Table 5). Two studies done in Third World

Table 5. Adverse Effects as Found in Hypothesis-Driven, Randomized Double-Blind Controlled Trials

• Inclusion	• Randomized controlled trials of CAM • Double blind • MEDLINE listed and tagged "adverse effects"
• Exclusion	• Psychotherapy • TENS • podophyllotoxin • electrical muscle stimulation • chemotherapy
• Study numbers	• Found—121 • Included—27
• CAM Topics	• plant products—22 • vitamins—2 • traditional Chinese medicine—2 • pulsed electromagnetic fields—1
• Study characteristics	• Mean duration—10.3 weeks (s.d. 11.4 weeks) • Mean size—n = 89 (s.d. 73.1)
• Adverse effects (AE)	• Total—17 out of 565 subjects for a 3% AE rate
• Comparative AEs	Direct comparisons with conventional medicine—9 studies • 6 of 9 CAM with decreased AE rates over conventional • 1 of 9 with CAM increased AE rate over conventional • 2 of 9 with no difference in AD rates

Adapted from (106).

countries using megadoses of vitamin A in healthy children are not included in this analysis. Both of these very large trials reported an increased rate of short-term (within 24 hours) vomiting, diarrhea, colds, rhinitis, and coughs among those receiving the megadose of vitamin A instead of placebo. Odds ratios were small, in the range of 1.02 to 1.18.

Assessing the use of complementary medical therapies under conditions that minimize indirect adverse effects and maximize an accurate estimate of attribution indicates an adverse effect rate of approximately 3%. It is important to note that the duration of these studies was short (mean 10.3 weeks), and the total numbers in each group were small (mean n = 45 per arm).

SUMMARY

Complementary medicine must deal seriously with the issue of safety and establish systems for addressing direct, indirect, and definitional issues that impact on the risk-benefit ratio of

these practices. Purity and standardization of both the products and the training (competence) in these practices are primary. Without assurance of a good product and a well-trained practitioner to deliver the therapy, the risk-benefit ratio will be higher than necessary. The prevalence of adverse effects in homeopathy, acupuncture, manipulation, herbal products, and mind-body therapies appears to be low, probably lower than comparable therapies in conventional medicine. These therapies are also at low risk for acute toxicity if used for short durations in the traditional manner or in controlled trials.

Important exceptions to this general rule exist, however. Especially of concern is possible heavy metal contamination of traditional herbal products. Almost no good data exist on the potential long-term adverse effects that might occur from chronic use of these practices. In addition to the issues of training and competence, it appears that many alternative diagnostic systems have been inadequately tested and may pose a real risk of exposing individuals to unnecessary anxiety, further testing, unnecessary treatment, and excessive costs. Misuse and poisonings do occur with symptomatic rates of approximately 12%. True attributable adverse effect rates appear to be in the range of 3%, especially for herbal and vitamin products, and probably less for practices such as homeopathy, acupuncture, and mind/body therapies. Safety testing is needed, using appropriate, hypothesis-generated prospective randomized methods with blinded evaluators.

Finally, methods for reporting toxicity and adverse effects need improvement. Current systems used in conventional medicine must be applied with a specific understanding of their use and limitations for obtaining accurate information about safety. Information from poison control centers, adverse effects-reporting hotlines, postmarketing surveillance studies, preclinical research, and phase I and II trials all have different purposes and limitations for determining the true attributable incidence and severity of adverse effects from complementary medical practices. Safety, as well as efficacy, must be evaluated under the conditions of proper use. Ultimately, only direct randomized comparative trials can give us the relative risk-benefit ratios needed for judging optimal therapy and the extent of misapplication. In the meantime, assessing the risks of misuse, educating the public about proper use, clarifying indications (versus claims) and precautions, and assuring competency of practitioners who use and refer for complementary and alternative medicine are the best ways to maximize the safety and benefit of these practices (106).

REFERENCES

1. Eisenberg DM, Kessler RC, Foster E, et al. Unconventional medicine in the United States—prevalence, costs, and patterns of use. N Engl J Med 1993;328:246–252.
2. Fisher P, Ward A. Complementary medicine in Europe. Br Med J 1994;309:107–111.
3. World Health Organization. Guidelines for safe acupuncture treatment. Geneva: World Health Organization, 1995.
4. MacLennan AH, Wilson DH, Taylor AW. Prevalence and cost of alternative medicine in Australia. Lancet 1996;347:569–573.
5. Ernst E. Bitter pills of nature: safety issues in complementary medicine. Pain 1995;60:237–238.
6. Ernst E. Competence in complementary medicine. Complement Therap Med 1995;6:179–186.
7. Ernst E. The risks of acupuncture. Int J Risk & Safety in Med 1995;6:179–186.
8. Turlings JDM, Feenstra MH. Aanbod en gebruik van voedingssupplementen. Een oriënterend onderzoek. 's-Gravenhage: Stichting Wetenschappelijk Onderzoek Konsumentenaangelegenheden, 1987.
9. Philen RM, Ortiz DI, Auerbach S, Falk H. Survey of advertising for nutritional supplements in health and body building magazines. JAMA 1992;268:1008–1011.
10. De Smet PAGM. Gezondheidsrisico's van voedingssupplementen. In: Anema PJ, Bemelmans K, Pieters JJL, eds. Voedingssupplementen. Aktueel Gezondheidsbeleid 14. Rijswijk: Ministerie van Welzijn, Volksgezondheid en Cultuur, 1992:23–34.
11. Wieringa NF, De Meijer AHR, Schutjens MDB, Vos R. The gap between legal rules and practice on advertising non-registered pharmaceutical products. Soc Sci Med 1992;35:1497–1504.
12. Furnham A, Smith C. Choosing alternative medicine: a comparison of the beliefs of patients visiting a general practitioner and a homoeopath. Soc Sci Med 1988;26:685–689.
13. Sutherland LR. Alternative medicine: what are our patients telling us? Am J Gastroenterol 1988;83:1154–1157.
14. Dorant E, Van den Brandt PA, Hamstra AM, et al. Gebruik van voedingssupplementen in Nederland. Ned Tijdschr Geneeskd 1991;135:68–73.
15. Moore J, Phipps K, Marcer D, Lewith G. Why do people seek treatment by alternative medicine? Br Med J 1985;290:28–29.
16. Jensen P. Alternative therapy for atopic dermatitis and psoriasis: patient-reported motivation, information source and effect. Acta Derm Venereol (Stockh) 1990;70:425–428.
17. Lloyd P, Lupton D, Wiesner D, Hasleton S. Choosing alternative therapy: an exploratory study of sociodemographic characteristics and motives of patients resident in Sydney. Aust J Publ Health 1993;17:135–144.
18. Danielson KJ, Stewart DE, Lippert GP. Unconventional cancer remedies. Can Med Assoc J 1988;138:1005–1011.
19. Lau BWK. Why do patients go to traditional healers? J R Soc Health 1989;109:92–95.
20. Furnham A, Bhagrath R. A comparison of health beliefs and behaviours of clients of orthodox and

complementary medicine. Br J Clin Psychol 1993;32:237–246.

21. Van der Ploeg HM, Molenaar MJ, Van Tiggelen CWM. Gebruik van alternatieve behandelwijzen door patiënten met multipele sclerose. Ned Tijdschr Geneeskd 1994;138:296–299.

22. Van der Zouwe N, Van Dam FSAM, Aaronson NK, Hanewald GJFP. Alternatieve geneeswijzen bij kanker: omvang en achtergronden van het gebruik. Ned Tijdschr Geneeskd 1994;138:300–306.

23. Visser GJ. Alternatieve geneeswijzen in de huisartspraktijk. Uitkomsten van een enquete. Huiarts Wet 1988;31:252–256.

24. Knipschild P, Kleijnen J, Ter Riet G. Geloof in alternatieve geneeswijzen. Med Contact 1990;45:421–412.

25. Foets M, Visser GJ. Het voorschrijven van homeopathische middelen in de Nederlandse huisartspraktijk. Med Contact 1993;48:683–687.

26. Taberner PV. Aphrodisiacs. The science and the myth. London: Croom Helm, 1985.

27. Barron RL, Vanscoy GJ. Natural products and the athlete: facts and folklore. Ann Pharmacother 1993;27:607–615.

28. Grunewald KK, Bailey RS. Commercially marketed supplements for bodybuilding athletes. Sports Med 1993;15:90–103.

29. Short SH, Marquart LF. Sports nutrition fraud. N Y State J Med 1993;93:112–116.

30. O'Conner BB. Healing traditions. Philadelphia: University of Pennsylvania Press, 1995.

31. Kerr HD, Saryan LA. Arsenic content of homoeopathic medicines. Clin Toxicol 1986;24:451–459.

32. Dossey L. Healing and the mind: is there a dark side? J Sci Explor 1994;8(1):73–90.

33. Linde K, Ramirez G, Mulroa CD, et al. St. John's Wort for depression—an overview and meta-analysis of randomized controlled trials. Br Med J 1996;313:253–258.

34. Baker CC. Report of the South Australian Working Party on Natural Nutritional Substances. South Australian Health Commission, 1990.

35. Blackburn JLC. Second Report of the Expert Advisory Committee on Herbs and Botanical Preparations to the Health Branch, Health Canada, Ministry of Health, Canada, 1993.

36. Blumenthal M, Klein ST, eds. Therapeutic monographs on medicinal plants for human use by commission E special expert committee of the German Federal Health Agency. Austin: American Botanicals Council, 1996.

37. Awang DDC. The information base for safety assessment of botanicals. OAM/FDA Sponsored symposium on Botanicals: A Role in U.S. Health Care. Washington, DC, 1994.

38. Harper P. Traditional Chinese medicine for eczema. Br Med J 1994;308:489–490.

39. Thomas KB. Temporarily dependent patients in general practice. Br Med J 1974;1:625–626.

40. Herbert V, Kasdan TS. Misleading nutrition claims and their gurus. Nutrition Today 1994;29(3):28–35.

41. Vorbach EU, Hubner WD, Arnoldt KH, et al. 1993. Nervenheilkunde 1993;12:290–296.

42. Gibson RG, Gibson S, MacNeill AD, Watson BW. Homeopathic therapy in rheumatoid arthritis: evaluation by double-blind clinical trial. Br J Clin Pharm 1980;9:453–459.

43. Cassir ZA. Endoscopic control trial of four regimes in the treatment of chronic duodenal ulceration. Irish Med J 1985;78:153–165.

44. Hammerschlag R. Survey of comparative outcomes research: clinical trials comparing acupuncture to standard medical treatment. Proceedings of the Society for Acupuncture Research, Washington, DC, SAR, 1994.

45. Knipschild P. Looking for gall bladder the disease in the patient's iris. Br Med J 1988;287:1578–1581.

46. Nores JM, Remy JM, Nenna AD, Reygagne P. Malpractice by nonphysician healers. NY State J Med 1987;87:473–474.

47. Robertson DA, Ayres RC, Smith CL, Wright R. Adverse consequences arising from misdiagnosis of food allergy. Br Med J 1988;297:719–720.

48. Labib M, Gama R, Wright J, et al. Dietary maladvice as a cause of hypothyroidism and short stature. Br Med J 1989;298;232–233.

49. Goodyear HM, Harper JI. Atopic eczema, hyponatraemia, and hypoalbuminaemia. Arch Dis Child 1990;65:231–232.

50. Southwood TR, Malleson PN, Roberts-Thomson PJ, Mahy M. Unconventional remedies used for patients with juvenile arthritis. Pediatrics 1990;85:150–153.

51. Benmeir P, Neuman A, Weinberg A, et al. Giant melanoma of the inner thigh: a homeopathic life-threatening negligence. Ann Plast Surg 1991;27:583–585.

52. Tsur M. Inadvertent child health neglect by preference of homeopathy to conventional medicine. Harefuah 1992;122:137–142.

53. Zimmer G, Miltner E, Mattern R. Lebensgefährliche Komplikationen unter Heilpraktikerbehandlung - Aufklärungsprobleme. Versicherungsmedizin 1994;46:171–174.

54. De Smet PAGM, Stricker BHCh, Nijman JJ. Indirecte risico's van alternatieve middelen - een oproep tot het rapporteren van concrete gevallen. Med Contact 1994;49:1593–1594.

55. Urban J, Blahova E, Smejkal V, et al. Lidovy lecitel jako pricina tezkeho diabetickeho komatu (folk healing causing severe diabetic coma). Casopis Lekaru Ceskych 1992;131:342–343.

56. Gill GV, Redmond S, Garratt F, Paisey R. Diabetes and alternative medicine: cause for concern. Diab Med 1994;11:210–213.

57. Püschel K, Lockemann U, Saukko P, et al. Scharlatanerie mit tödlichem Ausgang. "Alternative" Fehlbehandlung juveniler Diabetiker. Münch Med Wschr 1996;138:287–290.

58. Verrept H. Marokkaanse migranten en hun geneesmiddelen. Med Antropol 1992;4:184–198.

59. Verrept H, Schillemans L. Ziektegedrag van Marokkaanse migranten met vakantie in Marokko. Ned Tijdschr Geneeskd 1994;138:337–339.

60. Hoekstra DFJ. Onzorgvuldig handelen door alternatieve genezers en de wet. Med Contact 1988;43:711–714.

61. Boström H, Rössner S. Quality of alternative medicine—complications and avoidable deaths. Quality Assurance in Health Care 1990;2:111–117.

62. Dalvi SS, Nayak VK, Pohujani SM, et al. Effect of gugulipid on bioavailability of diltiazem and propranolol. J Assoc Physicians of India 1994;42:454–455.

63. Dandekar UP, Chandra RS, Dalvi SS, et al. Analysis of a clinically important interaction between phenytoin and Shankhapushpi, and Ayurvedic preparation. J Ethnopharmacol 1992;35:285–288.

64. Park BK, Pirmohamed M, Kitteringham NR. Idiosyncratic drug reactions: a mechanistic evaluation of risk factors. Br J Clin Pharmacol 1992;34:377–395.

65. Innes IR, Nickerson M. Atropine, scopolamine, and related antimuscarinic drugs. In: Goodman LS, Gilman A, Gilman AG, Koelle GB, eds. The pharmacological basis of therapeutics. 5th ed. New York: Macmillan Publishing Co., 1975:514–532.

66. Anonymous. ICH guidelines finalised for 2 further aspects of ADR reporting. Inpharma 1995;18:20–21.

67. Anonymous. Kommission E—Aufberereitungsmonographien. Dtsch Apoth Ztg 1993;133:2791–2794.

68. Bateman DN, Chaplin S. Adverse reactions. I. Br Med J 1988;296:761–764.

69. De Smet PAGM. *Teucrium chamaedrys*. In: De Smet PAGM, Keller K, Hänsel R, Chandler RF, ed. Adverse effects of herbal drugs. Volume 3. Heidelberg: Springer-Verlag, 1997:137–144.

70. De Smet PAGM. *Scutellaria* species. In: De Smet PAGM, Keller K, Hänsel R, Chandler RF, eds. Adverse effects of herbal drugs. Volume 2. Heidelberg: Springer-Verlag, 1993:289–296, 317.

71. De Smet PAGM. Health risks of herbal remedies. Drug Safety 1995;13:81–93.

72. Gordon DW, Rosenthal G, Hart J, et al. Chaparral ingestion. The broadening spectrum of liver injury caused by herbal medications. JAMA 1995;273:489–490.

73. Batchelor WB, Heathcote J, Wanless IR. Chaparral-induced hepatic injury. Am J Gastroenterol 1995;90:831–833.

74. Blumenthal M. Herb industry and FDA issue chaparral warning—experts unable to explain possible links to five cases of hepatitis. HerbalGram 1993;28:38–39,53,59,63,69.

75. Anonymous. "Natural" medicines: a Pandora's box. WHO Drug Information 1995;9:147–149.

76. Atawodi SE, Lamorde AG, Spiegelhalder B, Preussmann R. Nitrosation of Nigerian medicinal plant preparations under 'chemical' and 'simulated' gastric conditions. Food Chem Toxicol 1995;33:43–48.

77. De Smet PAGM. *Aristolochia* species. In: De Smet PAGM, Keller K, Hänsel R, Chandler RF, eds. Adverse effects of herbal drugs. Volume 1. Heidelberg: Springer-Verlag, 1992:79–89.

78. Cosyns J-P, Jadoul M, Squifflet J-P, et al. Urothelial malignancy in nephropathy due to Chinese herbs. Lancet 1994;344:188.

79. Vanherweghem JL, Tielemans C, Simon J, Depierreux M. Chinese herbs nephropathy and renal pelvic carcinoma. Nephrol Dial Transplant 1995;10:270–273.

80. De Smet PAGM. An introduction to herbal pharmacoepidemiology. J Ethnopharmacol 1993;38:197–208.

81. Oso BA. Mushrooms and the Yoruba people of Nigeria. Mycologia 1975;67:311–319.

82. De Smet PAGM. Ethnopharmacological art in perspective: enema scenes in black African sculpture. Int Pharm J 1992;6:197–202,239–244.

83. Yorston D, Foster A. Traditional eye medicines and corneal ulceration in Tanzania. J Trop Med Hyg 1994;97:211–214.

84. Courtright P, Lewallen S, Kanjaloti S, Divala DJ. Traditional eye medicine use among patients with corneal disease in rural Malawi. Br J Ophthalmol 1994;74:810–812.

85. Lewallen S, Courtright P. Peripheral corneal ulcers associated with use of African traditional eye medicines. Br J Ophthalmol 1995;79:343–346.

86. Anonymous. Ostrich fern poisoning—New York and Western Canada, 1994. MMWR 1994;43: 677–684.

87. Lai R-S, Chiang AA, Wu M-T, et al. Outbreak of bronchiolitis obliterans associated with the consumption of *Sauropus androgynus* in Taiwan. Lancet 1996;348:83–85.

88. Haynes RL. Carbon-monoxide poisoning from non-tobacco cigarettes. J Med Assoc Ga 1983; 72:553–555.

89. King M. Nontobacco cigarettes. Can Med Assoc J 1985;133:13.

90. Bloom JW, Kaltenborn WT, Paoletti P, et al. Respiratory effects of non-tobacco cigarettes. Br Med J 1987;295:1516–1518.

91. Sherrill DL, Kryzanowski M, Bloom JW, Lebowitz MD. Respiratory effects of non-tobacco cigarettes: a longitudinal study in the general population. Int J Epidemiol 1991;20:132–137.

92. Nahas G, Latour C. The human toxicity of marijuana. Med J Aust 1992;156:495–497.

93. Polen MR, Sidney S, Tekawa IS, et al. Health care use by frequent marijuana smokers who do not smoke tobacco. Western Medical Journal 1993; 158:596–601.

94. Jensen R, Closson W, Rothenberg R. Selenium intoxication—New York. MMWR 1984;33: 157–158.

95. Helzlsouer K, Jacobs R, Morris S. Acute selenium intoxication in the United States. Fed Proc 1985;44:1670.

96. Clark RF, Strukle E, Williams SR, Manoguerra AS. Selenium poisoning from a nutritional supplement. JAMA 1996;275:1087–1088.

97. Koch-Weser J, Sellers EM, Zachest R, et al. The ambiguity of adverse drug reactions. Eur J Clin Pharmacol 1977;11:75.

98. Reidenberg MM, Lowenthal DT. Adverse drug reactions. N Engl J Med 1968;279:678.

99. La Haba AF, Curet JO, Pelegia A, Bangdiwala I. Thrombophlebitis among oral and non-oral contraceptive users. Obstet Gynecol 1971;38:259.

100. De Smet PAGM. Health risks of herbal remedies. Drug Safety 1995;13(2):1995.

101. De Gerlache, Lans JM. Modulation of experimental rat liver carcinogenesis by ultra low doses of the carcinogens. Ultra low doses. C. Doutremepuich. Washington, DC: Taylor & Francis, 1991:17–27.

102. Huxtable RJ. Safety of botanicals: historical perspective. OAM/FDA Sponsored Symposium on Botanicals: A Role in U.S. Health Care. Washington, DC, 1994.

103. Peacher WC. Adverse reactions, contraindications and complications of acupuncture and moxibustion. Am J Chin Med 1975;335–346.

104. Sackett DL, Haynes RB, Guyatt GH, Tugwell P. Deciding whether your treatment does harm. In: Sackett DL, Haynes RB, Guyatt GH, Tugwell P, eds. Clinical epidemiology: a basic science for clinical medicine. Boston: Little, Brown & Co., 1993.

105. Perharic L, Shaw D, Colbridge M, et al. Toxicological problems resulting from exposure to traditional remedies and food supplements. Drug Safety 1994;11(4):264–294.

106. Jonas WB. Safety in complementary medicine. In: Ernst E, ed. Complementary medicine—an objective approach. Oxford: Butterworth-Heinemann, 1996:126–149.

CHAPTER 6

THE SAFETY OF HERBAL PRODUCTS

Peter A.G.M. De Smet

INTRODUCTION

A consumer of an officially licensed herbal medicine may not have to be concerned about the correct identity of the ingredients, but an individual who goes into the field to collect his or her own herbs should. Austrian physicians described a case of a young boy who developed venoocclusive disease of the liver after long-term consumption of a tea prepared from *Adenostyles alliariae*. The boy's parents had erroneously gathered this plant instead of coltsfoot (*Tussilago farfara*), and *A. alliariae* contains a much higher level of hepatotoxic pyrrolizidine alkaloids than does coltsfoot (1, 2). Botanical identity can also be problematic within the context of commercially available materials. For example, German researchers exposed that Sarothamni scoparii flos does not always originate from *Sarothamnus scoparius* (Besenginster) but may also come from *Spartium junceum* (Spanischer Ginster) (3). This adulteration could be clinically relevant because the flowers of *S. junceum* are rich in cytisine-type quinolizidine alkaloids (4, 5).

The botanical quality of prepackaged herbal products may also cause problems, especially in countries (such as the United States) that do not categorize these products as medicines (6). As a result, these products remain exempt from governmental approval processes, and their quality may remain essentially uncontrolled (7, 8). An example in the United States concerned a South American product labeled as "Paraguay Tea." This product was associated with an outbreak of anticholinergic poisoning. On chemical analysis, the product yielded belladonna alkaloids instead of the xanthine derivatives that were expected in a preparation from *Ilex paraguariensis* (8).

Herbal products should be free not only from toxic botanical adulterants, but also from other contaminants (Table 6.1) (9), such as substantial residues of pesticides (Table 6.2) (10). The need to prevent contamination with pathogenic microorganisms was illustrated by the case of a bone marrow transplant recipient, who probably acquired hepatic mycosis from the ingestion of a naturopathic medicine contaminated with a *Mucor* fungus (11). There is also evidence that medicinal plant materials from India and Sri Lanka can be contaminated with toxigenic fungi (*Aspergillus, Fusarium*). Because aflatoxin B has sometimes been recovered from these materials in potentially unsafe amounts, it is prudent to improve their storage conditions (9, 12, 13).

Another practical concern is the presence of toxic metals (e.g., lead, arsenic) or conventional pharmaceuticals (e.g., corticosteroids, nonsteroidal antiinflammatory drugs, benzodiazepines) in certain herbal medicines of Asian origin. These hazards have been denounced for more than two decades, but they continue to pose an occasional threat to public health (9). Although most of the recent reports on the undeclared presence of Western pharmaceuticals involve Chinese herbal medicines, the contamination of herbal medicines with pharmaceuticals is not necessarily limited to products of Oriental origin. We analyzed Dutch herbal drops for weight reduction that were declared to contain *Ephedra* and 14 other ingredients

Table 6.1. Potential Contaminants to Account for in Quality Control of Herbal Medicines

TYPE OF CONTAMINANT	EXAMPLES
Botanicals	*Atropa belladonna, Digitalis, Colchicum, Rauvolfia serpentina*, pyrrolizidine-containing plants
Microorganisms	*Staphylococcus aureus, Escherichia coli* (certain strains), *Salmonella, Shigella, Pseudomonas aeruginosa*
Microbial toxins	Bacterial endotoxins, aflatoxins
Pesticides	Chlorinated pesticides (e.g., DDT, DDE, HCH-isomers, HCB, aldrin, dieldrin, heptachlor), organic phosphates, carbamate insecticides and herbicides, ithocarbamate fungicides, triazin herbicides
Fumigation agents	Ethylene oxide, methyl bromide, phosphine
Radioactivity	Cs-134, Cs-137, Ru-103, I-131, Sr-90
Metals	Lead, cadmium, mercury, arsenic
Synthetic drugs	Analgesic and antiinflammatory agents (e.g., aminophenazone, phenylbutazone, indomethacin), corticosteroids, hydrochlorothiazide, diazepam
Animal drugs	Thyroid hormones

because a Dutch professional cyclist had tested positive for norpseudoephedrine at a doping control urinalysis. The level of norpseudoephedrine in the investigated product was substantially higher than that of ephedrine, which is normally not the case in Chinese *Ephedra* plants. The manufacturer later admitted that his product had been spiked (14).

Although the safety of herbal medicines can be compromised by deficient product quality, some herbal products become more dangerous when they have excellent quality. Yohimbe products rich in yohimbine will be less safe for over-the-counter use than products containing no or negligible amounts of this alkaloid (15, 16).

Nontraditional Hazards

Safety claims cannot always be based on long-standing traditional herbal experience: not all herbal medicines have firm roots in traditional practices, and this seems an underestimated issue. When traditional source plants are extracted in a nontraditional way (e.g., by resorting to a nonpolar solvent, such as hexane), the question can be raised whether this nontraditional extract is just as safe as the traditional one. Until recently, the ostrich fern (*Matteuccia struthiopteris*) was generally considered a nontoxic, edible plant with a history of use as a

spring vegetable that went back to the 1700s. However, recent observations of serious gastrointestinal toxicity following the consumption of lightly sauteed or blanched ostrich fern shoots suggest that this vegetable is safe only when thoroughly cooked before use (17). A similar example is the recent outbreak of bronchiolitis obliterans in Taiwan, which was associated with the ingestion of *Sauropus androgynus*. This herb normally is cooked before being eaten as a vegetable, but in this case the numerous victims had all consumed uncooked leaf juice as an unproven method of weight control (18).

It is also possible that an herbal ingredient may have no medicinal tradition at all, and its route of administration or dose level may be quite different from that used in a traditional setting. The question could be raised, for instance, to which extent the excellent oral safety record of certain traditional herbs is applicable to the herbal cigarettes, which are nowadays available in Western health food stores. After all, there is evidence to suggest that certain respiratory risks attributed to tobacco smoking may extend to the smoking of nontobacco herbal products, particularly marijuana (19–24).

Excipients

An inconspicuous source of adverse reactions to herbal medicines are the excipients (25). This

Table 6.2. Pesticide Residue Limits in Herbal Medicines*

SUBSTANCE	LIMIT (mg/kg)
Alachlor	0.02
Aldrin and Dieldrin (sum of)	0.05
Azinphos-methyl	1.0
Bromopropylate	3.0
Chlordane (sum of cis-, trans, and oyxchlordane)	0.05
Chlorfenvinphos	0.5
Chlorpyrifos	0.2
Chlorpyrifos-methyl	0.1
Cypermethrin (and isomers)	1.0
DDT (sum of p,p'-DDT, o,p'-DDT, p,p'-DDE, and p,p'-TDE)	1.0
Deltamethrin	0.5
Diazinon	0.5
Dichlorvos	1.0
Dithiocarbamates (as CS_2)	2.0
Endosulfan (sum of isomers and endosulphan sulphate)	3.0
Endrin	0.05
Ethion	2.0
Fenitrothion	0.5
Fenvalerate	1.5
Fonofos	0.05
Heptachlor (sum of heptachlor and heptachlorepoxide)	0.05
Hexachlorobenzene	0.1
Hexachlorocyclohexane isomers (other than gamma-)	0.3
Lindane (gamma-hexachlorocyclohexane)	0.6
Malathion	1.0
Methidathion	0.2
Parathion	0.5
Parathion-methyl	0.2
Permethrin	1.0
Phosalone	0.1
Piperonyl butoxide	3.0
Pirimiphos-methyl	4.0
Pyrethrins (sum of)	3.0
Quintozene (sum of quintozene, pentachloroaniline, and methyl pentachlorophenyl sulphide)	1.0

*As specified in the latest edition of the European Pharmacopoeia.

has been illustrated by the careful evaluation of a case of contact dermatitis caused by a commercial ointment containing a *Centella asiatica* extract. Instead of automatically assuming that this ingredient was responsible, the investigators decided to seek confirmation by patch testing with the individual components. It was thus discovered that the reactions were caused mainly by the presence of propylene glycol. A true allergic response to the botanical components remained unproven (26). Lanolin is among the notorious contact allergens that can be present as excipient in topical applications (27). In an evaluation of the contact sensitization potential of five commercial herbal ointments in 1032 consecutive or randomly selected visitors to patch test clinics, 2 of the 11 patients with a positive response had been sensitized by lanolin (28). There have also been reports about the presence of pesticide residues in lanolin (29, 30).

Another noteworthy excipient is alcohol. Psychological and physical dependence on herbal medicines with a high alcohol content seem rare, but they have been reported (31). There is also an association between a case of suspected fetal alcohol syndrome with a history of maternal ingestion of a herbal tonic (containing 14% alcohol) daily for the first two months (32). The U.S. Food and Drug Administration has ruled that the alcohol concentration in over-the-counter drug products intended for oral ingestion should not exceed 10% for adults and children over 12 year of age, 5% for children between 6 and 12 years of age, and 0.5% for children under 6 years of age (33).

CONSUMER-RELATED DETERMINANTS OF ADVERSE EFFECTS

The chance of an adverse reaction to an herbal medicine depends not only on the product's actual composition and manner of use, but also on consumer-bound parameters, such as age, genetics, and concomitant diseases. For instance, the risk that the alkaloid berberine in Chinese *Coptis* spp. elicits jaundice seems to be most substantial in infants who are deficient in glucose-6-phosphate dehydrogenase (34–36). Another example is that slow metabolizers of the quinolizidine alkaloid sparteine will be more prone to the oxytocic potential and other toxic effects of *Cytisus scoparius* than rapid metabolizers (35–37). This latter example illustrates the general principle that pharmacokinetic information can help to predict certain types of consumer-dependent adverse effects. However

complex the composition of an herbal medicine may be, its constituents are chemical entities which, besides having pharmacodynamic properties, must obey the same pharmacokinetic rules that apply to conventional drug molecules. In other words, insight into the ways in which the pharmacokinetics of complementary medicines are modified by factors such as hepatic or renal insufficiency provides a rational tool for predicting and avoiding dose-related adverse effects (38).

Another intriguing finding is that Chinese subjects are more sensitive to the effect of atropine on heart rate than are Caucasian subjects, who in their turn seem to be more sensitive than Black individuals (39). A theoretical implication of such interracial differences is that local experience with a traditional herbal remedy cannot always be extrapolated indiscriminately to societies with another ethnic make-up.

Concurrent use of other drugs must also be considered. For instance, consumers of caffeine-containing herbs (*Cola, Ilex,* and *Paullinia*) may have an increased risk of adverse effects, such as tremors or tachycardia, when they concurrently ingest pipemidic acid, ciprofloxacin, or enoxacin, because these antibacterial quinolones inhibit the hepatic metabolism of caffeine (40–43). Likewise, the oxidative metabolism of sparteine, a quinolizidine alkaloid in Scotch broom (*Cytisus scoparius*), can be inhibited by the simultaneous intake of haloperidol (44), moclobemide (45), or quinidine (46). This latter example shows that the interfering drug does not have to be a synthetic compound but can also come from nature. According to a comment on the numerous adverse events associated with Ma Huang (*Ephedra*) consumption in the United States, the adverse effects of combined ephedrine and caffeine may be greater than those from the consumption of either compound alone (47). Besides the possibility that the toxicity of an herbal compound is increased by a conventional drug, there is also the possibility that the effects of a conventional medicine are enhanced by an herbal medicine. For example, the Indian herbal drug karela (*Momordica charantia*) has hypoglycemic properties (48) and can thereby interfere with conventional antidiabetic treatment (49).

For an extensive overview of adverse drug interactions between conventional medicines and herbal products, the reader is referred to a publication elsewhere (50).

SITUATIONAL RISKS

Herbal medicines that are generally safe under normal conditions can be hazardous in specific circumstances. For example, psoralen-rich herbal preparations may produce phototoxic burns in visitors to tanning salons or in patients undergoing PUVA therapy (51, 52). Therefore, it is important to provide the consumer of herbal medicines with adequate product information, in which such situational hazards are clearly indicated.

Among the safety issues that need attention in this respect is the risk that herbal products make their consumers less fit for driving. This hazard should be taken into consideration for any plant-derived drug with central depressant activity, such as *Rauvolfia* (53) and tetrahydropalmatine (54).

An even more inconspicuous risk is that top athletes may unwittingly take a doping agent in the form of a herbal product because the list of doping substances, which is issued by the International Olympic Committee, comprises several substances that occur naturally in herbs (55). Among these doping agents are ephedrines and caffeine, which are regularly present in Western health food preparations (56–58).

ADVERSE EFFECTS

Individual Herbs

The following provides an overview of adverse effects of herbal preparations that have been reported in the literature. Unless otherwise specified, the presented data have been derived from previous reviews (59–61). For additional information about this subject, the reader is referred to a rapidly growing list of detailed textbooks on herbal medicines (62–75). Herbs, which are primarily used for recreational purposes, are re-

viewed separately, as are herbs primarily employed within the context of traditional Chinese and Indian medicine.

Sometimes, this review does not focus on the crude herb but on one or more components. This approach is acceptable because, in principle, the toxic potential of an herbal product does not depend on its natural origin but on the pharmacological characteristics and dose levels of its bioactive constituents. Although it is conceivable that the toxicity of an individual herbal constituent can be modified by one or more of the other constituents, this is by no means some iron-clad rule: a complex composition does not always protect the consumer against the toxicity of a single constituent, and it might also result in a more toxic remedy.

A potential hazard of most medicinal herbs is allergic contact dermatitis, but this risk is much more substantial for certain herbs (e.g., those containing sensitizing sesquiterpene lactones) than for others (27, 76). Another common adverse effect ascribed to various herbs is gastrointestinal disturbances (e.g., caused by the presence of tannins or irritating saponins). More serious problems can be elicited by herbs containing well-known botanical substances with toxic potential (e.g., cardiac glycosides, podophyllotoxin, reserpine). It should be noted that such classical drug substances may reside in a less familiar botanical source. For example, cardiac glycosides occur not only in such well-known source plants as foxglove (*Digitalis*) and oleander (*Nerium oleander*), but are also found in pleurisy root (*Asclepias tuberosa*) (77). Serious health risks are also possible with certain obsolete herbs, which were formerly employed in medicine but have now been superseded by other, less dangerous alternatives (e.g., chenopodium oil, male fern). In addition to such classical toxic agents, several herbs and herbal constituents have been repeatedly associated in recent years with new adverse effects of such a serious nature that their unrestricted internal use as phytotherapeutic agents no longer seems acceptable. *Aristolochia, Teucrium, Larrea tridentata*, and herbs rich in pyrrolizidine alkaloids all are part of this latter category.

The following is a summary of the known and reported adverse effects of medicinal herbs and products. When faced with a patient using these products, find the summary of known adverse effects of those products. This will provide an indication of the adverse effects known for that plant and help guide the practitioner in monitoring for possible adverse effects in that patient. It will also help the practitioner inform the patient about possible risks.

Alfalfa (*Medicago sativa*)

Prolonged ingestion of seeds or commercial tablets has been associated with a lupus-like syndrome (78, 79). Dermatitis has also been recorded (80).

Ammi fruit

Prolonged use or overdosing of the greater ammi (*Ammi majus*) may produce nausea, dizziness, obstipation, loss of appetite, headache, pruritus, and sleeping disorders. The psoralens in toothpick ammi (*Ammi visnaga*) can produce phototoxic reactions (81).

Amygdalin

The raw pits or kernels of certain *Prunus* species (e.g., apricot, bitter almond, choke cherry, peach) have been promoted as health foods. When ingested in sufficient quantity, they are poisonous because of the cyanogenic glycoside amygdalin, which yields hydrogen cyanide after ingestion. Teratogenicity has been observed in animals.

Anise fruit (*Pimpinella anisum*)

Occasionally allergic reactions.

Anthranoid derivatives

Anthranoid derivatives occur in various laxative herbs, such as aloe (*Aloe* spp.), buckthorn and cascara sagrada (*Rhamnus* spp.), medicinal rhubarb (*Rheum palmatum*), and senna (*Cassia* spp.). They are present in the form of free anthraquinones, anthrones, dianthrones and/or O- and C-glycosides derived from these substances. In the case of *Rhamnus*, the fresh drug contains anthrones and is strongly emetic; for this reason it must be stored for at least one year or be submitted to an artificial aging process. Anthranoid derivatives produce harmless discoloration of the urine. Depending on intrinsic activity and dose, they can also produce abdominal discomfort and cramps, nausea, violent purgation, and dehydration. They can be distributed into breast milk, but not always in sufficient amounts to affect the suckling infant. Long-term use may result in electrolyte disturbances and atony and dilation of the colon. Several anthranoid derivatives (notably the aglycones aloe-emodin, chrysophanol, emodin, and physcion) show genotoxic potential in bacterial and/or mammalian test systems (82), and two anthranoid compounds (the synthetic laxative danthrone and the naturally occurring 1-hydroxyanthraquinone) have shown carcinogenic activity in rodents (83). In one epidemiologic study, chronic abusers of anthranoid laxatives (identified by the detection of *pseudomelanosis coli*) showed an increased relative risk for colorectal cancer (84). More studies are needed to clarify this issue, if only to exclude the possibility that chronic constipation per se might increase the risk for colorectal cancer and would thus act as a confounding factor.

Pending the results of such studies, the German health authorities have restricted the indication of herbal anthranoid laxatives to constipation that is unresponsive to bulk-forming therapy (which rules out their inclusion in weight-reduction products). In addition, the German authorities have imposed restrictions to the laxative use of anthranoid-containing herbs (e.g., not to be used for more than 1 to 2 weeks without medical advice, not to be used in children under 12 years of age, and not to be used during pregnancy and lactation) (85–87).

Aristolochic acids

Plants belonging to the genus *Aristolochia* are rich in aristolochic acids and aristolactams.

continued on next page

For example, the roots of birthwort (*Aristolochia clematitis*) yield a substance called aristolochic acid, which is mainly a mixture of aristolochic acids I and II. Aristolochic acid passes into human breast milk. It is mutagenic and proved so highly carcinogenic in rats that the German health authorities have even banned homoeopathic *Aristolochia* dilutions up to D10 from the market. The closely related aristolactams are mutagenic as well (88).

It has been known for a long time that aristolochic acid is nephrotoxic in animals and humans (88). In 1993, the nephrotoxic effects of aristolochic acid in the rat were described in detail; histologically, there was evidence of necrosis of the epithelium of the renal tubules (89). In the same year, a human outbreak of renal toxicity of *Aristolochia* was reported from Belgium, where nephropathy was observed in more than 70 users of a slimming preparation, which had been substituted or contaminated with a Chinese *Aristolochia* species (see below for a detailed discussion). Subsequently, rapidly progressive interstitial renal fibrosis has also been associated with chronic intake of the European species *Aristolochia pistolochia* (90).

Arnica flower (*Arnica* spp.)

Skin-sensitizing sesquiterpene lactones are present. Ingestion of arnica tea can cause gastroenteritis, and large oral doses of undiluted tincture are said to produce various serious symptoms.

Asafetida (*Ferula assa-foetida*)

A case of methemoglobinemia in a 5-week-old infant treated with a gum asafetida preparation has been recorded (91).

Atractylis gummifera

Renal and hepatic toxicity have been reported (92, 93).

Basil (*Ocimum basilicum*)

Contains up to 0.5% of essential oil, which contains up to 85% of estragole. Estragole is mutagenic after metabolic activation and there is animal evidence to suggest carcinogenicity. The herb and essential oil should not be used during pregnancy and lactation or for prolonged periods. The German health authorities have no objection to the use of the herb as an admixture to herbal teas in levels up to 5%.

Bearberry leaf (*Arctostaphylos uva-ursi*)

Gastrointestinal disturbances. Reports of carcinogenicity of hydroquinone after prolonged administration of high doses to rats or mice raise a question about the long-term safety of bearberry and other medicinal herbs containing substantial amounts of arbutin. Arbutin is the monoglucoside of hydroquinone, and when it is administered orally to humans, it is hydrolyzed to hydroquinone and finally excreted in the urine as hydroquinone glucuronide and sulphate. These conjugates are also the major urinary metabolites, when rats are treated orally with hydroquinone (83). Bearberry should not be used for prolonged periods without consulting a physician.

Boldo leaf (*Peumus boldus*)

The essential oil and other preparations rich in ascaridole should not be used because of the toxicity of this constituent.

Broom, Scotch (*Sarothamnus scoparius = Cytisus scoparius*)

The herb contains sparteine and related quinolizidine alkaloids. Sparteine can reduce cardiac conductivity and stimulate uterine motility (38). Pharmacokinetic studies have shown that its metabolic oxidation exhibits genetic polymorphism and that about 6 to 9% of the Caucasian population are poor metabolizers (37). Inexpert self-medication with a broom tea has resulted in fatal poisoning with clinical symptoms of ileus, heart failure, and circulatory weakness (94). It is prudent to avoid broom preparations during pregnancy, not only because sparteine has abortifacient potential, but also because of preliminary information that the plant produces malformed lambs in feeding trials. According to the German health authorities, hydroalcoholic preparations of the herb should contain no more than 1 mg/mL of sparteine.

Broom flower contains only a low level of alkaloids but hypertension is a contraindication, and concurrent use with MAO-inhibitors should be avoided as over 2% of tyramine may be present. The German authorities have no objection to the addition of broom flower to herbal teas in levels up to 1%.

Bryony root (*Bryonia* spp.)
Drastic laxative and emetic properties due to the presence of cucurbitacins.

Burdock root (*Arctium* spp.)
Contact dermatitis (95).

Butcher's broan (*Ruscus aculeatus*)
Rarely gastric complaints, nausea. A case of enterocolitis caused by a preparation containing an extract of the rhizome of Butcher's broan has been reported (96). Topical use may lead to allergic contact dermatitis (97).

Caffeine
Occurs not only in coffee, tea, and cacao, but also in cola seeds (*Cola* spp.), mate leaves (*Ilex paraguariensis*), guayusa leaves (*Ilex guayusa*), yaupon leaves (*Ilex vomitoria*), guarana seeds (*Paullinia cupana*), and yoco bark (*Paullinia yoco*) (58). High doses of these herbs may therefore produce hyperexcitability, nervousness, and sleeping disturbances.

Canthaxanthin
This orange carotenoid has been promoted as a skin-tanning agent. It entails a risk of adverse effects when used in amounts exceeding the levels in which it is normally consumed as a food additive. Retinopathy with gold-yellow deposits around the macula has been reported, and there has also been a case of aplastic anaemia (98).

Caper plant (*Capparis spinosa*)
Allergic contact dermatitis following application of this plant in the form of wet compresses has been reported (99).

California poppy (*Eschscholtzia californica*)
It would be prudent to avoid use during pregnancy because the major alkaloid cryptopin has shown a stimulating effect on guinea pig uterus in vitro.

Camphor tree (*Cinnamomum camphora*)
Contact eczema is possible. Camphor preparations should not be applied near the nose of infants.

Cardiac glycosides
Occur in *Adonis vernalis* (pheasant's eye), *Asclepias tuberosa* (pleurisy root), *Convallaria majalis* (lily of the valley), *Digitalis* spp. (foxglove), *Nerium oleander* (oleander), *Strophanthus* spp., and *Urginea maritima* = *Scilla maritima* (squill). Although the cardiotoxic risks are well known, case reports continue to appear because plants rich in cardiac glycosides still serve as a folk remedy (100) or because they are erroneously mistaken for an innocuous herb (101, 102).

Cassia bark (*Cinnamomum aromaticum*)
Often allergic skin and mucosal reactions.

Castor oil (*Ricinus communis*)
When taken by mouth, especially in large doses, castor oil may produce violent purgation with nausea, vomiting, colic, and a risk of miscarriage.

continued on next page

Cayenne pepper (*Capsicum frutescens*)

Irritant properties and, rarely, allergic reactions.

Celandine (*Chelidonium majus*)

Warnings that use in children should be discouraged because fatal poisonings have been observed in children appear to go back to an unconvincing German case of fatal colitis in a 3-year-old boy. The original report does not provide conclusive evidence that celandine had been taken (103). A case of hemolytic anaemia following oral use has been reported (104).

Chamomile flower

Chamomile is an ambiguous vernacular name, as it can refer to *Chamomilla recutita* = *Matricaria chamomilla* (wild chamomile) and to *Anthemis nobilis* = *Chamaemelum nobile* (Roman chamomile). The latter herb is a more potent skin sensitizer than the former, presumably because it contains a higher level of the sesquiterpene lactone anthecotulid. This allergenic compound is present, at low levels, in only one of four chemotypes of wild chamomile.

Chamomile tea has been rarely associated with anaphylactic reactions (105) and its application as an eye wash can cause allergic conjunctivitis (106). When inhalation of steam from chamomile tea is used in children as a home remedy for inflammation of the upper respiratory tract, appropriate caution is needed to avoid serious burns (107).

Chaparral (*Larrea tridentata*)

At least nine cases of hepatotoxicity have been published (108–113), and in one of these cases inadvertent rechallenge led to recurrence within four weeks (109). Nordihydroguaiaretic acid (which is the major phenolic component) is able to produce lymphatic and renal lesions when given chronically in high doses to rodents (114–116). A possible human case of cystic renal cell carcinoma and acquired renal cystic disease associated with consumption of chaparral tea has been reported (117).

Chaste tree fruit (*Vitex agnus-castus*)

Skin reactions may occur. The herb has been associated with multiple follicular development in a female user (118).

Chenopodium oil (*Chenopodium ambrosioides*)

Formerly used as an anthelminthic but, because of the toxicity of its principle ascaridole, now superseded by less toxic alternatives.

Cinchona bark (*Cinchona* spp.)

Allergic skin reactions, fever; rarely thrombocytopaenia.

Cinnamon bark (*Cinnamomum verum* = *Cinnamomum zeylanicum*)

Often allergic skin reactions and mucosal reactions.

Coffee enemas

Two fatal cases related to therapy with voluminous coffee enemas have been described. These were assumed to be caused by electrolyte disturbances, because toxicological results in both cases indicated that not enough caffeine had been absorbed to cause a substantial toxic effect (119). The delivery of coffee enemas has also been associated with *Campylobacter* sepsis and amoebiasis (120).

Colocynth fruit (*Citrullus colocynthis*)

The dried pulp of the fruit is a drastic laxative because of the presence of toxic cucurbitacins. Colitis has been reported (121, 122).

Coumarin

This plant lactone is found in tonka beans (the seeds of *Dipteryx odorata* and *Dipteryx oppositofolia*), dried sweet clover (*Melilotus officinalis*), sweet vernal grass (*Anthoxanthum odoratum*), and woodruff (*Asperula odorata*). It has hepatotoxic potential in humans when taken in daily doses of 25 to 100 mg (123). Coumarin is not to be confused with coumarin anticoagulants because it is devoid of anticoagulant activity. However, the molding of sweet clover can increase the hemorrhagic potential of this herb by transforming coumarin to the anticoagulant dicoumarol. This transformation may explain a case of abnormal clotting function and mild bleeding after the drinking of an herbal tea prepared from tonka beans, sweet clover, and several other ingredients (124).

Croton oil (*Croton tiglium*)

The seeds, seed oil, and resin of *Croton tiglium* were formerly valued for purgative, abortifacient, and counterirritant properties. Their medicinal use has declined, however, after the isolation of skin irritant and tumor-promoting phorbol esters (diterpene esters of the tigliane type). Chronic exposure of humans to croton oil or croton tincture should be discouraged (125).

Dandelion root (*Taraxacum officinale*)

Gastric complaints are possible.

Dionaea muscipula

Reddening of the face, headache, dyspnea, nausea and vomiting; shivers, fever, and anaphylactic shock after intramuscular administration (126–128).

Diterpene esters

Several medicinal plants belonging to the Euphorbiaceae and Thymelaeaceae (such as *Croton tiglium*, *Euphorbia* spp., and *Daphne* spp.) contain diterpene esters of the tigliane, ingenane, or daphnane type. These substances cause irritation, inflammation, and blistering of the skin, and they are also tumor-promoting (i.e., capable of promoting

the growth of a tumor initiated by another trigger). Animal experiments have shown that a threshold dose is needed for the tumor-promoting activity (129).

Dyer's broom (*Genista tinctoria*)

Contains toxic quinolizidine alkaloids, such as anagyrin, cytisine, and N-methylcytisine. The latter two constituents have similar peripheral effects as nicotine, whereas their central activity may be different. Anagyrine is a suspected animal teratogen and cytisine has been shown to have teratogenic activity in rabbits.

Echinacea (*Echinacea* spp.)

Intravenous administration has been associated with anaphylactic reactions. It has been suggested that oral ingestion may also lead to allergic symptoms, such as skin reactions and respiratory reactions (130, 131).

Elfdock root (*Inula helenium*)

Allergic contact dermatitis is possible, and higher doses produce vomiting, diarrhea, cramps, and paralytic symptoms.

Ergot (*Claviceps purpurea*)

The sclerotium of this fungus (secale cornutum) is rich in toxic alkaloids.

Essential oils

Essential oils are capable of producing systemic toxicity, particularly when they are ingested in undiluted form. Among the reported effects are central depression, nephrotoxicity, hepatotoxicity, and abortion. Allergic contact dermatitis and phototoxic reactions are also possible (132, 133). Inhalation by infants and small children should be avoided.

A common way of using essential oils in complementary medicine is through aromatherapy, which involves the topical application (massage oils, oil baths, facial dressings), oral use (drops), or inhalation (aroma lamps)

continued on next page

of fragrances. Allergic airborne contact dermatitis has been described (134), as has occupational eczema in an aromatherapist (135).

Euphorbia cyparissias

This plant is one of the *Euphorbia* spp. containing skin irritant and tumor-promoting diterpene esters of the ingenane type (129). Chronic exposure of humans to the tincture should be discouraged (136).

Evening primrose oil
(*Oenothera biennis*)

The seeds yield evening primrose oil, which is used in various disorders, such as atopic eczema, premenstrual syndrome, and benign breast pain. When used as directed, it seems to produce no or only minor side effects, such as nausea, diarrhea, and headache. Allegations that evening primrose oil may make manifest undiagnosed temporal lobe epilepsy in patients receiving known epileptogenic drugs (e.g., phenothiazines) still need to be substantiated.

Fenugreek seed (*Trigonella foenum-graecum*)

Skin reactions to repeated external use.

Feverfew (*Tanacetum parthenium*)

Contact dermatitis is possible and is caused by allergenic sesquiterpene lactones, such as parthenolide. Mouth ulceration, inflammation of the oral mucosa and tongue, swelling of the lips, and loss of taste have also been reported.

Forking larkspur (*Delphinium consolida*)

The herb contains toxic diterpenoid alkaloids, but there are no reliable data on the alkaloid level in the flowers. The German health authorities have no objection to the use of the flowers as admixture to herbal teas in levels up to 1%.

Furocoumarins

Photosensitizing compounds, which are found in various medicinal plants, such as European angelica (*Angelica archangelica*) and rue (*Ruta graveolens*).

Garlic bulb (*Allium sativum*)

Gastrointestinal disturbances (rarely). Nondietary intake or excessive dietary intake may increase the risk of bleeding and postoperative hemorrhagic complications in patients undergoing surgery (137, 138). One case of spinal hematoma causing paraplegia in association with excessive ingestion was reported (139). Topical exposure can lead to contact dermatitis or burnlike skin lesions, and occupational inhalation may produce asthma (140–142).

Gentian root (*Gentiana* spp.)

Occasionally headache.

Ginkgo leaf (*Ginkgo biloba*)

Gastrointestinal complaints, headache, and allergic skin reactions. Recent case reports have associated the chronic ingestion of ginkgo with spontaneous bilateral subdural hematomas and increased bleeding time (143) and the combined use of ginkgo plus aspirin with spontaneous bleeding from the iris into the anterior chamber of the eye (144).

Ginseng

Ginseng is an ambiguous vernacular term; it may refer to *Panax* species, such as *P.ginseng* (Asian ginseng) and *P.quinquefolius* (American ginseng), *Eleutherococcus senticosus* (Siberian ginseng), *Pfaffia paniculata* (Brazilian ginseng), or unidentified material (e.g., Rumanian ginseng). Of all these sources, only the *Panax* species contain ginsenosides. Among the variety of adverse effects, which have been attributed in the literature to ginseng preparations, are hypertension, pressure headaches, dizziness, estrogenlike effects, vaginal bleeding, and mastalgia. Prolonged use has been associated with a "ginseng abuse syndrome," including symptoms of hypertension, edema, morning diarrhea, skin eruptions, insomnia, depression, and amenorrhea. Most reports are difficult to interpret, however, because of the absence of a control group, the simultaneous use of other agents, insufficient information about dosage, and, last but not least, the lack of botanical authentication. For example, when a case of neonatal androgenization was associated with maternal use of Siberian ginseng tablets during pregnancy (145), botanical analysis showed that the incriminated material almost certainly came from *Periploca sepium* (Chinese silk vine) (146).

Guar gum (*Cyamopsis tetragonolobus*)
Esophageal obstruction (58) and interference with the absorption of other drugs (50).

Haronga bark with leaf (*Harungana madagascariensis*)
Photosensitivity.

Hellebore (*Veratrum* spp.)
The rhizome and root of *Veratrum album* (white hellebore) and the rhizome of *Veratrum viride* (green hellebore) contain many alkaloidal constituents, including hypotensive ester alkaloids. Among the major toxic symptoms are hypotension and bradycardia (147). The related species *Veratrum californicum* has well-established teratogenic activity in livestock, due to the presence of the alkaloids cyclopamine, cycloposine, and jervine. The latter alkaloid is also found in white and green hellebore.

Horse chestnut seed (*Aesculus hippocastanum*)
Gastrointestinal disturbances (rarely).

Horseradish root (*Armoracia rusticana*)
Gastrointestinal disturbances. Convulsive syncope and abdominal discomfort have been observed following the ingestion of raw horseradish that had not been properly aired before use (148).

Ipecacuanha (*Cephaelis* spp.)
Ipecac syrup contains the toxic alkaloids cephaeline and emetine. When it is used as an emetic in accidental poisoning, serious adverse effects are usually absent, but misuse by anorectic and bulimic patients has resulted in severe myopathy, lethargy, erythema, dysphagia, cardiotoxicity, and even death (149).

Ispaghula seed and seedshell (*Plantago ovata*)
Allergic reactions are possible. Fatal bronchospasm after oral ingestion has been reported (150).

Jalap resin (*Exogonium purga*)
Drastic cathartic with irritant action, which has been superseded by less toxic laxatives.

Jessamine rhizome, yellow (*Gelsemium sempervirens*)
Narrow therapeutic window has resulted in many cases of poisoning, including fatal ones. Characteristic symptoms are dizziness, loss of speech, dysphagia, dry mouth, visual disturbances, trembling of extremities, muscular rigidity or weakness, and falling of the jaw.

Juniper berry (*Juniperus communis*)
The volatile oil distilled from the berries can act as a gastrointestinal irritant. It is said that excessive doses may result in renal damage, and use during pregnancy is discouraged because of a fear that this might stimulate not only the intestine, but also the uterus.

Kelp
General name for seaweed preparations obtained from different botanical species (*Fucus vesiculosus, Fucus serratus, Ascophyllum nodo-*
continued on next page

sum, Macrocystis pyrifera). Because kelp contains iodine, it occasionally produces hyperthyroidism, hypothyroidism, or extrathyroidal reactions, such as skin eruptions. The ingestion of kelp has been associated with a case of severe dyserythropoiesis and autoimmune thrombocytopenia (151).

Kombucha

The Kombucha "mushroom" is a symbiotic colony of several species of yeast and bacteria that are bound together by a surrounding thin membrane. Kombucha tea has been associated with hepatotoxicity (152, 153) and severe metabolic acidosis (154).

Levant wormseed (*Artemisia cina*)

Contains the toxic lactone santonin, which was formerly used as an anthelminthic, but has now been superseded by other less toxic anthelmintics. It should not be confused with American wormseed (*Chenopodium ambrosioides*). The latter yields chenopodium oil, which has caused numerous poisonings due to the presence of ascaridole.

Licorice root (*Glycyrrhiza glabra*)

Prolonged use and/or high doses may produce mineralocorticoid adverse effects and drug interactions due to the saponin glycoside glycyrrhizin, which is naturally present in liquorice root in the form of calcium and potassium salts of glycyrrhizinic acid. Most persons can consume 400 mg of glycyrrhizin daily without adverse effects, but some individuals will develop adverse effects following regular daily intake of as little as 100 mg of glycyrrhizin (155, 156).

Madder root (*Rubia tinctorum*)

The use of herbal medicines prepared from madder root is no longer permitted in Germany (157). Root extracts have shown genotoxic effects in several test systems, which are attributed to the presence of the anthraquinone derivative lucidin. One of the other main components, alizarin primeveroside, is transformed into 1-hydroxyanthraquinone, when given orally to the rat, and this metabolite shows carcinogenic activity in rats (158).

Male fern (*Dryopteris filix-mas*)

The rhizome was formerly used as an anthelmintic, but it is highly toxic and has been superseded by other less dangerous agents. Despite poor absorption, serious poisoning may occur (e.g., when absorption is increased by the presence of fatty foods).

Mandrake, American (*Podophyllum peltatum*)

The resin from the dried rhizome and roots contains podophyllotoxin, α-peltatin, and β-peltatin. When applied topically, it is a strong irritant to the skin and mucous membranes and may lead to poisoning because of systemic absorption. When taken orally, it has a drastic laxative action and produces violent peristalsis. Ingestion of large doses can result in severe neuropathic toxicity (159, 160). The oral and local use of the resin should be avoided during pregnancy because this has been associated with teratogenicity and fetal death. American mandrake should not be confused with the European mandrake (*Mandragora officinarum*), which contains belladonna alkaloids.

Marsh herb (*Ledum palustre*)

The essential oil is a potent gastrointestinal, renal, and urinary irritant. Other toxic effects include abortion.

Meadow windflower (*Pulsatilla vulgaris*)

Higher doses may irritate the kidneys and urinary tract, and pregnancy is considered a contraindication.

Meadow saffron (*Colchicum autumnale*)

Contains the toxic alkaloid colchicine.

Methylsalicylate

Constitutes more than 95% of the volatile oil of wintergreen leaves (*Gaultheria procumbens*). It has been associated with rare cases of allergic skin reactions, and accidental ingestion in young children has resulted in fatal salicylate poisoning. Methylsalicylate is also an important constituent of the red flower oil, which is used in Southeast Asia as a topical herbal analgesic. Some Southeast Asian users also take small amounts of the oil orally to enhance the analgesic effect. A suicide attempt by deliberate ingestion of a large dose ended in severe poisoning (161).

Mistletoe

This vernacular term is ambiguous; it may refer to *Phoradendron* species, such as *Phoradendrom flavescens* (American mistletoe) or to *Viscum album* (European Mistletoe). The stems and leaves of the latter plant have been reported to contain alkaloids, viscotoxins, and lectins. The viscotoxins and lectins have been found to be poisonous in animals when given parenterally, but the consulted literature has not provided experimental data on their oral toxicology profile. Parenteral preparations of *Viscum album* can give serious allergic reactions (162), and they should not be administered to patients with hypersensitivity to proteins or with a chronic progressive infection (e.g., tuberculosis). *Phoradendron* species contain phoratoxins (related to the viscotoxins). Teas prepared from unspecified plant parts or berries of *Phoradendron* have been associated with fatal intoxications.

Statements in the literature that mistletoe has hepatotoxic potential can be traced back to a single case report of hepatitis due to a herbal combination product claimed to have had mistletoe as one of its ingredients (163). However, because the incriminated product also contained skullcap, which has been repeatedly associated with hepatotoxic reactions, the attribution of this case to mistletoe is not acceptable.

Mugwort (*Artemisia vulgaris*)

This herb contains an essential oil with variable composition; depending on origin, 1,8-cineole, camphor, linalool, and thujone may all be major components. Allergic skin reactions (164) and abortive activity have been described.

Mustard (*Brassica* spp.)

White mustard seed (*Brassica alba* = *Sinapis alba*) should not be used externally for more than two weeks because skin and nervous damage can result from prolonged use. External application of black mustard (*Brassica nigra*) is also associated with prominent local reactions.

Myrrh gum-resin (*Commiphora* spp.)

The undiluted tincture may produce burning and local irritation.

Nettle (*Urtica dioica*).

The blister-raising properties of locally applied nettle extracts are well-known. They are said to subside by drying or heat-treatment. Oral use of root preparations occasionally gives rise to mild gastrointestinal complaints.

Nutmeg seed (*Myristica fragrans*)

Psychic disturbances by 5 g or more taken orally, atropinelike action by 9 teaspoons of seed powder, and abortion by higher doses. The essential oil contains the mutagenic and animal carcinogenic compound safrole. However, the use to correct smell or taste is considered acceptable.

Nux vomica seed (*Strychnos nux-vomica*)

Contains the toxic alkaloid strychnine.

Papain

Proteolytic enzyme or mixture of enzymes from the juice of the unripe fruit of *Carica*

continued on next page

papaya. Allergic reactions may occur after oral ingestion (165) and topical application (166). Cross-allergenicity with chymopapain has been documented (167).

Parsley (*Petroselinum crispum = Apium petroselinum*)

Phototoxicity and allergic reactions of skin and mucosae (rarely). The pure essential oil and its constituent apiole are toxic.

Pennyroyal oil (*Hedeoma pulegioides* and *Mentha pulegium*)

This volatile oil has a long history as a folk medicine for the induction of menses and abortion. Ingestion of large doses has resulted in serious symptoms including vomiting, abortion, seizures, hallucinations, renal damage, hepatotoxicity, shock, and death (168). The hepatotoxic potential of pulegone, the major constituent of the oil, has been confirmed in animal experiments. A case report describes serious pennyroyal toxicity in two Hispanic infants (one of whom died) who had been treated with teas brewed from home-grown mint plants. Both infants were positive for mentofuran, a toxic metabolite of pulegone, and one of them was also positive for pulegone (169).

Peru balsam (*Myroxylon balsamum* var. *pereira*)

Allergic skin reactions.

Poison oak (*Rhus toxicodendron*)

Allergic contact dermatitis (170).

Pokeweed (*Phytolacca americana*)

Severe emesis, diarrhea, and tachycardia may occur after ingestion of the raw leaves or after drinking tea prepared from the powdered root. A case of type I Mobitz heart block following the intake of uncooked pokeweed leaves has been reported (171).

Pollen

Gastrointestinal complaints (rarely). Anaphylactic reactions to oral ingestion have also been reported (172–174).

Poplar bud, black (*Populus nigra*)

External use is occasionally associated with allergic skin reactions.

Primrose flower and root (*Primula veris*)

Gastrointestinal disturbances (occasionally). Rarely contact allergy.

Psyllium seed (*Plantago afra* and *Plantago indica*)

Ingestion has been rarely associated with generalized urticarial rash and anaphylactic shock (175, 176).

Pyrrolizidine alkaloids

Pyrrolizidine alkaloids with a saturated necine base are nontoxic, but most of the pyrrolizidine alkaloids with an unsaturated necine base are hepatotoxic, mutagenic, and hepatocarcinogenic. Among the numerous plants, which contain the latter type, are *Adenostyles alliariae* (1), *Alkanna tinctoria*, *Anchusa officinalis*, *Borago officinalis*, *Crotalaria* spp., *Cynoglossum* spp., *Echium* spp., *Erechtites hieracifolia*, *Eupatorium* spp., *Heliotropium* spp., *Lithospermum officinale*, *Packera candidissima* (177), *Petasites* spp., *Pulmonaria* spp., *Senecio* spp., *Symphytum* spp., and *Tussilago farfara* (178–180). A venoocclusive disease of the liver can be produced with clinical features, such as abdominal pain with ascites, hepatomegaly and splenomegaly, anorexia with nausea, vomiting, and diarrhea. Sometimes damage to the pulmonary region occurs as well (178–183). Animal studies have shown transplacental passage and transfer to breast milk, and a human case of fatal neonatal liver injury has been associated with maternal use of a herbal cough tea containing pyrrolizidine alkaloids throughout the pregnancy (184, 185).

The German health authorities no longer permit herbal medicines providing more than 1 μg of unsaturated pyrrolizidine alkaloids internally or more than 100 μg externally per day; herbal medicines providing 0.1–1 μg internally or 10–100 μg externally per day, when used as directed, may be applied only for a maximum of 6 weeks per year and they should not be used during pregnancy or lactation (186, 187).

Radish, black (*Raphanus sativus var. niger*)

Urticarial manifestations from oral therapy have been reported (188). Consumption of several roots is said to have produced miosis, pain, vomiting, slowed respiration, stupor, and albuminuria. It is also claimed that poisoning secondary to the use of black radish sap for bile stones has occurred.

Rauwolfia root (*Rauvolfia serpentina*)

Contains numerous alkaloids, of which reserpine and rescinnamine are said to be the most active as hypotensive agents. Among the reported adverse effects of 0.25 to 0.50 mg/day of reserpine are lethargy, depression, nightmares, sexual dysfunction, anxiety, and gastrointestinal symptoms (189). Although depression has already been observed at a dose level of 0.25 mg/day (189, 190), this adverse effect mostly occurs at doses greater than 0.5 mg per day (191).

Rhatany root (*Krameria triandra*)

Rarely allergic mucosal reactions (local use in mouth). Undiluted tincture may produce burning and local irritation.

Rhododendron ferrugineum

Adverse effects have not been reported for herbal tea from the leaves, but toxic diterpenes may be present and chronic use might lead to hydroquinone poisoning (due to the presence of arbutin).

Rue (*Ruta graveolens*)

The essential oil not only can produce contact dermatitis and phototoxic reactions (due to the presence of furocoumarins), but can also induce severe hepatic and renal toxicity. Use as an abortive agent has resulted in fatal intoxications. Therapeutic doses can lead to melancholia, sleeping disorders, fatigue, dizziness, and cramps. The sap of the fresh leaf can give painful gastrointestinal irritation, fainting, sleepiness, weak pulse, abortion, swollen tongue, and cool skin.

Saffron stigma (*Crocus sativus*)

No risks have been documented for daily doses up to 1.5 g, but 5 g is toxic, 10 g is abortive, and 20 g may be lethal.

Sage leaf (*Salvia officinalis*)

The leaf contains 1 to 2.5% of essential oil consisting of 35 to 60% of thujone. This compound may produce toxicity, when the herb is taken in overdoses (more than 15 g per dose) or for a prolonged period. Pregnancy is listed as a contraindication for the use of the essential oil or alcoholic extracts.

Santalum album wood

Nausea, skin itching.

Saponins

Saponins with irritant properties occur, for example, in the rhizome of the German sarsaparilla (*Carex arenaria*), Senega snakeroot (*Polygala senega*), primrose flower and root (*Primula veris*), and soapwort (*Saponaria officinalis*).

Sassafras wood (*Sassafras albidum*)

Sassafras wood contains 1 to 2% of essential oil, which consists of about 80% of safrole. Some of the known or possible metabolites of this compound show mutagenic activity in bacterial testing, and it has been proven to have weak hepatocarcinogenic effects in rodents. Experiments in mice suggest the

continued on next page

possibility of transplacental and lactational carcinogenesis. All in all, prolonged internal use is to be discouraged. Of particular concern seems to be the uncontrolled availability of sassafras oil for so-called aromatherapy, which may result in a daily intake up to 0.2 g of safrole, when ingested as recommended (192). The German health authorities have proposed a withdrawal of sassafras-containing medicines from the market, including that of homoeopathic products up to D3 (193).

Saw palmetto fruit (*Serenoa repens = Sabal serrulata*)
Gastric complaints (rarely).

Scammony, Mexican
(*Convolvulus scammonia*)
The resin is a drastic purgative with irritant properties, which has been superseded by less toxic alternatives.

Senna (*Cassia* spp.)
Mutagenicity testing of sennosides has produced negative results in several bacterial and mammalian systems, except for a weak effect in *Salmonella typhimurium* strain TA102 (194, 195). A well-defined purified senna extract was not carcinogenic when administered orally to rats in daily doses up to 25 mg/kg for two years (196). No evidence of reproductive toxicity of sennosides has been found in rats and rabbits (197). When a standardized preparation containing senna pods (providing 15 mg/day of sennosides) was given to breast-feeding mothers, the suckling infants were only exposed to a nonlaxative amount of rhein, which remained a factor 10^{-3} below the maternal intake of this active metabolite (198). Considering these findings, the German health authorities do not forbid the use of senna fruit during pregnancy and lactation (163–165). Exceptional complications of senna abuse include hepatitis (199), finger clubbing, and hypertrophic osteopathy (200, 201).

Sesquiterpene lactones
Can produce allergic contact dermatitis. Among the medicinal herbs with moderate or strong sensitizing capacity due to the presence of sesquiterpene lactones are alant (*Inula helenium*), arnica (*Arnica* spp.), artichoke (*Cynara scolymus*), blessed thistle (*Cnicus benedictus*), costus root (*Saussurea lappa*), feverfew (*Tanacetum parthenium*), laurel (*Laurus nobilis*), pyrethrum (*Tanacetum cinerariifolium*), and sunflower (*Helianthus annuus*) (202). Sensitizing sesquiterpene lactones are also found in camomile (*Chamomilla recutita*), chicory (*Cichorium intybus*), dandelion (*Taraxacum officinale*), lettuce (*Lactuca* spp.), and yarrow (*Achillea millefolium*) (202, 203). Cross-sensitivity with other plants containing related allergenic sesquiterpene lactones is possible.

Silverweed (*Potentilla anserina*)
Gastrointestinal disturbances.

Skullcap
Herbal therapies comprising skullcap as one of their ingredients have been repeatedly associated with hepatotoxic reactions. One of these cases was originally attributed to mistletoe, although there were insufficient grounds for this allusion (163). Although Western skullcap preparations are supposed to come from *Scutellaria lateriflora*, it remains unclear whether this plant is responsible. In the United Kingdom, the American germander (*Teucrium canadense*) has been widely used to replace *S. lateriflora* in commercial skullcap materials and products. In one United Kingdom case of skullcap-associated hepatotoxicity, the material was found to come from *Teucrium canadense*, raising the possibility that other cases of skullcap toxicity may also have involved *Teucrium* rather than *Scutellaria* (83).

Snakeroot, black (*Cimicifuga racemosa*)
Occasionally gastric complaints.

Snakeroot, white (*Eupatorium rugosum*)

Can produce livestock poisoning as well as milk sickness. This latter syndrome can occur when humans ingest the milk from animals with abundant access to the plant. Symptoms include trembles, weakness, nausea and vomiting, prostration, delirium, and even death. Tremetol has long been considered to be the poisonous principle in white snakeroot, but chemically this substance is a mixture of many different compounds, including the ketones tremetone, hydroxytremetone, and dehydrotremetone. Tremetone seems to be the major toxic component but it is only toxic after microsomal activation. It readily decomposes to dehydrotremetone, which is not toxic, not even after microsomal activation (204).

Spindle tree, European (*Euonymus europaeus*)

The fruit is said to have cathartic and emetic activity.

Squirting cucumber (*Ecabalium elaterium*)

The fruit juice can cause severe skin irritation, inflammation, and Quincke's edema (205), and has also been associated with a fatal case of cardiac and renal failure (206). Among the isolated constituents is cucurbitacin B (207).

St. Mary's thistle fruit (*Silybum marianum = Carduus marianus*)

Occasionally slight laxative effect. A case of anaphylactic shock following the use of a herbal tea containing an extract of the fruit has been reported (208).

St. John's wort (*Hypericum perforatum*)

Gastrointestinal symptoms, allergic reactions, and fatigue (209). Ingestion of this herb by grazing animals can cause photosensitization, which effect is generally ascribed to the red-colored pigment hypericin.

Sunflower seed (*Helianthus annuus*)

Anaphylactic reactions have been recorded (210).

Sweet flag (*Acorus calamus*)

Mutagenic and carcinogenic β-asarone in volatile oil (high levels in tetraploid Indian plants, low levels in triploid Eastern European plants, and no detectable level in diploid North American plants) (82).

Tansy, common (*Chrysanthemum vulgare = Tanacetum vulgare*)

Contains essential oil with neurotoxic thujone in such amounts that normal doses may already be toxic.

Tea tree oil (*Melaleuca alternifolia*)

Topical use of the undiluted essential oil from the leaves can result in an allergic contact eczema, which is most commonly caused by the constituent d-limonene (211, 212). Internal use of half a teaspoonful of the oil may result in a dramatic rash (213), whereas half a tea cup may induce a coma followed by a semiconscious state with hallucinations (214). Less than 10 mL is sufficient to produce serious signs of toxicity in small children.

Temu lawak rhizome (*Curcuma xanthorrhiza*)

Gastrointestinal irritation from continued use.

Tobacco (*Nicotiana tabacum*)

The leaves contain the toxic alkaloid nicotine as major constituent and several other pyridine alkaloids as minor constituents. Although tobacco enemas have been abolished

continued on next page

in official medicine because of their life-threatening toxicity, self-medication has not completely died out. A case report in the 1970s described nausea and confusion, followed by hypotension and bradycardia, due to an enema prepared apparently from 5 to 10 cigarettes (215).

Tobacco, Indian (*Lobelia inflata*)

Because this herb contains the toxic alkaloid lobeline and other pyridine alkaloids, overdosing can result in serious toxicity. Lobeline has similar peripheral effects as nicotine, whereas its central activity may be different. Its use has been associated with nausea, vomiting, headache, tremors, and dizziness. Symptoms caused by overdosage include profuse diaphoresis, paresis, tachycardia, hypotension, Cheyne-Stokes respiration, hypothermia, coma, and death. Large doses are convulsant.

Tropane alkaloids

Tropane alkaloids occur naturally in various plants, such as *Atropa belladonna* (deadly nightshade), *Datura stramonium* (jimson weed), *Hyoscyamus niger* (henbane), *Mandragora officinarum* (European mandrake), and *Scopalia carniolica*. These alkaloids are powerful anticholinergic agents and can elicit peripheral symptoms (e.g., blurred vision, dry mouth) as well as central effects (e.g., drowsiness, delirium).

Valerian root (*Valeriana* spp.)

The valepotriates that occur in valerian roots have alkylating properties. Valtrate/isovaltrate and dihydrovaltrate are mutagenic in bacterial test systems in the presence of a metabolic activator, and their degradation products baldrinal (from valtrate) and homobaldrinal (from isovaltrate) are already mutagenic without metabolic activation. These latter compounds also show direct genotoxic activity in SOS-chromotesting. As far as is known, decomposition of didrovaltrate does not yield baldrinals.

The levels of valepotriates and baldrinals in valerian extracts depend on the botanical species: root extracts of *Valeriana officinalis* contain up to 0.9% of valepotriates, compared with 2–4% and 5–7% of valepotriates in root extracts of *Valeriana wallichii* and *Valeriana mexicana*, respectively. Another relevant parameter is the dosage form:

Herbal tea. When prepared by hot extraction from valerian root, up to 60% of the valepotriates remains in the root material, and only 0.1% can be recovered from the tea.

Tincture. A freshly prepared tincture contains 11% of the valepotriates originally found in the root material. Storage at room temperature rapidly reduces this level to 3.7% after one week and 0% after three weeks. In view of this rapid degradation, it is not surprising that commercially available tincture samples yield baldrinals when analyzed.

Tablets and capsules. Valerian-containing tablets and capsules may provide up to 1 mg of baldrinals per piece.

Valepotriates show poor gastrointestinal absorption, but 2% is degraded in vivo to baldrinals following the oral application of valtrate/isovaltrate to mice. In other words, a tablet with 50 mg of valepotriates may add 1 mg of baldrinals to the amount of baldrinals, which are already present before ingestion. In contrast to the valepotriates, the degradation product homobaldrinal is absorbed fairly well following oral application to mice. As much as 71% of the administered dose can be recovered from the urine in the form of baldrinal glucuronide. Because no unchanged homobaldrinal can be demonstrated in body fluids or liver samples following oral administration, the compound appears to undergo substantial first-pass metabolism. Because this glucuronidation leads to loss of the mutagenic properties, the primary target organs that may be at risk from valepotriates and baldrinals are the gastrointestinal tract and the liver (216).

The toxicological significance of these data is still not sufficiently clear because the carcinogenic potential of valerian preparations and their constituents has not yet been evaluated.

Vervain, European (*Verbena officinalis*)
Allergic contact dermatitis (217).

Wahoo bark (*Euonymus atropurpureus*)
Said to have cathartic and emetic activity.

Wall germander (*Teucrium chamaedrys*)
In France, numerous cases of hepatitis have been associated with the normal use of this herb. The frequency of this adverse effect has been estimated at 1 case in about 4000 months of treatment (218). Two additional cases were reported from Canada (219). Although most cases were not very serious, fatal outcome has been reported (220), and progression to liver cirrhosis has also been described (220). According to animal studies, the hepatotoxicity resides in one or more reactive metabolites of its furanoditerpenoids (221, 222).

The risk of *Teucrium*-induced hepatitis does not seem to be restricted to the single species *T. chamaedrys* because the related *T. canadense* (see the entry on skullcap) and *Teucrium polium* (223) have also been associated with this adverse effect.

Walnut fruit-shell (*Juglans regia*)
Fresh shells contain the naphthoquinone constituent juglone, which is mutagenic and possibly carcinogenic. The juglone content of dried shells has not been studied adequately.

Willow (*Salix* species)
The bark of various *Salix* species contains glycosides of saligenin (= salicylalcohol), namely the simple O-glycoside salicin and more complex glycosides like salicortin. When taken orally, these glycosides may undergo intestinal transformation to saligenin, which in its turn may be rapidly absorbed and then converted by the liver to salicylic acid. When willow bark preparations are used according to current dosage recommendations, they will not provide sufficient salicylic acid to produce acute salicylate poisoning. However, the risk of an idiosyncratic response (skin reactions, bronchospasm) in sensitive individuals cannot be excluded.

Witch hazel (*Hamamelis virginiana*)
Contact allergy has been reported (224).

Wolf's foot (*Lycopus europaeus*)
An increase in the size of the thyroid gland is possible, as is an initial increase of hyperthyreotic symptoms (e.g., nervousness, tachycardia, and loss of body weight). Interference with the thyroidal uptake of radioactive iodine has also been reported (225).

Wormwood (*Artemisia absinthium*)
The volatile oil is used to flavor the alcoholic liqueur absinthe, which can damage the nervous system and cause mental deterioration. This toxicity is attributed to thujone (a mixture of α- and β-thujone), which constitutes 3 to 12% of the oil, which in its turn reaches concentrations of 0.25 to 1.32% in the whole herb. Alcoholic extracts and the essential oil are forbidden in many countries.

Yohimbe bark (*Pausinystalia johimbe*)
A major alkaloid in yohimbe bark is yohimbine, which has α_2-adrenoreceptor antagonistic properties and can thereby counteract the effects of certain antihypertensives (e.g.,

continued on next page

guanabenz, the methyldopa metabolite α-methylnorepinephrine) An oral dose of 15 to 20 mg can increase blood pressure and induce anxiety in healthy volunteers, and hypertension may already be induced by 4 mg taken three times daily in patients on tricyclic antidepressants. The toxicity of yohimbine can also be enhanced by other drugs, such as phenothiazines. A dose of 5 mg is sufficient to produce adverse effects in patients with autonomic failure, and 10 mg can elicit maniclike symptoms in patients with bipolar depression. Bronchospasm and a lupuslike syndrome have also been reported (15, 16).

Yohimbine also occurs in other species of *Pausinystalia* (*P. angolensis* and *P. trillesii*) (226) and in the bark of *Corynanthe paniculata* (227).

Recreational Herbs

Western customers may purchase bioactive herbs not only for medicinal uses, but also for other purposes, such as mind-altering effects. Reported adverse reactions to some major source plants are reviewed below. The recreational use of botanical hallucinogens (other than marijuana) is showing signs of revival after a distinct decline during the 1970s and 1980s. Important examples are listed in Table 6.3 (228–230) on the basis of their hallucinogenic constituents. In addition to the general risk that consumers may overestimate their own abilities (233), specific toxic effects can result from plants such as *Datura* (234–237) and *Myristica fragrans* (238), which have a strong vegetative component besides their hallucinogenic activity.

The next page shows a summary of the known and reported adverse effects of recreational herbs and products.

Table 6.3. Botanical Hallucinogens and their Most Important Source Plants

TYPE OF HALLUCINOGEN	SOURCE PLANTS
Dimethyltryptamine and related alkaloids	*Anadenanthera* spp. *Phalaris arundinacea* (reed canarygrass)* *Virola* spp.
Harmine and related alkaloids	*Banisteriopsis* spp. *Peganum harmala* (Syrian rue)
Ibogaine	*Tabernanthe iboga* (iboga)
Lysergic acid derivatives	*Argyreia* spp. *Ipomoea* spp. (morning glories) *Turbina* spp. (morning glories)
Mescaline	*Lophophora williamsii* (peyote) *Trichocereus pachanoi* (San Pedro cactus) (= *Echinopsis pachanoi*)
Muscimol and ibotenic acid	*Amanita muscaria* (fly agaric)
Myristicin	*Myristica fragrans* (nutmeg)
Psilocybin and psilocin	*Conocybe* spp. *Copelandia* spp. *Panaeolus* spp. *Psilocybe* spp. *Stropharia* spp.
Scopolamine and related alkaloids	*Brugmansia* spp. (tree Daturas) *Datura* spp. (jimson weed)

*See refs. 231 and 232.

When faced with a patient using these products, the practitioner can find information on that product here. This section provides an indication of the adverse effects known for that plant and help guide the practitioner in monitoring for possible adverse effects in that patient. It will also help the practitioner inform the patient about possible risks.

Areca nut (*Areca catechu*)

A substantial part of the world's population chews betel nut quid, a combination of areca nut, betel pepper leaf (from *Piper betle*), lime paste, and tobacco leaf. The major alkaloid of the areca nut, arecoline, can produce cholinergic side effects such as bronchoconstriction (239) as well as antagonism of anticholinergic agents (240). Under the influence of the lime in the betel quid, arecoline hydrolyzes into arecaidine, a central nervous system stimulant which accounts, together with the essential oil of the betel pepper, for the euphoric effects of betel quid chewing. The use of the areca nut is widely implicated in the development of oral cancers, and it has been documented that the saliva of betel nut chewers contains nitrosamines derived from areca nut alkaloids (241).

Coca leaf (*Erythroxylum* spp.)

Coca leaves contain cocaine as the principal alkaloid and a variety of other minor alkaloids. Only decocainized coca products are legal in the United States, but some commercially available tea products were found to have a cocaine level normally found in coca leaves (about 5 mg of cocaine per tea bag of 1 gram). This level results in mild symptoms when package directions to drink a few cups per day are followed, but massive overdosing may result in severe agitation, tachycardia, perspiration, and elevated blood pressure (242).

Kava-kava rhizome (*Piper methysticum*)

South Pacific natives prepare a ceremonial beverage from this rhizome. The major constituents are nonalkaloidal pyrone derivatives, which produce sedation and centrally induced muscle relaxation in laboratory animals. This suggests that one should be aware of a potential effect on driving ability. Western case reports have described allergic skin reactions, yellow discoloration of the skin, sensory disturbances, sleepiness, and ataxia (243–245). Heavy chronic consumption of kava-kava can lead to a pellagroid dermopathy that appears to be unrelated to niacin deficiency (246).

Khat leaves (*Catha edulis*)

The chewing of khat leaves results in subjective mental stimulation, physical endurance, and increased self-esteem and social interaction. Until recently, this habit was confined to Arabian and East African countries, because only fresh leaves are active, but due to increased possibilities of air transportation, khat is now also chewed in other parts of the world. Tachycardia and increased blood pressure, irritability, psychosis, and psychic dependence have been described as adverse effects. Although cathine (= norpseudoephedrine) is quantitatively the main alkaloid, the amphetaminelike euphorigenic and sympathicomimetic cardiovascular effects of khat are primarily attributed to cathinone (247). Khat chewing by a breast-feeding mother can lead to the presence of cathine in the urine of the suckling child (248).

Ma Huang (*Ephedra* spp.)

The major alkaloid in commercial samples of Ma Huang and in its usual source plants is either the R(−)-isomer ephedrine or the S(+)-isomer pseudoephedrine (249–251). In high doses, ephedrine can produce serious peripheral and central adrenergic effects, such as palpitations, tachycardia, hypertension, coronary spasm, psychosis, convulsions, respiratory depression, coma, and death (47). The occurrence of pressor effects depends on factors such as specific isomer, dose, and consumer. In normotensive subjects, ephed-

continued on next page

rine can produce significant blood pressure elevation at oral doses of 60 mg or more. Infants and elderly patients are more susceptible, and the risk may also be greater in hypertensive patients. At oral doses of 60 mg, pseudoephedrine is considered to give a low incidence of blood pressure elevation in normotensive subjects. If blood pressure elevation does occur, this is likely to be due to idiosyncrasy (252).

Ma Huang and other ephedrine-containing dietary supplements have been associated in recent years with numerous adverse events, particularly in the United States. These products were marketed as legal producers of a "high," enhancers of sexual sensations, and increasers of energy and provided up to 45 mg of ephedrine and 20 mg of caffeine per tablet (47, 253). Among the reported effects were erythroderma (254), mania (255), psychosis (256), seizures, acute myocardial infarction, and fatal coronary artery thrombosis (47). The use of Ma Huang was also associated with a case of acute hepatitis, but given the lack of published cases of hepatotoxic reactions to Ma Huang or ephedrine, the reporting physicians rightly questioned whether the patient took a contaminated or misidentified product (257).

Poppy seed (*Papaver somniferum*)

The ingestion of poppy seeds can result in detectable urinary levels of morphine and codeine (258). There are rare cases of poppy dependence due to the frequent sucking of poppy seeds (259) or to the regular drinking of a tea infusion from poppy heads (260).

Traditional Chinese Medicines

The availability of traditional Chinese medicines for Western consumers appears to be increasing. Although herbal ingredients with potent pharmacological activity have become less and less common in Western phytotherapeutic medicines, a variety of potent herbs can still be encountered in traditional Chinese medicines (261–264). First, the Chinese materia medica comprises well-known toxic herbs, such as *Ephedra* and *Aconitum*. The latter continues to be associated with cases of serious heart failure (265, 266), although its cardiotoxicity can be substantially reduced by decocting the raw root (267). Second, there are familiar toxic constituents under the guise of unfamiliar Chinese or botanical names (Table 6.4) (268–271). Third, adverse effects can be produced by numerous unfamiliar Chinese herbs or their less familiar constituents. Finally, traditional Chinese medicines can contain, besides herbs, ingredients of animal and mineral origin, some of which make significant contributions to the adverse reaction potential of these medicines.

Botanical Quality

A potentially toxic Chinese herb that has drawn much attention in recent years is *Aristolochia fangchi*. In 1993 and 1994, Belgian researchers reported a human outbreak of nephropathy in

Table 6.4. Familiar Toxic Agents Contained in Unfamiliar Chinese Names

CHINESE NAME	LATIN BINOMIAL	TOXIC CONSTITUENT(S)
Bajiaolian	*Dysosma pleianthum*	Podophyllotoxin
Naoyanghua	*Rhododendron molle*	Scopolamine and atropine*
Shancigu	*Iphigenia indica*	Colchicine
Zangqie	*Anisodus tanguticus*	Hyoscyamine, scopolamine, and related alkaloids

*It should be noted, however, that this herb provides different toxins according to other sources [262, 263].

more than 70 users of a slimming preparation that supposedly contained the Chinese herbs *Stephania tetrandra* and *Magnolia officinalis* (272, 273). Analysis of the incriminated material showed that the root of *Stephania tetrandra* (Chinese name "Fangji") had in all probability been substituted or contaminated with the root of *Aristolochia fangchi* (Chinese name "Guang fangji") (274). In most cases, renal failure progressed despite the withdrawal of the slimming preparation, and 35 patients required renal replacement therapy. Renal biopsies showed extensive interstitial fibrosis with atrophy and loss of tubules (272, 273, 275, 276). The supposition that the renal interstitial fibrosis was immune-mediated was supported by the finding that the progression of the renal failure could be slowed by steroid therapy with prednisolone (277). At least two of the patients exposed to the slimming preparation rapidly developed urothelial malignancy (278, 279). This did not come as a great surprise, because the aristolochic acids in *Aristolochia* plants are extremely potent rodent carcinogens (88). Further evidence of the implication of aristolochic acid was provided by a report on aristolochic acid DNA adducts in renal tissue samples of some victims. The demonstration of the deoxyadenosine adduct of aristolochic acid I conclusively showed that aristolochic acid had been ingested in amounts sufficient to alter cellular DNA (280). Another *Aristolochia* species in traditional Chinese medicine is *Aristolochia manshuriensis*, which also provides toxic aristolochic acids (88). Because there is evidence that these compounds pass into human breast milk following maternal use (88), it is of concern that this herb is recommended for the improvement of mammary gland growth and function (281).

The *Stephania/Aristolochia* problem in Belgium illustrates that botanical quality assurance is as relevant for traditional Chinese medicines as it is for Western herbal products. A pharmacognostic study of crude materials imported into the United Kingdom suggests that there still is much room for improvement (Table 6.5) (282). Besides the presence of *Aristolochia fangchi* in Fang Ji (*Stephania tetrandra*), there was also the disturbing finding that *Akebia quinata* ("Mutong") had been substituted by *Aristolochia manshuriensis* ("Guanmutong") (283). Among the unexpected toxic botanicals that have been discovered in Chinese herbal medicines are also *Podophyllum emodi*, *Datura metel*, and *Mandragora officinarum* (284, 285). Not all practitioners of traditional Chinese medicine in the United Kingdom are experts in herb recognition (286).

Other Quality Issues

Quality control of traditional Chinese medicines is also important to exclude other contaminants (9), such as pathogenic microorganisms (287). Some recent chemical findings and toxicological observations concerning the presence of toxic metals in traditional Chinese medicines are provided in Tables 6.6 (288–290) and 6.7 (291–293), respectively. Not all of these data may refer to accidental contamination, because certain traditional Chinese herbal formulas intentionally contain toxic arsenic and/or mercury salts as ingredients (see the section on toxic metals in Chapter 7, "The Safety of Nonherbal

Table 6.5. Botanical Quality Problems with Certain Crude Chinese Plant Drugs Imported into the United Kingdom	
PLANT DRUG	QUALITY PROBLEM
Fang ji	Plant roots supplied under this name not only contained *Stephania tetrandra*, but also *Aristolochia fangchi*.
Mu Tong	Of two samples, one was *Clematis armandi* and the other was *Aristolochia manshuriensis*.
Zi Cao	One sample proved to be *Potentilla chinensis* rather than the required *Arnebia euchroma*. As a result, it contained no L-shikonin, the expected active ingredient.
Cheng Yiang	A sample imported from Hong Kong showed no characteristic signs of authentic *Aquilaria sinensis* and was in fact a piece of unidentified wood that had been dyed with black ink.

Table 6.6. Levels of Mercury and Arsenic (per product unit) Detected in Certain Traditional Chinese Medicines

PREPARATION	ANALYZED IN	MERCURY	ARSENIC	REFERENCE
Angong Niuhuang Wan	United Kingdom	47 mg	?	291
An Gong Niu Huang Wan	United States	up to 621 mg	up to 36.6 mg	292
Ba-Pao-Neu-Hwang-San	Taiwan	up to 6.57%	?	293
Da Huo Luo Wan	United States	up to 23 mg	up to 0.1 mg	292
Dendrobium Moniliforme Night Sight pills	United States	up to 28 mg	up to 0.6 mg	292
Niu Huang Chiang Ya Wan	United States	up to 45 mg	up to 9.5 mg	292
Niu Huang Ching Hsin Wan	United States	up to 182 mg	up to 9.9 mg	292
Tao Huo Lo Tan	United States	up to 99 mg	up to 22 mg	292
Tsai Tsao Wan	United States	up to 16 mg	up to 0.6 mg	292
Zhusha Aushen	United Kingdom	659 mg (as red mercuric sulfide)	?	291

Complementary Products"). Another concern involves the deliberate adulteration of certain traditional Chinese herbal medicines with conventional Western pharmaceuticals, such as corticosteroids, nonsteroidal anti-inflammatory agents, and benzodiazepines (83). Although this type of malpractice has been frequently denounced in the past decades (9), it continues to cause occasional problems (Table 6.8).

Kampo Medicines

Chinese herbal medicines are also widely used in Japan, where they are known as Kampoyaku. The number of case reports about the adverse reaction potential of these Kampo medicines is steadily growing. For instance, the use of Shosaiko-to (which consists of Bupleuri radix, Ginseng radix, Glycyrrhizae radix, Pinelliae tuber, Scutellariae radix, Zingiberis rhizoma, and Zizyphi fructus) has been repeatedly associated with cases of allergic pneumonitis and/or hepatitis (302–309).

Individual Herbs

The following is a summary of the known and reported adverse effects of some traditional Chinese medicinal herbs and products. See also the introductory part of this section for data on additional plants.

Table 6.7. Metal Poisoning by Traditional Chinese Medicines

PREPARATION	TOXIC METALS PRESENT	CLINICAL CASES (NO.)	REF.
Nutrien	3.05% thallium and 2.88% lead	Thallium poisoning (2)	294
Tse Koo Choy	Mercurous chloride (calomel)	Mercury poisoning (1)	295
Qing Fen	Mercurous chloride (calomel)	Fatal renal failure (2)	295
Chinese herbal medicine containing Hai Ge Fen (clamshell powder)	22.5% lead and 0.06% arsenic in Hai Ge Fen	Lead poisoning (1)	296

Table 6.8. Adulteration of Traditional Chinese Medicines with Western Pharmaceuticals

INCRIMINATED PRODUCT	PHARMACEUTICAL ADULTERANTS	CLINICAL FINDINGS	REFERENCE
Chuifong Toukuwan	Diazepam Mefenamic acid	Deterioration of blood pressure control	297
Chuifong Toukuwan	Dexamethasone Diazepam Diclofenac Hydrochlorothiazide Indomethacin Mefenamic acid	Cushingoid reaction, renal dysfunction	298
Gan Mao Tong Pian	Chlorpheniramine Diclofenac Phenylbutazone	Aplastic anemia	299
Miracle herb	Diazepam Mefenamic acid	Nausea and gastrointestinal pain	297
Tung Shueh	Diazepam Mefenamic acid	Positive urine drug screen	300
Tung Shueh	Diazepam Mefenamic acid	Somnolence	297
Tung Shueh	Diazepam Mefenamic acid	Acute interstitial nephritis	301
Tung Shueh	Diazepam Mefenamic acid	Acute renal failure	302
Unspecified black balls from China	Hydrocortisone	Remarkable therapeutic response	303
Unspecified cream obtained from Chinese practitioner in United Kingdom	Corticosteroid	Good therapeutic response	304
Unspecified product	Diazepam Mefenamic acid	Large gastrointestinal ulcer	297
Unspecified product	Diazepam Mefenamic acid	Acute exacerbation of chronic abdominal pain	297

When faced with a patient using these products, the practitioner should find the summary of known adverse effects of those products. This will provide an indication of the adverse effects known for that plant and help guide the practitioner in monitoring for possible adverse effects in that patient. It will also help the practitioner inform the patient about possible risks.

Alocasia macrorrhiza

Ingestion of the raw root tuber of this Chinese medicinal plant can result in neurological and gastrointestinal symptoms (e.g,. severe pain and numbness in the perioral area and throat, nausea, vomiting, and abdominal pain) (310).

Coptis spp.

Due to the presence of the alkaloid berberine, these medicinal herbs entail a risk of jaundice in infants who are deficient in glucose-6-phosphate dehydrogenase (34–36).

continued on next page

Dictamnus dasycarpus

This herb is among the common ingredients of the complex traditional Chinese herbal medicines that have been associated with liver damage, but a causal role remains to be established (311–314).

Gossypol

Occurs in certain *Gossypium* species, mostly in the seeds and root bark. Clinical studies have confirmed its efficacy as a male contraceptive agent. Reported side effects include fatigue, changes in appetite, transient elevation of ALT levels, and hypokalemia. Hypokalemic paralysis may occur with muscular weakness and severe fatigue as prodromal signs (315). Further assessment seems to be needed to determine to what extent gossypol entails a risk of irreversible sterility.

Lentinus edodes

This edible mushroom has been occasionally associated with skin reactions (316, 317).

Polygala spp.

Polygalae radix (the dry root of *Polygala tenuifolia* or *P. sibirica*) is known in traditional Chinese medicine under the name of Yuanzhi. It contains 1,5-anhydro-D-glucitol and can thus interfere with laboratory tests, which measure diabetes-related changes in the blood level of this compound (318).

Polygonum multiflorum

Shou-Wu-Pian (a proprietary Chinese medicine prepared from this herb) has been associated with a case of hepatitis (319).

Sauropus androgynus

An outbreak of bronchiolitis obliterans in Taiwan was associated with the ingestion of this herb. It is normally cooked before being eaten as a vegetable, but in this case the numerous victims had all consumed uncooked leaf juice as an unproven method of weight control (320).

Salvia miltiorrhiza

In China, the root (Danshen) has been used traditionally for the treatment of coronary diseases. A pharmacodynamic and pharmacokinetic study in rats suggests that this traditional agent may enhance the anticoagulant activity of warfarin when both drugs are taken together. This animal study was initiated because of observations in Hong Kong that patients on routine warfarin therapy experienced an adverse drug interaction when they self-medicated with a freely available Danshen preparation (321).

Sinomenium acutum

Ingestion of this Chinese herb (known in Japan as Boi) has been associated with a case of systemic edematous erythema with itching (322).

Taxus celebica

This plant, which contains the flavonoid sciadopitysin, is traditionally used in China as an herbal treatment of diabetes mellitus. In two cases, the ingestion of a massive dose was followed by acute renal failure. Both patients initially presented with gastrointestinal upset and fever (323).

Tetrahydropalmatine

l-Tetrahydropalmatine has been identified as the active constituent in Chinese Jin Bu Huan Anodyne tablets on the Western market. The package insert suggested *Polygala chinensis* as the source plant, but in reality this alkaloid comes from a *Stephania* species. Both *l*-tetrahydropalmatine and its racemic *dl*-form are used in Chinese medicine as analgesic and hypnotic agents. Reported side effects include vertigo, fatigue, nausea, and drowsiness, which could make users unfit for driving. Case reports have documented life-threatening bradycardia and respiratory depression in small children following unintentional overdosing and acute hepatitis in adult users (324–326).

Tripterygium wilfordii

Extracts from the root (Leigongteng) are used in China for the treatment of various disorders, such as rheumatoid arthritis, ankylosing spondylitis, systemic lupus erythematosus, and glomerulonephritis. The potential benefits in such serious diseases should be weighed carefully against a substantial risk of adverse reactions, including gastrointestinal disturbances, skin rashes, amenorrhea, leukopenia, and thrombocytopenia. In male users, prolonged use can induce oligospermia and azoospermia and a decrease in the size of the testis (327–329). In addition, the immuno- suppressive properties of Leigongteng may promote the development of infectious diseases (330).

Ziziphus jujuba

The fruit (Dazao) is often consumed in Eastern Asia as food or as a tonic and sedative. A case of angioneurotic edema following the oral ingestion of dazao preparations has been described (331).

Traditional Indian and Pakistani Medicines

Unani and Ayurvedic preparations are another type of non-Western herbal medicines increasingly being introduced into Western health markets. These preparations have a long tradition of medicinal use in India and Pakistan. A survey of the availability of such medicines in the United Kingdom identified as many as 320 different herbal ingredients (332). This inventory comprised several well-known potent herbs and herbs with well-known potentially toxic constituents (Table 6.9). Among the other Indian herbs with established toxic potential are *Androcephalus kadamba* (which contains salicylic acid) (333), *Canscora decussata* (a CNS depressant), and *Indigo tinctoria* (which causes headaches and is a known teratogen in rats) (336).

The botanical identity of herbal medicines from India may present problems (336, 337), and adulteration with Western pharmaceuticals is also occasionally reported (338–340). An even greater cause of concern is the accidental or intentional presence of toxic metals (336, 337), because this has repeatedly resulted in clinical poisonings (see the section on toxic metals in Chapter 7).

Table 6.9. Examples of Herbal Ingredients in Traditional Indian and Pakistani Medicines in the United Kingdom

BOTANICAL SOURCE	CONSTITUENTS
Aconitum heterophyllum	Diterpene alkaloids such as aconitine [333]
Acorus calamus	β-Asarone
Areca catechu	Arecoline and related alkaloids
Aristolochia rotunda	Aristolochic acids*
Atropa belladonna	Tropane alkaloids
Calotropis spp.	Cardiotoxic compounds
Cannabis sativa	Cannabinoids [333]
Cheiranthus cheiri	Cardioactive glycosides
Colchicum spp.	Colchicine
Cordia spp.	Pyrrolizidine alkaloids (?)
Dalbergia spp.	L-Dopa
Datura metel	Tropane alkaloids**
Echium spp.	Pyrrolizidine alkaloids

continued

Table 6.9. Examples of Herbal Ingredients in Traditional Indian and Pakistani Medicines in the United Kingdom (continued)

BOTANICAL SOURCE	CONSTITUENTS
Euphorbia resiniferia	Diterpene esters
Gossypium arboreum	Gossypol
Heliotropium indicum	Pyrrolizidine alkaloids
Helleborus niger	Cardioactive glycosides
Hemidesmus indicus	Coumarin
Hyoscyamus niger	Tropane alkaloids
Lagenaria siceraria	Cucurbitacins
Momordica charantia	Hypoglycemic principle(s) [48,49]
Mucuna pruriens	L-Dopa
Nerium spp.	Cardioactive glycosides [333]
Papaver somniferum	Morphine and related alkaloids
Peganum harmala	Harmine and related alkaloids
Psoralea corylifolia	Photosensitizing psoralens [334]
Rauvolfia serpentina	Reserpine and other alkaloids
Ricinus communis	Purgative seed oil
Rubia cordifolia	Alizarin derivatives
Strychnos nux-vomica	Strychnine [333]***
Terminalia arjuna	Cardiac stimulants

*Other *Aristolochia* spp. used in Indian folk medicine are *A. bracteata, A. tagala,* and *A. indica* [335].
**Another *Datura* sp. used in Ayurvedic medicine is *D. stramonium* [333].
***The seeds are often processed to remove this toxic alkaloid [332].

REFERENCES

1. Sperl W, Stuppner H, Gassner I, et al. Reversible hepatic veno-occlusive disease in an infant after consumption of pyrrolizidine-containing herbal tea. Eur J Pediatrics 1995;154:112–116.
2. De Smet PAGM. Drugs used in non-orthodox medicine. In: Dukes MNG, Beeley L, eds. Side effects of drugs - Annual 13. Amsterdam: Elsevier, 1989:442–473.
3. Schier W, Sachsa B, Schultze W. Aktuelle Verfälschungen von Arzneidrogen. 5. Mitteilung - Birkenblätter, Orthosiphonblätter, Besenginsterblüten, Wohlriechendes Gänsefusskraut und Isländisches Moos. Dtsch Apoth Ztg 1994;134:4569–4576.
4. Greinwald R, Lurz G, Witte L, Czygan F-C. A survey of alkaloids in *Spartium junceum* L. (Genisteae-Fabaceae). Z Naturforsch Sect C Biosci 1990;45:1085–1089.
5. Barboni L, Manzi A, Bellomaria B, Quinto AM. Alkaloid content in four *Spartium junceum* populations as a defensive strategy against predators. Phytochemistry 1994;37:1197–1200.
6. De Smet PAGM. Should herbal medicine-like products be licensed as medicines. Special licensing seems the best way forward. BMJ 310:1023–1024.
7. Tyler VE. Herbal remedies. J Pharm Technol 1995;11:214–220.
8. Hsu CK, Leo P, Shastry D, Meggs W, et al. Anticholinergic poisoning associated with herbal tea. Arch Intern Med 1995;155:2245–2248.
9. De Smet PAGM. Toxicological outlook on the quality assurance of herbal remedies. In: De Smet PAGM, Keller K, Hänsel R, Chandler RF, eds. Adverse effects of herbal drugs. Volume 1. Heidelberg: Springer-Verlag, 1992:1–72 .
10. Anonymous. European pharmacopoeia, 3rd ed. Strasbourg: Council of Europe, 1996.
11. Oliver MR, Van Voorhis WC, Boeck H, et al. Hepatic mucormycosis in a bone marrow transplant recipient who ingested naturopathic medicine. Clin Infect Dis 1996;22:521–524.
12. Abeywickrama K, Bean GA. Toxigenic *Aspergillus flavus* and aflatoxins in Sri Lankan medicinal plant material. Mycopathologia 1991;113:187–190.

13. Abeywickrama K, Bean GA. Cytotoxicity of *Fusarium* species mycotoxins and culture filtrates of *Fusarium* species isolated from the medicinal plant *Tribulus terrestris* to mammalian cells. Mycopathologia 1992;120:189–193.

14. Ros JJW, Pelders MG, De Smet PAGM. Positive doping case associated with the use of an ephedra-labeled health food product. Unpublished manuscript.

15. De Smet PAGM, Smeets OSNM. Potential risks of health food products containing yohimbe extracts. BMJ 1994;309:958.

16. De Smet PAGM. Yohimbe alkaloids—general discussion. In: De Smet PAGM, Keller K, Hänsel R, Chandler RF, eds. Adverse effects of herbal drugs. Volume 3. Heidelberg: Springer-Verlag, 1997:181–205.

17. Anonymous. Ostrich fern poisoning - New York and Western Canada, 1994. MMWR 1994;43:677–684.

18. Lai R-S, Chiang AA, Wu M-T, et al. Outbreak of bronchiolitis obliterans associated with the consumption of *Sauropus androgynus* in Taiwan. Lancet 1996;348:83–85.

19. Haynes RL. Carbon-monoxide poisoning from non-tobacco cigarettes. J Med Assoc Ga 1983;72:553-5

20. King M. Nontobacco cigarettes. Can Med Assoc J 1985;133:13

21. Bloom JW, Kaltenborn WT, Paoletti P, et al. Respiratory effects of non-tobacco cigarettes. BMJ 1987;295:1516-8

22. Sherrill DL, Kryzanowski M, Bloom JW, Lebowitz MD. Respiratory effects of non-tobacco cigarettes: a longitudinal study in the general population. Int J Epidemiol 1991;20:132-7

23. Nahas G, Latour C. The human toxicity of marijuana. Medi J Aust 1992;156:495-7

24. Polen MR, Sidney S, Tekawa IS, Sadler M, Friedman GD. Health care use by frequent marijuana smokers who do not smoke tobacco. West Med J 1993;158:596-601

25. Kumar A, Aitas AT, Hunter AG, Beaman DC. Sweeteners, dyes, and other excipients in vitamin and mineral preparations. Clin Pediatr 1996;35:443–450.

26. Eun HC, Lee AY. Contact dermatitis due to Madecassol. Contact Dermatitis 1985;13:310.

27. Cronin E. Contact dermatitis. Edinburgh: Churchill Livingstone, 1980.

28. Bruynzeel DP, Van Ketel WG, Young E, et al. Contact sensitization by alternative topical medicaments containing plant extracts. Contact Dermatitis 1992;27:278–279.

29. Ali SA, Blume H. Pestizidrückstände in Adeps Lanae anhydricus und Babycremes. Pharm Ztg 1986;131:1638–1640.

30. Coplenad CA, Raebel MA, Wagner SL. Pesticide residues in lanolin. JAMA 1989;261:242 .

31. De Jong CAJ. Melisana, voor uw broodnodige rust? Ned Tijdschr Geneeskd 1978;122:82–83.

32. Pradeepkumar VK, Tan KW, Ivy NG. Is 'herbal health tonic' safe in pregnancy, fetal alcohol syndrome revisited. Aust N Z J Obstet Gynaecol 1996;36:420–423.

33. Anonymous. Over-the-counter drug products intended for oral ingestion that contain alcohol. Fed Reg 1995;60:13590–13595.

34. Yeung CY, Lee FT, Wong HN. Effect of a popular Chinese herb on neonatal bilirubin protein binding. Biol Neonate 1990;58:98–103.

35. Chan E. Displacement of bilirubin from albumin by berberine. Biol Neonate 1993;63:201–208.

36. Chan TYK. The prevalence use and harmful potential of some Chinese herbal medicines in babies and children. Vet Hum Toxicol 1994;36:238–240.

37. Newton BW, Benson RC, McCarriston CC. Sparteine sulphate: a potent capricious oxytocic. Am J Obstet Gynecol 1996;94:234–241.

38. De Smet PAGM, Brouwers JRBJ. Pharmacokinetic evaluation of herbal remedies: basic introduction, applicability, current status and regulatory needs. Clin Pharmacokinet 1997;32:427–436.

39. Zhou H-H, Adedoyin A, Wood AJJ. Differing effects of atropine on heart rate in Chinese and white subjects. Clin Pharmacol Ther 1992;52:120–124.

40. Carbo M, Segura J, De la Torre R, et al. Effect of quinolones on caffeine disposition. Clin Pharmacol Ther 1989;45:234–240.

41. Harder S, Fuhr U, Staib AH, Wolff T. Ciprofloxacin-caffeine: a drug interaction established using in vivo and in vitro investigations. Am J Med 1989;87:89S-91S.

42. Healy DP, Polk RE, Kanawati L, et al. Interaction between oral ciprofloxacin and caffeine in normal volunteers. Antimicrob Agents Chemother 1989;33:474–478.

43. Mahr G, Soergel F, Granneman GR, et al. Effects of temafloxacin and ciprofloxacin on the pharmacokinetics of caffeine. Clin Pharmacokin 1992;22(Suppl 1):90–97.

44. Gram LF, Debruyne D, Caillard V, et al. Substantial rise in sparteine metabolic ratio during haloperidol treatment. Br J Clin Pharmacol 1989;27:272–275.

45. Gram LF, Brosen K, Danish University Antidepressant Group. Moclobemide treatment causes a substantial rise in the sparteine metabolic ratio. Br J Clin Pharmacol 1993;35:649–652.

46. Schellens JH, Ghabrial H, van der Wart HH, et al. Differential effects of quinidine on the disposition of nifedipine, sparteine, and mephenytoin in humans. Clin Pharmacol Ther 1991;50:520–528.

47. Anonymous. Adverse events associated with ephedrine-containing products—Texas, December 1993–September 1995. MMWR 1996;45:689–693.

48. Leatherdale BA, Panesar RK, Singh G, et al. Improvement in glucose tolerance due to *Momordica charantia* (karela). BMJ 1981;282:1823–1824.

49. Aslam M, Stockley IH. Interactions between curry in gredient (karela) and drug (chlorpropamide). Lancet 1979;1:607.

50. De Smet PAGM, D'Arcy PF. Drug interactions with herbal and other non-orthodox drugs. In: Wellington PJ, D'Arcy PF, eds. Drug interactions. Heidelberg: Springer-Verlag, 1996:327–352.

51. Ljunggren B. Severe phototoxic burn following celery ingestion. Arch Dermatol 1990;126:1334–1336.

52. Boffa MJ, Gilmour E, Ead RD. Celery soup causing severe phototoxicity during PUVA therapy. Br J Dermatol 1996;135:330–345.

53. De Smet PAGM. Alternatieve middelen en verkeersveiligheid. Arts en Auto 1987;53:1684–1686.

54. De Smet PAGM, Elferink F, Verpoorte R. Linksdraaiend tetrahydropalmatine in Chinese tablet. Ned Tijdschr Geneesk 1989;133:308.

55. Anonymous. Definition of doping and list of doping classes and methods. International Olympic Committee Medical Commission. Paris, September 5, 1994.

56. Hiller K. Ephedra. In: Hänsel R, Keller K, Rimpler H, Schneider G, eds. Hagers Handbuch der Pharmazeutischen Praxis. 5th edn. Fünfter Band: Drogen E-O. Berlin: Springer-Verlag, 1993:46–57.

57. Anonymous. Het eeuwige gevecht tegen de kilo's. Consumentengids 1995;5:296–300.

58. De Smet PAGM. Drugs used in non-orthodox medicine. In: Dukes MNG, Beeley L, eds. Side effects of drugs - Annual 14. Amsterdam: Elsevier, 1990:429–451.

59. De Smet PAGM. Drugs used in non-orthodox medicine. In: Dukes MNG, ed. Side effects of drugs. 11th ed. Amsterdam: Elsevier, 1992:1209–1232.

60. De Smet PAGM. Legislatory outlook on the safety of herbal remedies. In: De Smet PAGM, Hänsel R, Keller K, Chandler RF, eds. Adverse effects of herbal drugs. Volume 2. Heidelberg: Springer-Verlag 1993:1–90.

61. Ernst E, De Smet PAGM. Risks associated with complementary therapies. In: Dukes MNG, ed. Side effects of drugs. 13th ed. Amsterdam: Elsevier, 1996:1427–1454.

62. De Smet PAGM, Keller K, Hänsel R, Chandler RF, eds. Adverse effects of herbal drugs. Volume 1. Heidelberg: Springer-Verlag, 1992.

63. De Smet PAGM, Keller K, Hänsel R, Chandler RF, eds. Adverse effects of herbal drugs. Volume 2. Heidelberg: Springer-Verlag, 1993.

64. De Smet PAGM, Keller K, Hänsel R, Chandler RF, eds. Adverse effects of herbal drugs. Volume 3. Heidelberg: Springer-Verlag, 1997.

65. Tyler VE. The new honest herbal. A sensible guide to the use of herbs and related remedies. 3rd ed. Binghamton: Pharmaceutical Products Press, 1993.

66. Bisset NG, Wichtl M, eds. Herbal drugs and phytopharmaceuticals. A handbook for practice on a scientific basis. Stuttgart: Medpharm Scientific Publishers, 1994.

67. Newall CA, Anderson LA, Phillipson JD. Herbal medicines. A guide for health-care professionals. London: The Pharmaceutical Press, 1996.

68. Leung AY, Foster S. Encyclopedia of common natural ingredients used in food, drugs, and cosmetics. 2nd ed. New York: John Wiley & Sons, Inc., 1996.

69. Hänsel R, Keller K, Rimpler H, Schneider G, red. Hagers Handbuch der Pharmazeutischen Praxis. 5th edn. Vierter Band: Drogen A-D. Berlin: Springer-Verlag, 1992.

70. Hänsel R, Keller K, Rimpler H, Schneider G, red. Hagers Handbuch der Pharmazeutischen Praxis. 5th edn. Fünfter Band: Drogen E-O. Berlin: Springer-Verlag, 1993.

71. Hänsel R, Keller K, Rimpler H, Schneider G, red. Hagers Handbuch der Pharmazeutischen Praxis. 5th edn. Fünfter Band: Drogen P-Z. Berlin: Springer-Verlag, 1994.

72. Roth L, Daunderer M, Kormann K. Giftpflanzen - Pflanzengifte: Wirkung, Vorkommen, Wirkung, Therapie; allergische und phototoxische Reaktionen. 4. Auflage, Landsberg: Ecomed, 1994.

73. Teuscher E, Lindequist U. Biogene Gifte. Biologie - Chemie -Pharmakologie. 2. Auflage. Stuttgart: Gustav Fischer, 1994.

74. Wichtl M, red. Teedrogen und Phytopharmaka. Ein Handbuch für die Praxis auf wissenschaf-

tlicher Grundlage. 3. Auflage. Stuttgart: Wissenschaftliche Verlagsgesellschaft, 1997.

75. Frohne D, Pfänder HJ Giftpflanzen. Ein Handbuch für Apotheker, Ärzte, Toxikologen und Biologen. 4. Auflage. Stuttgart, Wissenschaftliche Verlagsgesellschaft, 1997.

76. Mitchell J, Rook A. Botanical dermatology. Plants and plant products injurious to the skin. Vancouver: Greengrass, 1979.

77. Longerich L, Johnson E, Gault MH. Digoxin-like factors in herbal teas. Clin Invest Med 1993;16:210–218.

78. Malinow MR, Bardana EJ Jr, Goodnight SH Jr. Pancytopenia during ingestion of alfalfa seeds. Lancet 1981;1:615.

79. Roberts JL, Hayashi JA. Exacerbation of SLE associated with alfalfa ingestion. N Engl J Med 1983;308:1361.

80. Kaufman WH. Alfalfa seed dermatitis. JAMA 1954;155:1058–1059.

81. Ossenkoppele PM, Van Der Sluis WG, Van Vloten WA. Fototoxische dermatitis door het gebruik van de Ammi majus-vrucht bij vitiligo. Ned Tijdschr Geneeskd 1991;135:478–480.

82. De Smet PAGM, Vulto AG. Drugs used in nonorthodox medicine. In: Dukes MNG, Beeley L, eds. Side effects of drugs - Annual 12. Amsterdam: Elsevier, 1988:402–415.

83. DeSmet PAGM. Heal risks of herbal remedies. Drug Safety 1995;13:81–93.

84. Siegers C-P, Von Hertzberg-Lottin E, Otte M, Schneider B. Antrhanoid laxative abuse—a risk for colorectal cancer? Gut 1993;34:1099–1101.

85. Kommission E. Aufbereitungsmonographien. Dtsch Apoth Ztg 1993;133:2791–2794.

86. Anonymous. Anthranoid-haltige Humanarzneimittel. Pharm Ztg 1994;139:2432.

87. Anonymous. Humanarzneimittel. Pharm Ztg 1996;141:2716–2717.

88. DeSmet PAGM. *Aristolochia* species. In: DeSmet PAGM, Keller K, Hansel R, Chandler RF, eds. Adverse effects of herbal drugs. Volume 1, Heidelberg: Springer-Verlag, 1992:79–89.

89. Mengs U, Stotzem CD. Renal toxicity of aristolochic acid in rats as an example of nephrotoxicity testing in routine toxicology. Arch Toxicol 1993;67:307–311.

90. Pena JM, Borras M, Ramos J, Montoliu J. Rapidly progressive interstitial renal fibrosis due to a chronic intake of a herb (*Aristolochia pistolochia*) infusion. Nephrol Dial Transplant 1996;11:1359–1360.

91. Kelly KJ, Neu J, Camitta BM, Honig GR. Methemoglobinemia in an infant treated with the folk remedy glycerited asafoetida. Pediatrics 1984;73:717–719.

92. Caravaca Magariños F, Cubero Gomez JJ, et al. Afectación renal y hepática en la intoxicación por Atractylis gummifera. Nefrologia 1985;5:205–210.

93. Nogue S, Sanz P, Botey A, et al. Insuffisance renale aigue due a une intoxication par le chardon a glu (Atractylis gummigera-L). Presse Méd 1992;21:130.

94. Müller AH. Über Vergiftung mit Besenginster (Sarothamnus scoparius). Dtsch Med Wschr 1951;75:1027.

95. Rodriguez P, Blanco J, Juste S, et al. Allergic contact dermatitis due to burdock (Arctium lappa). Contact Dermatitis 1995;33:134–135.

96. Widgren S, De Peyer R, Geissbühler P, Stalder H. Enterocolite due à un médicament contenant des saponines. Schweiz Med Wschr 1994; 124:313–318.

97. Landa N, Aguirre A, Goday J, et al. Allergic contact dermatitis from a vasoconstrictor cream. Contact Dermatitis 1990;22:290–291.

98. Bluhm R, Branch R, Johnston P, Stein R. Aplastic anemia associated with canthaxanthin ingested for 'tanning' purposes. JAMA 1990;264:1141–1142.

99. Angelini G, Vena GA, Filotico R, et al. Allergic contact dermatitis from *Capparis spinosa* L. applied as wet compresses. Contact Dermatitis 1991;24:382–383.

100. Tuncok Y, Kozan O, Cavdar C, et al. Urginea maritima (squill) toxicity. J Toxicol Clin Toxicol 1995;33:83–86.

101. Anonymous. Poisoning associated with herbal teas—Arizona, Washington. MMWR 1977;26: 257–259.

102. Bain RJI. Accidental digitalis poisoning due to drinking herbal tea. BMJ 1985;290:1624.

103. Koopmann H. Tödliche Schöllkraut-Vergiftung (Chelidonium majus). Vergiftungsfälle 1937;8: 93–98.

104. Pinto Garcỳa V, Vicente PR, Barez A, et al. Anemia hemolỳtica inducida por *Chelidonium majus*. Observación clỳnica. Sangre 1990;35:401–403.

105. Subiza J, Subiza JL, Hinojosa M, et al. Anaphylactic reaction after the ingestion of chamomile tea: a study of cross-reactivity with other composite pollens. J Allergy Clin Immunol 1989; 84:353–358.

106. Subiza J, Subiza JL, Alonso M, et al. Allergic conjunctivitis to chamomile tea. Ann Allergy 1990;65:127–132.

107. Balslev T, Moller AB. Forbraendinger hos born forarsaget af kamillete. Ugeskr Laeg 1990; 152:1384.

108. Gordon DW, Rosenthal G, Hart J, et al. Chaparral ingestion. The broadening spectrum of liver injury caused by herbal medications. JAMA 1995;273:489–490.

109. Batchelor WB, Heathcote J, Wanless IR. Chaparral-induced hepatic injury. Am J Gastroenterol 1995;90:831–833.

110. Katz M, Saibil F. Herbal hepatitis: subacute hepatic necrosis secondary to chaparral leaf. J Clin Gastroenterol 1990;12:203–206.

111. Anonymous. Chaparral-induced toxic hepatitis— California and Texas, 1992. MMWR 1992; 41:812–814.

112. Smith BC, Desmond PV. Acute hepatitis induced by ingestion of the herbal medication chaparral. Aust NZ J Med 1993;23:526.

113. Alderman S, Kailas S, Goldfarb S, et al. Cholestatic hepatitis after ingestion of chaparral leaf: confirmation by endoscopic retrograde cholangiopancreatography and liver biopsy. J Clin Gastroenterol 1994;19:242–247.

114. Grice HC, Becking G, Goodman T. Toxic properties of nordihydroguaiaretic acid. Food Cosmet Toxicol 1968;6:155–161.

115. Goodman T, Grice HC, Becking GC, Salem FA. A cystic nephropathy induced by nordihydroguaiaretic acid in the rat. Light and electron microscopic investigations. Lab Invest 1970;23: 93–107.

116. Gardner KD Jr, Evan AP, Reed WP. Accelerated renal cyst development in deconditioned germ-free rats. Kidney Int 1986;29:1116–1123.

117. Smith AY, Feddersen RM, Gardner Jr KD, Davis Jr CJ. Cystic renal cell carcinoma and acquired renal cystic disease associated with consumption of chaparral tea: a case report. J Urol 1994;152:2089–2091.

118. Cahill DJ, Fox R, Wardle PG, Harlow CR. Multiple follicular development associated with herbal medicine. Hum Reprod 1994;9:1469–1470.

119. Eisele JW, Reay DT. Deaths related to coffee enemas. JAMA 1980;244:1608–1609.

120. Green S. A critique of the rationale for cancer treatment with coffee enemas and diet. JAMA 1992;268:3224–3227.

121. Berrut C, Bisetti A, Widgren S, et al. Colite pseudomembraneuse causée par l'ingestion de coloquinte. Schweiz Med Wschr 1987;117:135–138.

122. Al Faraj S. Haemorrhagic colitis induced by Citrullus colocynthis. Ann Trop Med Parasitol 1995;89:695–696.

123. Cox D, O'Kennedy R, Thornes RD. The rarity of liver toxicity in patients treated with coumarin (1,2-benzopyrone). Hum Toxicol 1989;8: 501–506.

124. Hogan III RP. Hemorrhagic diathesis caused by drinking an herbal tea. JAMA 1983;249:2679.

125. Glaeser S, Hecker E. Drugs from Euphorbiaceae and Thymelaeaceae as possible health hazards: phytotherapeutics derived from Croton tiglium—an iatrogenic risk of cancer? Planta Med 1991;57(Suppl.2):A50–A51.

126. Stadler HW, Dietzel U, Sauer R. Erfahrungen mit einem "Onkophytotherapeutikum". Dtsch Med Wchschr 1985;110:1184–1185.

127. Dietzel U, Sauer R, Reichardt U. Erfahrungen mit Carnivora. Fortschr Med 1985;103:760–761.

128. Anonymous. Carnivora(R)—Masznahmen des Bundesgesundheits amtes. Pharm Ztg 1986; 131:109–110.

129. Hecker E, Gläser S, Gminski R. Konditionalkanzerogene als eine neuartige Kategorie vorn Krebsrisikofaktoren am Beispiel der Tumorpromotoren des Diterpenestertyps. Pharm Ztg Wiss 1991;4(5/6):1–16.

130. Anonymous. Immunallergische Reaktionen nach Echinacea-Extrakten (Echinacin, Esberitox N u.a.). Arznei-Telegramm 1991;4:39.

131. Anonymous. Wie verträglich sind Echinacea-haltige Präparate? Deutsches Ärzteblatt 1996; 93:2723.

132. Schilcher H. Ätherische Öle—Wirkungen und Nebenwirkungen, Dtsch Apoth Ztg 1984; 124:1433.

133. Tisserand R, Balacs T. Essential oil safety. A guide for health care professionals. Edinburgh: Churchill Livingstone, 1995.

134. Schaller M, Korting HC. Allergic airborne contact dermatitis from essential oils used in aromatherapy. Clin Exp Dermatol 1995;20:143–145.

135. Bilsland D, Strong A. Allergic contact dermatitis from the essential oil of French marigold (Tagetes patula) in an aromatherapist. Contact Dermatitis 1990;23:55–56.

136. Gminski R, Hecker E. Drugs from Euphorbiaceae and Thymelaeaceae as possible health hazards: homeopathics derived from Euphorbia cyparissias and Daphne mezereum—an iatrogenic risk of cancer? Planta Med 1991;57(Suppl.2):A50.

137. German K, Kumar U, Blackford HN. Garlic and the risk of TURP bleeding. Br J Urol 1995;76:518.

138. Burnham BE. Garlic as a possible risk for postoperative bleeding. Plast Reconstruct Surg 1995; 95:213.

139. Rose KD, Croissant PD, Parliament CF, Levin MB. Spontaneous spinal epidural hematoma with associated platelet dysfunction from excessive garlic ingestion: a case report. Neurosurgery 1990;26:880–882.

140. Lee TY, Lam TH. Contact dermatitis due to topical treatment with garlic in Hong Kong. Contact Dermatitis 1991;24:193–196.

141. Garty B-Z. Garlic burns. Pediatrics 1993;91: 658–659.

142. Canduela V, Mongil I, Carrascosa M, et al. Garlic: always good for the health? Br J Dermatol 1995;132:161–162.

143. Rowin J, Lewis SL. Spontaneous bilateral subdural hematomas associated with chronic Ginkgo biloba ingestion. Neurology 1996;46:1775–1776.

144. Rosenblatt M, Mindel J. Spontaneous hyphema associated with ingestion of *Ginkgo biloba* extract. N Engl J Med 1997;336:1108.

145. Koren G, Randor S, Martin S, Danneman D. Maternal ginseng use associated with neonatal androgenization. JAMA 1990;264:2866.

146. Awang DVC. Maternal use of ginseng and neonatal androgenization. JAMA 1991;266:363.

147. Quatrehomme G, Bertrand F, Chauvet C, Ollier A. Intoxication from *Veratrum album*. Hum Exp Toxicol 1993;12:111–115.

148. Rubin HR, Wu AW. The bitter herbs of Seder: more on horseradish horrors. JAMA 1988; 259:1943.

149. De Smet PAGM, Vulto AG. Drugs used in nonorthodox medicine. In: Dukes MNG, ed. Side effects of drugs - Annual 11. Amsterdam: Elsevier, 1987:422–431.

150. Hulbert DC, Thorpe PJ, Winning AJ, Beckett MW. Fatal bronchospasm after oral ingestion of isphagula. Postgrad Med J 1995;71:305–306.

151. Pye KG, Kelsey SM, House IM, Newland AC. Severe dyserythropoiesis and autoimmune thrombocytopenia associated with ingestion of kelp supplements. Lancet 1992;339:1540.

152. Perron AD, Patterson JA, Yanofsky NN. Kombucha "mushroom" hepatotoxicity. Ann Emerg Med 1995;26:660–661.

153. Anonymous. Kombucha tea. Aust Adv Drug React Bull 1997;16(2):6.

154. Currier RW, Goddard J, Buechler K, et al. Unexplained severe illness possibly associated with consumption of kombucha tea—Iowa 1995. MMWR 1995;44:892–900.

155. Stormer FC, Reistad R, Alexander J. Glycyrrhizic acid in liquorice—evaluation of health hazard. Food Chem Toxicol 1993;31:303–312.

156. Chandler RF. *Glycyrrhiza glabra*. In: De Smet PAGM, Keller K, Hänsel R, Chandler RF, eds. Adverse effects of herbal drugs. Volume 3. Heidelberg: Springer-Verlag, 1997:67–87.

157. BGA-Pressedienst. Widerruf der Zulassung für Krappwurzelhaltige Arzneimittel angeordnet. Berlin: Bundesgesundheitsamt, 1993.

158. De Smet PAGM, Stricker BHC. Meekrapwortel in Duitsland niet langer toegestaan. Pharm Weekbl 1993;128:503.

159. Cassidy DE, Drewry J, Fanning JP. Podophyllum toxicity: a report of a fatal case and a review of the literature. Clin Toxicol 1982;19:35–44.

160. Dobb GJ, Edis RH. Coma and neuropathy after ingestion of herbal laxative containing podophyllin. Med J Aust 1984;140:495–496.

161. Chan TH, Wong KC, Chan JCN. Severe salicylate poisoning associated with the intake of Chinese medicinal oil (Red Flower Oil). Aust NZ J Med 1995;25:57.

162. Pichler WJ, Angeli R. Allergie auf Mistelextrakt. Dtsch Med Wschr 1991;116:1333–1334.

163. Harvey J, Colin-Jones DG. Mistletoe hepatitis. BMJ 1981;282:186–187.

164. Kurz G, Rapaport MJ. External/internal allergy to plants (Artemisia). Contact Dermatitis 1979;5:407–408.

165. Mansfield LE, Ting S, Haverly RW, Yoo TJ. The incidence and clinical implications of hypersensitivity to papain in an allergic population, confirmed by blinded oral challenge. Ann Allergy 1985;55:541–543.

166. Bernstein DI, Gallagher JS, Grad M, Bernstein IL. Local ocular anaphylaxis to papain enzyme contained in a contact lens cleansing solution. J Allergy Clin Immunol 1984;258–260.

167. Sagona MA, Bruszer GV, Lin L, et al. Evaluation of papain/chymopapain cross allergenicity. J Allergy Clin Immunol 1985;76:776–781.

168. Anderson IB, Mullen WH, Meeker JE, et al. Pennyroyal toxicity: measurement of toxic metabolite levels in two cases and review of the literature. Ann Intern Med 1996;124:726–734.

169. Bakerink JA, Gospe Jr SM, Dimand RJ, Eldridge MW. Multiple organ failure after ingestion of pennyroyal oil from herbal tea in two infants. Pediatrics 1996;98:944–947.

170. Sasseville D, Nguyen KH. Allergic contact dermatitis from Rhus toxicodendron in a phytotherapeutic preparation. Contact Dermatitis 1995; 32:182–183.

171. Hamilton RJ, Shih RD, Hoffman RS. Mobitz type I heart block after pokeweed ingestion. Vet Hum Toxicol 1995;37:66–67.

172. Dechamp C. Anaphylaxis following pollen ingestion. Allerg Immunol (Paris) 1986;18:2.

173. Mirkin G. Can bee pollen benefit health? JAMA 1989;262:1854.

174. Chivato T, Juan F, Montoro A, Laguna R. Ana-

phylaxis induced by ingestion of a pollen compound. J Investig Allergol Clin Immunol 1996;6:208–209.

175. Suhonen R, Kantola I, Björksten F. Anaphylactic shock due to ingestion of psyllium laxative. Allergy 1983;38:363–365.

176. Lantner RR, Espiritu BR, Zumerchik P, Tobin MC. Anaphylaxis following ingestion of a psyllium-containing cereal. JAMA 1990;264:2534–2536.

177. Bah M, Bye R, Pereda-Miranda R. Hepatotoxic pyrrolizidine alkaloids in the Mexican medicinal plant *Packera candidissima* (Asteraceae: Senecioneae). J Ethnopharmacol 1994;43:19–30.

178. Mattocks AR. Chemistry and toxicology of pyrrolizidine alkaloids. New York: Academic Press, 1986.

179. Anonymous. Pyrrolizidine Alkaloids. Environmental Health Criteria 80. Geneva: World Health Organization, 1988.

180. Westendorf J. Pyrrolizidine alkaloids—general discussion. In: De Smet PAGM, Keller K, Hänsel R, Chandler RF, eds. Adverse effects of herbal drugs. Volume 1. Heidelberg: Springer- Verlag, 1992:193–205.

181. Stuart KL, Bras G. Veno-occlusive disease of the liver. Quart Med J 1957;26:291–315.

182. McGee J, Patrick RS, Wood CB, Blumgart LH. A case of veno-occlusive disease of the liver in Britain associated with herbal tea consumption. J Clin Pathol 1976;29:788–794.

183. Ortiz Cansado A, Crespo Valades E, Morales Blanco P, et al. Enfermedad venooclusiva hepatica por ingestion de infusiones de *Senecio vulgaris*. Gastroenterol Hepatol 1995;18:413–416.

184. Roulet M, Laurini R, Rivier L, Calame A. Hepatic veno-occlusive disease in newborn infant of a woman drinking herbal tea. J Pediatr 1988;112:433–436.

185. Spang R. Toxicity of tea containing pyrrolizidine alkaloids. J Pediatrics 1989;115:1025.

186. Anonymous. Vorinformation Pyrrolizidinalkaloidhaltige Humanarzneimittel. Pharm Ztg 1990;135:2532–2533,2623–2624.

187. Anonymous. Aufbereitungsmonographien Kommission E. Pharm Ztg 1990;135:2081–2082.

188. El Sayed F, Manzur F, Marguery MC, et al. Urticarial manifestations due to *Raphanus niger*. Contact Dermatitis 1995;32:241.

189. Participating Veterans Administration Medical Centers. Low doses *v* standard dose of reserpine. A randomized, double-blind, multiclinic trial in patients taking chlorthalidone. JAMA 1982;248:2471–2477.

190. Freis ED. Mental depression in hypertensive patients treated for long periods with large doses of reserpine. N Engl J Med 1954;251:1006–1008.

191. Goodwin FK, Bunney Jr WE. Depressions following reserpine: a reevaluation. Sem Psychiatry 1971;3:435–448.

192. De Smet PAGM. Een alternatieve olie met een luchtje. Pharm Weekbl 1994;129:258.

193. Arzneimittelkommission der Deutschen Apotheker. Vorinformation Sassafras-haltige Arzneimittel. Dtsch Apoth Ztg 1995;135:366–368.

194. Mengs U. Toxic effects of sennosides in laboratory animals and in vitro. Pharmacology 1988;36(Suppl.1):180–187.

195. Sandnes D, Johansen T, Teien G, Ulsaker G. Mutagenicity of crude senna and senna glycosides in *Salmonella typhimurium*. Pharmacol Toxicol 1992;71:165–172.

196. Lydén-Sokolowski A, Nilsson A, Sjöberg P. Two-year carcinogenicity study with sennosides in the rat: emphasis on gastro-intestinal alterations. Pharmacology 1993;47(Suppl 1):209–215.

197. Mengs U. Reproductive toxicological investigations with sennosides. Arzneim Forsch 1986;36:1355–1358.

198. Faber P, Strenge-Hesse A. Relevance of rhein excretion into breast milk. Pharmacology 1988;36(Suppl.1):212–220.

199. Beuers U, Spengler U, Pape GR. Hepatitis after chronic abuse of senna. Lancet 1991;337:372–373.

200. Prior J, White I. Tetany and clubbing in a patient who ingested large quantities of senna. Lancet 1978;2:947.

201. Armstrong RD, Crisp AJ, Grahame R, Woolf DL. Hypertrophic osteoarthropathy and purgative abuse. BMJ 1981;282:1836.

202. Hausen BM. Sesquiterpene lactones. In: De Smet PAGM, Keller K, Hänsel R, Chandler RF, eds. Adverse effects of herbal drugs. Volume 1. Heidelberg: Springer-Verlag, 1992:227–260.

203. Hausen BM, Breuer J, Weglewski J, Rücker G. α-Peroxyachifolid and other new sensitizing sesquiterpene lactones from yarrow (*Achillea millefolium* L., Compositae). Contact Dermatitis 1991;24:274–280.

204. Beier RC, Norman JO, Reagor JC, et al. Isolation of the major component in white snakeroot that is toxic after microsomal activation: possible explanation of sporadic toxicity of white snakeroot plants and extracts. Natural Toxins 1993;1:286–293.

205. Plouvier B, Trotin F, Deram R, et al. Concombre

d'ane (*Ecabalium elaterium*) une cause peu banale d'oedème de Quincke. Nouv Presse Méd 1981;10:2590.

206. Vlachos P, Kanitsakis NN, Kokonas N. Fatal cardiac and renal failure due to *Ecbalium elaterium* (squirting cucumber). J Toxicol Clin Toxicol 1994;32:737–738.

207. Yesilada E, Tanaka S, Sezik E, Tabata M. Isolation of an anti-inflammatory principle from the fruit juice of *Ecballium elaterium*. J Nat Prod 1988;51:504–508.

208. Geier J, Fuchs T, Wahl R. Anaphylaktischer Schock durch einen Mariendistel-Extrakt bei Soforttyp-Allergie auf Kiwi. Allergologie 1990; 13:387–388.

209. Woelk H, Burkard G, Grünwald J. Benefits and risks of the Hypericum extract LI 160: drug monitoring study with 3250 patients. J Geriatr Psychiatry Neurol 1994;7(suppl 1):S34-S38.

210. Axelsson IGK, Ihre E, Zetterström O. Anaphylactic reactions to sunflower seed. Allergy 1994; 49:517–520.

211. Knight TE, Hausen BM. Melaleuca oil (tea tree oil) dermatitis. J Am Acad Dermatol 1994; 30:423–427.

212. Anonymous. Kontaktallergie gegen Teebaumöl (MELALEUKA u.a.). Arznei-Telegramm 1997; 2:23.

213. Elliott C. Tea tree oil poisoning. Med J Aust 1993;159:830–831.

214. Seawright A. Tea tree oil poisoning. Med J Aust 1993;159:830–831.

216. Garcia-Estrad H. Fischman CM. An unusual case of nicotine poisoning. Clin Toxicol 1977; 10:391–393.

216. Dieckmann H. Untersuchungen zur Pharmakokinetik, Metabolismus und Toxikologie von Baldrinalen. Inaugural-Dissertation. Berlin: Freie Universität, 1988.

217. Del Pozo MD, Gastaminza G, Navarro JA, et al. Allergic contact dermatitis from *Verbena officinalis*. Contact Dermatitis 1994;31:200–201.

218. Castot A, Larrey D. Hépatites observées au cours d'un traitement par un médicament ou une tisane contenant de la germandrée petit-chêne. Bilan des 26 cas rapportés aux Centres Régionaux de Pharmacovigilance. Gastroenterol Clin Biol 1992; 16:916–922.

219. Laliberté L, Villeneuve J-P. Hepatitis after the use of germander, a herbal remedy. Can Med Assoc J 1996;154:1689–1692.

220. Mostefa-Kara N, Pauwels A, Pines E, et al. Fatal hepatitis after herbal tea. Lancet 1992;340:674.

221. Loeper J, Descatoire V, Letteron P, et al. Hepatotoxicity of germander in mice. Gastroenterology 1994;106:464–472.

222. Kouzi SA, McMurtry RJ, Nelson SD. Hepatotoxicity of germander (Teucrium chamaedrys L.) and one of its constituent neoclerodane diterpenes teucrin A in the mouse. Chem Res Toxicol 1994;7:850–856.

223. Mattei A, Rucay P, Samuel D, et al. Liver transplantation for severe acute liver failure after herbal medicine (*Teucrium polium*) administration. J Hepatol 1995;22:597.

224. Granlund H. Contact allergy to witch hazel. Contact Dermatitis 1994;31:195.

225. Winterhoff H. *Lycopus* species. In: De Smet PAGM, Keller K, Hänsel R, Chandler RF, red. Adverse effects of herbal drugs. Volume 2. Heidelberg: Springer-Verlag, 1993:245–251.

226. De Smet PAGM. Yohimbe alkaloids—*Pausinystalia* species. In: De Smet PAGM, Keller K, Hänsel R, Chandler RF, eds. Adverse effects of herbal drugs. Volume 3. Heidelberg: Springer-Verlag, 1997:211–214.

227. De Smet PAGM. Yohimbe alkaloids—*Corynanthe* species. In: De Smet PAGM, Keller K, Hänsel R, Chandler RF, eds. Adverse effects of herbal drugs. Volume 3. Heidelberg: Springer-Verlag, 1997:207–209.

228. Schultes RE, Hofmann A. The botany and chemistry of hallucinogens. 2nd ed. Springfield: Charles C.Thomas Publisher, 1980.

229. De Smet PAGM. Ritual enemas and snuffs in the Americas. Ph.D. Thesis. Latin America Studies no.33, Centro de Estudios y Documentacion Latinoamericanos, Amsterdam. Dordrecht: Foris Publications, 1985.

230. Spoerke DG, Hall AH. Plants and mushrooms of abuse. Emerg Med Clin North Am 1990; 8:579–593.

231. Hovin AW, Marten GC. Distribution of specific alkaloids in reed canarygrass cultivars. Crop Science 1975;15:705–707.

232. Gander JE, Marum P, Marten GC, Hovin AW. The occurrence of 2-methyl-1,2,3,4,-tetrahydro-β-carboline and variation in alkaloids in *Phalaris arundinacea*. Phytochemistry 1976;15:737–738.

233. Grinspoon L, Bakalar JB. Psychedelic drugs reconsidered. New York: Basic Books, 1981.

234. Guharoy SR, Barajas M. Atropine intoxication from the ingestion and smoking of jimson weed (Datura stramonium). Vet Hum Toxicol 1991; 33:588–589.

235. Coremans P, Lambrecht G, Schepens P, et al.

Anticholinergic intoxication with commercially available thorn apple tea. Clin Toxicol 1994; 32:589–592.

236. Anonymous. Jimson weed poisoning—Texas, New York, and California. MMWR 1995; 44:41–44.

237. Koevoets PFM, Van Harten PN. Doornappel-intoxicatie. Ned Tijdschr Geneeskd 1997; 141:888–889.

238. Abernethy MK, Becker LB. Acute nutmeg intoxication. Am J Emerg Med 1992;10:429–430.

239. Taylor RFH, Al-Jarad N, John LME. Betel-nut chewing and asthma. Lancet 1992;339:577–578.

240. Deahl M. Betel nut-induced extrapyramidal syndrome: an unusual drug interaction. Mov Disord 1989;4:330–333.

241. Pickwell SM, Schimelpfening S, Palinkas LA. 'Betelmania'. Betel quid chewing by Cambodian women in the United States and its potential health effects. West J Med 1994;160:326–330.

242. Siegel RK, Elsohly MA, Plowman T, et al. Cocaine in herbal tea. JAMA 1986;255:40.

243 Siegel RL. Herbal intoxications: psychoactive effects from herbal cigarettes, tea, and capsules. JAMA 1976;236:473–476.

244. Levine R, Taylor WB. Take tea and see. Arch Dermatol 1986;122:856.

245. Suess R, Lehmann P. Haematogenes Kontaktekzem durch pflanzliche Medikamente am Beispiel des Kavawurzel-extraktes. Hautarzt 1996;47: 459–461.

246. Ruze P. Kava-induced dermopathy: a niacin deficiency? Lancet 1990;335:1442–1445.

247. Widler P, Mathys K, Brenneisen R, et al. Pharmacodynamics and pharmacokinetics of khat: a controlled study. Clin Pharmacol Ther 1994; 55:556–562.

248. Kristiansson B, Abdul Ghani N, Eriksson M, et al. Use of khat in lactating women: a pilot study on breast-milk secretion. J Ethnopharmacol 1987;21:85–90.

249. Zhang JS, Zhen T, Zhi-cen L. Simultaneous determination of six alkaloids in Ephedrae Herba by high performance liquid chromatography. Planta Med 1988;54:69–70.

250. Zhang JS, Tian Z, Lou ZC. Quality evaluation of twelve species of Chinese Ephedra (Ma huang). Acta Pharm Sin 1989:24:865–871.

251. Liu Y-M, Sheu S-J, Chiou S-H, et al. A comparative study on commercial samples of Ephedrae herba. Planta Med 1993;59:376–378.

252. Chua SS, Benrimoj SI. Non-prescription sympa-

thomimetic agents and hypertension. Adverse Drug Exp 1988;3:387–417.

253. Anonymous. Botanical ephedrine supplements cause alarm. Scrip OTC News 1996;28:8.

254. Catlin DH, Sekera M, Adelman DC. Erythroderma associated with ingestion of an herbal product. West J Med 1993;159:491–493.

255. Capwell RR. Ephedrine-induced mania from an herbal diet supplement. Am J Psychiatry 1995;152:647.

256. Doyle H, Kargin M. Herbal stimulant containing ephedrine has also caused psychosis. BMJ 1996;313:756.

257. Nadir A, Agrawal S, King PD, Marshall JB. Acute hepatitis associated with the use of a Chinese herbal product, Ma-Huang. Am J Gastroenterol 1996;91:1436–1438.

258. ElSohly HN, ElSohly MA, Stanford DF. Poppy seed ingestion and opiates urinalysis. A closer look. J Anal Toxicol 1990;14:308–310.

259. Kaplan R. Poppy seed dependence. Med J Aust 1994;161:176.

260. Unnithan S, Strang J Poppy tea dependence. Br J Psychiatry 1993;163:813–814.

261. Chang H-M, But PP-H, eds. Pharmacology and applications of Chinese materia medica. Volume 1. Singapore: World Scientific Publishing, 1986.

262. Chang H-M, But PP-H, eds. Pharmacology and applications of Chinese materia medica. Volume 2. Singapore: World Scientific Publishing, 1987.

263. Tang W, Eisenbrand G. Chinese drugs of plant origin. Chemistry, pharmacology, and use in traditional and modern medicine. Heidelberg: Springer-Verlag, 1992.

264. Bensoussan A, Myers SP. Towards a safer choice. The practice of traditional Chinese medicine in Australia. Campbelltown: University of Western Sydney Macarthur, 1996.

265. Tai YT, But PP, Young K, Lau CP. Cardiotoxicity after accidental herb-induced aconite poisoning. Lancet 1992;340:1254–1256.

266. Chan TY, Tomlinson B, Critchley JA. Aconitine poisoning following the ingestion of Chinese herbal medicines: a report of eight cases. Aust NZ J Med 1993;23:268–271.

267. Hikino H, Yamada C, Nakamura K, et al. Change of alkaloid composition and acute toxicity of *Aconitum* roots during processing. Yakugaku Zasshi 1977;97:359–366.

268. Kao W-F, Hung D-Z, Lin K-P, Deng J-F. Podophyllotoxin intoxication: toxic effect of Bajiaolian in herbal therapeutics. Hum Exp Toxicol 1992;11:480–487.

269. Chan JCN, Chan TYK, Chan KL, et al. Anticholinergic poisoning from Chinese herbal medicines. Aust NZ J Med 1994;24:317–318.

270. Deji D, Qingtian Z. Shancigu. In: Chang H-M, But PP-H, eds. Pharmacology and applications of Chinese materia medica. Volume 1. Singapore, World Scientific Publishing Co, 1986:117–123.

271. Songbai Y. Zangqie. In: Chang H-M, But PP-H, eds. Pharmacology and applications of Chinese materia medica. Volume 2. Singapore, World Scientific Publishing Co, 1987:1250–1255.

272. Vanherweghem JL, Depierreux M, Tielemans C, et al. Rapidly progressive interstitial renal fibrosis in young women: association with slimming regimen including Chinese herbs. Lancet 1993;341:387–391.

273. Vanherweghem JL. Une nouvelle forme de nephropathie secondaire a l'absorption d'herbes chinoises. Bull Mem Acad Roy Med Belg 1994;149:128–135.

274. Vanhaelen M, Vanhaelen-Fastre R, But P, Vanherweghem JL. Identification of aristolochic acid in Chinese herbs. Lancet 1994;343:174.

275. Van Ypersele De Strihou C, Vanherweghem JL. The tragic paradigm of Chinese herbs nephropathy. Nephrol Dial Transplant 1995;10:157–160.

276. Depierreux M, Van Damme B, Vanden Houte K, Vanherweghem JL. Pathologic aspects of a newly described nephropathy related to the prolonged use of Chinese herbs. Am J Kidney Dis 1994;24:172–180.

277. Vanherweghem J-L, Abramowicz D, Tielemans C, Depierreux M. Effects of steroids on the progression of renal failure in chronic interstitial renal fibrosis: a pilot study in Chinese herbs nephropathy. Am J Kidney Dis 1996;27:209–215.

278. Cosyns J-P, Jadoul M, Squifflet J-P, et al. Urothelial malignancy in nephropathy due to Chinese herbs. Lancet 1994;344:188.

279. Vanherweghem JL, Tielemans C, Simon J, Depierreux M. Chinese herbs nephropathy and renal pelvic carcinoma. Nephrol Dial Transplant 1995;10:270–273.

280. Schmeiser HH, Bieler CA, Wiessler M, et al. Detection of DNA adducts formed by aristolochic acid in renal tissue from patients with Chinese herbs nephropathy. Cancer Res 1996;56:2025–2058.

281. Wu G, Yamamoto K, Mori T, et al. Improvement by Guan-mu-tong (Caulis aristolochiae manshuriensis) of lactation in mice. Am J Chin Med 1995;23:159–165.

282. Anonymous. Drug development from natural products. Pharm J 1995;255:430–431.

283. Quansheng C. Mutong. In: Chang H-M, But PP-H, eds. Pharmacology and applications of Chinese materia medica. Volume 1. Singapore: World Scientific Publishing, 1986:195–198.

284. But PP. Herbal poisoning caused by adulterants or erroneous substitutes. J Trop Med Hyg 1994;97:371–374.

285. Chan TY. Anticholinergic poisoning due to Chinese herbal medicines. Vet Hum Toxicol 1995;37:156–157.

286. Jin Y, Berry MI, Chan K. Chinese herbal medicine in the United Kingdom. Pharm J 1995;255:R37.

287. Liu XM, Meng ZH. Pseudomonas contamination of Chinese herbal drug, Tremella fuciformis. Chin J Prev Med 1993;27:227–229.

288. Shaw D, House I, Kolev S, Murray V. Should herbal medicines be licensed? BMJ 1995;311:451–452.

289. Espinoza EO, Mann M-J, Bleasdell B. Arsenic and mercury in traditional Chinese herbal balls. N Engl J Med 1995;333:803–804.

290. Chi Y-W, Chen S-L, Yang M-H, Hwang R-C, Chu M-L. Heavy metals in traditional Chinese medicine: Ba-Pao-Neu-Hwang-San. Acta Paediatr Sin 1993;34:181–190.

291. Schaumburg HH, Berger A. Alopecia and sensory polyneuropathy from thallium in a Chinese herbal medication. JAMA 1992;268:3430–3431.

292. Kang-Yum E, Oransky SH. Chinese patent medicine as a potential source of mercury poisoning. Vet Hum Toxicol 1992;34:235–238.

293. Markowitz SB, Nunez CM, Klitzman S, et al. Lead poisoning due to Hai Ge Fen. The porphyrin content of individual erythrocytes. JAMA 1994;271:932–934.

294. Gertner E, Marshall PS, Filandrinos D, et al. Complications resulting from the use of Chinese herbal medications containing undeclared prescription drugs. Arthritis Rheum 1995;38:614–617.

295. Van der Stricht BI, Parvais OE, Vanhaelen-Fastré RJ, Vanhaelen MH. Remedies may contain cocktail of active drugs. BMJ 1994;308:1162.

296. Nelson L, Shih R, Hoffman R. Aplastic anemia induced by an adulterated herbal medication. J Toxicol Clin Toxicol 1995;33:467–470.

297. Floren AE, Fitter W. Contamination of urine with diazepam and mefenamic acid from an Oriental remedy. J Occup Med 1991;33:1168–1169.

298. Diamond JR, Pallone TL. Acute interstitial nephritis following use of Tung Shueh pills. Am J Kidney Dis 1994;24:219–221.

299. Abt AB, Oh JY, Huntington RA, Burkhart KK.

Chinese herbal medicine induced acute renal failure. Arch Intern Med 1995;155:211–212.

300. Joseph AM, Biggs T, Garr M, et al. Stealth steroids. N Engl J Med 1991;324:62.

301. Graham-Brown RAC, Bourke JF, Bumphrey G. Chinese herbal remedies may contain steroids. BMJ 1994;308:473.

302. Kubo K, Watanabe F, Sakuma S, et al. Hypersensitive hepatic injury induced by Shosaikoto, a liver-supporting herb medicine. IRYO (Jap J Nat Med Serv) 1986;40:205–206,257–260.

303. Tsukiyama K, Tasaka Y, Nakajima M, et al. A case of pneumonitis due to Sho-saiko-to. Jap J Thoracic Dis 1989;27:1556–1561.

304. Daibo A, Yoshida Y, Kitazawa S, et al. A case of pneumonitis and hepatic injury caused by a herbal drug (Sho-saiko-to). Jap J Thoracic Dis 1992;30:1583–1588.

305. Imokawa S, Sato A, Taniguchi M. A case of Sho-Saiko-to induced pneumonitis and the review of literature. Jap J Chest Dis 1992;51:53–58.

306. Takada N, Arai S, Kusuhara N, et al. A case of Sho-Saiko-to-induced pneumonitis, diagnosed by lymphocyte stimulation test using bronchoalveolar lavage fluid. Jap J Thorac Dis 1993;31:1163–1169.

307. Itoh S, Marutani K, Nishijima T, et al. Liver injuries induced by herbal medicine, Syo-saiko-to (xiao-chai-hu-tang). Dig Dis Sci 1995;40:1845–1848.

308. Kawasaki A, Mizushima Y, Kunitani H, et al. A useful diagnostic method for drug-induced pneumonitis: a case report. Am J Chin Med 1994;22:329–336.

309. Tojima H, Yamazaki T, Tokudome T. Two cases of pneumonia caused by Sho-saiko-to. Jap J Thorac Dis 1996;34:904–910.

310. Chan TY, Chan LY, Tam LS, Critchley JA. Neurotoxicity following the ingestion of a Chinese medicinal plant, *Alocasia macrorrhiza*. Hum Exp Toxicol 1995;14:727–728.

311. Pillans P, Eade MN, Massey RJ. Herbal medicine and toxic hepatitis. NZ Med J 1994;107:432–433.

312. Kane JA, Kane SP, Jain S. Hepatitis induced by traditional Chinese herbs; possible toxic components. Gut 1995;36:146–147.

313. Vautier G, Spiller RC. Safety of complementary medicines should be monitored. BMJ 1995;311:633.

314. Perharic L, Shaw D, Leon C, et al. Liver damage associated with certain types of traditional Chinese medicines used for skin diseases. Vet Hum Toxicol 1995;37:562–566.

315. Woerdenbag HJ. Gossypol. In: De Smet PAGM, Keller K, Hänsel R, Chandler RF, eds. Adverse effects of herbal drugs. Volume 2. Heidelberg: Springer-Verlag, 1993:195–208.

316. Nakamura T, Kobayashi A. Toxikodermie durch den Speisepilz Shiitake (*Lentinus edodes*). Hautarzt 1985;36:591–593.

317. Nakamura T. Shiitake (*Lentinus edodes*) dermatitis. Contact Dermatitis 1992;27:65–70.

318. Kato C, Morishita Y, Fukatsu T. False-positive increase in 1,5-anhydro-D-glucitol due to Kampo (Japanese herbal) medicine. Jap J Clin Pathol 1996;44:396–399.

319. But PP, Tomlinson B, Lee KL. Hepatitis related to the Chinese medicine Shou-wu-pian manufactured from *Polygonum multiflorum*. Vet Hum Toxicol 1996;38:280–282.

320. Lai R-S, Chiang AA, Wu M-T, et al. Outbreak of bronchiolitis obliterans associated with the consumption of *Sauropus androgynus* in Taiwan. Lancet 1996;348:83–85.

321. Lo ACT, Chan K, Yeung JHK, Woo KS. The effects of Danshen (*Salvia miltiorrhiza*) on pharmacokinetics and pharmacodynamics of warfarin in rats. Eur J Drug Metab Pharmacokin 1992;17:257–262.

322. Okuda T, Umezawa Y, Ichikawa M, et al. A case of drug eruption caused by the crude drug Boi (Sinomenium stem/Sinomeni caulis et Rhizoma). J Dermatol 1995;22:795–800.

323. Lin JL, Ho YS. Flavonoid-induced acute nephropathy. Am J Kidney Dis 1994;23:433–440.

324. Horowitz RS, Gomez H, Moore LL, et al. Jin Bu Huan toxicity in children—Colorado 1993. MMWR 1993;42:633–636.

325. Woolf GM, Petrovic LM, Rojter SE, et al. Acute hepatitis associated with the Chinese herbal product Jin Bu Huan. Ann Intern Med 1994;121:729–735.

326. Horowitz RS, Feldhaus K, Dart RC, et al. The clinical spectrum of Jin Bu Huan toxicity. Arch Int Med 1996;156:899–903.

327. Yu D-Y. Clinical observation of 144 cases of rheumatoid arthritis treated with glycoside of Radix Tripterygium wilfordii. J Tradit Chin Med 1983;3:125–129.

328. Tao X-L, Sun Y, Dong Y, et al. A prospective, controlled, double-blind, cross-over study of *Tripterygium wilfordii* Hook f in treatment of rheumatoid arthritis. Chin Med J 1989;102:327–332.

329. Qian SZ. *Tripterygium wilfordii*, a Chinese herb effective in male fertility regulation. Contraception 1987;36:335–345.

330. Guo J-L, Yuan S-X, Wang X-C, et al. *Tripterygium wilfordii* Hook f in rheumatoid arthritis and ankylosing spondylitis. Preliminary report. Chin Med J 1981;94:405–412.

331. Chan TYK, Chan AY, Critchley JA. Hospital admissions due to adverse reactions to Chinese herbal medicines. J Trop Med Hyg 1992; 95:296–298.

332. Aslam M. Asian medicine and its practice in Britain. In: Evans WC, ed. Trease and Evans' Pharmacognosy. 14th edn. London: WB Saunders Company Ltd, 1996:488–504.

333. Thatte UM, Rege NN, Phatak SD, Dahanukar SA. The flip side of Ayurveda. J Postgrad Med 1993;39:179–182.

334. Maurice PDL, Cream JJ. The dangers of herbalism. BMJ 1989;299:1204.

335. Vanherweghem J-L. *Aristolochia* sp. and chronic interstitial nephropathies in Indians. Lancet 1997;349:1399.

336. Aslam M, Shaw J. A case study—dangers of transcultural medicine in the U.K. J Clin Pharm Ther 1995;20:345–347.

337. Aslam M, Shaw J. Problems of identity with traditional Asian remedies. Pharm J 1992;248:20–23.

338. Barnes AR, Paul CJ, Secrett PC. Adulteration of an Asian alternative medicine. Pharm J 1991;247:650.

339. Thatte U, Ucchil D, Dahanukar S. Screening Ayurvedic drugs. Essential Drugs Monitor 1996;22:12.

340. Raman A, Jamal J. 'Herbal' hay fever remedy found to contain conventional drugs. Pharm J 1997;258:105–106.

CHAPTER 7

THE SAFETY OF NONHERBAL COMPLEMENTARY PRODUCTS

Peter A.G.M. De Smet

GENERAL INTRODUCTION

Many general concerns reviewed in the previous chapter on the safety of herbal products also apply to nonherbal complementary products. For instance, product quality is an important issue of nonherbal products because the risk of contamination with a toxic substance is not always limited to herbal products. There have been reports about unacceptably high levels of lead in propolis capsules (1) and in dietary calcium supplements (2). A human case of lead poisoning has been published, in which the source of lead was a dietary calcium supplement made from horse bone (3). The possibility also exists that animal products transmit an infectious disease due to the presence of a pathogenic microbe (4, 5) or another pathogenic organism (6).

The risk of adverse reactions to nonherbal products can also depend on consumer-bound parameters, such as concomitant diseases or concurrent drug use. Acute hepatitis B was reported to induce acute hypervitaminosis A in a 42-year-old man who had taken 25,000 IU of vitamin A without ill effects for 10 years (7). Vitamin E may increase cyclosporin toxicity by improving its absorption (8), and it can also enhance the action of oral anticoag- ulants by increasing vitamin K requirements (9, 10).

Finally, situational risks should also be taken into consideration when it comes to nonherbal complementary products. For instance, the rec- reational substance gamma-hydroxybutyrate can make its consumers less fit for driving (11).

This chapter reviews information on the ad- verse effects of animal preparations, toxic met- als, diets, vitamins and trace elements, amino acids, and various other products.

ANIMAL PREPARATIONS

Substances of animal origin can produce ana- phylactic or anaphylactoid reactions, particu- larly after parenteral administration (12).

The following is a summary of the known and reported adverse effects of some animal preparations and products. When faced with a patient using these products, find the summary of known adverse effects of those products. This will provide an indication of the adverse effects known for that animal substance and help guide the practitioner in monitoring for possible ad- verse effects in that patient. It will also help the practitioner inform the patient about possible risks.

Arumalon

Chondroprotective agent containing an extract of cartilage and of red bone marrow of calves. Parenteral use has been associated with local reactions at the site of the injection and with allergic symptoms (e.g., fever, malaise, symptoms of pronounced inflammation, nephrotic syndrome). Allegedly, polymyositis and fatal dermatomyositis are also possible (13).

Arteparon

Chondroprotective agent prepared from bovine lung and tracheal cartilage. Mucopolysaccharide polysulfuric acid ester (also known as glycosaminoglycan polysulfate) is declared its major principle. This substance resembles heparin in its molecular structure and can have the same increasing effect on platelet aggregation. Cross-reactivity with heparin is possible. The use of arteparon has been associated with life-threatening thromboembolic complications (e.g., myocardial infarction, pulmonary embolus, hemiplegic apoplexia, cerebral hemorrhage, death). Other reported side effects include local reactions at the site of the injection, serious allergic symptoms, arthropathy, subcutaneous fat necrosis, and reversible alopecia (13).

Bee-sting therapy

The development of persistent nodular lesions from bee-sting therapy has been reported (14). Anaphylaxis in allergic individuals is, of course, of concern.

Bile preparations

The raw bile of the grass carp (*Ctenopharyngodon idellus*) is believed in Asia to be good for health. However, eating this substance can result in hepatic failure and renal toxicity. The former reaction may resolve within a few days, but the latter is more serious, culminating in acute renal failure within 2 to 3 days after ingestion. The toxic component of the bile is probably 5-α-cyprinol (15, 16). Likewise, the ingestion of sheep bile as a traditional remedy for diabetes mellitus is associated with hepatic and renal toxicity (17).

Cell therapy

Cell therapy consists of the parenteral or enteral administration of cells or cell parts obtained from animal organs and/or tissues of bovine donors, sheep, pigs, or rabbits. Two different types of cell preparations are in use: fresh cells, which are administered in fresh form, and dried cells or so-called sicca cells, which are worked up for later use. The most prevailing risk of cell therapy seems local and generalized allergic reactions (e.g., fever, nausea, vomiting, urticaria, and anaphylactic shock). Other untoward consequences include fatal and nonfatal encephalomyelitis, polyneuritis, Landry-Guillain-Barré syndrome, fatal serum sickness, perivenous leucoencephalitis, and immune-complex vasculitis (18–20).

Fish oil

Fish oil supplements rich in long chain polyunsaturated omega-3 fatty acids (eicosapentaenoic acid, docosahexaenoic acid) can reduce plasma levels of triglycerides and very low-density lipoproteins, decrease platelet aggregation, prolong bleeding time, and affect leukotriene production. Reported side effects include fullness and epigastric discomfort, diarrhea, and a fishy taste after burping. In addition, some more serious problems have been identified (18):

- There is a potential risk that the favorable changes in plasma lipids could be offset by a deleterious increase in low-density lipoprotein (LDL) cholesterol or LDL apoprotein B.
- The capacity to increase bleeding time and to reduce platelet aggregation could have untoward consequences, especially in patients with preexisting bleeding and platelet abnormalities, and in those taking other antithrombotic agents.

continued on next page

- Preliminary evidence suggests that a deteriorating effect on patients with aspirin-sensitive asthma is possible.
- There is also the risk that the metabolic control of patients with type 2 diabetes mellitus may be adversely affected when these patients are not being treated with a sulfonylurea derivative (21).

Gangliosides

Gangliosides extracted from bovine brain tissue have been widely used in Western Europe and South America for several neurological disorders. In addition to discomfort at the injection site, reported side effects include motoneuron diseaselike illness, cutaneous erythema (with or without fever and nausea), and anaphylaxis. After evaluating reported associations between the use of gangliosides and Guillain-Barré syndrome (22, 23), the Committee for Proprietary Medicinal Products (CPMP) of the European Commission recommended in 1994 that marketing authorizations for mixtures of gangliosides for the treatment of peripheral neuropathies should be withdrawn (24).

Ghee

Ghee is the clarified butter from the milk of water buffaloes or cows. Although the butter is heated enough to eliminate non-sporulating organisms, the process is unlikely to kill *Clostridium tetani* spores. This may explain why its traditional use as an umbilical cord dressing is sometimes identified as a risk factor for the development of neonatal tetanus (25).

Green-lipped mussel

An extract of the New Zealand green-lipped mussel (*Perna canaliculus*) is advocated for the treatment of arthritic symptoms. Reported side effects include flare-up of the disease, epigastric discomfort, flatulence, and nausea (26). A case of jaundice appearing

weeks after starting treatment has been reported (27).

Imedeen

Imedeen is the trade name of an oral health food product containing freeze-dried proteins from the cartilage of deep-sea fish, which is advocated as an antiwrinkling agent. Its use has been associated with generalized skin reaction and extensive Quincke's edema (28).

Liver extracts

Products derived from animal liver may contain levels of vitamin A that are far greater than nutritional levels (e.g., up to 48,000 IU per tablet). As a result, indiscriminate use of such products carries a risk of hypervitaminosis A and birth defects (29). Anaphylactic reactions to parenteral forms of liver extracts have been rarely reported (30, 31).

Orgotein

Orgotein (also known as Cu Zn superoxide dismutase) is obtained from bovine liver. It has been advocated as an antiinflammatory agent. Parenteral administration has been associated with anaphylactic reactions (32, 33).

Oyster extract

A food supplement consisting of oyster extract, ginseng, taurine, and zinc has been associated with a case of Quincke's facial edema. The reaction developed immediately after intake of the food supplement, and the oyster extract was considered its most likely cause (34).

Propolis

Propolis, or bee-glue, is a resinous material used by bees to seal hive walls and to strengthen the borders of the combs as well as the hive entrance. It is increasingly associated with cases of allergy following use of the substance in biocosmetics and in self-treatment of various diseases. Although most cases involve allergic contact dermatitis arising from topical application, a few reports describe an allergic reaction to oral ingestion (35). The poplar bud constituent 1,1-dimethylallyl caffeic acid ester has been identified as its main contact allergen (36).

Rattlesnake meat

Dried rattlesnake meat is a well-known Mexican folk remedy that can be purchased without prescription in Mexico, El Salvador, and the southwestern part of the United States. It is available as such and in the form of powder, capsules, or pills, which may be labeled in Spanish as *víbora de cascabel, pulvo de víbora,* or *carne de víbora.* Because the rattlesnake is a well-established reservoir for *Salmonella arizona,* such products can cause serious systemic infections. Typically, victims are Hispanic patients with a medical illness undermining their immunological integrity (e.g., systemic lupus erythematosus, AIDS). Although most patients respond well to intravenous therapy with ampicillin or cotrimoxazole, fatalities have been observed (13, 37, 38).

Royal jelly

Royal jelly is a viscous secretion produced by the pharyngeal glands of the worker bee, *Apis mellifera,* and is widely used in alternative medicine as a health tonic. Its internal use by atopic individuals can induce severe, sometimes even fatal, asthma and anaphylaxis (39, 40). Topical application can lead to contact dermatitis (41).

Shark cartilage

The use of shark cartilage is promoted as a potential treatment for malignant disease, although there is no conclusive evidence of efficacy (42). A case of hepatitis, which was possibly caused by this form of therapy, has been reported (43).

Spanish fly

Spanish fly (also known as cantharides) is the dried blistering beetle (*Cantharis vesicato-*

ria and related species), which contains cantharidin as the major active constituent. A related drug, which serves as an alternative cantharidin source in the East, is the Chinese blistering beetle (*Mylabris* species). Spanish fly has gained a considerable reputation as an aphrodisiac agent after it was observed that nearly toxic doses could cause priapism in men and pelvic congestion with occasional uterine bleeding in women. These effects are caused by an irritant effect on the genitourinary tract, which can be misinterpreted as increased sensuality. Cantharidin was formerly used medicinally as a counterirritant and vesicant, but this use has been abandoned because of its high toxicity. Manifestations of cantharidin poisoning range from local vesicobullous formation to gross hematuria, hepatotoxicity, myocardial damage, denudation of the gastrointestinal tract, and, occasionally, death. The lethal dose is not well established. One patient died after the ingestion of only 10 mg, while another patient survived the intake of 50 mg (44–46).

Squalene

Squalene is a popular over-the-counter Asian folk remedy derived from shark liver oil. Oral capsules are readily available in Asian health food stores, and the substance is also widely used in cosmetics. Ingestion of squalene capsules has been associated with a case of severe lipoid pneumonia due to aspiration; the patient also had abnormal liver function, which raised the possibility of hepatotoxicity (47).

Thyroid hormones

Thyroid hormones continue to be found in unconventional medicines for weight reduction (47, 48) and in health food capsules (49). Although it is well recognized that these hormones can help reduce weight, primarily by increasing metabolic rate, they have no place in the therapy of obese euthyroid patients. When dietary intake of protein and

continued on next page

calcium is inadequate, use of these hormones may induce worrisome catabolic losses of these muscular and skeletal components, and the weight loss is not sustained after termination of therapy. Furthermore, the large doses needed for weight reduction may suppress endogenous thyroid function and have potentially dangerous effects on the heart, such as tachyarrhythmias and cardiomegaly (50, 51).

Toad venom

The dried venom of the Chinese toad (*Bufo bufo gargarizans*) is a traditional ingredient (Ch'an Su) of Chinese medicine. It contains bufalin and cinobufaginal, which are structurally related to digoxin. Deliberate and accidental overdosing with preparations containing Ch'an Su has been associated with serious, sometimes fatal, cardiotoxicity (52–55). Interference with digoxin immunoassays is also possible. By a cross-reaction with the digoxin antibodies, a false impression of high plasma digoxin levels is created (56). A digoxin immunoassay that avoids cross-reactivity with Chinese medicine has been developed (57).

TOXIC METALS

Toxic metals, such as arsenic, cadmium, lead, and mercury, can occur in herbal medicines and in other traditional preparations, not only as accidental contaminants, but also as intentional ingredients (58). In a given case, the potential intake of the toxic metal can be calculated based on its level in the product and the recommended or estimated dosage of the product. This potential exposure can then be put into a toxicological perspective by comparison with the so-called Provisional Tolerable Weekly Intake values for toxic metals, which have been established by the Food and Agriculture Organization of the United Nations (FAO) and the World Health Organization (WHO) (Table 7.1).

In various parts of the world, toxic metal salts or oxides are also deliberately put in medicines and cosmetics (Table 7.2). Of particular concern is the intentional presence of toxic metals in traditional medicines from India and Pakistan, which have been associated with a risk of serious poisoning (Table 7.3). In the case of traditional Chinese medicines, it is often difficult to find out whether the metals are there by accident or on purpose (see Chapter 6). The latter possibility is illustrated in Table 7.4.

Toxic metal salts or oxides are also found among the ingredients used for homeopathic medicines, and they may be present in these medicines in potentially unsafe levels (59). For instance, normal doses of cadmium sulfuricum D3 drops (i.e., 0.1% of cadmium sulfate) will provide a daily amount of 160 to 320 μg cadmium (60). This exposure exceeds the tolerable limit of 1 μg/kg of cadmium per day, which has been provisionally set by the Joint FAO/WHO Expert Committee on Food Additives.

Table 7.1. Provisional Tolerable Weekly Intake (PTWI) Values for Toxic Metals, as Established by FAO and WHO

METAL	PTWI VALUE (μg/kg/week)	REFERENCE
Arsenic (inorganic)	15*	61
Cadmium	7	62
Lead	25	62
Mercury	5**	63

*This PTWI does not refer to organoarsenicals, as the organoarsenic compounds naturally occurring in marine products are considerably less toxic than inorganic arsenicals.
**But no more than 3.3 μg/kg/week in the form of methyl mercury.

Table 7.2. Ethnic Medicines and Cosmetics Known or Suspected to Contain Intoxicating Metal Compounds as Intentional Ingredients*

MEDICINE	ORIGIN	DETAILS
Al Kohl	Kuwait	Lead poisonings have resulted from the use of this traditional preparation in children. It is applied as an eye cosmetic (in a manner similar to surma) or as a pack on the raw unbilical stump. The principal component is lead sulphide; lead levels up to 91.8% have been recovered.
Azarcón	Mexico	This folk remedy consists of lead tetra-oxide (over 90% lead by weight). It is used among Hispanic populations in the United States for relief of abdominal distress in children. It has been associated with several cases of lead poisoning. In at least one case, it was the suspected cause of fatal encephalopathy.
Bhasam	India	Bhasams are medicines prepared by repeated oxidation of ores, which are commonly used by Ayurvedic practitioners. Arsenic contents up to 67 μg/g have been reported.
Crema de Belleza	Mexico	This cream was marketed in the United States for skin cleansing and prevention of acne. After it had been associated with three cases of mercury poisoning in the United States, it was discovered that calomel (mercurous chloride) was a listed ingredient and that the cream contained 6%–10% mercury [64, 65].
Ghasard	India	This brown powder may be given as a tonic. A lead concentration of 1.6% was found in a sample that (together with two other lead-containing Indian folk remedies) was associated with fatal lead poisoning in a 9-month-old boy [66].
Greta	Mexico	This remedy resembles azarcón, both in its folk uses and health risks. It consists of lead oxide (over 90% lead by weight).
Kushta	India, Pakistan	Kushta medicines are often used as aphrodisiacs. Their composition is mainly oxidized metals (e.g., lead, mercury, arsenic, zinc) ground together with various herbs. Lead contents up to 72.8% have been reported. Because Kushta medicines are directly ingested, they are potentially more hazardous than surma powders.
Pay-loo-ah	Laos	Pay-loo-ah preparations are used by Laotian Hmong and Mien refugees living in the United States. They can have arsenic levels of 70%–80% and lead levels up to 90%. Their consumption has been associated with arsenic poisonings and lead poisonings.
Sikor	Asia	This mineral clay substance is relatively rich in lead and arsenic and may also contain cadmium, mercury, and other metals. It is traditionally taken by many Asians living in Britain as a remedy for indigestion and as a tonic during pregnancy.
Surma	India, Pakistan	Surma powders are brought into the United Kingdom, where they are used by Asian families. They can contain over 80% lead as lead sulphide. They are applied as a cosmetic to the conjunctival surface of infants and children, who may transfer the powder to the mouth by wiping the eyes and then sucking the fingers. This can result in abnormally high blood lead concentrations and has been associated with fatal encephalopathy.
Tiro	Nigeria	This preparation has lead sulphide as its major ingredient and may contain up to 81.1% lead. It is used as an eye medicine and cosmetic similar to surma and al kohl in other parts of the world.
Unspecified	Oman	Mercury and its salts are frequently used in the native medicine of Oman. A case of mercury poisoning was attributed to exposure to the inhalation of smoke created by burning a mixture of substances on an open fire. This therapy had been initiated by a native doctor [67].

*Adapted from Table 33 in ref. [68] unless specified otherwise.

Table 7.3. Occurrence of Arsenic and Mercury Salts in Chinese Herbal Formulas [69]

FORMULA	SALT(S)	PROVIDING*
An-Kung-Niu-Huang-Wan (Bezoar Resurrection pills)	Arsenic disulfide Red mercuric sulfide	48 mg/g As 45 mg/g Hg
Chen-Ling-Tan (Pills for Shocking the Spirits)	Red mercuric sulfide	37 mg/g Hg
Chi-Chu-Wan (Sedative Pills with Magnetite and Cinnabar)	Red mercuric sulfide	97 mg/g Hg
Chi-Li-San (Antibruises Powder)	Red mercuric sulfide	60 mg/g Hg
Chih-Pao-Dan (The Most Precious Pellets)	Arsenic disulfide Red mercuric sulfide	16 mg/g As 20 mg/g Hg
Chou-Che-Wan (The Boat and Carriage Pills)	Mercurous chloride	8 mg/g Hg
Chu-Sha-An-Shen-Wan (Cinnabar Sedative Pills)	Red mercuric sulfide	12 mg/g Hg
Liu-Shen-Wan (Pills of Six Miraculous Drugs)	Arsenic disulfide	NC
Niu-Huang-Chieh-Tu-Pian (Antiphlogistic Pills with Bos Calculus)	Arsenic disulfide	NC
Shu-Ching-Huo-Hsieh-Tang (Decoction for Removing Blood Stasis in the Channels)	Red mercuric sulfide	10 mg/g Hg
Tien-Wang-Pu-Hsin Tan (The King's Mind-easing Tonic Pills)	Red mercuric sulfide	13 mg/g Hg
Tzu-Hsueh-Tan (Purple Snowy Powder)	Red mercuric sulfide	12 mg/g Hg

*Expressed as mg of As or Hg per g of total active ingredients; NC = not calculable.

Germanium

The daily intake of germanium through food-stuffs is estimated to be between 0.4 and 3.5 mg. In past years, germanium preparations supplying much larger amounts have hit the health food markets of Japan and Europe. Various case reports have shown that a daily intake of 30 to 700 mg of germanium for months or years (corresponding to a cumulative dose varying from 8.5 g to more than 300 g of germanium) can lead to serious renal failure, which is not always reversible. Neuropathy, myopathy, and hepatic damage may also occur. Some patients ultimately died of gastrointestinal bleeding, cardiogenic shock, or multiple organ failure. Most cases involved the use of inorganic germanium dioxide or an unidentified germanium compound. However, carboxyethylgermanium sesquioxide and germanium-lactate-citrate have also been incriminated (70, 71).

DIETS

Strict, injudicious adherence to certain dietary restrictions may result in nutritional deficiencies of protein, vitamins, electrolytes, and/or trace elements. For example, an injudicious vegetarian diet can result in vitamin B_{12} deficiency. Infants seem to be at particular risk of developing dietary deficiencies (72–76). Unbalanced diets can also lead to an excessive intake of certain nutrients, which can cause adverse reactions, interference with conventional treatment, or both. For example, there was a case of myocardial infarction in a patient on warfarin therapy. The patient's special diet provided excessive amounts of vitamin K and had apparently induced resistance to the warfarin treatment (77). In addition to a risk of pharmacodynamic problems, there is also the possibility that a dietary change induces pharmacokinetic changes (78). For example, a balanced diet with adequate pro-

Table 7.4. Metal Poisoning by Traditional Preparations of Asian Origin

CLINICAL FINDING (NO. OF CASES)	INCRIMINATED PREPARATION(S)	ORIGIN	REFERENCE
Lead poisoning (1)	Yellow-white powder containing lead oxide, lead sulfate, and lead nitrate, with a total lead content of 84%	Asia*	[79]
Lead poisoning (1)	Grayish-white powder with 49% lead	India	[80]
Lead poisoning (1)	Brown Maha Yogran Guggulu pills containing 17 mg of lead per pill	India	[81]
Lead poisoning (1)	Pushap tablets containing 79 mg of lead, 0.75 mg of arsenic and >10 mg of mercury per tablet *plus* Shakti tablets containing 56 mg of lead, 5.4 mg of arsenic, and >10 mg of mercury per tablet	India	[82]
Arsenic poisoning (1)	Mixed white and orange-brown powder with 105 mg of arsenic trioxide and 654 mg of mercuric sulfide per dose	India	[83, 84]
Mercury poisoning (1)	Red-brown pills containing 30–42 mg of mercuric sulfide per dose	India	[83]
Mercury poisoning (1)	Product containing 37% arsenic and 54% mercury	Asia	[84]
Haemolytic anaemia (1)	Product containing 0.9% arsenic and 1.9% lead	Asia	[84]
Lead poisoning (1)	Product containing 16.7% lead	Asia	[84]
Lead poisoning (1)	Pale brown powder containing 19% lead	India	[85]
Lead poisoning (1)	Maya Yograj Guggul tablets containing 0.9 mg of arsenic, 1 mg of lead, and 18 mg of mercury per tablet *plus* Chandraprabha tablets providing lower amounts of arsenic, lead, and mercury *plus* a tonic, which also contained arsenic and lead	India	[86]
Lead poisoning (1)	Brown tablets containing 10% lead	India	[87]
Lead poisoning (1)	Orange powder containing 55% lead	Asia**	[87]
Lead poisoning (1)	Ayurvedic brown tablets containing 6% lead	India	[87, 88]
Lead poisoning (1)	White Deshi Dewa powder with 12% lead	Asia	[87–89]
Lead poisoning (1)	Yellow powder containing 60% lead	Asia**	[87]
Lead poisoning (1)	Powder containing 16.7% lead	Asia	[90]
Lead poisoning (5)	Ayurvedic capsules containing 22–30 mg of lead per capsule	Asia	[91]

*Pakistani patient treated by a "traditional Asian practitioner"
**Patient treated by a traditional "hakim" healer

tein causes an acidic urine, whereas a low protein diet or a strict vegetarian diet may cause an alkaline urine. Consequently, diet-induced shifts in urinary pH may alter the rate of excretion of both weakly acidic and basic drugs (92, 93).

VITAMINS AND TRACE ELEMENTS

Vitamins and minerals are not harmful in nutritional doses (Table 7.5) (94, 95), but it is well established that some vitamins and minerals can cause serious adverse effects when taken in megadoses. Although regulations for vitamin preparations are increasing, minerals seem to be regulated less commonly, despite the fact that such regulations would be just as relevant as they are for vitamin preparations.

The following is a summary of the known and reported adverse effects of vitamins and trace elements.

Table 7.5. United States Recommended Dietary Allowances (RDA) for Vitamins and Minerals

NUTRIENT	RDA FOR ADULTS
Vitamins	
Vitamin A (retinol)	2667–3333 IE (800–1000 RE)
Vitamin B_1 (thiamin)	1.0–1.5 mg
Vitamin B_2 (riboflavin)	1.2–1.7 mg
Provitamin B_3 (niacin)	13–19 mg
Vitamin B_5 (pantothenate)	4–7 mg*
Vitamin B_6 (pyridoxine)	1.6–2.0 mg
Vitamin B_{11} (folic acid)	0.18–0.20 mg
Vitamin B_{12} (cyanocobalamin)	2 μg
Vitamin C (ascorbic acid)	60 mg
Vitamin D (cholecalciferol)	200–400 IE (5–10 μg)
Vitamin E (α-tocopherol)	8–10 mg
Vitamin K (phytomenadione)	60–80 μg
Minerals	
Calcium	800–1200 mg
Phosphorus	800–1200 mg
Magnesium	280–350 mg
Iron	10–15 mg
Zinc	12–15 mg
Iodine	150 μg
Selenium	55–70 μg
Copper	1.5–3.0 mg*
Manganese	2–5 mg*
Chromium	50–200 μg*
Molybdenum	75–250 μg*

*This is not an RDA but a suggested safe and adequate daily intake for adults.

When faced with a patient using these products, find the summary of known adverse effects of those products. This will provide an indication of the adverse effects known for that substance and help guide the practitioner in monitoring for possible adverse effects in that patient. It will also help the practitioner inform the patient about possible risks.

Vitamin A (retinol) and Provitamin A (beta carotene)

Acute toxic reactions to vitamin A have become rare after megadose supplementation (0.5–4 million IU) to infants has been abandoned. Chronic toxicity occurs more often but is rare at doses below 100,000 IU/day. The risk is increased by low body weight, protein malnutrition, liver disease, renal disease, hyperlipoproteinemia, alcohol consumption, and vitamin C deficiency. For an adult, the mean time to intoxication is estimated to be 7.5 months at doses of 300,000 IU/day and 3.5 months for 500,000 IU/day. Reported symptoms include skin changes (e.g., dryness, fissures, depigmentation, and pruritus), hair loss, bone and joint pain with marked tenderness, hepatotoxicity, neurological complaints (e.g., benign intracranial hypertension), and psychiatric symptoms (96–99).

Of particular concern are the teratogenic effects of vitamin A (e.g., craniofacial, central nervous system, heart, neural tube, musculoskeletal, and urogenital). In one study, an increased frequency of defects was concentrated among babies born to women who had consumed high levels of vitamin A before the seventh week of gestation. The apparent threshold for this effect was near 10,000 IU/day of supplemental vitamin A. About 1 in 57 babies born to mothers exceeding this threshold had a malformation attributable to vitamin A supplementation (100). Women of reproductive age should not take supplements providing more than 8,000 IU/day of vitamin A (101).

Unlike vitamin A, beta carotene (provitamin A) is generally considered devoid of serious adverse effects. Except for yellowing of the skin after prolonged consumption of more than 30 mg/day, only questionable cases of adverse reactions have been reported (96, 99). Although its teratogenicity in humans has not been specifically studied, animal experiments do not indicate that it is teratogenic (100). A question about this impeccable safety record was raised when two clinical trials showed that beta carotene supplementation (20 or 30 mg/day) was associated with an increased relative risk of lung cancer in Finnish male smokers (102) and in American smokers, former smokers, and workers exposed to asbestos (103). The estimated excess risks observed were small, however, and it could not be concluded with certainty that beta carotene was truly harmful (104).

Vitamin D (cholecalciferol)

Excessive intake (e.g., 50,000–60,000 IU or more daily) of vitamin D for months or years can lead to hypercalcemia and its associated symptoms and complications, such as nausea, vomiting, weakness, headache, bone pain, hypercalciuria, renal calcinosis, metastatic calcification, and hypertension (94, 97, 98, 105–107).

Vitamin E (tocopherols)

Case reports are few at dosages less than 3,200 mg/day (96). In large doses, vitamin E increases the vitamin K requirement severalfold. Although this increase does not lead to bleeding diathesis in otherwise healthy individuals who are taking sufficient dietary amounts of vitamin K, coagulopathy can be produced in vitamin K–deficient patients. Therefore, it seems prudent to avoid substantial vitamin E supplementation in patients taking oral anticoagulants (96, 99, 108). Intravenous administration of vitamin E to neonates has been associated with hepatotoxicity in necrotizing enterocolitis (99).

Provitamin B₃ (niacin = nicotinic acid)

Niacin is transformed into nicotinamide (vitamin B₃) by the liver. Because of its vasodilator properties, niacin can produce flushing and hypotension headaches when taken in substantial doses. Other reported effects of high doses include pruritus, abdominal pain, diarrhea, peptic ulcer, skin rash, hepatotoxicity, hyperuricemia, hyperglycemia, and arrhythmias (100, 101). There is evidence to suggest that users of sustained-release products are more prone to hepatotoxic reactions than are consumers of unmodified products (109, 110).

Vitamin B₆ (pyridoxine)

Prolonged administration can lead to severe peripheral sensory neuropathy and ataxia. Although this risk is primarily associated with large doses (2–6 g/day), it has also been observed following 500 mg/day (94, 97, 111–113). Pyridoxine reduces the effects of levodopa, but this does not occur if a dopa decarboxylase inhibitor is also given (94).

continued on next page

Vitamin B₁₁ (folic acid)

The principal risk of folic acid supplementation is the masking or precipitation of clinical symptoms related to vitamin B_{12} deficiency; strict vegetarians need to be informed that they are at risk of this deficiency (114, 115).

Vitamin C (ascorbic acid)

Adverse reactions to vitamin C are rare at dosages less than 4 g/day. Gastrointestinal symptoms (e.g., diarrhea, esophagitis) have been observed, and vitamin C has also been associated with the formation of renal oxalate stones. Although this latter problem was reportedly caused by high oral doses, most reports involved either intravenous administration or chronic renal failure. Vitamin C can alter the results of various laboratory tests because it is a reducing agent and can thus interfere with colorimetric redox assays (96).

Chromium

No adverse effects were seen in 30 patients with type 2 diabetes mellitus who received 200 μg of chromium picolinate for 2 months (116). However, there have been reports on dichromate toxicity among urbanized South African blacks who have started to replace the herbal ingredients of their traditional purgative enemas with sodium or potassium dichromate. This replacement can result in serious poisoning, characterized by acute renal failure, gastrointestinal hemorrhage, and hepatocellular dysfunction (117, 118).

Copper

One case described a patient who developed acute liver failure and cirrhosis resembling Wilson's disease due to chronic overdosing of a dietary copper supplement (10–20 times the maximum recommended dose of 3 mg/day for years) (119).

Selenium

No cases of selenium toxicity were observed in a clinical trial that involved oral treatment of hundreds of patients with a history of basal or squamous cell carcinoma with 200 μg/day of selenium for several years (120). A level of 0.5–0.6 mg of selenium has been repeatedly proposed as the maximum acceptable daily intake level (121–123). Some reports have described toxicity due to health food tablets that contained many times more selenium (5–31 mg per tablet) than was stated on their label. Among the observed symptoms were nausea and vomiting, abdominal cramps, watery diarrhea, nail changes, alopecia, dryness of hair, fatigue, irritability, and paraesthesias (124–126).

Zinc

The risk of copper deficiency and anemia due to prolonged use of excessive doses has been occasionally reported (127–130). Treatment of 11 healthy men with 150 mg of elemental zinc twice a day for 6 weeks was associated with a reduction in lymphocyte stimulation response to phytohemagglutinin as well as chemotaxis and phagocytosis of bacteria by polymorphonuclear leukocytes (131). However, the clinical relevance of these findings remains to be established. Because of concern for possible toxicity, it is recommended that chronic use of zinc supplements exceeding 15 mg/day should be undertaken only under medical supervision (94).

AMINO ACIDS

Amino acids are not devoid of adverse effects when consumed in excessive amounts (132). The following is a summary of the known and reported adverse effects of some amino acids. When faced with a patient using these products, the practitioner should find the summary of known adverse effects of those products. This will provide an indication of the adverse effects known for that amino acid and help guide the practitioner in monitoring for possible adverse effects in that patient. It will also help the practitioner inform the patient about possible risks.

Carnitine

The natural amino acid L-carnitine functions in the transport of fatty acids into mitochondria, and its therapeutic value in the treatment of primary carnitine deficiencies (and some secondary deficiencies) is well established. Its direct toxicity seems negligible, and only minor adverse effects (e.g., gastrointestinal discomfort) have been observed in its consumers (133, 134). According to one case report, the addition of L-carnitine (1 g/day orally) to long-term acenocoumarol therapy may result in marked potentiation of this anticoagulant (135).

DL-Carnitine has been advocated in health food stores as a means to improve athletic performance. It competitively inhibits L-carnitine and can thus cause symptoms of carnitine deficiency. An exemplary case involved an athlete who took 500 mg of DL-carnitine for 2 days before running a long-distance race. No problems were encountered during the race, but later he developed muscle weakness and urinary discoloration suggestive of myoglobinuria (136).

Tryptophan

L-tryptophan (LT) is a naturally-occurring essential amino acid that has been advocated as an innocuous health food for the treatment of depression, insomnia, stress, behavioral disorders, premenstrual syndrome, and so on. At the end of 1989, LT-containing health food products were associated with an epidemic in the United States of the so-called eosinophilia-myalgia syndrome (EMS). This syndrome was characterized by an eosinophil count of $\geq 10^9/l$ and intense generalized myalgia. Other relatively frequent signs and symptoms were reports of fatigue, arthralgia, skin rash, cough and dyspnea, edema of the extremities, fever, sclerodermalike skin abnormalities, increased hair loss, xerostomia, pneumonia or pneumonitis with or without pulmonary vasculitis, and neuropathy. About one third of the cases required hospitalization, and a substantial number of patients died. Although there is good evidence that the epidemic was triggered by a contaminant, the responsible substance has not been identified (137).

In 1994, LT was reintroduced on the United Kingdom market under the strict condition that it should only be prescribed by hospital specialists for patients with long-standing resistant depression (138).

OTHER PRODUCTS

The following is a summary of the known and reported adverse effects of various other complementary products. When faced with a patient using these products, the practitioner should find the summary of known adverse effects of those products. This will provide an indication of the adverse effects known for that product and help guide the practitioner in monitoring for possible adverse effects in that patient. It will also help the practitioner inform the patient about possible risks.

Baking soda

Life-threatening complications developed following the use of baking soda (sodium bicarbonate) as a home remedy intended to help a 6-week-old infant burp (139).

Edetate

The parenteral administration of edetate disodium is advocated as chelation therapy for cardiovascular diseases. Serious adverse effects have been reported, such as renal tubular necrosis, acute renal failure, and death. Rapid infusions have been associated with acute hypocalcemia, tetany, and cardiac arrhythmias. Less commonly, vasculitis, bone marrow depression, and exfoliative dermatitis have occurred in association with chelation therapy. Few adverse effects have been reported when a protocol using 50 mg/kg per infusion was followed as recommended (140–142).

Fumaric acid esters

Monoethyl and dimethyl fumarate are being used in some countries to treat psoriasis. The major risk is nephrotoxicity. This effect can take the form of an acute renal failure, which is only partially reversible (143); osteomalacia due to renal tubular toxicity has been reported (144). Other side effects include gastrointestinal disturbances, skin reactions, flushing, reversible elevation of transaminases, reversible lymphopenia, and eosinophilia (145, 146). Consequently, the use of fumaric acid esters requires regular hematological control as well as periodic renal and hepatic function determinations.

Gamma-hydroxybutyrate

Gamma-hydroxybutyrate (GHB, or sodium oxybate) has been illicitly promoted for body building, weight control, treatment of insomnia, and recreational use as a euphoric agent ("liquid ecstasy"). Ingestion of 0.5–3 teaspoons can produce vomiting, drowsiness, hypotonia and/or vertigo, loss of consciousness, irregular respiration, tremors, or myoclonus. Seizure-like activity, bradycardia, hypotension, and/or respiratory arrest have also been reported. Severity and duration of symptoms depend on the dose of GHB and on the presence of other CNS depressants, such as alcohol (147–150). A recent case suggests that GHB may cause impairment of the psychomotor skills required for safe operation of a motor vehicle (151). Prolonged use of high doses may lead to a withdrawal syndrome (e.g., insomnia, anxiety, and tremor), which takes 3 to 12 days to resolve (152).

D-Glucosamin

Parenteral administration of this chondroprotective agent may produce a local reaction at the injection site as well as serious allergic reactions. Other reported side effects include nausea, vomiting, stupor, and isolated cases of blood disorders. It is likely that these reactions are partly due to the presence of lidocaine in the injection fluid (153).

Hydrogen peroxide

Intravenous injection of hydrogen peroxide as an unconventional therapy for cancer or AIDS has resulted in acute hemolytic anemia, which can be followed by fatal complications, such as cardiopulmonary arrest (154) or progressive renal impairment (155).

Lorenzo's Oil

This oil (20% erucic acid and 80% oleic acid) has been advocated as a miracle cure for adrenoleukodystrophy. Prolonged treatment has been associated with thrombocytopenia (156).

Ozone

Ozone therapy involves the foaming up of citrated autologous blood with oxygen, subsequent treatment of the blood in a quartz-glass container with UV-B radiation, and, finally, reinjection of the ozone-enriched blood. This treatment has been repeatedly associated with transmission of viral hepatitis (157, 158). A possible case of pancytopenia has also been reported (159).

Ubidecarenone

Ubidecarenone (coenzyme Q_{10}) not only is an investigational cardiovascular drug, but it is also widely available as an unconventional over-the-counter product. Several cases have been described in which a reduced effect of warfarin was observed after adding nonorthodox ubidecarenone to the patients' warfarin regimens. Ubidecarenone is chemically closely related to menaquinone (vitamin K_2), but the exact mechanism of this interaction remains to be identified (160, 161).

References

1. Anonymous. Propolis—recalled because of lead contamination. WHO Pharmaceuticals Newsletter 1995;1:3.

2. Diment M, Melnyk P, Coote C. Lead content of calcium supplements. Can Pharm J 1995; 128:21, 52.

3. Crosby WH. Lead-contaminated health food. Association with lead poisoning and leukemia. JAMA 1977;237:2627–2629.

4. Grave W, Sturm AW. Brucellosis as a result of cosmetic treatment. Neth J Med 1983;26: 188–190.

5. Miller L, Mangione E, Beebe J, et al. Infection with *Mycobacterium abscessus* associated with intramuscular injection of adrenal cortex extract - Colorado and Wyoming, 1995–1996. MMWR 1996;45:713–715.

6. Yu ZQ, Fu WB, Hua HM, Feng CT. Viper's blood and bile. Lancet 1997;349:250.

7. Hatoff DE, Gentler SL, Miyai K, et al. Hypervitaminosis A unmasked by acute viral hepatitis. Gastroenterology 1982;82:124–128.

8. Sokol RJ, Johnson KE, Karrer KE, et al. Improvement of cyclosporin absorption in children after liver transplantation by means of vitamin E. Lancet 1991;338:212–215.

9. Corrigan J, Marcus FI. Coagulopathy associated with vitamin E ingestion. JAMA 1974;230:1300–1301.

10. Meyers DG, Maloley PA, Weeks D. Safety of antioxidant vitamins. Arch Intern Med 1996;156:925–935.

11. Stephens BG, Baselt RC. Driving under the influence of GHB? J Anal Toxicol 1994;18:357–358.

12. De Smet PAGM, Pegt GWM, Meyboom RHB. Acute circulatoire shock na toepassing van het niet-reguliere enzympreparaat Wobe-Mugos. Ned Tijdschr Geneeskd 1991;135:2341–2344.

13. De Smet PAGM. Drugs used in non-orthodox medicine. In: Dukes MNG, Beeley L, eds. Side effects of drugs - Annual 14. Amsterdam: Elsevier, 1990:429–451.

14. Veraldi S, Raiteri F, Caputo R, Alessi E. Persistent nodular lesions caused by "bee-sting therapy." Acta Derm Venereol 1995;75:161–162.

15. Chan DWS, Yeung CK, Chan MK. Acute renal failure after eating raw fish gall bladder. BMJ 1985;290:897.

16. Anonymous. Acute hepatitis and renal failure following ingestion of raw carp gallbladders— Maryland and Pennsylvania, 1991 and 1994. MMWR 1995;44:565–566.

17. Al-Qahtani MS. Hepatic and renal toxicity among patients ingesting sheep bile as an unconventional

remedy for diabetes mellitus. MMWR 1996; 45:941–943.

18. De Smet PAGM. Drugs used in non-orthodox medicine. In: Dukes MNG, Beeley L, eds. Side effects of drugs - Annual 13. Amsterdam: Elsevier, 1989:442–473.

19. Anonymous. Sondersitzung nach Stufenplan Injizierbare Arzneimittel zur Zellulartherapie. Pharm Ztg 1988;133:7, 80.

20. De Ridder M, Dienemann D, Diamann W, et al. Zwei Todesfälle nach Zelltherapie. Dtsch Med Wschr 1987;112:1006–1009.

21. Sorisky A, Robbins DC. Fish oil and diabetes. The net effect. Diabetes Care 1989;12:302–304.

22. Anonymous. Ganglioside (Cronassial u.a.) und neurologische Erkrankungen. Arznei-Telegramm 1992;12:126.

23. Nobile-Orazio E, Carpo M, Scarlato G. Gangliosides: their role in clinical neurology. Drugs 1994;47:576–585.

24. Committee for Proprietary Medicinal Products. Pharmacovigilance Opinion No.17. Ganglioside containing products. Brussels, September 14, 1994.

25. Traverso HP, Bennett JV, Kahn AJ, et al. Ghee applications to the umbilical cord: a risk factor for neonatal tetanus. Lancet 1989;1:486–488.

26. Li Wan Po A. Green-lipped mussel. Pharm J 1990;244:640–641.

27. Ahern MJ, Milazzo SC, Dymock R. Granulomatous hepatitis and Seatone. Med J Aust 1980;2:151–152.

28. Anonymous. Imedeen[R], bron der eeuwige jeugd? Gebu Prikbord 1993;27:68.

29. Anonymous. Vitamin A and birth defects. Aust Adv Drug React Bull 1996;15(4):14–15.

30. Dahm K. Schwerer anaphylaktischer Schock bei Leberhydrolysatbehandlung. Med Klin 1967; 62:1510–1511.

31. Vatutin NT, Tverskaia ShN. Anafilakticheskii shok ot sirepara. Klin Med (Mosk) 1973; 51:112–113.

32. Díez-Gómez ML, Hinojosa M, Moneo I, Losada E. Anaphylaxis after intra-articular injection of orgotein. Detection of an IgE-mediated mechanism. Allergy 1987;42:74–76.

33. Anonymous. Schock, Kollaps und andere Komplikationen nach Orgotein (Peroxinorm). Arznei-Telegramm 1988;2:24.

34. Anonymous. Quincke's oedeem bij gebruik van oesterextract in Ostrin plus GTZ 611[R]. Gebu Prikbord 1994;28:67.

35. Hausen BM, Wollenweber E, Senff H, Post B. Propolis allergy (I). Origin, properties, usage and literature review. Contact Dermatitis 1987;17: 163–170.

36. Hausen BM, Wollenweber E, Senff H, Post B. Propolis allergy - (II). The sensitizing properties of 1,1-dimethylallyl caffeic acid ester. Contact Dermatitis 1987;17:171–177.

37. Kraus A, Guerra-Bautista G, Alarcon-Segovia D. Salmonella arizona arthritis and septicemia associated with rattlesnake ingestion by patients with connective tissue diseases. A dangerous complication of folk medicine. J Rheumatol 1991; 18:1328–1331.

38. Cortes E, Zuckerman MJ, Ho H. Recurrent Salmonella arizona infection after treatment for metastatic carcinoma. J Clin Gastroenterol 1992; 14:157–159.

39. Bullock RJ, Rohan A, Straatmans JA. Fatal royal jelly-induced asthma. Med J Aust 1994;160:44.

40. Peacock S, Murray V, Turton C. Respiratory distress and royal jelly. BMJ 1995;311:1472.

41. Takahashi M, Matsuo I, Ohkido M. Contact dermatitis due to honeybee royal jelly. Contact Dermatitis 1983;9:452–455.

42. Markman M. Shark cartilage: the Laetrile of the 1990s. Cleve Clin J Med 1996;63:179–180.

43. Ashar B, Vargo E. Shark cartilage-induced hepatitis. Ann Intern Med 1996;125:780–781.

44. Till JS, Majmudar BN. Cantharidin poisoning. South Med J 1981;74:444–447.

45. Heepe J, Kristek J, Ahlmann J, et al. Makrohämaturie nach Cantharidin-Einnahme. Med Welt 1991;42:243–245.

46. Kok-Choi C, Hee-Ming L, Bobby SSF, David YCP. A fatality due to the use of cantharides from Mylabris Phalerata as an abortifacient. Med Sci Law 1990;30:336–340.

47. Asnis DS, Saltzman HP, Melchert A. Shark oil pneumonia. An overlooked entity. Chest 1993;103:976–977.

48. Anonymous. Gefährliche und irrationale Zusammensetzungen bei Magistralrezepturen gegen Übergewicht. Schweiz Apoth Ztg 1989;127:353.

49. Cooper N, Palmer B. Thyroid hormone in a health food capsule. N Z Med J 1994;107:231.

50. Rivlin RS. Therapy of obesity with hormones. N Engl J Med 1975;292:26–29.

51. American Medical Association Department of Drugs, Division of Drugs and Technology. AMA Drug Evaluations. 6th ed. Chicago: American Medical Association, 1986.

52. Lin C-S, Lin M-C, Chen K-S, et al. A digoxin-like immunoreactive substance and atrioventricular block induced by a Chinese medicine "kyushin'. Jap Circul J 1989;53:1077–1080.

53. Kwan T, Paiusco AD, Kohl L. Digitalis toxicity caused by toad venom. Chest 1992;102:949–950.

54. Burbacher J, Hoffman RS, Bania T, et al. Deaths associated with a purported aphrodisiac—New York City, February 1993 - May 1995. MMWR 1995;44:853–861.

55. Ko RJ, Greenwald MS, Loscutoff SM, et al. Lethal ingestion of Chinese herbal tea containing ch'an su. West J Med 1996;164:71–75.

56. Fushimi R, Koh T, Iyama S, et al. Digoxin-like immunoreactivity in Chinese medicine. Ther Drug Monit 1990;12:242–245.

57. Fushimi R, Yamanishi H, Inoue M, Iyama S, Amino N. Digoxin immunoassay that avoids cross-reactivity from Chinese medicines. Clin Chem 1995;41:621.

58. De Smet PAGM. Toxicological outlook on the quality assurance of herbal remedies. In: De Smet PAGM, Keller K, Hänsel R, Chandler RF, eds. Adverse effects of herbal drugs. Volume 1. Heidelberg: Springer-Verlag, 1992:1–72 .

59. Kerr HD, Saryan LA. Arsenic content of homeopathic medicines. Clin Toxicol 1986;24: 451–459.

60. De Smet PAGM. Giftige metalen in homeopathische preparaten. Pharm Weekbl 1992;127: 26,125–126.

61. Anonymous. Evaluation of certain food additives and contaminants. 33rd Report of the Joint FAO/ WHO Expert Committee on Food Additives. Technical Report Series 776. Geneva: World Health Organization, 1989.

62. Anonymous. Evaluation of certain food additives and contaminants. 41st Report of the Joint FAO/ WHO Expert Committee on Food Additives. Technical Report Series 776. Geneva: World Health Organization, 1993.

63. Anonymous. Evaluation of certain food additives and contaminants. 22nd Report of the Joint FAO/ WHO Expert Committee on Food Additives. Technical Report Series 776. Geneva: World Health Organization, 1978.

64. Villanacci JF, Beauchamp R, Perrotta DM, et al. Mercury poisoning associated with beauty cream—Texas, New Mexico, and California, 1995–1996. MMWR Morb Mortal Wkly Rep 1996;45:400–403.

65. Villanacci JF, Beauchamp R, Perrotta DM, et al. Update: mercury poisoning associated with beauty cream—Texas, New Mexico, and California, 1996. MMWR Morb Mortal Wkly Rep 1996;45:633–635.

66. Anonymous. Lead poisoning-associated death from Asian Indian folk remedies—Florida. MMWR Morb Mortal Wkly Rep 1984; 33:638–645.

67. Mohan SB, Tamilarasan A, Buhl M. Inhalational mercury poisoning masquerading as toxic shock syndrome. Anaesth Intens Care 1994;22: 305–306.

68. De Smet PAGM. Toxicological outlook on the quality assurance of herbal remedies. In: De Smet PAGM, Keller K, Hänsel R, Chandler RF, eds. Adverse effects of herbal drugs. Volume 1. Heidelberg: Springer-Verlag, 1992:1–72.

69. Yeung H-C. Handbook of Chinese herbs and formulas. Volume 2. Los Angeles, 1985.

70. De Smet PAGM. Drugs used in non-orthodox medicine. In: Dukes MNG, Beeley L, eds. Side effects of drugs – Annual 13. Amsterdam: Elsevier, 1989:442–473.

71. van der Spoel JI, Stricker BHC, Schipper MEI, et al. Toxische beschadiging van nier, lever en spier toegeschreven aan het gebruik van germaniumlactaat-citraat. Ned Tijdschr Geneeskd 1991; 135:1134–1137.

72. Labib M, Gama R, Wright J, et al. Dietary maladvice as a cause of hypothyroidism and short stature. BMJ 1989;298:232–233.

73. Tripp JH, Francis DEM, Knight JA, Harries JT. Infant feeding practices: a cause for concern. BMJ 1979;2:707–709.

74. Grüttner R. Die alternative Ernährung des Kindes. Ihre Vorzüge und ihre Risiken. Monatsschr Kinderheilkd 1988;136:222–227.

75. Kühne T, Bubl R, Baumgartner R. Maternal vegan diet causing a serious infantile neurological disorder due to vitamin B12 deficiency. Eur J Pediatr 1989;150:205–208.

76. Prakken ABJ, Veenhuizen L, Bruin MCA, et al. Vitamine B_{12}-deficiëntie bij 2 kinderen door afwijkende voedingsgewoonte. Ned Tijdschr Geneeskd 1994;138:474–476.

77. Walker FB. Myocardial infarction after diet-induced warfarin resistance. Arch Intern Med 1984;144:2089–2090.

78. Alvares AP. Environmental influences on drug biotransformations in humans. Wld Rev Nutr Diet 1984;43:45–59.

79. Dolan G, Jonas AP, Blumsohn A, et al. Lead poisoning due to Asian ethnic treatment for impotence. J Roy Soc Med 1991;84:630–631.

80. Smitherman J, Harber P. A case of mistaken identity: herbal medicine as a cause of lead toxicity. Am J Industr Med 1991;20:795–798.

81. Saryan LA. Surreptitious head exposure from an

Asian Indian medication. J Anal Toxicol 1991;15:336–338.

82. Dunbabin DW, Tallis GA, Popplewell PY, Lee RA. Lead poisoning from Indian herbal medicine (Ayurveda). Med J Aust 1992;157:835–836.

83. Kew J, Morris Cl Aihie A, et al. Arsenic and mercury intoxication due to Indian ethnic remedies. BMJ 1993;306:506–507.

84. Perharic L, Shaw D, Colbridge M, et al. Toxicological problems resulting from exposure to traditional remedies and food supplements. Drug Safety 1994;11:284–294.

85. Kenn RW, Deacon AC, Delves HT, et al. Indian herbal remedies for diabetes as a cause of lead poisoning. Postgrad Med J 1994;70:113–114.

86. Sheerin NS, Monk PN, Aslam M, Thurston H. Simultaneous exposure to lead, arsenic, and mercury from Indian ethnic remedies. Br J Clin Pract 1994;48:332–333.

87. Bayly GR, Braithwaite RA, Sheehan TMT, et al. Lead poisoning from Asian traditional remedies in the West Midlands—report of a series of five cases. Hum Exp Toxicol 1995;14:24–28.

88. Kulshrestha MK, Newey SE, Ferner RE. A radiographic lead in lead poisoning. Hum Exp Toxicol 1994;13:369–370.

89. Kulshrestha MK. Lead poisoning diagnosed by abdominal X-rays. J Toxicol Clin Toxicol 1996;34:107–108.

90. Brown S, Ede R. Occult lead poisoning. Br J Hosp Med 1995;53:469.

91. Prpic-Majic D, Pizent A, Jurasovic J, et al. Lead poisoning associated with the use of Ayurvedic metal-mineral tonics. Clin Toxicol 1996;34:417–423.

92. Wesley-Hadzija B. a note on the influence of diet in West Africa on urinary pH and excretion of amphetamine in man. J Pharm Pharmacol 1971;23:366–368.

93. Pierpaoli PG. Drug therapy and diet. Drug Intell Clin Pharm 1972;6:89–99.

94. Reynolds JEF, ed. Martindale The Extra Pharmacopoeia. 31th ed. London: The Pharmaceutical Press, 1996;1349–1396.

95. McEvoy GK, ed. AHFS Drug Information 97. Bethesda: American Society of Hospital Pharmacists, 1997:2389.

96. Meyers DG, Maloley PA, Weeks D. Safety of antioxidant vitamins. Arch Intern Med 1996;156:925–935.

97. Evans CDH, Lacey JH. Toxicity of vitamins: complications of a health movement. BMJ 1986;292:509–510.

98. Brown GR, Greenwood JK. Megavitamin toxicity. Can Pharm J 1987;120:80–87.

99. Diplock AT. Safety of antioxidant vitamins and beta-carotene. Am J Clin Nutr 1995;62(6 Suppl):1510S-1516S.

100. Rothman KJ, Moore LL, Singer MR, et al. Teratogenicity of high vitamin A intake. N Engl J Med 1995;333:1369–1373.

101. Oakley Jr GP, Erickson JD. Vitamin A and birth defects. Continuing caution is needed. N Engl J Med 1995;333:1414–1415.

102. Alpha-Tocopherol, Beta Carotene Cancer Prevention Study Group. The effect of vitamin E and beta carotene on the incidence of lung cancer and other cancers in male smokers. N Engl J Med 1994;330:1029–1035.

103. Omenn GS, Goodman GE, Thornquist MD, et al. Effects of a combination of beta carotene and vitamin A on lung cancer and cardiovascular disease. N Engl J Med 1996;334:1150–1155.

104. Hennekens CH, Buring JE, Manson JE, et al. Lack of effect of long-term supplementation with beta carotene on the incidence of malignant neoplasms and cardiovascular disease. N Engl J Med 1996;334:1145–1149.

105. Kerstens PJSM, Van Ditzhuijsen TJM, Van Tongeren JHM. Megadoses vitamine D: progressieve geneeskunde? Ned Tijdschr Geneeskd 1990;134:1959–1961.

106. Allen SH, Shah JH. Calcinosis and metastatic calcification due to Vitamin D intoxication. Horm Res 1992;37:68–77.

107. Jacobus CH, Holick MF, Shao Q, et al. Hypervitaminosis D associated with drinking milk. N Engl J Med 1992;326:1173–1177.

108. Corrigan J, Marcus FI. Coagulopathy associated with vitamin E ingestion. JAMA 1974;230:1300–1301.

109. Henkin Y, Johnson KC, Segrest JP. Rechallenge with crystalline niacin after drug-induced hepatitis from sustained-release niacin. JAMA 1990;264:241–243.

110. Rader JI, Calvert RJ, Hathcock JN. Hepatic toxicity of unmodified and time-release preparations of niacin. Am J Med 1992;92:77–81.

111. Schaumburg H, Kaplan J, Windebank A, et al. Sensory neuropathy from pyridoxine abuse. A new megavitamin syndrome. N Engl J Med 1983;309:445–448.

112. Berger A, Schaumburg HH. More on neuropathy from pyridoxine abuse. N Engl J Med 1984;311:986–987.

113. Cohen M, Bendich A. Safety of pyridoxine. A

review of human and animal studies. Toxicol Lett 1986;34:129–139.

114. Campbell NR. How safe are folic acid supplements? Arch Intern Med 1996;156:1638–1644.

115. Tucker KL, Mahnken B, Wilson PWF, et al. Folic acid fortification of the food supply. JAMA 1996;276:1879–1885.

116. Lee NA, Reasner CA. Beneficial effect of chromium supplementation on serum triglyceride levels in NIDDM. Diab Care 1994;17:1449–1452.

117. Wood R, Mills PB, Knobel GJ, et al. Acute dichromate poisoning after use of traditional purgatives. A report of 7 cases. S Afr Med J 1990; 77:640–642.

118. Dunn JP, Krige JE, Wood R, et al. Colonic complications after toxic tribal enemas. Br J Surg 1991;78:545–548.

119. O'Donohue JW, Reid MA, Varghese A, et al. Micronodular cirrhosis and acute liver failure due to chronic copper self-intoxication. Eur J Gastroenterol Hepatol 1993;5:561–562.

120. Clark LC, Combs GF, Turnbull BW, et al. Effects of selenium supplementation for cancer prevention in patients with carcinoma of the skin. A randomized controlled trial. JAMA 1996; 276:1957–1963.

121. Anonymous. Selenium. Environmental Health Criteria 58. Geneva: World Health Organization, 1987.

122. Yang G, Zhou R. Further observations on the human maximum safe dietary selenium intake in a seleniferous area of China. J Trace Elem Electrolytes Health Dis 1994;8:159–165.

123. Yang GQ, Xia YM. Studies on human dietary requirements and safe range of dietary intakes of selenium in China and their application in the prevention of related endemic diseases. Biomed Environ Sci 1995;8:187–201.

124. Jensen R, Closson W, Rothenberg R. Selenium intoxication - New York. MMWR 1984; 33: 157–158.

125. Helzlsouer K, Jacobs R, Morris S. Acute selenium intoxication in the United States. Fed Proc 1985;44:1670.

126. Clark RF, Strukle E, Williams SR, Manoguerra AS. Selenium poisoning from a nutritional supplement. JAMA 1996;275:1087–1088.

127. Simon SR, Branda RF, Tindle BF, Burns SL. Copper deficiency and sideroblastic anemia associated with zinc ingestion. Am J Hematol 1988;28:181–183.

128. Ramadori G, Meyer Zum Büschenfelde KH. Anemia with zinc therapy. Gastroenterology 1988;95:849–850.

129. Hoffman HN 2nd, Phyliky RL, Fleming CR. Zinc-induced copper deficiency. Gastroenterology 1988;94:508–512.

130. Patterson WP, Winkelmann M, Perry MC. Zinc-induced copper deficiency: megamineral sideroblastic anemia. Ann Intern Med 1985;103: 385–386.

131. Chandra RK. Excessive intake of zinc impairs immune responses. JAMA 1984;252:1443–1446.

132. Benvenga NJ, Steele RD. Adverse effects of excessive consumption of amino acids. Ann Rev Nutr 1984;4:157–181.

133. Anonymous. Carnitine. Med Lett 1986; 28: 88–89.

134. Goa KL, Brogden RN. l-Carnitine. A preliminary review of its pharmacokinetics, and its therapeutic use in ischaemic cardiac disease and primary and secondary carnitine deficiencies in relationship to its role in fatty acid metabolism. Drugs 1987;34:1–24.

135. Martinez E, Domingo P, Roca-Cusachs A. Potentation of acenocoumarol action by L-carnitine. J Intern Med 1993;233:94.

136. Keith RE. Symptoms of carnitinelike deficiency in a trained runner taking DL-carnitine supplements. JAMA 1986;255:1137.

137. De Smet PAGM. Drugs used in non-orthodox medicine. In: Dukes MNG, Aronson JK, red. Side effects of drugs - Annual 15. Amsterdam: Elsevier, 1991:514–531.

138. D'Arcy PF. L-tryptophan (Optimax): limited availability for resistant depression. Int Pharm J 1994;8:56.

139. Nichols MH, Wason S, Gonzalez del Rey J, Benfield M. Baking soda: a potentially fatal home remedy. Ped Emerg Care 1995;11:109–111.

140. Collet JT. EDTA-chelatiebehandeling. Ned Tijdschr Geneeskd 1992;136:191–192.

141. Anonymous. EDTA chelation therapy for atherosclerotic cardiovascular disease. Med Lett 1994;36:48.

142. Welter EA, Coote C. Chelation therapy for coronary atherosclerosis. J Can Pharm Hosp 1995;48:305–306.

143. Roodnat JI, Christiaans MHL, Nugteren-Huying WM, et al. Akute Nierinsuffizienz bei der Behandlung der Psoriasis mit Fumarsäure-Estern. Schweiz Med Wschr 1989;119:826–830.

144. Spiegel P, Fliegner L, Delling G. Osteomalazie infolge Fumarsäure-induzierten Tubulus-Defektes (sekundäres DeToni-Debré-Fanconi-Syndrom). Nieren- und Hochdruckkrankheiten 1991;20:280–288.

145. Nieboer C, Van Loenen AC. Fumaarzuurtherapie

bij psoriasis - Wat is het waard? Geneesmiddelen-bulletin 1987;21:57–60.

146. Nugteren-Huying WM, Van der Schroeff JG, Hermans J, Suurmond D. Fumaarzuurtherapie tegen psoriasis; een dubbelblind, placebo-gecontroleerd onderzoek. Ned Tijdschr Geneeskd 1990;134:2387–2391.

147. Anonymous. Multistate outbreak of poisonings associated with illicit use of gamma hydroxy butyrate. MMWR 1990;39:861–863.

148. Steele MT, Watson WA. Acute poisoning from gamma hydroxybutyrate (GHB). Missouri Med 1995;92:354–357.

149. Stell IM, Ryan JM. Ecstasy and neurodegeneration: gamma-hydroxybutyrate is a new recreational drug that may lead to loss of consciousness. BMJ 1996;313:424.

150. Thomas G, Bonner S, Gascoigne A. Coma induced by abuse of gamma-hydroxybutyrate (GBH or liquid ecstasy): a case report. BMJ 1997; 314:35–36.

151. Stephens BG, Baselt RC. Driving under the influence of GHB? J Analyt Toxicol 1994;18: 357–358.

152. Galloway GP, Frederick SL, Staggers FE Jr, et al. Gamma-hydroxybutyrate: an emerging drug of abuse that causes physical dependence. Addiction 1997;92:89–96.

153. De Smet PAGM. Drugs used in non-orthodox medicine. In: Dukes MNG, Beeley L, eds. Side effects of drugs - Annual 14. Amsterdam: Elsevier, 1990:429–451.

154. Hirschtick RE, Dyrda SE, Peterson LC. Death from an unconventional therapy for AIDS. Ann Intern Med 1994;120:694.

155. Jordan KS, Mackey D, Garvey E. A 39-year-old man with acute hemolytic crisis secondary to intravenous injection of hydrogen peroxide. J Emerg Nurs 1991;17:8–10.

156. Zinkham WH, Kickler T, Borel J, Moser HW. Lorenzo's oil and thrombocytopenia in patients with adrenoleucodystrophy. N Engl J Med 1993;328:1126–1127.

157. Anonymous. Infektionsgefahr durch Ozontherapie. Arznei-Telegramm 1991;6:56.

158. Gabriel C, Blauhut B, Greul R, et al. Transmission of hepatitis C by ozone enrichment of autologous blood. Lancet 1996;347:541.

159. Frankum B, Katelaris CH. Ozone therapy in AIDS - truly innocuous? Med J Aust 1993; 159:493.

160. Spigset O. Reduced effect of warfarin caused by ubidecarenone. Lancet 1994:344:1372–1373.

161. Anonymous. Coenzym Q10 (Qumin Q10 u.a.) stört orale Antikoagulation. Arznei-Telegramm 1994;12:120.

CHAPTER 8

THE SAFETY OF HOMEOPATHY

Wayne B. Jonas and Edzard Ernst

INTRODUCTION

Homeopathy involves the application of extremely small doses of substances diluted in a serial fashion and succussed, or agitated, between dilutions. These preparations are administered to healthy individuals to illicit symptoms to produce "drug pictures," which are then matched to those with similar symptoms who are ill.

Originally, the founder of homeopathy, Samuel Hahnemann (1755–1843), began diluting the drugs of his era to reduce their toxic side effects. He and others claimed that when these drugs were carefully matched to patients, these serial-agitated dilutions (SADs) lost their toxic effects, yet still retained stimulatory and therapeutic effects. It was subsequently discovered that many homeopathic preparations no longer have the possibility of any original molecules left in them. The assumptions from this are that they can have no specific effects at all; they are either therapeutic or toxic, and therefore are at least harmless. This attitude is reflected in the approach taken by the Food and Drug Administration of the United States, which generally classifies homeopathic preparations as over-the-counter drugs approved for sale without the standard toxicity and safety testing required of other medications.

Recent evidence indicates that homeopathic medications may not work in identical fashion to placebo (1, 2). If these claims are substantiated and homeopathic remedies are thought to produce specific effects, then the possibility that they also may produce specific adverse effects exists. In this regard, their evaluation will require the same assessment of risk-benefit ratio as any other drug.

RISKS

Direct Risks

Direct risks refer to direct toxic effects from a drug itself or adverse reactive effects to a drug. Homeopathic drug pictures are produced by a process called "provings," in which homeopathic preparations are given to healthy individuals and the symptoms produced are recorded. This is analogous to a Phase I trial and assumes direct adverse effects from stimulation by homeopathic remedies. Little animal research has been done to test whether such adverse effects occur in an objective way. However, when this has been done, it has not indicated an innocuous nature assumed from low dilutions. Here are some examples:

- Stearnes, in 1928, examined the effects of low dilutions of *Naturum muriticum* on several generations of guinea pigs. He reported that, compared to a control group, guinea pigs given repeated doses of low dilutions of *Naturum muriticum* became unhealthy, lost their hair, were less alert, lost weight, and began to stop breeding (3).
- Dwarakanath reported a study in 1979 in which the homeopathy remedy *China*, in the 200 C and 1000 C potency, produced acute reductions in body temperature measured

rectally in rats compared to a control group (4).

- Chandrasekhar reported that high potencies of *Pulsatilla* M and 10 M (very low dilutions) administered to rats immediately before and after mating induced lymphocytic infiltration of the implanted fetus and a higher frequency of fetal reabsorption compared to controls (5).

- Kumar reported that high potencies of *Caulophytum* retarded uterine ovarian cell maturation and stimulated endometrial proliferation in rats. Similar results have been reported in other animal experiments (6).

These studies are few and often of low methodological quality. Still, they indicate that one cannot assume that high potencies of homeopathic remedies have no direct toxic effects. This brings into question the nontoxicity homeopathy in which the perceived minimum toxic dose in a potency is assumed to be safe under all conditions.

Under normal use, homeopathic remedies appear too diluted to bring about toxic effects. This is not true for all dilutions, however. When toxic metals are used as homeopathic remedies, unsafe concentrations of arsenic (7), cadmium (8), and mercury (9) can result from the use of low potencies. For example, regular doses of *Cadmium sulfuricum* D_3 would exceed the daily tolerable dose of cadmium in a human of average size by two- to fourfold. There has been concern about potentially carcinogenic effects of low homeopathic potencies of *Aristolochia* (10). Low potencies of most homeopathic remedies can also cause allergic reactions. Several such adverse effects have been reported (11, 12). In cases of concomitant drug treatments, interactions with homeopathic remedies are conceivable, although as yet there seems to be no documented evidence of this. Finally, homeopathic remedies have on occasion been adulterated with potent allopathic medicaments (13, 14).

Adverse effects from homeopathic medications are assumed to be rare. In a survey of 386 users of complementary medicine, 10% of those who employed homeopathy had experienced adverse effects at some time (15). Reilly, in a systematic study of high dilutions of allergens, showed that approximately 24% of patients reported adverse aggravations. This resulted in about a 6% dropout rate from the study due to such adverse effects (16). Until reliable prevalence figures exist, we cannot conclude that homeopathic remedies are entirely risk-free.

HOMEOPATHIC AGGRAVATION

The term homeopathic "aggravation" describes the concept that symptoms may get initially worse if the optimal remedy has been administered. Homeopathic physicians see aggravations as a positive sign on the correct route to recovery. Patients, however, may view aggravation as an adverse effect. In our survey (15), about half of the adverse effects reported by users of homeopathy were associated with aggravation of symptoms. Sensitive patients are said to often produce severe aggravations. One of the authors (WJ) has seen a case of sudden severe aggravation of asthma necessitating hospitalization from homeopathic treatment. A recent placebo-controlled trial of homeopathy showed that homeopathic aggravation happened in the placebo group roughly as frequently as in the verum group (17), casting doubts on the existence of the phenomenon.

Homeopathic aggravation is a complex issue. Until more evidence is available to demonstrate the existence of homeopathic aggravation, it may be best to view it as a potential for adverse events.

The fact that homeopaths believe it does may significantly increase the risk of delaying mainstream treatments. Thus, the issue of homeopathic aggravation could be relevant in terms of both direct and indirect risks of homeopathy.

DOSE-DEPENDENT REVERSE EFFECTS

Dose-dependent reverse effects may also be an example of indirect effects from homeopathic preparations. Doutremepuich has demonstrated in several models that serially agitated preparations of aspirin can induce rather than inhibit thrombosis (18). Animal studies have shown that high potencies of arsenic can accelerate the elimination of arsenic when subsequently given in toxic dose (19, 20). One must consider whether homeopathic preparations of essential minerals and nutrients might also stimulate the elimination of such nutrients. If dose-dependent reverse effects occur for other substances, one wonders whether cytotoxic drugs, when given in homeopathic preparations, might stimulate cellular proliferation and carcinogenesis rather than inhibit it.

Indirect Risks

A second category of adverse effects in homeopathy relates to indirect effects. If an effective therapy exists, then treatment with ineffective therapy, be it homeopathy or conventional treatment, may result in unnecessary progression of the disease, which is an indirect adverse effect. These are "neglect" effects. An extreme example would be an attempt to use homeopathy in place of setting a fracture or getting emergency care. More subtle "neglect" effects can also occur, however. Comparing a drug to placebo is insufficient to assess the difference in adverse effects between two active drug treatments. A drug response over one placebo may not be the same as another drug over another placebo. Only direct comparison of two interventions gives information about optimal therapies, and thus the degree of "neglect" effects that occur through the administration of a suboptimal therapy.

Other indirect effects in homeopathy can occur because of its philosophy of healing. Homeopathy stimulates the healing response, which may be slow in some patients.

For example, some homeopaths claim there is a duration of action from particular potencies, even up to a year after a single dose. One of the authors (WJ) has seen cases where individuals with chronic illness, such as gingivitis and gall bladder disease, have been told to wait for the full duration of action of the remedy, often for very long periods, resulting in continued suffering. Homeopaths also claim that the return of old symptoms is a good sign during the action of the remedy, but for most individuals this is not desirable. These symptoms would also be classified as indirect adverse effects.

Symptom control without resolution of the underlying problem is another indirect adverse effect. The only evidence for this in homeopathy comes from case reports. For example:

- A woman with staples inadvertently left in the skin of her scalp postoperatively was taking the homeopathic remedy *Hypericum* to treat the pain. This resulted in the staples being undiscovered for longer than would have without such treatment.
- A woman was treating what she thought were menstrual cramps with a homeopathic remedy. Later it was discovered that she had a ruptured ovarian cyst and was bleeding internally.

These adverse effects, of course, can occur with any kind of misdiagnosis and symptom control. There are certain conditions, such as acute myocardial infarction, fractures, bacterial meningitis, and so on, which require immediate conventional attention for managing. The attempt to use homeopathic medications in these conditions can result in adverse outcomes.

Even if homeopathic remedies were totally safe, the homeopath might not always be. In all professions, there should be proper training and competence for scope of practice (21). If a homeopathic practitioner takes over full medical responsibility for a patient, he or she should be medically competent to dose, including full diagnostic and management skills. If competence is insufficient, disasters may occur. A review of the medical literature indicates that these indirect risks are not merely an academic issue. There are distressing case reports, some with fatal outcomes (22–24).

In this context, vaccination is a particularly relevant and clear example (25, 26). Some homeopaths (as well as some chiropractors and naturopaths) hinder access to immunization by advocating a homeopathic vaccination (27), which is not documented to be effective (28), or by advising their clients not to comply with immunization programs. Our own survey shows that none of the nonmedically qualified homeopaths recommended orthodox vaccination, whereas the majority of physician–homeopaths do (29). Certainly, there can be adverse effects from immunizations and these vary depending on the type of immunization. In view of their potential benefit, however, a general rejection of immunization puts the individual patient and the population at large at risk.

Illness Fabrication and Misclassification

Adverse effects in homeopathy also can arise from misclassification through the creation of false-positive syndromes. The classical homeopathic approach requires assessing the "totality" of symptoms in the assessment and treatment of a case. A homeopath may spend 60 to 90 minutes getting all the symptoms of a patient and prescribe a remedy for this "totality." Six weeks later, the vast majority of these systems are likely to have regressed due to spontaneous remission or statistical regression to the mean or other factors. In this situation, the remedy will appear to have been successful, thus giving a false sense of efficacy. Repeated experiences such as this can result in a kind of treatment addiction to these false syndromes. The patient returns to have further symptoms assessed and apparently resolved through such nonspecific means. This also risks turning the therapeutic interaction into worry management. The patient attempts to resolve all symptoms or reduce all risk, resulting in repeated visits to the physician. This then is an adverse effect.

A similar phenomenon may occur when practitioners use electrodermal diagnostic techniques that apply homeopathic remedies for treatments. In this technique, electrical potential changes on acupuncture points of the fingers and toes are said to be related to premorbid health problems. These electrodermal changes then become diagnostic categories in themselves, requiring treatment with repeated visits and unnecessary medication. This results in the fabrication of illness. The assumption is that "treatment" of these electrical potentials will prevent health problems in the future. If patients then neglect well-known lifestyle and other prevention activities, such as exercise, appropriate diet, and smoking cessation, they may assume they are protected, when they are not.

This may result in adverse effects from failure to take concrete steps to prevent illness. A number of other safety issues related to homeopathy are beyond the scope of this chapter but have been reviewed in detail elsewhere (30).

CONCLUSIONS

The risks of any type of medicine should not be evaluated in isolation. Whenever a practitioner prescribes a treatment, he or she should weigh its risks against its benefits. If the former is small, the latter should be minute so that, on balance, the benefits clearly outweigh the risks. Both homeopathy's benefits and its potential risks need to be established with a much higher degree of certainty before definitive answers to the complex question of safety can be given. Safety in homeopathy cannot be assumed without empiricalal testing and verification. Systematic evaluation of the direct, indirect, misclassification, and paradigmatic issues of homeopathic treatment is necessary.

REFERENCES

1. Linde K, Jonas WB, Melchart D, et al. Critical review and meta-analysis of serial agitated dilutions in experimental toxicology. Hum Exper Toxicol 1994;13:481–492.
2. Linde K, Clausius N, Ramirez G, et al. Are the clinical effects of homeopathy all placebo effects? A meta-analysis of randomized, placebo controlled trials. Lancet 1997;350:934–843.
3. Stearns G. Completion of the experiment with high dilutions of natrium muriaticum given to guinea pigs. J Am Inst Hom 1925;18(790):790–792.
4. Dwarkanath SK, Stanley MM. Short term observations on the effect of China in relation to the rectal temperature of albino rats. Hahn Glean 1979; 46(37):37–41.
5. Chandrasekhar K, Sarma GHR. Effect of caulophyllum 200 and 10,000 potencies on the ovaries, the uteri and the thyroids of rats. Ind J Zootomy 1975;16(199):199–204.
6. Kumar S, Srivastava AK, Chandrasekhar K. Effects of caulophyllum on the uteri and ovaries of adult rats. Br Homoeop J 1981;70(135):135–138.
7. Kerr HD, Saryan LA. Arsenic content of homeopathic medicines. Clin Toxicol 1986;24:451–459.

8. De Smet PAGM. Giftige metalen in homeopathische preparaten. Pharm Weekbl 1992;127: 26,125–126.

9. Montoya-Cabrera MA, Rubio-Rodriguez S, Valazquez-Gonzalez E, Avila Montoya S. Intoxicacion mercurial causada por un medicamento homeopatico. Gaceta Med Mex 1991;127:267–270.

10. Oepen I. Kritische Argumente zur Homöopathie. Dtsch Apoth Ztg 1983;123:1105.

11. Van Ulsen J, Stolz E, Joost T. Chromate dermatitis from a homoeopathic drug. Contact Derm 1988;18:56–57.

12. Forsman S. Homeopati kan vara farling vid hudsjukdomar och allergier. Läkartidningen 1991; 88:1672.

13. Morice A. Adultered "homoeopathic" cure for asthma. Lancet 1986;1:862–863.

14. Goulon M, Combes A. Crise thyrotoxique médicamenteuse. Des dangers d'une préparation prétendue homéopathique. Nouv Press Med 1977; 6:3729–3731.

15. Abbot NC, White AR, Ernst E. Complementary medicine. Nature 1996;381:361.

16. Reilly DT, Taylor MA, McSharry C, Aitchinson T. Is homeopathy a placebo response? Controlled trial of homeopathic potency, with pollen in hayfever as model. Lancet 1986;2(8512):881–885.

17. Walach H, Haeusler W, Lowes T, et al. Classical homeopathic treatment of chronic headaches. Cephalalgia 1997;17:119–126.

18. Doutremepuich C, DeSéze O, LeRoy D, et al. Aspirin at very ultra low dosage in healthy volunteers: effects on bleeding time, platelet aggregation and coagulation. Haemostasis 1990;20:99–105.

19. Cazin JC, Cazin M, Boiron J. A study of the effect of decimal and centesimal dilutions of arsenic on the retention and mobilization of arsenic in rats. Hum Toxicol 1987;135(6):315–320.

20. Boiron J. Comparaison de l'action de Arsenicum album 7 CH normal et chauffe a 120_C sur l'intoxication arsenicale provoquee. Homeopathie 1985; 2(5):49–53.

21. Ernst E. Competence in complementary medicine. Comp Ther Med 1995;3:6–8.

22. Goodyear HM, Harper JI. Atopic eczema, hyponatraemia, and hypoalbuminaemia. Arch Dis Child 1990;65:231–232.

23. Tsur M. Inadvertent child health neglect by preference of homeopathy to conventional medicine. Harefuah 1992;122:137–142.

24. De Smet PAGM, Stricker BHCh, Nijman JJ. Indirecte risico's van alternatieve middelen - een oproep tot het rapporteren van concrete gevallen. Med Contact 1994;49:1593–1594.

25. Fisher P. Enough nonsense on immunization. Br Homoeop J 1990;79:198–200.

26. English J. The issue of immunization. Br Homoeop J 1992;81:161–163.

27. Ernst E. The attitude against immunisation within some branches of complementary medicine. Eur J Pediatr 1997;156:513–515.

28. Burgess M. Homoeopathy and vaccination. Lancet 1994;344:1168.

29. White AR, Ernst E. Homoeopathy and immunization. Br J Gen Pract 1995;48:629–630.

30. Jonas WB: Safety in homeopathy. In: Ernzt E, ed. Homeopathy: a critical appraisal. London: Butterworth, 1998.

CHAPTER 9

ADVERSE EFFECTS OF ACUPUNCTURE

Edzard Ernst

Acupuncture is one of the most popular complementary therapies worldwide. Contrary to claims made by some authors, acupuncture is not free of adverse effects or complications. Most of these are mild and transient (e.g., aggravation of symptoms, pain during needling, fainting). However, serious complications, including 45 deaths (1–4), are on record.

INFECTIONS

Inadequate use of acupuncture needles carries an obvious risk of infection. One overview identified 126 published cases of hepatitis associated with acupuncture (5). One outbreak of hepatitis B was traced back to an acupuncturist who infected 36 patients by reusing needles (6). Six patients were infected through acupuncture treatments at a chiropractic institution (7). In a further instance, 35 patients of one acupuncturist tested positive for hepatitis B (8). Five cases of hepatitis B were reported in Israel, and an additional six people were infected but remained asymptomatic (9). Four similar cases have been documented in Europe (10, 11).

Epidemiologic studies contribute further important evidence. Kiyosawa and associates investigated two areas of Japan, one of which was endemic for hepatitis C. Acupuncture was significantly more prevalent in the region endemic with hepatitis C (12). During a screening program for hepatitis B, 651 individuals tested positive, 4 of whom had a history of acupuncture (13). Other Japanese researchers investigated 262 hepatitis C carriers. They found that in 20% of cases, the most likely route of infection was via acupuncture (14). Finally, a survey in Singapore (15) revealed that the prevalence of hepatitis B in acupuncture patients was 8.7%, which was slightly less than for tattooing (10.9%) or blood transfusions (12.8%).

Even HIV infections have been linked to acupuncture. A Frenchman became HIV positive eight weeks after having being treated with acupuncture for six weeks (16). No other plausible origin of the infection could be identified. In a study of 148 AIDS patients, two individuals with no other recognized risk factor had previously used acupuncture (17).

Other serious infections include subacute bacterial endocarditis due to *Propionibacterium acnes* infection after ear-acupuncture (18). Similar cases had been reported previously in which the causal agents were *Pseudomonas aeruginosa* (19) and *Staphylococcus aureus* (20). All patients thus infected recovered with antibiotic therapy.

Two fatalities have been reported in which acupuncture led to *Staphylococcus* septicemia (21). Two further cases of septicemia are on record (22, 23). A dramatic incident was described (19) in which a patient received acupuncture treatment in the lumbar paraspinal region for low back pain and subsequently contracted bilateral psoas abscesses infected with *S. aureus*. He fortunately survived a severe and protracted illness.

Obviously, these infections are preventable. A survey of 500 Japanese acupuncturists showed that, in 1993, 60% of these therapists used disposable needles (24). It seems that use of sterile needles and correct handling of these needles are preconditions for safe acupuncture (25). If this precondition would be universally adhered to, such complications would be a thing of the past.

serted into the paraspinal musculature and penetrate as far as the spinal cord.

Traumatic injury of a blood vessel often results in a hematoma, which is a frequent complication of acupuncture (5). However, hematomas are rarely severe. A recent report described a case in which an acupuncture needle caused a false aneurysm of the popliteal artery (38). The patient presented with rupture of the aneurysm and was saved by arterial repair.

TRAUMA

The insertion of an acupuncture needle represents a tissue trauma. Depending on the anatomic site, this may lead to serious complications or, as in the majority of cases, be of no consequence at all.

Numerous cases of pneumothorax have been reported. In total, well over 100 cases have been published (2, 5, 26). In most cases, a direct causal link to acupuncture is indisputable. In Germany, one well-documented fatality through pneumothorax is on record (3). A 63-year-old woman suffering from asthma went to a *heilpraktiker* (i.e., a nonmedically trained complementary therapist) who had a reputation as an acupuncturist. He used acupuncture points on the thorax to treat the chronic asthma. During therapy, the patient felt acute breathlessness and died within 20 minutes. The postmortem diagnosis was bilateral pneumothorax.

There are also several reports of cardiac tamponade through acupuncture (27–29). One patient's heart was pierced by an acupuncturist through a foramen in the sternum (30). The patient died within 2 hours, and cardiac tamponade was confirmed at autopsy. Congenital sternal foramina can be found in 10% of the male and 4% of the female populations. Others have commented on this case that the acupoint in question must be punctured obliquely to the sternum, which would prevent cardiac tamponade (31).

Several authors have reported trauma of the spinal cord by acupuncture needles (32–36). Recently, a rare case of transverse myelopathy after acupuncture was published (37). These complications can occur when needles are in-

OTHER ADVERSE EFFECTS OF ACUPUNCTURE

Other adverse effects of acupuncture range across a wide array of conditions and symptoms (39). A fatality was observed in Japan (40) in which a patient received acupuncture for his chronic asthma. An acute asthma attack was triggered by acupuncture, and the patient died during treatment. As is often the case with anecdotal reports, it is difficult to decide whether the fatality was causally related to acupuncture or whether this was a mere temporal coincidence. In one report (41), the electromagnetic interference of an electroacupuncture device suppressed a demand cardiac pacemaker; in another report, manual needle acupuncture was apparently followed by cardiac arrhythmias in a 70-year-old woman who carried a cardiac pacemaker (42).

In addition to these rare and serious adverse effects, there are more frequent but less serious problems (Table 9.1). In our own survey, 13% of acupuncture users reported mild adverse effects of which the most frequent was "aggravation of symptom" (43). In a much larger Australian survey of approximately 2000 practitioners, a total of 3177 adverse events of acupuncture were reported; the most frequent was fainting during treatment (2).

Although these surveys represent first attempts to estimate the size of the problem, we cannot yet give reliable prevalence figures at present. Thus, all we can state with certainty is that properly delivered acupuncture seems relatively safe but does lead to adverse effects which, at times, can be severe and even life-threatening.

Table 9.1. Frequent Complications of Acupuncture

NATURE OF EVENT DOCUMENTED	NUMBER OF CASES*
Drowsiness, syncope, fainting	1429
Increased pain	1129
Nausea, vomiting	540
Infections (endocarditis, osteomyelitis, septicemia, perichondritis, skin infection)	228
Pneumothorax	129
Hepatitis	127
Psychiatric complications	112
Convulsions	80
Cardiac trauma	7

* Combined data from the published literature. A total of 45 fatalities are on record.

REFERENCES

1. Ernst E, White AR. Life threatening adverse reactions after acupuncture? A systematic review. Pain 1997;71:123–126.
2. Bensoussan A, Myers SP. Towards a safer choice. Sydney, Australia: Southern Cross University, 1996.
3. Brettel HF. Akupunktur als Todesursache. Münch Med Wschr 1981;123:97–100.
4. Huang K Ch. Acupuncture. The past and the present. New York: Vantage Press, 1997.
5. Rampes H, James R. Complications of acupuncture. Acupunct Med 1995;11:26–33.
6. Boxall EH. Acupuncture hepatitis in the West Midlands. J Med Virol 1978;2:377–379.
7. Stryker WS, Gunn RA, Francis DP. Outbreaks of hepatitis B associated with acupuncture. J Fam Pract 1986;22(2):155–158.
8. Kent GP, Brondum J, Keenlyside RA, et al. A large outbreak of Acupuncture-Associated Hepatitis B. Am J Epidemiol 1988;127(3):591–598.
9. Slater PE, Ben-Ishai P, Leventhal A, et al. An acupuncture-associated outbreak of hepatitis B in Jerusalem. Eur J Epidemiol 1988;4(3):322–325.
10. Hussain KK. Serum hepatitis associated with repeated acupunctures. Br Med J 1974;3:41–42.
11. Kobler E, Schmutziger P, Hartmann G. Hepatitis nach akupunktur. Schweiz Med Wschr 1979; 109(46):1828–1829.
12. Kiyosawa K, Tanaka E, Sodeyama T. Transmission of hepatitis C in an isolated area in Japan. Gastroenterol 1994;106:1596–1602.
13. Kiyosawa K, Gibo Y, Sodeyama T, et al. Possible infectious causes in 651 patients with acute viral hepatitis during a 10-year period (1976–1985). Liver 1987;7:163–168.
14. Shimoyama R, Sekiguchi S, Suga M, et al. The epidemiology and infection route of asymptomatic HCV carriers detected through blood donations. Gastroenterol Japan 1993;28:1–5.
15. Phoon WO, Fong NP, Lee J. History of blood transfusion, tattooing, acupuncture and risk of hepatitis B surface antigen among Chinese men in Singapore. AJPH 1988;78(8):958–960.
16. Vittecoq D, Mettetal JF, Rouzioux C, et al. Acute HIV infection after acupuncture treatments. N Engl J Med 1989;320(4):250–251.
17. Castro KG, Lifson AR, White CR. Investigation of AIDS patients with no previous identified risk factors. JAMA 1988;259:1338–1342.
18. Scheel O, Sundsfjord A, Lunde P, Andersen BM. Endocarditis after acupuncture and injection treatment by a natural healer. JAMA 1992;267:56.
19. Jeffreys DB, Smith S, Brennand-Roper DA, Curry PVL. Acupuncture needles as a cause of bacterial endocarditis. Br Med J 1983;287:326–327.
20. Lee RJE, Mc Ilwain JC. Subacute bacterial endocarditis following ear acupuncture. Int J Cardiol 1985;7:62–63.
21. Pierik MG. Fatal staphylococcal septicemia following acupuncture: report of two cases. RI Med J 1982;65:251–253.
22. Izatt E, Fairman M. Staphylococcal septicaemia with DIC associated with acupuncture. Postgrad Med J 1977;53:285–286.
23. Doutscu Y, Tao Y, Sasayama K. A case of staphylococcus aureus septicemia after acupuncture therapy. Kansenshogaku Zasshi 1986;60:911–916.
24. Hirose K, Tajimak I, Fujikira N, et al. AIDA/HIV related knowledge, attitude and behaviour of acupuncturists in Aichi Prefecture. Jap J Publ Health 1995;42:269–279.
25. Ernst E, White A. Acupuncture: safety first. Training programmes should include basic medical knowledge and experience. Br Med J 1997;314:1362.
26. Norheim AJ, Fonnebo V. Adverse effects of acupuncture. Lancet 1995;345:1576.
27. Schiff AF. A Fatality due to acupuncture. Medical Times 1965;93(6):630–631.
28. Nieda S, Abe T, Kuribayashi R, et al. Cardiac trauma as complication of acupuncture treatment; a case report of cardiac tamponade resulting from a broken acupuncture needle. Japan J Thorac Surg 1973;26:881–883.
29. Hasegawa J, Noguchi N, Yamasaki J, et al. Delayed cardiac tamponade and hemothorax induced by an acupuncture needle. Cardiology 1991;78:58–63.

30. Halvorsen TB, Anda SS, Levang OW. Fatal cardi-actamponade after acupuncture through congenital sternal foramen. Lancet 1995;345:1175.

31. Carneiro NM, Shih-Minl. Acupuncture technique. Lancet 1995;345:1577.

32. Kataoka H, Sakata M. Nerve injury due to an acupuncture treatment. Geka 1958;20:578–82.

33. Kondo A, Koyama T, Ishikaway K. Injury to the spinal cord produced by acupuncture needle. Surg Neurol 1979;11:155–156.

34. Shiraiski S, Goto I, Kuroiwa Y. Spinal cord injury as a complication of an acupuncture. Neurology 1979;229:1180–1182.

35. Isu T, Iwasaki Y, Sasaki H. Spinal cord and root injuries due to glass fragments and acupuncture needles. Surg Neurol 1985;23:255–260.

36. Sato M, Yamane K, Ezima M. A case of transverse myelopathy caused by acupuncture. Rinsko Shin-keigaku 1991;31:717–719.

37. Ilhan A, Alioglu Z, Adanir M. Transverse myelopa-thy after acupuncture therapy. Acupunct Electro Therap Res Int J 1995;20:191–194.

38. Lord RV, Schwartz P. False aneurism of the popli-teal artery complicating acupuncture. Austr New Zealand J Surg 1996;66:645–647.

39. Ernst E. The risks of acupuncture. Int J Risk Safety Med 1995;6:179–186.

40. Ogata M, Kitamura O, Kubo S, Nakasono Q. An astmatic death while under Chinese acupuncture and moxibustion treatment. Am J Forensic Med Pathol 1992;13:338–341.

41. Fujiwara H, Taniguchi K, Ikezono E. The influence of low frequency acupuncture on a demand pace-maker. Chest 1980;78:96–97.

42. White AR, Abbot NC, Ernst E. Self-reports of adverse effects of acupuncture included cardiac ar-rhythmia. Acup Med 1996;14:121.

43. Abbot NC, White AR, Ernst E. Complementary medicine. Nature 1996;381:361.

CHAPTER 10

ADVERSE EFFECTS OF SPINAL MANIPULATION

Edzard Ernst

SPINAL MANIPULATIVE THERAPIES

Osteopathy and chiropractic can be categorized as spinal manipulative therapies (SMT), which are aimed at restoring spinal joint function through adjustments of spinal motion segments. Chiropractic often involves high-velocity thrusts that seem to be particularly burdened with serious complications.

Direct Adverse Effects

Recent narrative (1) and systematic reviews (2) report a multitude of direct adverse reactions to SMT. The latter located 295 case reports, including 165 vertebrobasilar accidents (25 of which were fatal), 61 cases of disk herniation or progression to cauda equina syndrome, 13 cerebral complications other than vertebrobasilar accidents, and 56 other types of complications. Of the documented 295 adverse events, 135 had occurred at the hands of chiropractors. Vertebrobasilar accidents occurred most frequently after upper cervical spinal manipulation with a rotational component (3). Their cause is usually arterial dissection at the atlantoaxial joint with intimal tear, intramural bleeding, or pseudoaneurysm that leads to thrombosis or embolism (4). Cauda equina syndrome seems to occur considerably less frequently, typically after lumbar SMT (5). The risk factors for these complications are summarized in Table 10.1. The list comprises entities that are not normally detectable by chiropractors.

Estimations as to the incidence rates of adverse events after SMT are inconsistent and widely variable (Table 10.2). The variation can only partly be explained by the differences in type of adverse reactions. Obviously, mild adverse effects are more frequent than serious ones.

Several other complications of SMT have been recorded (Table 10.3). They all seem to be extremely rare events (1, 6–9), and some have been observed only after cranial-sacral treatment, a variation of SMT.

There are no systematic investigations of the adverse effects of SMT; most of our knowledge is based on case reports (10). However, several published surveys have shed more light on this issue. In our own survey (11), 16% of users of SMT reported having experienced adverse effects; fortunately, most were mild. When United States neurologists were asked whether they had seen complications of SMT during the last 2 years, a large proportion claimed to have witnessed mostly serious complications, including 50 cases of stroke (12). Based on the results of a survey of 226 members of the Danish Chiropractors' Association, it was calculated that cerebrovascular accidents occurred 1 in 120,000 cervical treatment sessions (13).

Comparative Safety

Chiropractors are keen to point out that SMT is much safer than other (conventional) treatment options for the same complaint (14). It should be stressed, however, that such comparisons

Table 10.1. Risk Factors for Complications of SMT

Upper cervical manipulation

Misdiagnosis by manipulator

Presence of a bleeding disorder

Presence of a herniated nucleus pulposus

Improper technique

(Adapted from Shekelle PG. Spine update: Spinal manipulation. *Spine* 1994;19(7):858–6.)

are problematic on methodological grounds. First, they compare one treatment (e.g., nonsteroidal antiinflammatory drugs [NSAIDs]), for which proper postmarketing surveillance techniques (often unreliable in themselves) are in place, with SMT, for which no such systems exist. Thus, it is to be expected that relatively fewer adverse effects are on record for SMT. Second, they compare incidence rates of adverse effects following a single SMT treatment with incidence rates related to prolonged drug therapy (14). This could be an unfair comparison—for example, contrasting one tablet of aspirin with one series of SMT. Third, they compare SMT for which the benefit is far from established (15) with treatments of documented efficacy. Thus, comparative evaluations of risk–benefit ratios are highly complex issues that are not resolved by the data available to date and will be extremely difficult to resolve in the future.

Indirect Risks

IMMUNIZATION

Some chiropractors advise their clients against immunization of their children (16). If this were to happen on a large scale, not only would it put the child at risk, but it could endanger the herd immunity of entire populations. This is a good example of how complementary practitioners can hinder their clients' access to effective orthodox treatments.

USE OF X-RAYS

Another indirect risk is the excessive use of x-rays by chiropractors. A survey of 48 members of the British Chiropractic Association showed that 82% of them had x-ray facilities in their clinics. Of 1598 patients with low back pain, 71% had been x-rayed (17). A more recent survey from the same source recorded that 74% of chiropractors had their own x-ray equipment, but no data on the frequency of x-ray use were provided (18). Pederson sent questionnaires to all chiropractors working in the European Union (19). X-rays were used in 72% of the patients with low back pain. Of all the patients seen by chiropractors, 64.4% were x-rayed. A survey of a random sample of members of the American Chiropractic Association suggested that 96.3% of new patients and 80% of patients at follow-up visits were x-rayed (20). A 1992 survey of 60 licensing boards in the United

Table 10.2. Estimated Incidence Rates of Complications and Adverse Effects after SMT

RATE (CASE: TREATMENTS)	SEVERITY/TYPE OF ADVERSE EFFECT	SOURCE
1:10	Mild and transient	Abbot, Nature 1996;381:361
1:40,000	Serious	Dvorak, Man Medizin 1985;2:1
1:120,000	Cerebrovascular incident	Klougart, J Man Physiol Ther 1996;19:563
1:400,000	Serious	Gutman, Man Medizin 1983;21:2
1:1,000,000	Serious	Patijn, J Man Med 1991;6:89
1:2,000,000	Serious	Shekelle, Am J Public Health 1991;81:439
1:3,300,000	Death	Hurwitz, Spine 1996;15:1746
1:4,000,000	Serious	Carey, J Can Chiroprac Ass 1993;37:104
1:100,000,000	Cauda equina syndrome	Shekelle, Spine 1994;7:858

Table 10.3. Rare Complications of SMT

Brainstem dysfunction*	Ophthalmoplegia
Confusion*	Opisthotonus*
Depression*	Phrenic nerve palsy
Diplopia*	Plexus paralysis
Disc herniation	Seizures*
Dissection of internal carotid artery	Tetraplegia
Fainting*	Trigeminal nerve damage*
Headache*	Vertebral dislocations
Hypopituitarism*	Vertebral fractures
Long thoracic nerve palsy	Vertigo*
Miscarriage*	Vomiting*
Nausea*	

* Described after cranial-sacral treatment.

States and Canada (21) showed that full spine, skull, soft tissue, barium, and topography studies were permitted in 100%, 98.1%, 96.2%, 36.0%, and 56.3%, respectively, by the boards. A survey of all the members of the Netherlands' Chiropractors Association indicated that 80% of chiropractors would often or always use x-rays for a new patient (22). Only 6% would employ it seldom or never, and virtually all thought that it was "desirable" or "absolutely desirable" to have access to x-ray equipment. In a recent clinical trial of various treatments of back pain, 208 practitioners of various types were randomly selected from six strata (23). Plain spine x-rays were used more frequently by the chiropractors (in 67% of all patients) than by any other profession.

Within the chiropractic profession, "there is currently no agreement regarding indications for taking x-rays" (19). Osteoporosis is a relative contraindication for several chiropractic techniques (Table 10.4). Plain x-rays of the spine (the type usually taken by chiropractors) do not help in diagnosing osteoporosis unless it is in very advanced stages (24, 25). Chiropractors could therefore use x-rays to detect malignancies, fractures, infections, inflammatory spondylarthropthies, and other contraindications (19). Yet, "bone disease is not immediately revealed by X-rays" (26), and unsuspected pathological findings on routine lumbar radiographs are as infrequent as 1 in 2500 (27). Many chiropractors employ x-rays for diagnosing misalignment or subluxation of the spine (28). Yet "subluxation of the vertebra as defined by chiropractic. . . . does not occur" (29) and "minor misalignments of vertebrae are normal and not necessarily a sign of trouble" (30) and such irregularities "show up on almost anyone's X-ray" (31). Thus, the question of why chiropractors so frequently use x-rays amounts to a serious safety issue that needs addressing.

Table 10.4. Contraindications of SMT

Absent odontoid process
Coagulant medication
Disc lesions
Gross segment instability
Neoplasm
Osteoporosis
Postoperative states in children
Rheumatoid arthritis
Spinal tuberculosis
Upper respiratory tract infections

(Adapted from Grieve GP. Incidents and accidents of manipulation and allied techniques. In: Grieve's modern manual therapy. Edinburgh: Churchill Livingstone, 1994:679.)

CONTRAINDICATIONS TO SMT

The list of contraindications of SMT in Table 10.4 is impressive. It raises questions as to the validity of these items, particularly because there seems to be no agreement among authors as to what constitutes a contraindication of SMT. It also raises questions regarding the ability and competence of nonmedically trained practitioners to diagnose these conditions.

In conclusion, SMT does produce adverse effects, some of which are serious. Their incidence is not completely known, and estimates vary enormously. In addition, important indirect safety issues need to be addressed, particularly in relation to the chiropractic profession.

REFERENCES

1. Ernst E. Cervical manipulation: is it really safe? Int J Risk Safety Med 1994;6:145–149.
2. Assendelft WJJ, Bouter LM, Knipschild PG. Complications of spinal manipulation: a comprehensive review of the literature. J Fam Pract 1996;42: 475–480.
3. Terrett AGJ. Vascular accidents from cervical spine manipulation: report on 107 cases. J Aust Chiropractors Assoc 1987;17:15–24.
4. Frisoni GB, Anzola GP. Vertebrobasilar ischemia after neck motion. Stroke 1991;22:1452–1460.
5. Malmivaara A, Pohjola R. Cauda equina syndrome caused by chiropraxis on a patient previously free of lumbar spine symptoms. Lancet 1982;2:986–987.
6. Segal DH, Lidov MW, Camins MB. Cervical epidural hematoma after chiropractic manipulation in healthy young women: case report. Neurosurgery 1996;39(5):1043–1045.
7. McPartland JM. Craniosacral iatrogenesis. Side-effects from cranial-sacral treatment: case reports and commentary. J Bodywork Movement Ther 1996;1(1):2–5.
8. Oware A, Herskovitz S, Berger AR. Long thoracic nerve palsy following cervical chiropractic manipulation. Muscle-Nerve 1995;18(11):1351.
9. Peters M, Bohl J, Thömke F, et al. Dissection of the internal carotid artery after chiropractic manipulation of the neck. Neurology 1995;45:2284–2286.
10. Shekelle PG. Spine update: spinal manipulation. Spine 1994;19(7):858–861.
11. Abbot NC, White AR, Ernst E. Complementary medicine. Nature 1996;381:361.
12. Lee KpH, Carlini WG, McCormick GF, Albers GW. Neurologic complications following chiropractic manipulation. Neurology 1995;45:1213–1215.
13. Klougart N, Leboeuf-Yde C, Rasmussen LR. Safety in chiropractic practice. Part II: treatment to the upper neck and the rate of cerebrovascular incidents. J Manipulative Physiol Ther 1996;19(9): 563–569.
14. Dabbs V, Lauretti WJ. A risk assessment of cervical manipulation vs NSAIDs for the treatment of neck pain. J Manipulative Physiol Ther 1995;18(8): 530–536.
15. Ernst E. Complementary medicine: the facts. Phys Ther Rev 1997;2:49–57.
16. Ernst E. The attitude against immunisation within some branches of complementary medicine. Eur J Pediatr 1997;156:513–515.
17. Breen AC. Chiropractors and the treatment of back pain. Rheumatol Rehabil 1977;6: 207–218.
18. Huisman M. Chiropractic practice in Britain. Undergraduate project, Anglo-European College of Chiropractic, Bournemouth, 1989.
19. Pedersen P. A survey of chiropractic practice in Europe. Eur J Chiropractic 1994;42:3–28.
20. Plamindon RL. Summary of 1994 ACA statistical study. J Am Chiropractic Ass 1995;32:57–63.
21. Lamm LC, Wegner E, Collord D. Chiropractic scope of practice: what the law allows. J Manipulative Physiol Ther 1995;18:16–20.
22. Assendelft WJJ, Pfeifle ChE, Bouter LM. Chiropractic in the Netherlands: a survey of Dutch chiropractors. J Manipulative Physiol Ther 1995;18:129–139.
23. Carey T, Garrett J, Jackman A, et al. The outcome and costs of care for acute low back pain among patients seen by primary care practitioners, chiropractors, and orthopaedic surgeons. N Engl J Med 1995;333:913–917.
24. Kane WJ. Osteoporosis, osteomalacia, and Paget's disease. In: Frymoyer JW, ed. The adult spine. New York: Raven Press, 1991:637–659.
25. Michel BA, Lanc NE, Jones HH. Plain radiographs can be used in estimating lumbar bone density. J Rheumatol 1990;17:528–531.
26. Grieve GP. Incidents and accidents of manipulation and allied techniques. In: Grieve, GP, ed. Grieve's modern manual therapy. Edinburgh: Churchill Livingstone, 1994:679.
27. Brodin I. Product control of lumbar films. Läkartidningen 1975;72:1793–1795.
28. Sanders M. Take it from a D.C. Med Econ 1990;67:31–32.
29. Crelin ES. A scientific test of the chiropractic theory. Am Scientist 1973;61:574–580.
30. Chiropractors. Consumer Reports 1994;59:383–390.
31. Fultz O. Chiropractic, what can it do for you? Am Health 1992;11:41–43.

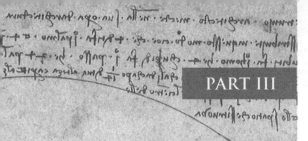

PART III

OVERVIEWS OF COMPLEMENTARY
AND ALTERNATIVE
MEDICINE SYSTEMS

INTRODUCTION: COMMON ASPECTS OF TRADITIONAL HEALING SYSTEMS ACROSS CULTURES

Stanley Krippner

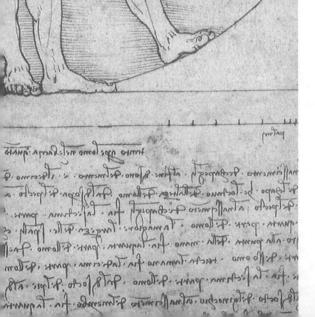

INTRODUCTION

Second only to the diversity of approaches to health, healing, and sickness around the world are their resemblances. Despite diverse languages, cultures, and concepts about the nature of reality, spirituality, humanity, and the human body, there are some remarkable similarities in how both traditional ethnomedical practices and allopathic biomedical practices approach wellness and illness. Attempts to relieve suffering and distress can be labeled *treatments;* they typically involve a relationship between a practitioner and a client. Frank and Frank (1) have identified three historical traditions of these treatments: the religio-magical (e.g., shamanism, faith healing); the rhetorical (e.g., affirmations, psychodrama); and the empirical (e.g., allopathic biomedicine, behavior therapy).

According to the United Nations' World Health Organization (WHO), more than 70% of the world's population relies on non-allopathic systems of healing. Determined to ensure that medical care would be available to all the people of the earth by the end of the twentieth century, WHO staff members realized that this goal was beyond the scope of personnel trained in Western biomedicine. As a result, WHO initiated a program to prepare native practitioners to serve as health care auxiliaries. A former director-general of WHO pointed out that the great number of traditional (i.e., indigenous to a particular region or environment) practitioners should not be overlooked. He noted that traditional healers and local midwives could, at a very moderate expense, be trained to the level at which they could provide adequate and acceptable health care and treatment under suitable supervision (2).

At the same time, physicians in the industrialized countries are encountering clients whose ethnic backgrounds and/or belief systems challenge the physicians' limited contact with other world views and categories of illness as well as presumed causal agents thereof. At the same time, biomedicine has attained such a degree of primacy throughout the world that the adjective *Western* is superfluous. As a result, biomedicine is often poorly prepared to meet the challenge posed by its encounter with different cultures and their systems of health and healing.

The term *ethnomedicine* refers to the comparative study of indigenous (or native) medical systems. Typical ethnomedical topics include causes of sickness, medical practitioners and their roles, and specific treatments used. The abundance of ethnomedical literature has been stimulated by an increased awareness of the consequences of the forced displacement and/or acculturation of indigenous peoples, the recognition of indigenous health concepts as means of maintaining ethnic identities, and the search for new medical treatments and technologies. In addition, Kleinman (3) finds ethnographic studies an "appropriate means of representing pluralism . . . and of drawing upon those aspects of health and suffering to resist the positivism, the reductionism, and the naturalism that biomedicine and, regrettably, the wider society privilege." In other words, biomedicine gives priority to a world view that extols rationality to the near-exclusion of intuition, that focuses on "parts" rather than "wholes," and that constructs a mechanistic model of humanity that frequently ignores potential spiritual and metaphysical components.

In his exhaustive study of cross-cultural practices, Torrey (4) concluded that *effective treatment* inevitably contains one or more of four fundamental principles:

1. A shared world view that makes the diagnosis or naming process possible.
2. Certain personal qualities of the practitioner that appear to facilitate the client's recovery.
3. Positive client expectations that assist recovery.
4. A sense of mastery that empowers the client.

Because Kleinman (5) has referred to Torrey's comparisons as *superficial*, this list will be used as a structure to provide examples rather than an attempt to distill universal essences of cross-cultural healing.

The necessity to individualize treatment can be seen cross-culturally. The nature of the ailment determines what treatment options are available. The nature of the client's condition determines whether the ailment should be cured or healed. The nature of the environment establishes how much of a cultural and familial support system is available to assist the client's recovery, growth, or integration. These factors, singly or in combination, will ascertain how many of the four fundamental healing principles described by Torrey can be brought to bear.

A Shared World View

Reaching an agreement on the name of a client's condition demonstrates that someone understands, that the client is not the only person who has ever had the condition, and that there is a way to get well. Identifying the offending factor may activate a series of associated ideas in the client's belief system that produce contemplation, relief, and general catharsis. A physician can prescribe an antibiotic for a client who has a certain kind of infection, and that client will probably recover. The use of antibiotics does not depend upon a common language or shared world view for its effectiveness. However, the world views of some cultural groups posit etiological factors that biomedicine and psychotherapy, with their reliance on biological explanations of sickness, do not accept. For example, various *cultures* postulate an imbalance between *dark* and *light forces* of energy, a punishment for the violation of taboos, or various types of *soul loss* and *spirit possession* as the underlying causes of illness. Levi-Strauss (6) has observed that many shamans, physicians, and therapists attempt to bring to a conscious level the conflicts and resistances that have remained in the client's unconscious. The naming process involves the use of words as symbols for what is wrong; the process is effective not only because of the knowledge that the words convey, but also because this knowledge permits a specific experience to take place, in the course of which the client may begin to recover.

Depending on the culture, illness is thought to be caused by one or more of three factors: biological events, experiential events, and metaphysical events. The third factor, which is ridiculed by biomedicine, is the *very foundation* of many other traditions. Thus, not only must the ailment be named, but the diagnosis must reflect the shared world view of the practitioner and client to be maximally effective. For example, there is no North American equivalent for *wagamama*, which is an emotional disorder reported in some parts of Japan that is characterized by childish behavior, emotional outbursts, apathy, and negativity. Nor is there a counterpart to *susto*, which is a *loss of soul* in certain parts of Latin America thought to be caused by a shock or fright, often connected with breaking a spiritual rule, sorcery, or a physical accident. Even within a specific culture, there can be different world views that interfere with treatment: for example, differences between upper-class practitioners and lower-class clients, or between practitioners whose gender or ethnic backgrounds differ from their clients.

Frank and Frank (1) explain how shamans supply their clients with a conceptual framework for making sense out of feelings and experiences that are often chaotic and mysterious, suggesting a plan of action that helps the clients gain a sense of direction and competence. Shamans have represented and transmitted their community's unified, all-encompassing world view—a role not possible in today's pluralistic societies. Nevertheless, health care practitioners still collaborate with the client to construct a treatment program, and this construct involves a *hermeneutic circle* (i.e., the interpretation of the latent meanings and understandings embod-

ied in treatment). This circle involves both practitioner and client as they attempt to understand why the client's health status is unsatisfactory, and endeavor to construct a new direction.

The Practitioner's Personal Qualities

There is a consensus among healers, psychotherapists, and medical doctors that some practitioners have personality characteristics that are therapeutic, whereas others do not. Not only are the actual personal qualities of the practitioners important, but those projected onto them by the client are crucial. This process of projection often is termed *transference* by psychotherapists and can be a salient factor in a treatment's success.

Carl Rogers observed that, although a practitioner's intellectual training and acquiring of information have many valuable effects, it is not necessarily associated with the practitioner's success in producing positive outcomes. In his studies of psychotherapy, Rogers (7) found that a therapist's accurate empathy, nonpossessive warmth, and personal genuineness were the factors that most closely related to a client's behavior change. Personal qualities that foster recovery from sickness may differ from culture to culture. Levy (8), after observing the Yakut healers of Tahiti at work, reported that these healers feel an *inner force* that does not offend clients yet is conscious of its power. The shamanic claim to communicate with spirits, which is valued in the individual tribes, would be considered deviant in most Western cultures. However, Boyer, Klopfer, Brawer, and Kawai (9) observed that Apache shamans received higher scores on tests of mental health than did the average members of their society who, in turn, scored more favorably than the individuals who claimed to be shamans but were not recognized as such by their community.

Positive Client Expectation

There is abundant evidence that demonstrates the importance of client expectation. What a person *expects* to happen during treatment often *will* occur if the anticipation is strong enough. Frank and Frank (1) describe the *symbolic message* of the placebo and its ability to evoke hope. At least 50% of people who receive a placebo will report significant relief (1). Such remedies as lizard blood and swine teeth have no known medicinal property, but they seem to have worked well for centuries, apparently because clients and their healers have expected them to work.

Torrey (4) has identified several factors that produce client expectations—hope, faith, trust, and emotional arousal. Frank and Frank (1) have noted that most psychotherapies use emotional arousal as part of the treatment, either at the beginning of therapy, followed by systematic reinforcement of newly developed skills and attitudes, or in the latter parts of therapy, when gains of the preceding therapeutic sessions can be crystallized.

A Sense of Mastery

A client's emerging sense of mastery equips him or her with knowledge about what to do in the future to cope with life's adversities. After recovery from a physical illness, a client may feel better and return to work. In addition, the client may have learned self-regulation procedures, dietary and exercise regimens, and other preventive techniques to forestall a recurrence of the ailment. If there are psychological problems, the client may have learned the proper prayers that counteract malevolent spirits, the healthy attitudes that counteract depression and anxiety, or the dream interpretation procedures that provide for personal empowerment. Each of these practices has the potential to bolster the client's sense of mastery and self-efficacy by providing a *myth* or conceptual scheme that explains deleterious symptoms and supplies a *ritual* or procedure for overcoming them (1). These myths and rituals combat demoralization by strengthening the therapeutic relationship, arousing hope, inspiring expectations of assistance, and affording opportunities for rehearsal and practice in facing life's difficulties.

Learning and mastery are important components of treatment. In addition, they are impor-

tant factors in both *curing* (removing the symptoms of an ailment and restoring a client to health) and *healing* (attaining wholeness of body, mind, emotions, and/or spirit). Some clients might be incapable of being *cured* because their illness is terminal. Yet those same clients could be *healed* mentally, emotionally, and/or spiritually as a result of being taught by the practitioner to review their lives in search of meaning, and thus become reconciled to death. Clients who have been *physically cured,* however, may learn healing procedures that will prevent a relapse or recurrence of their symptoms.

Proper medicinal remedies can also empower a client, even one who distrusts the practitioner. For example, a patient may not trust the nurse or physician administering an antibiotic but will probably recover from the illness nevertheless.

THE CULTURAL CONTEXT OF HEALING SYSTEMS

Western perspectives of health emanated principally from the age of enlightenment and the philosophy of elementalism that divided the human being into body *(soma)*, mind *(psyche)*, and spirit *(pneuma)*. Elementalism's assumption that sickness within one component could be treated without regard to the other component laid the groundwork for allopathic biomedicine, and the elevation of rationality in eighteenth century Western Europe made *spiritual* concerns irrational and irrelevant. Allopathic biomedicine adheres both to this rational approach and to empirical methodology, whereas many alternative medical systems are empirical without being rational in the Western sense, even though they work with world views that are internally consistent.

In 1925, a Nigerian *babalawo,* or *father of mysteries,* was summoned to England to treat an eminent Nigerian who had experienced a psychotic breakdown. The babalawo successfully treated his client with rauwolfia root, which was better medicine than any English psychiatrist had available; it was not until 1950 that this herb was introduced into biomedicine as the tranquilizer reserpine. Further, many Native American treatment procedures have been remarkably effective, even when judged by current standards. Native American practitioners lanced boils, removed tumors, treated fractures and dislocations, and cleaned wounds in ways that were more hygienic that those of the European invaders. The Hurons used evergreen needles, which are rich in vitamin C, to treat scurvy; the Shoshone used stoneseed to produce spontaneous abortions; several tribes used the bark of willow or poplar trees, whose active ingredient, salicin, resembles today's aspirin for musculoskeletal aches. Of the herbs used by the Rappahannock tribe, 60% were later found to have had unquestioned medicinal value—a record somewhat higher than that for the medicines brought by the Europeans to America. The first United States pharmacopoeia, which was published in 1820, listed 296 substances, 130 of which were originally used by Native Americans. Pharmacological analyses of the herbs used in Chinese, Tibetan, and Ayurvedic medicine, and that of other traditions, reveal that a significant number have active medical properties (10).

MODELS OF TREATMENT

For several decades, social and behavioral scientists have been collecting data that reflect the wide variety of humankind's healing systems. Sicknesses and injuries are universal experiences, but each social group implicitly or explicitly classifies them as to cause and cure in its own way. Furthermore, each person has a belief system that provides an explanation of how he or she can maintain health and overcome sickness. For example, Chicano (Mexican-American) *curanderos* (i.e., healers) often attribute a sickness to an *agent* whose existence must be taken on faith because it cannot be detected with medical instruments. For example, the *mal ojo,* or *evil eye,* has no status in allopathic biomedicine, but the *curanderos* claim it is caused by a person staring intently at someone else, usually with envy or desire and can bring on various disorders. This condition is often treated by forming three crosses on the victim's body with an egg while the practitioner recites the Apostle's Creed. An Apache ailment, *nitsch,* is said to

result from the neglect of natural entities. If an Apache does not properly salute an owl, he or she may suffer from heart palpitations, anxiety, sweating, and shaking. Shamanic prayers and songs are needed to treat this condition, which, it is believed, can lead to suicide.

Frank and Frank (1) have conjectured that the first healing model was built around the prehistoric belief that the etiology of sickness was either metaphysical (e.g., possession by a malevolent spirit) or magical (e.g., the result of a sorcerer's curse). Treatment consisted of appropriate rituals that supposedly undid or neutralized the cause. These rituals typically required the active participation not only of the sufferer but also family and community members. Spirits were believed to facilitate the healing process (9). Some perceived causes and cures were seen to operate from the world of nature through the use of herbs, exercises, and fasts.

There are both similarities and differences between allopathic biomedical medicine models and traditional medical models that have originated and developed in a specific place among members of a particular ethnic group (i.e., ethnomedicine). However, many anthropologists have proposed that the kind of logic developed by tribal people is as rigorous and complete as that of Western medicine; it is not the quality of the intellectual process that differs but the mode of its expression and application. For example, the cultural myths of pre–Columbian Mexican and Central American societies not only provided comprehensive guides to daily conduct but also explained the mysteries of the universe. Each mythic episode can be interpreted in several ways according to the context and the listener's understanding. The symbols used are manipulated with such economy that each serves a wide range of philosophical and religious ideas. For many Meso-Americans, Quetzalcoatl was the *feathered serpent* (who symbolized the transformation of matter into spirit), as well as the god of the winds, the Lord of Dawn, the spirit of the sacred ocelot (a fierce jungle cat), the last king of the Toltecs, and (following the Spanish conquest) Jesus Christ.

The complexity of many traditional treatment systems can be demonstrated by evaluating them on the basis of a 12-faceted healing

Table 1. Comparison of 12 Facets of Healing Models

	PIMAN MODEL	CURANDERISMO MODEL	KALLAWAYA MODEL	CHINESE MODEL	ALLOPATHIC MODEL
Practitioners	Shaman, herbalist, allopathic physician, or nurse	Curandero(a), herbolaria, medica, herbalista, señora; parchera, espiritisa, medium	Spiritual healers, midwives, various types of herbalists	Physician, apprentice, shaman, herbalist, masseur	Physician, nurse, rehabilitationist
Diagnosis	Shaman, with assistance by benevolent spirits	Curandero(a): initially may be made by patient, family member, or neighbor; may involve natural, psychological, and spiritual procedures	Taking pulse and blood pressure; examining tongue, eyes, breath, urine, feces; using coca leaves for divination	Examines *yin* and *yang* forces; pulse diagnosis; physician observation	Physician, with or without input from patient; family input rare; no community input
Cause of problem	Impurities that wander through body; improper behavior towards power objects	Natural, psychological, or spiritual	Lack of harmony between client and community and/or nature, except for metaphysical intervention	Blockage of *qi*	Natural
Treatment	For wandering illness—usually herbs, sometimes allopathic agents; for staying illness—changing, singing, oratory, sand paintings	Incantations, manipulation, suggestion, confession, persuasion; group activities, church functions, visit to holy shrine; herbs, praying, chanting, holy water, incense, candles	Highly individualized, but emphasizes balanced diet; medicinal plants (e.g., coca, quinine, corn fungus); rituals; dancing; amulets; healing songs, steam boxes	Acupuncture, herbs, moxibustion, diet, massage; unblock flow of *qi*	Usually medical or surgical; specific for diagnosis; may occur before diagnosis
Client behavior	Provides important clues for diagnosis and treatment	Used to make diagnosis	Calm client is healthy; crying and screaming are signs of soul loss or other problems	Important part of diagnosis	Patient reports symptoms; examination of body yields signs
Client priority and role	Treatment—cooperate with practitioner	Work closely with curandero(a); follow directions	Obtain treatment; cooperation with practitioner	Relax, don't resist; avoid tension; obey physician; follow regimen	Assume sick role (receive care, not assume responsibilities); obey practitioner
Family priority and role	Obtain treatment; avoid violation of dangerous objects and their dignity	Accompany patient to sessions; ensure patient's compliance with regimen	Obtain diagnosis and treatment for family member; provide emotional support and practical assistance	Seek help; reflect laws of nature; cooperate with physician	Seek help, sympathy; receive information about patient's condition and progress; cooperate with practitioner

Table 1. *Continued*

	PIMAN MODEL	CURANDERISMO MODEL	KALLAWAYA MODEL	CHINESE MODEL	ALLOPATHIC MODEL
Societal priority and role	Guarantee availability of practitioners; obey traditional spiritual laws; keep members *proper*	Support patient's recovery; protect social cohesiveness	Maintain a balanced environment in harmony with nature, expelling members who endanger this balance	Encourage teaching and practice of healing arts; mirrors both entire universe and individual's body	Be protected from people who are ill and therefore dangerous; provide medical care
Prognosis	Hopeful if treatment is appropriate, prompt, powerful	Favorable if patient follows regimen	Dependent on severity of sickness, cooperation of clients and their families, confidence and faith of client	Positive if patient follows instructions	Positive if diagnosis is correct
Premature death	Inadequate treatment or severe ailment	Failure of patient to comply with treatment; severity of malevolent forces	Suicide brings dishonor to family and is rare; early death represents imbalance or metaphysical intervention	Severe imbalance of bodily forces	Failure of medical system, but more often the result of aging or serious physical or psychiatric disorder
Goal of model	Uphold *ways* or customs	Assist recovery of patient; restore balance, hereby preserving traditions of family and culture	Maintain and restore harmonious relationships among community members, the community as a whole, and natural environment	Relieve and prevent pain and tension; promote harmony within body and between patient and environment	Treat patients for illness; restore function; accumulate medical knowledge
Function of institution	Healing	Reflect divine order; thereby facilitating recovery	Diagnosis and treatment in clinic or client's home	Provide quiet, comfortable place for diagnosis and treatment	Provide care for patient

Modified from Krippner S. A cross-cultural comparison of four healing models. Altern Therap Health Med 1995; 1:21–29.

model proposed by Siegler and Osmond (11) (Table 1). In the social and behavioral sciences, *models* are explicit or implicit explanatory structures that underlie a set of organized group behaviors. The use of models in science attempts to improve understanding of the processes they represent. Certain models have been constructed to describe human conflict, competition, and cooperation, whereas other models have been proposed to explain communicable diseases, mental illnesses, personality dynamics, and family interactions. Greenfield (12) has pro-

posed an information flow-based model to explain Brazilian spiritistic surgeries, whereas Russek and Schwartz (13) have propounded a systems model to examine interpersonal relationships across the domains of cardiology, heart-brain physiology, and social psychology. The Siegler and Osmond model is applicable to both *physical* and *mental* disorders, although non-Western traditions usually do not differentiate between the two. Krippner (14) has modified this model, attempting to eliminate some terms that suggest a Western bias, and substituting terms that lend themselves to a more useful cross-cultural comparison (see Table 1).

It is beyond the scope of this introduction to describe how each system described in this book uses these fundamental aspects of healing. What follows is a description of how five different healing systems (including biomedicine) approach these aspects.

Example 1: The Pima Indian Healing Model

Pima Indian shamanism, still active in the Southwest United States, is often regarded as subtle and sophisticated as any Western medical theory and practice. The principles of Piman shamanism have been recorded in some detail as a result of a study in which an anthropologist, Donald Bahr, collaborated with a shaman, a Pima Indian translator, and a linguist (15). Some previous anthropological studies have been flawed because tribal respondents lied to the investigators, played jokes on them, or told them what they wanted to hear. Apparently, the anthropologists did not think that the natives they were studying had the intelligence to give information that was incorrect! In this case, the involvement of the shaman and translator provided for greater accuracy.

Practitioners

It is the task of the shaman to make an accurate diagnosis and then to turn the client over to other practitioners for treatment. In doing this, shamans purportedly are assisted by *benevolent spirits;* it is believed that shamans are recruited, trained, and ordered into action by these spirits.

Diagnosis

Because of its elegance, the Piman theory of health and sickness lends itself to analysis in terms of the Siegler-Osmond model. Among the Pimas, *diagnosis* is as crucial as treatment and is carried out by the shaman. A client's body is seen as the stratified repository of a lifetime's acquisitions of strengths and weaknesses.

Cause

Etiology, or cause of the sickness, depends on the type of problem that is being treated. Some types of indispositions are untreatable because the body's self-healing capacities will deal with them (e.g., constipation, indigestion, venomous bites), or because treatment is futile (e.g., mental retardation, infant deformities). Other types of ailments are amenable to treatment: *wandering sickness* (problems caused by impurities that *wander* through the body) or *staying sickness* (problems caused by improper behavior toward such *power objects* as buzzard feathers, jimson weed, or roadrunners). For the Pimans, there was no separation between *physical* and *mental*; therefore, problems could be mental/behavioral and/or physical in nature. When the Europeans arrived, the Pimas noted that their visitors did not fall victim to staying sicknesses. However, the Pimas did not lose faith in their model, merely concluding that the objects in question were not sacred to the Europeans; hence the newcomers could not be punished for treating these objects with disrespect.

Client Behavior

The client's behavior provides important clues for diagnosis and treatment. Wandering sickness entails such symptoms as fever, hives, piles, or sores. Staying sickness can be identified by compulsive or erratic actions and by lethargy or self-destructive activities. The former ailments (wandering sickness) can be passed from one person to another, in contrast to the latter (staying sickness).

Treatment

The treatment for wandering sickness usually entails herbs; once allopathic medical substances were encountered, they were added to the list of curative agents for wandering sickness, as the native shamans observed the positive effects of many of the new medicines. The treatment for staying sickness involves singing, speaking in public, blowing the harmful agents away from the client, sucking the harmful agents from the client's body, eating the flesh of the dangerous object whose violation caused the problem, or placing the client on a sand painting. In the case of staying sickness, some treatment implements (such as crystals, tobacco smoke, and eagle feathers) are used to connect the shaman's power (or *heart*) with the client's self-healing capacities, whereas other implements (such as rattles and the shaman's voice) are directed toward the spirits. Herbalists can also appeal to spirits when treating wandering sickness by requesting that they bless the various plant remedies.

Treatment Setting

Treatment is attempted in an environmental setting created by the shaman or other healing practitioner. It is usually out-of-doors and often around a fire. For some types of wandering sickness, the shaman may refer the client to an allopathic physician's office or a hospital, both of which would then serve as the environment for treatment. Thus, the *function of the institution* is for healing whether it represents the Piman tradition or allopathy. The *practitioners* involved in healing can range from the allopathic physician or nurse to the Piman shaman or herbalist. Staying sickness is primarily treated by shamans, whereas wandering sickness is treated by herbalists or referred to allopathic physicians.

Prognosis

Prognosis, or anticipated outcome, is hopeful if the treatment is appropriate, prompt, and powerful. If the treatment does not meet any of these criteria, or if the client's condition is of such a nature that it cannot be successfully treated, premature death may result, or the indisposition may continue. Suicide can result from staying sickness, whereas fatal heart attacks from *horned toad sickness* (i.e., circulatory disorders) are common.

Client Role

In the Piman system, the clients' first priority is that of treatment, and they assume the role of cooperating with the practitioner; for example, when they are told to refrain from further violating the dangerous objects that cause staying sickness, they obey. Each person has internal capacities, or *strengths*, located in specific parts of the body. In staying sickness, the strength of each dangerous object interfaces with the victim's strength. Thus, the victim's strength can serve as the repository of the ailment; once the shaman has located it, such treatments as massaging the muscles or sucking out the impurities can be initiated.

Family Role

The major priority of the client's family is to obtain treatment for its indisposed family members. The parents take on the role of avoiding the violation of dangerous objects and their dignity; this might not only result in their own affliction but in that of their children. Parental misdemeanors are considered to be a frequent cause of infant birth defects. The Piman society places a high priority on the availability of healing practitioners for its members. Society also plays the role of obeying traditional spiritual laws so that its people will be protected from plagues and epidemics.

Goal of the Model

The goal of this healing model is to uphold the *way*—that is, the Piman customs that were given to the tribe at the time of creation. The Piman tradition attempts to assist the lives of individuals and keep the society proper. This propriety results in health and happiness; failure to follow the traditional commandments is thought to result in sickness. The strength of the Piman model is exemplified by their response to the allopathic description of how germs can cause communicable diseases: the Pima Indians simply subsumed this new information under their category of wandering sickness because germs were described as invisible microorganisms that appeared to wander through the body.

Example 2: The Curanderismo Healing Model

Curanderismo, or Mexican-American folk healing, is a coherent, comprehensive system of healing that primarily derives from the synthesis of

Mayan and Aztec teachings along with Mexico's heritage of Spanish Catholicism. However, traces of Arabic medicine and European witchcraft can be discerned as well. Its underlying concept is the spiritual focus of the healing; the typical *curandera* (female practitioner) and *curandero* (male practitioner) who subscribe to this world view place the religious element at the center of their practice (16).

PRACTITIONERS

The practitioners will vary depending on location; a practitioner who is referred to as a *curandera* in San Jose, California, may correspond to a *señora* in San Antonio, Texas; a *medica* in New Mexico; and a *parchera* in parts of Guatemala. Most practitioners of Curanderismo are women, but the proportion varies geographically. *Curanderas* typically are *called* to their profession by spiritual entities; they apprentice themselves to a friend or relative until they are considered ready to practice. Most of them are part-time practitioners who do not charge a specific fee, but are given a small offering or gift. *Curanderos* (male practitioners) have similar powers. The setting is often the home of the practitioner; the function is diagnosis and treatment.

DIAGNOSIS

Diagnosis is based on the history of the malady, the symptoms, and (retrospectively) on the response to treatment. Diagnosis may involve natural, psychological, and spiritual procedures. On the natural level, a practitioner can observe the client and ask questions. On the psychological level, a *curandera* may claim that she can *see* her client's *aura,* or energy body; the size, color, and shape of this aura can be an important diagnostic sign. Some *curanderas* claim that diagnosis can be carried out at a distance through what is often called *mental telepathy.* On the spiritual level, the nature of a client's problem is often revealed to the practitioner in dreams by a spirit guide. Initial diagnoses often are carried out by the clients themselves or by family members and neighbors.

CAUSE

Etiology, like diagnosis, can be natural, psychological, or metaphysical. The role of bacteria and viruses is taken for granted as a possible causal factor. Another alleged natural cause of a client's difficulty is *empacho*—indigestion due to a ball of food being lodged in the intestine, or food sticking to the wall of the stomach. Psychological causes are thought to be behind *bilis* (caused by anger or fear), *envidia* (caused by jealousy), *mal aire* (caused by imbalances in relationships or personal qualities), and *caida de mollera*—the perception that an infant's fontanel is too low because of the mother's neglect. Metaphysical etiologies abound; *embrujada,* an illness caused by sorcery, involves the participation of demonic spirits, whereas *mal puesto* (a mental/behavioral disorder in which the client engages in bizarre conduct) results from a hex. Sometimes there is a combined etiology; *empacho* can be brought about when a mother forces her child to eat too much or to consume food the child dislikes.

CLIENT BEHAVIOR

The client's behavior is used to make a diagnosis; for example, if diarrhea, crying, vomiting, and sunken eyes accompany a fallen fontanel, the diagnosis of *caida de mollera* is confirmed. One form of envidia is *mal ojo,* which occurs when someone with an evil eye stares at the victim because of envy or desire. Symptoms include fever, headaches, vomiting, and drooping eyes. In contrast, gas, constipation, a bitter taste in the mouth, and a *dirty white tongue* accompany *bilis.*

TREATMENT

Treatment is generally carried out by specialists. Herbal treatments are supervised by the *herbolaria, médica,* and *herbalista,* whereas the *señora* prescribes home remedies. The client's *vibrating energy* may need to be modified by incantations or manipulation. Suggestion, confession, and persuasion are employed; the practitioner may increase clients' self-esteem by getting them involved in group activities and church functions, or asking them to visit a holy shrine. The *mágica* combines herbs with spiritual practices, such as praying, chanting, sprinkling holy water, burning incense, and lighting candles. Exorcisms are done by an *espiritista,* or medium, who is adept at enlisting the help of benevolent spirits and ridding the client of malevolent ones. The etiology must be accurately made to ensure both the proper type of treatment and the most appropriate practitioner.

Regional Differences

Important regional differences exist within the system of Curanderismo. For example, its model of health emphasizes balance in relationships and behavior. But a balance of emotional *humors* and the avoidance of an excess of either *hot* or *cold* foods is important as well. An exception is found in Southern Texas, where the consideration of hot and cold foods as treatment is virtually absent. The role thought to be played by witchcraft in causing a malady also varies from location to location.

Prognosis

Prognosis is favorable if the treatment regimen is closely followed up. However, failure to comply may lead to a worsening of the condition or, in the case of such problems as *caida de mollera* and *mal puesto*, to premature death. Suicide can result from metaphysical sources or from failure to find a spiritual approach to life's problems. The function of the *institution*, whether it is the *curandera's* home, the home of the client, a church, or a hospital, is to reflect the divine order and, in so doing, to facilitate the client's recovery.

Client, Family, and Societal Roles

The client's priorities and roles are to work closely with the *curandera*, following her directions carefully, especially those of a spiritual nature. The family's priorities and roles are of great importance because familial allegiance and obligation are overriding cultural values. Family members generally accompany the client to the Curanderismo sessions and assist the client's

compliance with the regimen. The society's priorities and roles are to support the client's recovery because the entire community is concerned and affected when a member becomes ill.

Goal of the Model

The goal of the Curanderismo model is to assist the recovery of the client, restoring his or her balance within a social framework that preserves the traditions of the family and the Mexican-American subculture. Suffering and infirmity are seen as an inevitable part of life and as part of God's plan to instruct human beings and lead them to salvation. Sickness is not seen as a punishment from God, but as a challenge.

Example 3: The Kallawaya Healing Model

The Kallawaya practitioners of Bolivia trace their tradition back to the legendary Tiahuanaco cultures of 400 to 1145 AD, continuing through the eras of other pre-Inca cultures, the Inca empire, and the Spanish conquest, to present times.

Practitioners

Kallawaya practitioners often travel to parts of Argentina, Chile, and Peru, but always in small groups rather than alone (17). Most Kallawaya practitioners are males, but talented females are admitted to the profession as well.

The practitioners involved among the Kallawaya represent various skills and functions. *Herbalarios* collect plants; *yerbateros* prepare medicines from the plants; *curanderos* apply the herbs and other medicines; *yatiris* (also known as *amautas*) are spiritual healers; and *partidas* are midwives. Over time, Kallawaya practitioners began to perform more than one function; hence, many of these traditional divisions have become less rigid. Nevertheless, all practitioners mediate between the environment and the client (and, in some cases, the community at large). If a Kallawaya healer cannot help a client, there may be a referral to an allopathic physician, especially if surgery is needed; it is a common practice for referrals to go in both directions because some allopathic physicians send clients to Kallawaya healers.

DIAGNOSIS

Among the Kallawaya, diagnosis is as important as treatment. A client's body is seen as the microcosm of the natural environment. The healer's task is to make an accurate diagnosis, and an initial decision must be made as to whether the client should be referred to an allopathic physician, who serves as a resource for infectious diseases, broken bones, internal injuries, and other problems in which Kallawaya healers feel they tend to be less effective. Another decision involves whether the sickness can be treated by the person doing the diagnosis, or if another Kallawaya healer should be consulted. After making the first decision, and before making the second decision, the practitioner must determine the problem.

A common diagnostic tool is the *casting* of coca leaves, in which the healer holds several leaves high above his or her head and drops them onto the ground or onto a ceremonial *mesa* (a cloth that purportedly has spiritual powers and on which various objects are displayed). Each aspect of the leaf is instructive—the side of the leaf exposed, the orientation of the leaf, its resemblance to the Christian cross, and its relative location to other leaves. The practitioner also takes the client's pulse (at the heart, left arm, and right arm) and blood pressure and makes direct observations of the tongue, eyes, breath, urine, and feces. An irregular pulse is an immediate sign of disharmony. The color of the tongue and iris are observed carefully as is the dilation of the client's pupil.

It is important that the practitioner and client come to an agreement. Family members often are present when the diagnosis is announced, and they may be given tasks to perform. The clients and their families are fully informed and are advised to share the diagnosis with the entire community—except in the case of *kharisiri* (i.e., sorcery), which the practitioner might treat privately to keep others from being alarmed. In general, liver, stomach, and respiratory problems are the most commonly diag-

nosed sicknesses, but Kallawaya healers also diagnose and treat most other conditions, both physical and psychological, that are familiar to allopathic biomedicine. In addition, they work with spiritual problems such as *susto*, the loss of one's *haio* (i.e., soul), which is often conceptualized as a vital fluid that animates each human being. Each person has a major and a minor *haio*, and maintaining harmony between them is a crucial life task.

CAUSE

Etiology is seen as a disintegration of harmony between the clients and their community and/or natural environment, except when there is a direct metaphysical intervention (as in *kharisiri*). Thunder is perceived as capable of bringing affliction to both humans and animals. *Susto* has several possible etiologies—sorcery, traumas, shocks, or an inclement wind that captures a baby's soul (which is why the birth process occurs indoors). Sometimes it is the major *haio* that is lost, and sometime the minor *haio*; in either instance, the individual loses balance.

CLIENT BEHAVIOR

This factor provides important clues for diagnosis and treatment. In general, a calm client is healthy; crying and screaming may be signs of soul loss. The symptoms of *susto* vary, but include depression, anxiety, laziness, loss of appetite, shaking, fever, nausea, hearing noises in the ears, and passing gas. Folk tradition in Bolivia defines being sick operationally as someone who is unable to work.

TREATMENT

Treatment is highly individualized, but the importance of a balanced diet is emphasized by many practitioners who tell clients to "eat food from the area and during its season." The Kallawaya healers employ more than 1,000 medicinal plants, approximately one-third of which have demonstrated their effectiveness by Western biomedical standards, and another third of which have been judged to be probably effective (18). These plants redivided according to the three distinct *weathers* that the gods Pachamama (the great Earth Mother) and Tataente (Father Sun, the Creator) have given to their district—namely, hot, mild, and cold.

Coca leaves play a major role in many of the healing procedures because the plant is said to grow between the world of human beings and the world of the spirits. A coca and quinine mixture has been used to treat malaria—most notably, as the Kallawaya tell the story, during the digging of the Panama Canal, which is a triumph that brought these native people worldwide attention. The fungus of corn or bananas produces a type of penicillin used to treat local infections. More serious infections are treated by a tetramycin preparation yielded from fermented soil, which is also used to treat various chronic ailments.

Kallawaya medicine generally is accompanied by rituals involving prayers, amulets, and *mesas*. Llama fetuses are commonly used in the preparation of *mesas* because the llama is a sacred animal to these people. Amulets are placed on the *mesa* or worn around the client's neck, giving him or her confidence and spiritual power. Different amulets represent health, love, wealth, or equilibrium with the deities Pachamama and Tataente. *Mesas* also are used to prevent sickness or imbalance, often for the entire community.

Herbal preparations usually are ingested, but occasionally they are used in conjunction with a *steam box;* the nude client enters the receptacle that is filled with steam created from the medicinal mixture. The active ingredients of the herbs enter the pores of the client, and the sweat eliminates the toxins. Also, there is an armamentarium of procedures that do not involve herbs, including healing songs (especially for treating insomnia) and dances (particularly to renew the client's supply of energy).

Treatment Setting

The setting depends on the client's mobility; if the client cannot go to the healer, the healer will go to the client. However, female Kallawaya practitioners typically do not leave their homes; thus, their clients must come to them. In La Paz and other large cities, there are clinics where clients can visit a Kallawaya practitioner. The function of the institution is for diagnosis and treatment regardless of its location, but the client's preference usually is home visitation, which is far from the influence of hostile spirits and unfamiliar surroundings and near to familiar animals, plants, and land. Hospitals are dreaded, in part because the color white, in folk traditions, is associated with the death and burial of infants.

Prognosis

Prognosis, or anticipated outcome, depends on many factors—the sickness itself, its severity, and the cooperation of clients and their families. The confidence and the faith of the client are key factors because herbal treatment is a slow process that requires a great deal of patience. Belief is thought to activate the self-healing mechanisms that are fundamental to recovery.

If the treatment does not work, or if the client's problem occurs where no practitioner is available (e.g., a serious industrial or traffic accident), premature death may result. There are few suicides among the Kallawaya; such an act would bring dishonor to the family. Death, however, is a natural process that can be prepared for and confronted with valor; after death, one or both of one's souls rejoins Pachamama, the great Earth Mother. Premature death, however, is often attributed to metaphysical intervention.

Client and Family Role

In the Kallawaya system, the client's first priority is that of treatment, and he or she assumes the role of cooperating with the practitioner. The major priority of the client's family is to obtain diagnosis and treatment for its indisposed family members. The parents take on the role of providing emotional support for the client, maintaining his or her faith, and providing practical assistance, for example, helping administer medicinal herbs. The family receives an accurate and honest diagnosis (with the exception of instances of sorcery) and is informed of the client's progress or deterioration, as would be the case if the condition is incurable; for example, acquired immunodeficiency syndrome–related conditions or terminal cancer.

SOCIETAL ROLE

It is the priority of the Kallawaya society to maintain a balanced environment that exists in harmony with nature. The community, at times, plays the role of expelling members who endanger this balance. Another role is to support clients by bringing them food, money, music, and anything else that will maintain their faith and motivation to recover; this community process is referred to as *ayni*. A festive ceremony for offering group assistance is referred to as *apreste* and is frequently used to treat *susto*. Society places a high priority on the availability of healing practitioners for its members. There is a vigorous attempt to train students to become effective practitioners. It is the duty of the eldest son of a healer to become a healer himself, and the boy will spend some 14 years in preparation before he will be allowed to assist his mentor (17).

GOAL OF THE MODEL

The goal of the Kallawaya model is to maintain and restore the harmonious relationship of community members, the community as a whole, and the natural environment. The Kallawaya practitioner needs to guarantee the availability of medicinal plants and proficient healers who are conversant with health, sickness, the natural realm, and the world of spirits. Prevention involves the practice of moderation in daily life and of the maintenance of trust among members of the community.

Example 4: The Chinese Healing Model

PRINCIPAL CONCEPTS/DIAGNOSIS

The model of traditional Chinese medicine is based on the belief that health problems reflect disharmony between the individual and the environment, or within individuals themselves. A practitioner will conduct the diagnosis in a way that examines an imbalance in the *yin* and *yang* (i.e., "dark" and "light") forces that impinge upon the client's inner forces. Pulse diagnosis is a common diagnostic method, supplemented by keen observation, including the practitioner's use of smell and taste. Etiology focuses on the interruption or blockage of *qi*, the driving force of both the cosmos and human life; this is the *energy* that has two manifestations—*yin* and *yang*. *Qi* flows along its own bodily channels, or *meridians*. It can be blocked by environmental stress, faulty eating habits, or careless behavior patterns. Indeed, learning about the client's behavior is an important part of the diagnosis; key symptoms of *qi* blockage or imbalance are irritability, anxiety, depression, and insomnia (19).

PRACTITIONERS

Medical practitioners include physicians and their apprentices. In some areas, a shaman is the sole practitioner available; in other areas, a client might prefer a shaman to a physician. A few shamanic practitioners still implement their own version of traditional Chinese medicine, intermingling the notion of *qi* with their own traditional rituals. There are also practitioners who specialize in herbal treatment or massage; the latter often use their fingernails, knuckles, and elbows to unblock the flow of *qi*.

TREATMENT/PROGNOSIS

Treatment can involve acupuncture, herbal medicine, moxibustion (applying cones of herbal substances to the skin and igniting them), diet, and massage. The prognosis is usually positive if the instructions are followed diligently, especially when changing one's lifestyle is involved. Considerable emphasis is placed upon follow-up after the treatment and on prevention of further problems. Death is seen as part of the life cycle and is accepted gracefully. However, a premature death or suicide can be the result of continued or extreme imbalance.

Traditional Chinese physicians treat clients in an office setting but will sometimes visit clients in their homes. The function of the institution is to provide a quiet, comfortable place for diagnosis and treatment. Often, the site will be selected on the basis of the surrounding *qi*, especially that believed to exist in the natural environment.

CLIENT/FAMILY/SOCIETAL ROLE

The client is expected to cooperate with the practitioner. His or her priority is to relax and not resist; by *flowing* with the treatment, tension is avoided that would hamper the movement of *qi*. Clients are also assigned the role of obeying their physician; for example, a diet may be prescribed that will help to balance a client's *yin* and *yang* qualities.

The family of the client has the priority to seek help. Family members are told about the client's condition and are asked to cooperate with the physician. At its best, the family will reflect the laws of nature. For example, the *law of the mother and child* enacts itself in the family as well as in the environment, where earth is seen as the *mother of metal*; metals melt into water, and water condenses on metal—its *mother*. Water nurtures wood which, in turn, is the *mother of fire*. These five *elements* interact harmoniously, serving as an example for the family. The family enacts the *role* given them not only by the physician but by nature itself.

Society is also a part of nature, and one of its priorities must be to encourage the teaching and practice of the healing arts. Society plays the role of mirroring both the macrosystem of the universe and the microsystem of the body. Each bodily organ has its counterpart in society; for example, the heart (a *fire* organ) is the *supreme master*, whereas the gallbladder (a *wood* organ) corresponds to the official who makes decisions and judgments. The time of day and time of year are important for treating the client's ailments, just as they are important for decision making by the society's rulers.

GOAL OF THE MODEL

The goal of the traditional Chinese medical model is to relieve the pain and tension of the client's disorders and prevent their recurrence. On a broader level, however, the goal is to promote harmony within the body—and among the client, family, community, and environment.

Example 5: The Allopathic Biomedical Model

The allopathic biomedical model exhibits both similarities and differences when compared with the traditional models of the Piman shamans, the *curanderos*, the Kallawaya practitioners, and the traditional Chinese physicians. As practiced in Western and Western-influenced societies, allopathic biomedicine typically deals with urgent matters at a rapid pace; Siegler and Osmond call the emergency ward "a microcosm of the hospital as a whole" (11). A client usually comes to the hospital, clinic, or physician's office voluntarily (or is brought by others, but rarely against his or her consent), agrees to be called a *patient*, and is referred to as a *case*. The patient is frequently handled by *physicians* who use physically invasive procedures to determine what the patient *has* rather than what the patient *is*. On the basis of this procedure, treatment begins, and it is often "unpleasant, disgusting, painful, expensive, life-threatening, or sometimes all of these" (10), but not always so. Nevertheless, the procedure usually works well enough for people to repeat it when they again believe that their health, or their very lives, are threatened, and for them to advocate it to family and friends.

DIAGNOSIS

A diagnosis is usually made by the physician and follows logical procedures that may be carried out with or without input from the client; in the allopathic diagnostic process, extensive input from the family is rarely requested, and input from the client's community is almost never involved. Etiology is always considered natural rather than metaphysical. However, treatment sometimes proceeds in the absence of a diagnosis, a clear etiology, or even a favorable prognosis (11).

CLIENT BEHAVIOR

The client's behavior is connected to the diagnosis through symptoms (the client's reported experiences) and signs (the results of examinations of the client's body). The treatment of symptoms and signs sometimes proceeds in the absence of a known etiology. For example, a physician will often prescribe medication to lower a client's fever before identifying the cause of the fever.

TREATMENT

Treatment is usually medicinal or surgical and specific for each condition, but when a diagnosis is unclear, it may proceed by trial and error.

Treatment is oriented toward specific objectives and is adjusted to the response of the client. Prognosis, which is the physician's perspective on the course of the client's problem, is based on diagnosis. The physician will discuss such matters as the chances of recovery, the probable length of time needed for recovery, and the chances of a relapse. The physician offers hope, but often cannot promise a cure. Premature death is seen as a failure of the diagnostic and treatment system or as a result of a serious ailment that is unresponsive to the best treatment currently available. Suicide typically is seen as an extreme outcome of a psychiatric disturbance or reaction to the illness.

FUNCTION OF THE INSTITUTION

The function of the institution, whether the setting is the physician's office or a hospital, is to provide care for clients. Some physicians are based at a hospital, whereas others may work at an office. Practitioners in the allopathic medical system include physicians (who treat the clients), nurses (who assist physicians in caring for the clients), and various rehabilitationists (who teach clients how to regain lost or damaged bodily functions). These personnel are subject to formal regulative and licensure procedures to maintain standards of quality.

GOAL OF THE MODEL

The allopathic biomedical model holds that its clients can assume the *sick role*. While assuming this role, they can receive care and are not expected to assume their ordinary responsibilities. Clients are expected to obey their physician, nurse, and/or rehabilitationist. The client's family is expected to seek help. Family members are permitted to receive information about the client's condition and progress. Their role is to cooperate with medical personnel in carrying out the treatment. The client's society is expected to protect its other members from ill people who are a danger to them. Society/government is also expected to protect clients against incompetent practitioners.

The goal of this model is to treat clients for health problems. Allopaths attempt to restore clients to the greatest degree of functioning possible, or to at least prevent the problem from getting worse. A secondary goal is to accumulate medical knowledge so that more ailments can be cured and treatment can become increasingly effective (11).

TREATMENT MODELS IN CROSS-CULTURAL PERSPECTIVE

The allopathic biomedical model, the Piman model, the Kallawaya model, the Curanderismo model, and the traditional Chinese medical model are all comprehensive, yet each presents its adherents with very different world views. The Piman, Curanderismo, Kallawaya, and Chinese models are, in part, spiritual because they demonstrate an awareness of a broader life meaning that transcends the immediacy of everyday physical expediency, as well as an *otherworldly* transcendent reality that interfaces with ordinary reality. An individual allopathic practitioner might work spiritual aspects into his or her world view and practice, but this effort is not intrinsic to the medical model as it is widely taught and promulgated. *Spirituality*, however, is part and parcel of the other healing systems; their treatment modalities would change radically if they were to lose their spiritual components.

The diversities of these models are important when a differentiation is made between *disease* and *illness*. One can conceptualize disease as a mechanical difficulty of the body resulting from injury or infection, or from an organism's imbalance with its environment. Illness, however, is a broader term implying dysfunctional behavior, mood disorders, or inappropriate thoughts and feelings. These behaviors, moods, thoughts, and feelings can accompany an injury, infection, or imbalance—or can exist without them. Thus, English-speaking people refer to a *diseased brain* rather than an *ill brain*, but to *mental illness* rather than *mental disease*. Cassell (20) goes so far as to claim that allopathic biomedicine treats disease but not illness: "physicians are trained to practice a technologic medicine in which disease is their sole concern and in which technology is their only weapon." Shamans often have been described as "technicians of the sacred" (21), but their technology involves the entry into *other worlds* so that the spiritual aspects of their clients' problems can be addressed. Dimensions similar to these may start to be reintroduced into Western medicine.

The fourth edition of the American Psychiatric Association's *Diagnostic and Statistical Manual of Mental Disorders* (22) is the first allopathic biomedicinal reference to mention "religious or spiritual problems" (23). The manual also includes material concerning cultural factors related to mental illness and treatment. First, there is a statement about culture and ethnicity in the manual's introduction. Second, the text of the manual mentions cultural variations in idioms of distress, symptom patterns, social-cultural correlates of mental illnesses, and courses of disorders.

Third, new cultural annotations point out the following:

- Possible cultural factors should be listed for the client being assessed.
- Cultural factors are especially important in assessment because normative ideas about personality development and behavior are culture-based to a significant extent.
- Medical conditions are differentially distributed across various cultural and ethnic groups.
- Minority and non-Western cultural groups often suffer under extreme social, economic, and political conditions in comparison to middle-class American groups.

Fourth, there is a "Cultural Formulation Guideline" in the manual's appendix that attempts to instruct clinicians how to make an assessment of an illness within the cultural context of the client's experience and judge the implications that assessment has for clinical treatment. Fifth, the appendix also contains a glossary of culture-bound syndromes and idioms of distress. This is a collection of non-Western, folk, or popular psychiatric syndromes that are standard forms of mental illness in indigenous cultures, but are also found with increasing frequency in the American multicultural society. *Susto* is one of the syndromes included, but it should be pointed out that *anorexia nervosa* is found only in Western cultures (24).

The inclusion of culturally sensitive material in the fourth edition of the *Diagnostic and Statistical Manual of Mental Disorders* is an important step toward recognizing alternative models of psychotherapy and medicine. Implicitly, this move necessitates education and training for practitioners whose focus has been biomedicine and Western psychotherapy, a world view that is clearly inappropriate for many clients and several disorders.

POSTMODERN PERSPECTIVES

Many traditional people, especially those in the developing world, recognize the advantages of allopathic biomedicine. Its effectiveness in surgery and in treating infections, fractures, and trauma is apparent, as is its success in preventing epidemics. Yet these indigenous groups are often wary of how biomedicine can be used as a political instrument to discriminate against ethnic groups and socioeconomic classes, and create dependency relations with the industrialized countries who supply (and profit from) allopathic biomedicines and implements (18). In this way, the contrast of traditional healing models with that of allopathic biomedicine enters what has been called the *postmodern* discourse (25), in which the role played by power in mediating paradigms and world views becomes more apparent. (25). *Official* medicine (i.e., biomedicine) has more sources of political and financial power than does *traditional medicine* (i.e., ethnomedicine), and the latter has had to struggle for legitimacy against influential forces. In general, it is a constant struggle for traditional practitioners to preserve their ways of living, feeling, and thinking, which all emphasize balance, harmony, and community support (3).

Biomedical technology often determines what is considered authoritative knowledge and, in turn, establishes a particular domain of power. Biomedicine typically extends this privileged position to economics, politics, and class relationships; its power is jealously guarded by legislation, medical schools, licensing regulations, and medical terminology. Biomedical practitioners generally act out of good faith and noble motives in using their power, but traditional people frequently view biomedicine with suspicion (18). Rather than supporting the extremist view, which sees any use of biomedicine by indigenous people as a form of colonization, postmodernity simply requests that traditional ethnomedicine be allowed to join the medical dialogue—what Anderson (25) refers to as the "belief basket of the world"—and be assured of a fair hearing. Testing, experimentation, replication, scientific methods, and disciplined inquiry are major contributions of biomedicine and are just as important in the postmodern world as they ever were. Possible explanations for health and affliction need to compete, but these explanations must be tempered with a revitalized awareness of the role that vested interests and entrenched authority typically play in the outcome of the dialogue (25).

Cross-cultural studies have described the ways in which social and cultural forces shape human behavior (26) and how natural settings produce classification systems that are often remarkably adaptive for indigenous people (27). Kleinman (5) has drawn upon these findings in describing the way treatment by traditional practitioners moves through: 1) the labeling of the problem with an appropriate and culturally sanctioned category; 2) the treatment of the client on the basis of that label (including the label's ritual manipulation); and 3) the application of a new label (e.g., *healed, cured*) that is sanctioned as a meaningful symbolic form.

Postmodernists use the term *privileged* to describe a standard or style that is preeminent in a given time, place, or world view. Biomedicine privileges scientific methodology, even though it sometimes applies this methodology in a biased manner. Nevertheless, it is necessary to use outcome measures to determine the extent to which ethnomedicine is effective, even on its own terms. Kleinman (5) observed that Taiwanese shamans were most successful when dealing with what Westerners would term acute, self-limited sicknesses, secondary somatic manifestations of psychological disorders, and chronic ailments that were not life threatening; and Finkler (28) observed that diarrhea, simple gy-

necological disorders, somatic manifestations, and psychological disorders were most amenable to treatment by Mexican spiritists. In her description of Malay shamanism, Laderman (29) described how practitioners use ritual, dialogue, and music to provide intense personal experiences that mobilize the immune system. Also, various aspects of Chinese medicine (e.g., pain control, asthma) have been evaluated using Western scientific methodology, often yielding positive results (30). It is to the credit of biomedicine that the accumulation of such medical knowledge is an important goal. Granted that empirical scientific methods are *privileged* styles; but at their best, they can produce standards by which other models of healing can be evaluated, thus enhancing the effectiveness of procedures by which ailments can be treated. As the practitioner learns about the systems of healing described in the chapters that follow, keep in mind the cultural context of all healing systems. These systems may shed light on understanding of biology and provide approaches to benefit our patients, just as science may help these systems become more evidence-based and generally applicable.

WHO has launched initiatives to support traditional healers whose expertise is needed if worldwide health care is to become a reality. The value of a plethora of medical plants used in ethnomedicine has now been confirmed by pharmacological research, and their cost effectiveness also argues in their favor. The value of ethnomedical practitioners and their incorporation into biomedical systems has also become widely heralded since their advocacy by WHO. However, the high cost of training folk healers, the reluctance of the medical bureaucracy to accept them, and the decline of ethnomedicine in many parts of the world have frustrated such incorporation. The objective of available medical care for all people of the earth by early in the twenty-first century depends upon granting traditional practitioners some professional autonomy and educating them in abandoning worthless (and sometimes harmful) practices (31). It also involves teaching them and their communities about effective public health measures. But this educational process needs to be mutual. Many traditional practitioners use adaptive strategies that involve dynamic systems subject to change in response to the community and the environment. Biomedicine can learn a great deal by observing how quickly these adaptations are often made, especially during times of emergency. In a world on the brink of ecological disaster, these resourceful tactics may be important skills for thoughtful people concerned with both local and global survival.

REFERENCES

1. Frank JD, Frank JB. Persuasion and healing. 3rd ed. Baltimore: Johns Hopkins University Press, 1991:139, 140.
2. Mahler W. The staff of Aesculapius. World Health [Organization], Geneva, Switzerland, Nov 1977:3.
3. Kleinman A. Writing at the margin: discourse between anthropology and medicine. Berkeley: University of California Press, 1995:195–196.
4. Torrey EF. Witchdoctors and psychiatrists. New York: Harper & Row, 1986.
5. Kleinman A. Patients and healers in the context of culture. Berkeley: University of California Press, 1980:33, 372.
6. Levi-Strauss C. Structural anthropology. New York: Basic Books, 1963.
7. Rogers CR. The necessary and sufficient conditions of therapeutic personality change. J Consult Psychol 1957;21:95–103.
8. Levy RI. Tahitian folk psychotherapy. Int Public Health Res Newslett 1967;9(4):12–15.
9. Boyer LB, Klopfer B, Brawer FB, Kawai H. Comparisons of the shamans and pseudoshamans of the Apaches of the Mescalero Indian reservation: a Rorschach study. J Projective Techniques 1964; 28:172–180.
10. Krippner S, Welch P. Spiritual dimensions of healing. New York: Irvington Publishers, 1992.
11. Siegler M, Osmond H. Models of madness, models of medicine. New York: Macmillan, 1974:23–27.
12. Greenfield SM. A model explaining Brazilian spiritist surgeries and other unusual, religious-based healings. Subtle Energies 1994;5(2):109–141.
13. Russek LG, Schwartz GE. Interpersonal heart-brain registration and the perception of parental love: a 42-year follow-up of the Harvard Mastery of Stress study. Subtle Energies 1994;5(3):195–208.
14. Krippner S. A cross-cultural comparison of four healing models. Altern Therap Health Med 1995; 1:21–29.
15. Bahr DM, Gregorio J, Lopez DI, Alvarez A. Piman shamanism and staying sickness. Tucson: University of Arizona Press, 1974.
16. Trotter RT III, Chavira JA. Curanderismo. Athens, GA: University of Georgia Press, 1981.
17. Bastien JW. Healers of the Andes. Salt Lake City, UT: University of Utah Press, 1987.
18. Bastien JW. Drum and stethoscope. Salt Lake City, UT: University of Utah Press, 1992:17, 47.
19. Beinfield H, Korngold E. Between heaven and earth. New York: Ballantine, 1991.
20. Cassell EJ. The healer's art. Middlesex, England: Penguin, 1979:18.
21. Elinde, M. Shamanism: archaic techniques of ecstasy. New York: Pantheon, 1964:7.
22. American Psychiatric Association. Diagnostic and statistical manual of mental disorders. 4th ed. Washington, DC: American Psychiatric Association, 1994.
23. Lukoff D, Lu F, Turner R. Toward a more culturally sensitive DSM-IV: psychoreligious and psychospiritual problems. J Nerv Ment Dis 1992;180: 673–682.
24. Bletzer KV. Biobehavioral characteristics of a culture-bound syndrome perceived as life-threatening illness. Qualitative Health Res 1991;1:200–233.
25. Anderson WT. Reality isn't what it used to be. San Francisco: Harper, 1990:77, 188.
26. Parker I. Discourse and power. In: Shotter J, Gergen K, eds. Texts of identity. Newbury Park, CA: Sage, 1989.
27. Kim U, Berry JW. Introduction. In: Kim U, Berry JW, eds. Indigenous psychologies. Newbury Park, CA: Sage, 1993.
28. Finkler K. Spiritualist healers in Mexico: successes and failures of alternative therapeutics. New York: Praeger, 1985.
29. Laderman C. Taming the winds of desire: Psychology, medicine, and aesthetics in Malay shamanistic performance. Berkeley: University of California Press, 1991:297–298.
30. Kleijnen J, Rietter G, Knipschild P. Acupuncture and asthma: a review of controlled trials. Thorax 1991;46:799–802.
31. Edgerton RB. Sick societies. New York: Free Press, 1992.

CHAPTER 11

AYURVEDIC MEDICINE

D. Vasant Lad

BACKGROUND INFORMATION

Definition

Ayurveda is an ancient system of healing that has its roots in the Vedic knowledge of ancient India. It is thought by many scholars to be the oldest healing system in existence. The knowledge contained in Ayurveda deals with the nature, scope, and purpose of life. This system of healing embraces the metaphysical and physical, health and disease, happiness and sorrow, and pain and pleasure. It defines life as the expression of cosmic consciousness (sometimes called God, the Divine, Universal Awareness, or the Creator) manifest as the entire sphere of creation. In Vedic knowledge, the purpose of life is to know or realize the Creator (cosmic consciousness) and to express this divinity in one's daily life.

Ayur means life, and *veda* means knowledge. Systematized knowledge becomes a science, and so Ayurveda is considered the science of life. According to this system, individual life is a microcosm of the cosmos—an indivisible, unique phenomenon. Ayurveda evolved from practical, philosophical, and spiritual illumination, rooted in the understanding of creation. The ancient seers, or *rishis*, were highly evolved, spiritual human beings who came to understand creation through deep meditation and other spiritual practices. In their search for an understanding of the creation of all things, Ayurveda was evolved. It helps each person understand one's unique body, mind, and the nature of daily operating consciousness. According to Ayurveda, this basic knowledge of body, mind, and consciousness is the foundation of health and happiness.

History and Development

Ayurveda dates back more than 5000 years. Of the seven ancient philosophies that it incorporates, the Sankhya model of creation and evolution is a system for use in daily life. The ancient sages who evolved this philosophy perceived how energy and the laws of nature manifest in all living, nonliving, gross, and subtle things, and they developed these precepts into a system of thought.

There are many ancient texts on Ayurveda, all originally written in Sanskrit. Although these works exist in English translation, their format may not be familiar or easily translatable into Western concepts. These texts are written in the form of *sutras*, which express the essence of the information in poetic form only. In the Ayurvedic tradition, it is essential for each student to have a mentor who can expand the student's understanding of Ayurveda and, in essence, provide the keys that unlock the layers of meaning contained within these ancient writings.

THREE IMPORTANT AYURVEDIC TEXTS

The *Caraka Samhita*, the *Susruta Samhita*, and the *Astanga Hrdayam Samhita* are probably the most important Ayurvedic texts. The *Caraka Samhita,* which is believed to have been written between 200 BC to 400 BC is the oldest and most important ancient writing on Ayurveda. This work is based on an even older oral tradition. It presents most of the theoretical edifice of Ayurveda and concentrates on the branch of Ayurveda called *kayacikitsa,* or internal medicine. The English translation by P. V. Sharma (Chaukhambha Orientalia: Varanasi, India, 1981) is available in four volumes; two volumes are original text and two are commentary about the original work. Sharma's translation includes numerous appendices and an index. The translation by Bhagwan Dash and Ram Karan Sharma (Chowkhamba Sanskrit Series Office: Varanasi, India, 1992) has commentary incorporated in the original text. Both translations contain the original Sanskrit prose and poetry.

The *Susruta Samhita* presents the field of Ayurvedic surgery called *salakya,* meaning foreign body. This work is also believed to be based on oral material passed down from generation to generation. It is thought to have been written soon after the *Caraka Samhita.* Although the *Susruta Samhita* deals with the practice and theory of surgery, it is also an important source of Ayurvedic aphorisms. For example, the most commonly quoted definition of health is from Susruta. Translated from the Sanskrit, it reads: The person whose *doshas* (physiology) and digestion are balanced, whose tissue formation, elimination, and bodily processes are proper, and who experiences bliss in spirit, sense, and mind is a healthy person. The three-volume translation by K. L. Bhishagratna is the only English version available (Chowkhamba Sanskrit Series Office: Varanasi, India, 1991).

The *Astanga Hrdayam Samhita* is the work of a person named Vagbhata and also dates back to 200 BC to 400 BC. Vagbhata's use of the Sanskrit language is poetic and melodious, making it easy for students to commit to memory. This exposition deals primarily with *kayacikitsa* (internal medicine). Emphasis is placed on treating the physiology of the body and on suggestions for therapeutic use of metals and minerals. K. R. Srikantha Murthy has provided an English translation (Krishnadas Academy: Varanasi, India, 1991).

OTHER IMPORTANT TEXTS

The *Sarngadhara Samhita* is a concise exposition of Ayurvedic principles. This treatise is thought to have originated in the fourteenth century. Its subject matter is *kayacikitsa.* The *Sarngadhara Samhita* is prized for its enumeration and description of numerous pharmacologic formulations and contains perhaps the first textual reference to diagnosis by means of the pulse. The work is available in English translation by K. R. Srikantha Murthy (Chaukhambha Orientalia: Varanasi, India, 1995).

Madhava Nidanam, available in English translation by K. R. Srikantha Murthy (Chaukhambha Orientalia: Varanasi, India), deals with the Ayurvedic classification of diseases. This work is dated around 700 AD and covers a wide range of diseases. Although this treatise provides detailed descriptions of disease prodroma and cardinal signs and symptoms, it does not provide etiologies or suggestions for treatment. *Madhava Nidanam* is a book of practical, clinical medicine.

PRINCIPAL CONCEPTS

Creation of the Universe: Five Elements

Kapila, the founder of Sankhya philosophy, outlined five elements in the creation of the universe: *Purusha, Prakruti, Mahad, Buddhi,* and *Ahamkar.*

According to Sankhya, *Purusha* is male energy. *Prakruti* is female energy. *Purusha* is formless, colorless, beyond attributes, and it takes no active part in creation. This energy is choiceless, passive awareness. *Prakruti* yields form, color, and attributes in the field of action. It is awareness with choice, Divine Will, the One who desires to become many. The universe is the child born out of the womb of *Prakruti,* the Divine Mother. *Prakruti* creates all forms in the universe, whereas *Purusha* is the witness to this creation. *Purusha* and *Prakruti* merge together to bring cosmic order, or *Mahad* (also called universal intelligence). Within *Mahad,* or universal intelligence, a center arises and from that center, *Buddhi*, the individual's intellect, is created. Intelligence is a universal phenomenon; intellect is individual. The radius from the *Buddhi* center creates a small enclosure, a circle. The center of that circle is called *Ahamkar*—the ego, the feeling of "I am."

This feeling of "I am" further manifests through three universal qualities that pervade all creation:

1. *Sattva* is the pure essence of light, right action, and spiritual purpose. On the universal level, *sattva* is vast clear space in the universe; on the individual level, *sattva* is the clarity of perception.
2. *Rajas* is the principle of movement. On the universal level, *rajas* is atmosphere; on the individual level, *rajas* is the movement of perception, which becomes attention.
3. *Tamas* is the principle of inertia and darkness. On the universal level, *tamas* is the body of the planet solidity in all of nature; on the individual level, *tamas* is precipitation of perception, which is experience. Without *tamas*, there is no experience.

According to Ayurveda, these three universal qualities influence both our minds and bodies. *Rajas* is the active vital life force in the body that moves both the organic and inorganic universal aspects to *sattva* and *tamas*, respectively. Therefore, *sattva* and *tamas* are inactive potential energies that require the active kinetic force of *rajas*. As a result of the influence of the three universal qualities, the five senses (hearing, touch, vision, taste, and smell), the five motor organs (mouth, hands, feet, reproductive organs, and excretory organs), and the mind are differentiated as parts of the organic universe. The five objects of perception (sound, touch, sight, taste, and smell) and the five basic elements (space, air, fire, water, and earth) are parts of the inorganic universe.

Inorganic Universe

An Ayurvedic principle states that all organic and inorganic substances are made up of the five basic elements: space, air, fire, water, and earth.

SPACE

Within the body, each cell occupies space. Through the cellular space, cells communicate with one another. There is a continuous flow of intelligence between every cell. Every cell is a center of awareness; every cell has a mind and has the ability to choose what it ingests and what it expels. Therefore, space, which is the first expression of consciousness, is the basic need of the bodily cells. Even modern physics states that matter is that which occupies space. Thus, the development of matter begins with space.

AIR

The flow of consciousness, from one cell to another cell in the form of intelligence, is called *prana*, the principle of the air element. *Prana* is a vital life force that is essential for communication on all levels of body, mind, and spirit. The air element is necessary for all subtle and gross movement within the cell, within each organ, and within the physical body as a whole. In other words, sensory stimuli and motor responses are the subtle movements of the air principle. Even the movements of the heart, respiration, peristalsis, and other involuntary movements are governed by *prana*.

FIRE

The fire element manifests as the metabolic processes regulating the transformation of food into energy. All transformative processes are governed by the fire element. The fire element is responsible for governing body temperature and the processes of digestion, absorption, and assimilation of food. Essential to these transformation processes are gastric action, hydrochloric acid, digestive enzymes, liver enzymes, and the amino acids present in every cell. Even within each of the doors of perception—eyes, ears, nose, tongue, skin—there is a subtle fire component that is necessary for sensory perception and processing these perceptions into knowledge.

WATER

Water is necessary in the human body for assimilation and for maintaining electrolyte balance.

The blood in our bodies is composed of 90% water, and this water carries nutrients from one part of the body to the other. Oxygen, food particles, and the molecules of minerals are carried from one cell into another cell, from one system to another system, by this continuous river of fluid, the blood plasma. This is the Water of Life.

EARTH

From Earth, all organic living bodies, including humans, are created. The solid structures of the body—hard, firm, and compact tissues (e.g., bones, cartilage, nails, hair, teeth, and skin)—are derived from the Earth. Earth also contains the inorganic substances that constitute the mineral kingdom.

Types of Energy: Vata, Pitta, and Kapha

In addition to the five basic elements of the inorganic universe, Ayurveda identifies three basic types of energy, or functional principles, that are present in everybody and everything. There are no single words in English to describe these principles, so we use the original Sanskrit words: *vata, pitta,* and *kapha.* These three *doshas—vata, pitta,* and *kapha*—are the active forms of the five elements. They are forces of energy, patterns, and movements, not substances and structures.

DEFINITIONS

Energy is required to create movement so that fluids and nutrients get to the cells, enabling the body to function. Energy is also necessary to metabolize the nutrients in the cells and is needed to create and maintain cellular structure. *Vata* is the energy of movement; *pitta* is the energy of digestion or metabolism; and *kapha* is the energy that forms the body's structure and holds the cells together. All people have a unique combination of *vata, pitta,* and *kasha.* Some individuals have one *dosha* predominant; others have a predominance of two *doshas;* still others might have the equal involvement of all three. Although each *dosha* is composed of all five basic elements, two of these elements are

predominant. The cause of disease in Ayurveda is viewed as the lack of proper cellular function because of an excess or deficiency of *vata, pitta,* or *kapha* and/or the presence of toxins that interfere with *dosha* balance.

BALANCING THE THREE ENERGIES

According to Ayurveda, at the moment of fertilization, we are endowed with a certain genetic code and unique psychophysiological constitution, which is determined by the proportional combination of *vata, pitta,* and *kapha* of our biological parents. This constitution is called an individual's *prakruti.* It governs the individual's responses to events and life circumstances, both mental and physiological. It is believed that if one is aware of one's basic constitution and its concomitant tendencies, one can take actions—including changing diet, behavior patterns, and emotional responses—to maintain equilibrium with one's constitution, thereby living a balanced, happy, and fulfilled life.

In Ayurveda, body, mind, and consciousness work together in maintaining balance. They are simply viewed as different facets of one's being. To learn how to balance the body, mind, and consciousness requires an understanding of how *vata, pitta,* and *kapha* work together. According to Ayurvedic philosophy, the entire cosmos is an interplay of the energies of the five basic elements—space, air, fire, water, and earth. *Vata, pitta,* and *kapha* are combinations of these five elements that manifest as patterns in all creation.

According to Ayurveda, there are seven body types. There are monotypes in which one *dosha* is predominant, either *vata, pitta,* or *kapha.* There are dual types in which two *doshas* are equally dominant, either *vata-pitta, pitta-kapha,* or *kapha-vata.* And, very rarely, there are equal types, in which all three *doshas* are present in equal proportions. Every individual has a unique combination of these three *doshas.*

Vata

In the body, *vata,* which is principally composed of space and air, is the subtle energy associated with movement. It governs breathing, blinking, muscle and tissue movement, heartbeat, and all movement in the cytoplasm and cell membranes. In balance, *vata* promotes creativity and flexibility in a person; out of balance, *vata* produces fear and anxiety. In the external world, *vata* types tend to earn and spend money quickly. They are not good planners and, consequently, may suffer economic hardship. On the physical level, *vata* people are more susceptible to diseases involving the air principle, such as emphysema, pneumonia, and arthritis. Other common disorders caused by imbalanced *vata* include flatulence, tics, twitches, aching joints, dry skin and hair, nervous system disorders, constipation, and mental confusion. The energy of *vata* tends to increase with age, regardless of the individual's basic constitution.

Pitta

Pitta, principally made up of fire and water, is expressed as the body's metabolic system. *Pitta* governs digestion, absorption, assimilation, nutrition, metabolism, and body temperature. In balance, *pitta* promotes understanding and intelligence in a person; out of balance, *pitta* arouses anger, hatred, and jealousy. In the external world, *pitta* people like to be leaders and planners and seek material prosperity. *Pitta* people tend to have diseases involving the imbalanced fire principle, such as fevers, inflammatory diseases, and jaundice. Common symptoms include skin rashes, burning sensations, ulcers, fever, and inflammations or irritations (e.g., conjunctivitis, colitis, sore throats). *Pitta* is predominant during adulthood.

Kapha

Kapha, principally comprised of earth and water, is the energy that forms the body's structure—bones, muscles, tendons—and holds the cells together. *Kapha* supplies the water for all body parts and systems. It lubricates joints, moisturizes the skin, and maintains immunity. In balance, *kapha* is expressed as the action of love, calmness, and forgiveness. Out of balance, it leads to attachment (e.g., to family, job, lifestyle, possessions), greed, and possessiveness. In the external world, *kapha* tendencies toward groundedness, stability, and attachment help *kapha* people earn and hold onto money. They tend to have diseases connected to the water principle, such as influenza, sinus congestion,

and other mucus-involving diseases. Sluggishness, excess weight, diabetes, water retention, and headaches are also common. *Kapha* is predominant during the years of rapid development, from infancy through late childhood.

PROVIDER–PATIENT/CLIENT INTERACTIONS

Patient Assessment Procedures

There are eight classical clinical modalities that Ayurveda uses for examination. These clinical barometers are the pulse, urine, feces, tongue, speech and voice, examination by touch, examination of the eyes, and general physical examination (Table 11.1).

These eight important limbs are based on *darshanam* (observation), *sparshanam* (examination by tactile experience), and *prashnam* (inquiry or questioning). Every patient is like a living book: to read that book, a physician must develop the ability to use these clinical barometers to properly perceive the diagnosis.

The Ayurvedic physician should have a basic understanding of how the inner organizations of *vata, pitta,* and *kapha* are acting in and reacting to the patient's lifestyle, diet, emotions, job, and stress. According to Ayurveda, each constitutional type has an inclination toward certain disorders. For example, *vata* individuals or those with *vata* imbalance have a tendency toward constipation, bloating, arthritic changes, sciatica, insomnia, and degenerative arthritis. *Pitta* individuals, when out of balance, may have conditions such as hyperacidity, peptic ulcer

Table 11.1. Physical Examination
Nadi: examination of the pulse
Mutra: examination of the urine
Mala: examination of feces
Jihva: observation of the tongue
Shabda: observation of the person's speech and voice
Sparsha: tactile examination by palpation
Druga: examination of eyes
Akruti: the general physical examination of the entire body

disease, ulcerative colitis, or other inflammatory and infectious diseases. Metabolic disorders, such as slow metabolism, underactive thyroid, obesity, diabetes, hypertension, and high cholesterol, are associated with *kapha* imbalance. A physician should know the signs and symptoms of the aggravation of *vata, pitta,* and *kapha.* Then, when a clinical assessment is made, the examiner asks questions to confirm which *dosha* is out of balance. These observations are also confirmed by examination of pulse, tongue, and general physical examination.

The constitutional imbalances and their causes are understood on clinical grounds, identified through the eight classical modalities discussed previously in this chapter. Ayurveda is not only a metaphysical science, it is also a practical clinical science. The Ayurvedic understanding of health, imbalance, and disease is based on an understanding of the unique constitution of the individual, the aggravating or debilitating causes, the present imbalance if any, and the resulting pathogenesis.

Etiology

The Ayurvedic physician understands the pathogenesis and etiologic factors of the individual's problem by asking the patient about his/her diet, lifestyle, and relationships. The causative factors of the same disease may vary according to what aspect of the individual is imbalanced. Every disease has its origin. For example, all *vata* disorders have their root in the colon. *Pitta* disorders begin in the small intestine. *Kapha* diseases have their foundation in the stomach and gastric mucosal secretions. The condition of these organs is checked.

To help understand the causes of disease, that is, those factors which have weakened the system's ability to defend itself, Ayurveda has classified causes into groups:

- Acute versus chronic
- Genetic or hereditary
- Traumatic
- Habitual
- Dietary, including food poisoning and wrong food combining
- Seasonal

- Climate
- Lifestyle
- Age
- Metabolic condition
- Emotional and psychological makeup
- Supernatural and planetary disposition
- Acts of God

Certainly bacteria and viruses cause disease, but the physician also asks what affects the patient's ability to defend himself against them. Ayurveda is about physiology, not pathogens. The question asked is whether the body is protected by its balanced physiology or is in a state of imbalance and therefore open to disease. The body has its own protective mechanism, the *doshas*. The *doshas* respond to these causes in an attempt to fight off disease.

Stages of Disease

According to Ayurveda, there are six progressive stages of disease resulting from uncontrolled aggravating causes: accumulation, provocation, spread, deposition, manifestation, and differentiation.

ACCUMULATION

During the first stage, the aggravated *dosha* begins to accumulate in its respective location: *kapha* in the stomach, *pitta* in the small intestine, and *vata* in the colon. The *dosha* that accumulates is the result of one or more of the various causes previously listed. This beginning stage is the ideal time to begin therapy; the *dosha* is more easily removed before the condition spreads beyond its primary location. For this reason, Ayurveda strongly advises seasonal purification at the juncture of the seasons to eliminate the accumulation of *doshas* that tend to occur during the season.

PROVOCATION

During the second stage, *vata, pitta,* or *kapha* continue to accumulate in their respective locations and begin to affect the function of these and surrounding organs. This stage is also relatively easy to treat, although attention must be taken to strengthen the organs under pressure after the increased *doshas* are removed from the body. Excess *dosha* is removed by the traditional Ayurvedic cleansing therapy called *panchakarma*. The organ systems are strengthened through herbal supplements and modification of diet and lifestyle.

SPREAD

The third stage is spread. At this stage, the aggravated *dosha* moves from its primary location and begins to circulate in the body. The *doshas* may move in any direction. If *vata* moves upward, it can cause nausea, vomiting, or a feeling of light-headedness. If it moves downward too rapidly, diarrhea may result.

The tissues and organs of the body are divided into three *margas*, or pathways, through which the *doshas* flow. When a *dosha* enters this third stage of spread, it begins to travel along one of these pathways. These *margas* are as follows:

1. The internal, or gastrointestinal, pathway, which includes the entire alimentary canal.
2. The intermediate pathway, which includes *rasa* (plasma) and *rakta dhatus* (blood tissues).
3. The deep, or vital, pathway, which includes all the other *dhatus* (*mamsa*, muscle tissue; *meda*, fat tissue; *asthi*, bone tissue; *majja*, nerve tissue; and *shukra/artava*, reproductive tissue). This pathway also encompasses the essential organs and major vessels and nerves.

DEPOSITION

During the fourth stage, deposition, the aggravated *dosha* settles in a weak area in the bodily tissues and begins to accumulate. It is during this stage that the disease's prodromal symptoms begin. The physician must recognize these symptoms so that treatment can be initiated. By stopping the disease process at this stage, the body can heal itself more rapidly with less danger of lasting effects.

MANIFESTATION AND DIFFERENTIATION

In the fifth stage of manifestation, the diagnosis of the disease and the cardinal signs and symptoms are readily apparent. In Sanskrit, the sixth stage of disease is called *bheda*, which means

destruction or differentiation (i.e., tissue damage). When the disease process reaches the sixth stage, it is fully manifest with structural changes and complications involving other tissues and systems. The disease is also more difficult to treat at this stage.

THERAPY AND OUTCOMES

Treatment Options

Ayurveda has eight traditional specialities, or branches: surgery, internal medicine, gynecology, pediatrics, ear-nose-throat, psychiatry, toxicology, and geriatrics. Ayurveda uses surgery if there is a need. Ayurveda uses gemstones, crystals, metals, even *mantra* and sound for the purpose of healing. *Marma* therapy, pressing points to send energy to the organs and connective tissue, is also used. Ayurveda has a wide scope of practice, including related disciplines such as *jyotisha* (Vedic astrology), meditation, *yoga asanas* (yoga), and *pranayama* (cleansing).

According to Ayurveda, treatment is an action that creates balance among the components of constitution—*dosha, dhatu* (tissues), and *mala* (excretas: urine, feces, sweat). Ayurveda starts this action through prevention, which involves attention to maintaining the balance of the constitution. Living a proper, preventive lifestyle involves knowledge of one's unique constitution (*prakruti*) and of how to maintain its balance in the face of all outer and inner challenges and stresses. Strengthening the organs and tissues and eliminating toxins from the body before they reach the stage of producing symptoms of disease are equally important. The first line of treatment is to remove the cause of the disease. If this is not possible, a basic guideline is to control the *doshas* at the stage of accumulation by following an anti-*doshic* regimen.

All Ayurvedic treatment attempts to reestablish the person's unique constitutional balance. As discussed, disease develops when the person's immune function is low and the aggravated *doshas* settle in a weak area and begin to affect the functions of that system. Treatment of symptoms often makes the patient feel better; however, this does not address the fundamental cause of the illness, and the problem will likely reappear in the same or another form.

Treatments may be applied to the physical, emotional, and spiritual levels. Looking at the emotional level, most people learn in childhood not to express negative emotions (e.g., anger, fear, anxiety, nervousness, jealousy, possessiveness, and greed). As a result, these emotions become repressed and unprocessed. Ayurveda proposes that if these negative emotions remain repressed and are not dealt with, emotional toxins and unhealthy behavioral patterns will accumulate in the system. Ayurveda teaches a technique of dealing with negativity by observation and release. Recognize the emotion as it arises, observe it without judgment, and then release it. This technique helps to transform the unprocessed emotions into processed form. Negative emotions can be dealt with in this way through this awareness of emotion and release of it. Fear, anxiety, and apprehension are associated with *vata*; anger, hate, and jealousy with *pitta*; and greed, attachment, and possessiveness with *kapha*. Each of these three aspects of the body can influence and affect the others. For example, if a person represses fear, the kidneys tend to be disturbed; anger affects the liver; greed and possessiveness settle in the heart and spleen. Therefore, the emotional makeup of the patient is assessed and taken seriously.

PALLIATION

A basic Ayurvedic principle states that *jathar agni*, the gastric fire, and *dhatu agni*, the metabolic and regulatory component of each tissue, must be in harmony. If *agni* is low, food is not properly digested; undigested food becomes nonhomogenous, toxic, and morbid, and produces *ama* (or toxins) in the system. *Ama* is the root cause of disease. This *ama* must be eliminated, and *panchakarma* (Ayurvedic cleansing therapy) is the best treatment for this process. However, *panchakarma* should only be done with a person who has sufficient energy and strength. If a person is debilitated, tired, or weak, he or she cannot bear *panchakarma* and it could further complicate his or her condition. For these people, palliation is a better choice. Palliation involves the use of herbs, such

as ginger, black pepper, Piper longum, or *chitrak,* in addition to a specific diet appropriate for the person's constitution and condition.

Palliation helps not only to kindle digestive fire, but also to burn the *ama*. A person should drink no more than seven or eight cups of water daily because it will only slow down digestion, add to the *ama*, and create more congestion. Instead of cold water, a person should drink ginger tea, cinnamon tea, or certain herbal teas (e.g., mint tea or cumin-coriander-fennel tea). These teas kindle fire, detoxify *ama*, and cleanse the *srotas*, the subtle channels of the body. After this treatment, mild laxatives, such as *triphala,* are given to remove toxins from the colon.

The process of palliation still involves the removal of toxins from the system. However, the approach is more gentle and involves several aspects: herbal medication to digest accumulated toxins (*ama*) and to strengthen the digestive fire (*agni*); fasting from food and/or liquids; and sunbathing or windbathing. As this treatment continues, proper lifestyle, diet, and exercise must also be employed to sustain the benefits of treatment. With many conditions, treatment by palliation is used first and then, when the patient is stronger and the toxins have been moved from the tissues to the hollow organs, purification is appropriate to finish the removal of the toxins from the body.

PANCHAKARMA

To remove aggravated *doshas* and *ama* (toxins), Ayurveda suggests *panchakarma*. *Pancha* means five, and *karma* means action. The five actions associated with *panchakarma* are therapeutic vomiting, purgatives or laxatives, medicated enemas, nasal administration of medication, and purification of the blood. *Panchakarma* is indicated as a therapy *only* in cases in which the patient has sufficient strength and health to tolerate the removal of excess *doshas* and toxins. Even then, it should only be administered by trained personnel under the supervision of a qualified Ayurvedic physician.

Before the actual operation of purification begins, the body must be prepared to release the toxins. The two preparatory procedures are *snehana* (oil massage) and *swedana* (sweat therapy). With *snehana,* oil is applied to the entire body with a particular type of massage. This procedure helps the toxins to move from the deep tissues to the gastrointestinal tract. Oil massage also makes the superficial and deep tissues soft and supple, thus helping to remove stress and to nourish the nervous system. *Snehana* is given daily for three to seven days. *Swedana,* sweating, is given every day immediately following the *snehana.* An herbal concoction may be added to the steam to further loosen the toxins. After three to seven days of *snehana* and *swedana,* the *doshas* become well ripened. A particular *panchakarma* method is then given according to the individual's constitution and disorder.

Vamana: Therapeutic Vomiting

Therapeutic vomiting (*vamana*) is used to treat excess accumulations of *kapha* in the stomach. After three or four glasses of special herbs or salt water administered in the early morning, the tongue is rubbed to induce vomiting. The release of mucus through this therapy can bring immediate relief to congestion, wheezing, bronchitis, or breathlessness, and the sinuses will clear. Therapeutic vomiting is also indicated for skin diseases, chronic asthma, diabetes, chronic cold, lymphatic obstruction, chronic indigestion, edema, chronic sinus problems, and repeated attacks of tonsillitis. All of these conditions are associated with an imbalance of *kapha.*

Virechana: Purgatives and Laxatives

The use of purgatives (*virechana*) is helpful in treating *pitta* imbalance, which involves inflammation or irritation. Excess secretion of bile accumulated in the gallbladder, liver, or small intestine may cause allergic rash or skin inflammation (e.g., acne, dermatitis) as well as chronic fever or jaundice. A number of substances can be used for this treatment, including triphala, senna, psyllium, castor oil, or even cow's milk with *ghee* (clarified butter). Purgatives should not be given to persons with acute fever, diarrhea, severe constipation, or bleeding from the rectum or lungs. Other contraindications include patients with emaciation, weakness, or prolapsed rectum.

Basti: Therapeutic Enema

The third action is treatment with therapeutic enema (*basti*), which involves introducing medicinal oils or herbal decoctions into the rectum. Medicated enema is the action of choice for *vata* disorders. This treatment alleviates constipation, distention, chronic fever, sexual disorders, kidney stones, heart pain, vomiting, backache, and neck pain. Other *vata* disorders, including sciatica, arthritis and gout, also respond well to this therapy. Unlike colonics, which are popular with many therapies today, the principle reason for use of the enema in Ayurveda is for absorption of medicated oils and herbs through the colon wall. Of course, cleansing does take place when the enema is expelled. Oil or decoction enemas should be retained for a minimum of ten minutes, longer if possible.

Nasya: Nasal Administration of Medication

The fourth action, nasal administration of medicated oils and powders, is called *nasya.* The nose is a doorway to the brain and to consciousness, and life energy (*prana*) enters the body through breath taken in through the nose. Nasal medication helps to correct the disorders of *prana,* which affect the higher cerebral, sensory, and motor functions. This treatment is also used for dryness of the nose, sinus congestion, hoarseness, migraine headache, and certain eye and ear problems. Nasal medication is contraindicated following a bath, ingestion of food, sex, or alcohol consumption.

Rakta Moksha: Purification of the Blood

The fifth action of *panchakarma* is purification of the blood (*rakta moksha*). Literally, *rakta moksha* means liberation of blood, or bloodletting; a more liberal interpretation is the cleansing or purification of the blood. In Ayurveda, both historically and in modern times, bloodletting is used in certain cases, either directly or by the application of leeches. *Rakta moksha* is to remove toxins from the blood in conditions such as skin disorders, enlarged liver and spleen, and gout. However, in most Western countries, bloodletting is either illegal or considered to be quackery. Hence various other procedures, usually herbal, are used to cleanse the blood. For blood-carried disorders, such as allergy, rash, or acne, the patient could take burdock root tea as a blood purifier.

Ayurveda believes that toxins absorbed into the bloodstream through the gastrointestinal tract create toxemia, the cause of many disorders, such as eczema, rheumatoid arthritis, and even the common cold. These toxins circulate throughout the body and may manifest under the skin or in the joint spaces, creating disease. Skin disorders, such as urticaria, rash, eczema, acne, scabies, leucoderma, and hives also respond well to blood cleansing, as do cases of gout and enlarged liver and spleen. Excess *pitta* circulating as a waste product in the blood creates these disorders. Therefore, for many *pitta* ailments, using herbal blood cleaners or extracting a small amount of blood from the vein relieves the tension created by the toxins in the blood. This type of treatment is contraindicated in cases of anemia, edema, and weakness, and is not recommended for young children or the elderly. Although the above treatment should only be administered by a physician with Ayurvedic training, in some cases the symptoms of excess *pitta* are relieved by the donation of blood at a blood bank.

ROUTINE, REJUVENATION, AND VIRILIZATION

After the cleansing process occurs, a program of rejuvenation is recommended with specific herbs appropriate to the *dosha* imbalance. For *vata*, *guggulu* is used. If the person is *pitta*, *shatavari* or *guduchi* are used. For *kapha*, *punarnava*, *gokshura*, or *shilajit* are appropriate. In this approach, treatment is determined by looking at the entire process—what the person's strength is, which *dosha* is out of balance, and which *dhatu* (tissue) is affected.

According to Ayurveda, all substances have medicinal properties. Ayurveda's knowledge and usage of herbs and other substances were gained from long experience and observation and date from early times. In addition to most substances, there are hundreds of herbs commonly used in Ayurvedic preparations, in addition to those commonly used for food, such as cinnamon and turmeric. Many different modes of preparation are required and each substance, according to its properties, is appropriate for treatment of different imbalances. For example, the common cold has the properties of *kapha*—mucus, congestion, thick, and lethargic. The antidote is herbs with opposite qualities, such as hot ginger tea.

Once the body, mind, and spirit are essentially free from disease and back in balance, maintaining the vitality of the body and its systems through *rasayana*, rejuvenation therapy, and *vajikarana*, virilization therapy, is essential for health and longevity. *Ojas, tejas,* and *prana* are protected by virilization therapy. *Ojas*, the superfine essence of *kapha*, is a necessary factor for maintaining immunity. *Tejas*, the superfine essence of *pitta*, maintains cellular metabolism. *Prana*, the superfine essence of *vata*, is responsible for maintaining the continuous flow of information, intelligence, and communication of cells and is necessary for maintaining the life force. Specific routines and herbal products are available to assist in maintaining the vital function of these three life-giving forces. Ayurveda contains a science of longevity.

CHROMOTHERAPY

Ayurveda includes chromotherapy as a mode of treatment. Chromotherapy involves the use of specific colored light beamed directly on various parts of the body, water placed in the sunlight with specific colored cellophane attached to the jar, or wearing specific colors of clothing. Colors have psychological and physiological effects. Red, orange, and yellow are connected with *pitta*. Red improves circulation; orange acts as an antiseptic and antibacterial agent; yellow acts as a decongestant. These three colors are *pitta*-promoting and pacify *vata* and *kapha*. Ayurveda also uses the other colors of the rainbow, which are present in sunlight. Green is grounding and nourishing, so it is associated with *kapha*. Blue is cooling. In India, if a child is jaundiced, the child is put under blue light. The liver heals faster and the jaundice is relieved. Blue pacifies *pitta* and promotes liver function. Purple and indigo are cosmic colors associated with the higher spectrum and they relate to *vata dosha*.

Treatment Evaluation

Ayurveda addresses the causes of disease and the individual's personal response to these causes. Because each patient is evaluated according to his or her unique constitution, any aggravating causes, the present state of imbalance, and the stage of the disease process, there is less emphasis on standard treatments or remedies according to presenting symptoms. In Ayurveda, there is less emphasis on treating someone according to the name of the disease and more emphasis on treating the subject's imbalance and aggravating causes. Ayurveda goes deeply to the root cause of disease, and the treatment protocol for any given disease may vary from person to person and according to the stage and specifics of the disease process. Because of this approach, Ayurvedic treatments are generally not standardized. Individuals with similar Western diagnoses may often receive different Ayurvedic treatments.

There is a 5000-year tradition of the success and usefulness of Ayurveda, and there are many articles and studies reported. Ayurveda has developed and is used as an integrated system of medicine in which a unified theory guides the assessment and treatment of the patient. Its theory of health and disease, disease classifications, language and, in some cases, outcomes are different from those in the West and therefore are difficult (but not impossible) to investigate using modern Western approaches. At this point, however, there is no organization of the available literature, and finding studies on a specific area is difficult. There is an interest in testing Ayurveda as a medical system, using accepted Western medical style protocols. These studies are in the beginning stages at several university medical centers in the United States. For thousands of years, thousands of physicians and millions of patients have believed in and practiced Ayurveda. The question is, can this efficacy be proven by Western medicine?

One problem with proving efficacy according to Western protocols is the issue of double-blind trials and the placebo effect. The healing effects caused by the spiritual strength of the physician and placebos are acknowledged by Ayurveda and considered significant in many Eastern health care systems. However, these elements are generally difficult to quantify and may not be reproducible by every practitioner. In clinical studies to date, it seems that either the Western clinical protocols are compromised to allow for the satisfaction of the alternative/complementary side or the alternative/complementary side is unhappy with the changes necessary to satisfy Western clinical trial protocols. Many Western clinical trial studies are based on drugs and medicines formulated from a synthetically produced compound that can be quantified and standardized. Many of the Eastern approaches to health care, like Ayurveda, have a substantial pharmacopeia that uses only whole herbs. These herbs may be processed into tinctures, powders, or combinations, but active ingredients are not separated from the whole; the entire herb is used and is therefore difficult to standardize. Despite these difficulties, the benefits of a number of Ayurvedic products and practices have been studied and are summarized in the next section.

USE OF THE SYSTEM FOR TREATMENT

Ayurveda in the West

Currently in the West, there is no unification and standardization of Ayurvedic medicine, and there is only a small number of traditionally trained Ayurvedic physicians. Although Ayurveda as a medical system is uniquely applicable in almost all medical conditions, the lack of access to fully trained practitioners limits its use for primary care. The laws regulating the practice of medicine of course prevent any Ayurvedic physician, no matter how qualified, from practicing medicine in the United States without an acceptable license. In addition, the practice of Ayurveda in the United States is limited even for licensed practitioners because of restrictions placed on many of its therapies, such as bloodletting and compounds containing specially prepared metals considered toxic in the West (e.g., arsenic or mercury). For this reason, many problems are not treated with Ayurvedic medicine in the United States as they are in India.

Major Indications

CHRONIC CONDITIONS

Allopathic medicine uses powerful medications and has the technology to deal with acute emergencies. However, in chronic conditions, such as rheumatoid arthritis, stroke paralysis, or multiple sclerosis, allopathic medicine has less success. Ayurveda believes it can effectively treat these conditions with diet and lifestyle recommendations, cleansing programs, Ayurvedic massage, and rejuvenation. Ayurvedic treatment for any condition requires a commitment from the patient, and the patient needs to be questioned about his or her willingness to follow through with diet and lifestyle changes. A significant component of the treatment process is the patient's personal responsibility as well as a genuine desire on the part of the patient to heal.

There has been no study that we know of using the Western clinical trial method on Ayurveda as an entire *system* of medicine. There are a number of studies on specific treatments and considerable literature on the pharmacological action of Ayurvedic herbs and their active ingredients. An example is guggulipid, a traditional Ayurvedic herb demonstrated to lower serum cholesterol in clinical studies (1). By consulting with experienced Ayurvedic practitioners, conventional researchers in India have discovered a number of useful herbs and have done so more rapidly and economically than those that have been discovered using the usual drug-screening and development strategies (2, 3). Laboratory and human experimental studies have indicated benefits of Ayurvedic products in conditions such as Alzheimer's disease (4), Parkinson's disease (5), and rheumatoid arthritis (6). These studies have also helped to identify potentially toxic substances (7) and drug–herb interactions (8), requiring knowledge and careful use of Ayurvedic products.

Transcendental meditation (TM) is a specialized meditation technique adapted from Ayurvedic traditions and is widely taught in Western countries. It has been shown to produce beneficial effects on a number of conditions, including reduction of blood pressure (9, 10); posttraumatic stress syndrome (11); anxiety (12); alcohol, nicotine, and drug abuse (13); and for general improvement in psychological health (14). Physiological effects of TM were reported three decades ago (15), and long-term practice may include electroencephalogram changes that persist during sleep (16). Meditation techniques derived from Ayurveda, with their emphasis on changing consciousness, may produce greater health benefits than those that simply teach relaxation (17). For example, a carefully controlled trial of TM demonstrated reductions in blood pressure in hypertensive, elderly African Americans who practiced the technique (9, 10).

Recently, data collected on the costs and health outcomes of individuals who regularly engage in the lifestyle and preventive practices of Ayurveda have shown considerably cost reductions because of less use of conventional health care services (18). When people take responsibility for their health and consciously engage in health-promoting behaviors, chronic disease is often mitigated or eased.

PERSONAL RESPONSIBILITY

Identifying the cause of one's disorder is the beginning of the process of returning to balance. An important step is the client taking responsibility for dealing with the issues that are causing the undesirable effects and eventually doing something about these issues. Although classical Ayurveda has powerful techniques and an extensive pharmacopoeia, its more limited contemporary practice in the West is generally more effective when there is time for recovery (e.g., when the disease is in the early stage or is not life-threatening). If a patient persists in habits and behaviors identified as causative for his or her health problems, the Ayurvedic approach will only be partially effective. Ayurveda is most effective when the individual faces the cause of his or her condition and applies remedies according to his or her own constitution.

Ayurveda is a philosophy and system that encompasses the body, mind, emotions, and spirit. Many medical systems are held within this philosophy—from herbology and diet to surgery and drugs. What medicines to use, when to use them, and in what combination and for whom is the strength and great contribution of Ayurveda.

Preventive Value

Modern medicine is just beginning to address the importance of preventive measures. Because of Ayurveda's emphases on the balance of body, mind, and consciousness and on the importance of appropriate diet, lifestyle, and exercise for one's constitution, it is called the Science of Life. Following this approach, it seeks to bring one to a state of perfect health and to enhance longevity.

ORGANIZATION

Training

In ancient times, the Vedic tradition in India passed this knowledge from *guru* to disciple, teacher to student, and continued for many thousands of years as an oral tradition. Approximately 2000 years ago, much of this knowledge was recorded in print, Ayurvedic medical colleges were established, and training became more formalized. This ancient Vedic tradition can still be sought out.

Today there are approximately 200 Ayurvedic colleges and schools in India connected to universities in every state. An Ayurvedic specialist in India has an educational and internship requirement similar to physicians (MDs) in the United States. The title is Master of Ayurvedic Science (MASc). The course of study for the bachelors degree (Bachelor of Ayurvedic Medicine and Surgery; BAMS) is five years, plus a two-year internship. The curriculum is established according to the basic principles of Ayurveda. In the second year, the students begin clinical work in a hospital under experienced Ayurvedic physicians. After finishing the requirements for the BAMS, a student may elect graduate study. During the intern years, the student's guidance counselor helps the student decide a research topic, which culminates in a thesis. After the thesis is accepted, there is a series of examinations, both oral and written.

If the student passes, he or she is declared an Ayurvedic specialist and is granted the MASc degree. It typically takes nine to ten years to obtain an MASc. In recent years the MASc degree has been changed to Doctor of Medicine in Ayurveda (MD in Ayurveda).

There is wide variance in how Ayurveda is practiced in the West. Because it is not yet recognized as a legitimate health care practice in the United States, there are only a handful of fully trained Ayurvedic physicians here. Although there are a growing number of schools in the West that teach Ayurvedic principles, the curriculum is limited and there is no consensus as to curriculum or requirements for graduation. These schools vary from small private schools, solely dedicated to Ayurveda, to a number of universities now beginning to develop programs of study. Ayurvedic physicians from India are sometimes brought to lecture for these new programs. However, a fully developed curriculum similar to those in India is not yet available in the West. Similarly, there is no licensing of Ayurvedic physicians, even for fully qualified Ayurvedic physicians trained in India. In the United States, licensed health care professionals, such as physicians, nurses, acupuncturists, and chiropractors, can incorporate Ayurvedic principles into their practice to the extent of their training and understanding. However, this practice becomes problematic in the West when a health care professional attends only a weekend seminar or other short course of study in Ayurvedic medicine, begins an Ayurvedic practice, and then has no further Ayurvedic medical training. An understanding of Ayurveda takes time and, although basic principles can be incorporated after some serious study, a thorough understanding of its proper application requires extensive study and commitment.

Quality Assurance

In most Western countries, health care is regulated by the government. The laws govern not only what a practitioner can call oneself or claim to be, but also whether one can practice at all. The language of modern health care law is based on scope of practice. When a practitioner wishes to diagnose and recommend specific treatment, it is considered to be the practice of medicine and hence requires a license that allows for that—MD, DO, ND, DC, and so on. Also, in most Western countries, the educational institution and the awarded degree are separate from the licensing and governing body that regulates the profession. Rather than endorse certain professions and practitioners, these licensing boards effectively control which health care options are available to people.

This regulation of health care in many Western countries affects Ayurveda in a dramatic manner. Even well-qualified and respected Ayurvedic physicians, those with a BAMS or MASc, who are approved to practice medicine in India are unable to practice in most Western countries. It is almost impossible for a person seeking professional Ayurvedic health care in most Western countries to obtain it. For an Ayurvedic physician to be able to practice medicine in most Western countries, he or she would literally need to go back to an approved medical school and obtain a degree in one of the licensable professions; all of this could take four to six years. This situation forces people who want Ayurvedic care to seek care from practitioners who are less knowledgeable in the Ayurvedic practice.

Currently, people in Western countries who want Ayurvedic care have two options: to choose a qualified and licensed medical doctor who has some training and understanding of Ayurveda, or to choose a unlicensed person with probably little or no formal medical education. The first choice will undoubtedly provide the patient with good medical care, but not necessarily expert Ayurvedic care. The second choice, although well intentioned, may not be able to provide the patient with good medical care.

There is a potential third option: a clinic with a licensed medical doctor, in the role of coordinating physician, who supervises the health care program of the patient and uses another person in the office who can provide expert Ayurvedic assessment and recommendations for treatment. However, there are few doctors or clinics currently providing this type of practice.

Reimbursement

For the patient who wants or needs insurance reimbursement, the best choice is to choose a doctor who is incorporating Ayurveda into his or her practice and whose services are covered by insurance. There are one or two new, smaller insurance companies that will provide coverage for alternative health care. The question for the consumer is how to find these companies and how to judge their stability. The costs of modern health care and health insurance make these decisions a difficult task.

Relations with Conventional Medicine

Modern allopathic medicine uses powerful and effective drugs, such as antibiotics, steroids, tranquilizers, and muscle relaxants. These drugs may have significant side effects. Knowledge of Ayurvedic principles can help an individual deal with some of these side effects. Ayurveda can complement conventional medicine by bringing insights to treatment of the patient, so that a drug can be selected for the person's *prakruti* (i.e., unique constitution).

For example, some people may be sensitive to penicillin. Because, according to Ayurvedic principles, penicillin is *hot, sharp,* and *penetrating,* it is *pitta*-provoking. Knowing this, a physician would carefully consider whether to prescribe penicillin to a *pitta* person. The same approach applies to aspirin. A *pitta* person is sensitive to aspirin. In that case, the doctor can suggest that aspirin be taken with bicarbonate of soda or *shanka bhasma,* an Ayurvedic preparation. With this combination, the aspirin will still work but will not burn the wall of the stomach.

Steroids should not be given to a *kapha* person because steroids have a *kapha*-type of action. They slow down metabolism and can create steroid toxicity, resulting in a moon-face and water retention. Therefore, steroids should be given only in emergency and for a short period of time to a *kapha* person.

In addition, Ayurveda can alleviate some of the side effects of modern pharmaceuticals. For example, when a cancer patient on chemotherapy loses his or her hair, which is a *pitta* symptom, the patient can apply Bhringraj Oil to the scalp and take *shatavari* and *guduchi*. These herbs help prevent hair loss and *pitta* provocation, and the person can more easily bear chemotherapy with reduced side effects.

PROSPECTS FOR THE FUTURE

Ayurveda has great prospects in the West, and the future of this system is bright. The medicine of the twenty-first century will incorporate the best of East and West, and the time-proven truths of Ayurveda will be a gift for all generations to come. Studying Ayurveda will give modern physicians additional tools for their practice, and the incorporation of Ayurvedic principles will bring improved health—to the body, mind, and consciousness.

SUGGESTED READINGS

Frawley D. Ayurvedic healing. Salt Lake City: Morson Publishing, 1989.

Frawley D, Lad V. The yoga of herbs. Santa Fe: Lotus Press, 1986.

Lad V. Ayurveda: the science of self-healing. Santa Fe: Lotus Press, 1986.

Lad V. Secrets of the pulse: the ancient art of ayurvedic pulse diagnosis. Albuquerque: The Ayurvedic Press, 1996.

Lad V, Lad U. Ayurvedic cooking for self-healing. Albuquerque: The Ayurvedic Press, 1994.

Morrison JH. The book of Ayurveda: a holistic approach to health and longevity. New York: Simon & Schuster, Inc., 1995.

Svoboda RE. Ayurveda: life, health and longevity. London: Penquin, 1992.

Svoboda RE. The hidden secret of Ayurveda. Pune, India, 1980; reprint, Albuquerque: The Ayurvedic Press, 1994.

Svoboda RE. Prakruti: your Ayurvedic constitution. Albuquerque: Geocom Limited, 1989.

REFERENCES

1. Satyarati GU. Gum guggul (Commiphoral makal): the success of an ancient insight leading to a modern discovery. Indian J Med Res 1998;87:327–335.
2. Jain SK. Ethnobotany and research on medicinal plants in India. Ciba Found Symp 1994;153–164.
3. Chaudhury RR. Herbal medicine for human health. World Health Organization monograph. New Dehli, 1991.
4. Effect of Trasina, an Ayurvedic herbal formulation, on experimental models of Alzheimer's disease and central cholinergic markers in rats. J Altern Complement Med 1997;3(4):327–336.
5. An alternative medicine treatment for Parkinson's disease: results of a multicenter clinical trial. HP-200 in Parkinson's Disease Study Group. J Altern Complement Med 1995;1(3):249–255.
6. Studies on the mechanism of action of Semecarpus anacardium in rheumatoid arthritis. J Ethnopharmacol 1989;25(2):159–164.
7. Arsenic and Ayurveda. Leuk Lymphoma 1993; 10(4–5):343–345.
8. Scientific evidence on the role of Ayurvedic herbals on bioavailability of drugs. J Ethnopharmacol 1981;4(2):229–232.
9. Schneider RH, Staggers F, Alexander CN, et al. A randomized controlled trial of stress reduction for hypertension in older African Americans. Hypertension 1995;26(5);820–827.
10. Alexander CN, Schneider RH, Staggers F, et al. Trial of reduction for hypertension in older African Americans II: sex and risk subgroup analysis. Hypertension 1996;28;228–237.
11. Brooks JS, Scarano T. Transcendental meditation in the treatment of post-Vietnam adjustment. J Counsel Devel 1986;64:212–215.
12. Eppley K, Abrams A, Shear J. The differential effects of relaxation techniques on trait anxiety: a meta-analysis. J Clin Psychol 1989;45:957–974.
13. Alexander CN, Robinson P, Rainforth M. Treating and preventing alcohol, nicotine, and drug abuse through Transcendental Meditation: a review and statistical meta-analysis. Alcoholism Treatment Quarterly 1994;11:13–87.
14. Alexander CN, Rainforth MV, Gelderloos P. Transcendental Meditation, self actualization and psychological health: a conceptual overview and statistical meta-analysis. J Soc Behav Pers 1991;6: 189–247.
15. Wallace RK. Physiological effects of Transcendental Meditation. Science 1970;167:1751–1754.
16. Mason L, Alexander CN, Travis FT, et al. Electrophysiological correlates of higher states of consciousness during sleep in long-term practitioners

of the Transcendental Meditation program. Sleep 1997;20(2):102–110.

17. Orme-Johnson DW, Walton K. All approaches to preventing or reversing effects of stress are not the same. Am J Health Prom 1998;March/April:12[4].

18. Orme-Johnson DW, Herron RE. An innovative approach to reducing medical care utilization and expenditures. Am J Managed Car 1997;3(1): 135–144.

CHAPTER 12

TRADITIONAL CHINESE MEDICINE

Lixing Lao

BACKGROUND

Description

Traditional Chinese medicine (TCM) is a well-developed, coherent system of medicine that has been practiced in China for thousands of years. The system views the human body as a whole and as part of nature. Harmony must be maintained within body functions and between the body and nature to remain healthy. Disease occurs when this harmony is disrupted. To restore the state of harmony, several therapeutic approaches are commonly used: Chinese herbal medicine, acupuncture/moxibustion, *Tui Na* (Chinese massage and acupressure), mind/body exercise, and Chinese dietary therapy. Disease prevention is an integral part of TCM.

History and Development

The origins of Chinese medicine are linked to three legendary emperors: Huang Di, the Yellow Emperor (2697 BC), known as the originator of the traditional medicine of China; Shen Nong (2698–2598 BC), the divine husbandman, considered to be the founder of agriculture and the originator of Chinese herbal medicine; and Fu Xi, the Ox tamer, known as the creator of acupuncture needles (1). Huang Di is said to be the author of the first classic work on traditional Chinese medicine, the *Yellow Emperor's Inner Classic (Huang Di Nei Jing)*. This text is divided into two parts: *Simple Questions (Su Wen)*,

which delineates the theory of Chinese medicine, and the *Spiritual Axis (Ling Shu)*, which describes the practices of acupuncture and moxibustion (a method in which a moxa herb is burned above the skin to apply heat to the acupuncture points for the alleviation of symptoms). Although the *Yellow Emperor's Inner Classic* is believed to have been compiled by unknown authors circa 200 BC, long after the time of Huang Di, it has remained the most respected text of Chinese medical society throughout the long history of TCM.

Several key historical figures contributed to the development of TCM. During the Han dynasty (25–220 AD), a well-known physician, Zhang Zhongjing (150–219 AD), wrote *Treatise on Febrile and Miscellaneous Diseases (Shang Han Za Bing Lun)* (1–3). In this book, he established the principle that treatment should be based on the differentiation of symptoms. This principle is considered a milestone in the development of TCM. The earliest book exclusively about acupuncture and moxibustion was written by Huangfu Mi in the second century AD, between the Wei and Jin dynasties (1, 2, 4). This book described the meridians, the names and locations of acupuncture points, needling techniques and contraindications, and the detailed acupuncture treatment of many symptoms and diseases. It recorded 349 acupoints, far more than the 160 recorded in the *Yellow Emperor's Inner Classic*. During the same time period, *The Classic of Difficult Issues (Nan Jing)* emphasized the reinforcing and reducing methods that are considered important components of needling technique (1, 2, 5). Thirteen centuries later, during the Ming dynasty (1368–1644), Yang Jizhou (1522–1620) further developed the theory and practice of acupuncture. He summarized all of the previous important acupuncture literature and described 361 acupuncture points. This book became a very important textbook for the study of acupuncture (1, 2, 6).

The first Chinese herbal classic, written by an unknown author, is the *Divine Husbandman's Classic of Materia Medica (Shen Nong Ben Cao Jing)* (25–220 AD). This book records 365 individual herbs (2). In 1578, Li Shizhen, a well-known herbalist in Chinese medical history, completed the *Grand Materia Medica (Ben Cao Gang Mu),* which elaborated on the properties and functions of 1892 herbs (1, 2). By 1977, the number of Chinese herbal medicines identified increased to 5767 (1, 7).

Other Chinese medical techniques have also been practiced for centuries. Yi Yin, an emperor's chef who lived in the eleventh century BC, was the founding father of Chinese dietary therapy (2, 8). The earliest Chinese massage (*Tui Na*) techniques were recorded in *The Ten Volumes of Huang Di and Qi Bo's Massage (Huang Di Qi Bo An Mo Shi Juan)* during the Qin and Han dynasties (221 BC–220 AD) (8). Chinese mind-body exercise (e.g., *QiGong*) can be traced back more than 2000 years. A silk manuscript discovered in 1972 from a Han dynasty tomb, the *Ma Wang Tui* tomb, recorded the movements of the early form of *Qi Gong* technique (2).

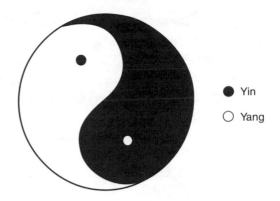

FIGURE 12.1. The *Yin-Yang* symbol.

verse and the phenomena of nature, including human beings.

Yin-Yang Theory

According to TCM, the universe is a whole that is made up of the unity of two opposite components (Fig. 12.1). *Yin* usually represents things relatively inactive, descending, internal, cold, and dark; *yang* usually represents things relatively active, ascending, external, hot, and bright (Table 12.1). All physiological functions of the body, as well as the signs and symptoms of pathological change, can be differentiated on the basis of *yin* and *yang* characteristics (Table 12.2). However, the natures of *yin* and *yang* are not absolute—they are relative concepts. *Yin* and *yang* are interdependent and can transform into each other. The equilibrium of *yin* and *yang* ensures that the harmony of the body is maintained. Normally, a healthy person with no symptoms of illness is considered to have equilibrium between *yin* and *yang*. A typical *yin* deficiency syndrome may be exemplified by menopause syndrome (e.g., hot flashes, night sweats). A typical *yang* deficiency syndrome may

PRINCIPAL CONCEPTS AND BASIC THEORIES

The fundamental concepts of TCM are *yin-yang* and the five element theory (*Wu Xing*). These two concepts explain changes in the uni-

Table 12.1. Examples of *Yin-Yang* Opposite Characters									
Yang	Up	Sun	Day	Fire	Heat	Movement	Exterior	Brightness	Function
Yin	Down	Moon	Night	Water	Cold	Stillness	Interior	Darkness	Structure

Adapted with modifications from Liu G, Hyodo A, eds. *Fundamentals of Acupuncture and Moxibustion.* Tianjin: Tianjin Science and Technology Translation and Publishing Corporation, 1994, p 12.

Table 12.2. Syndrome Differentiation According to *Yin* and *Yang*

SYNDROMES OF *YANG*	SYNDROMES OF *YIN*
Fever, perspiration, hyperfunction	Chills or aversion to cold, hypofunction
Raised basal metabolic rate	Reduced basal metabolic rate
High temperature	Low temperature
Profuse perspiration	Reduced perspiration
Increased gastric peristalsis	Reduced gastric peristalsis
Sympathetic hyperactivity	Parasympathetic hyperactivity
Intolerance of heat	Intolerance of cold
Red or rosy complexion	Pale complexion
Desire for cold drink and food	Desire for hot drink and food
Yellow urine	Clear urine

Adapted with modifications from Liu G, Hyodo A, eds. *Fundamentals of Acupuncture and Moxibustion.* Tianjin: Tianjin Science and Technology Translation and Publishing Corporation, 1994, p 13.

be exemplified by hypothyroidism, with symptoms including pale color, cold limbs, or edema.

Wu Xing (Five Element Theory)

The five element theory (also known as the five phase theory) in TCM developed from an ancient Chinese philosophy that views the universe as consisting of five basic elements: wood, fire, earth, metal, and water. The theory explains the relationships between the human body and the external environment as well as the physiological and pathological relationships among the internal organs within the human body (Table 12.3).

The dynamic physiological relationships among these five elements are shown in Figure 12.2. *Interpromotion* (see Fig. 12.2A) means that one element promotes or generates the other element in the order of wood, fire, earth, metal, and water. For example, wood promotes or gen-

Table 12.3. Classification According to *Wu Xing*: Five Elements Theory

FIVE ELEMENTS	WOOD	FIRE	EARTH	METAL	WATER
Seasons:	Spring	Summer	Late summer	Autumn	Winter
Directions:	East	South	Middle	West	North
Weather:	Wind	Summer Heat	Dampness	Dryness	Cold
Colors:	Green	Red	Yellow	White	Black
Tastes:	Sour	Bitter	Sweet	Acrid	Salty
Development:	Germination	Growth	Transformation	Reaping	Storing
Zang organs:	Liver	Heart	Spleen	Lung	Kidney
Fu organs:	Gallbladder	Small intestine	Stomach	Large intestine	Urinary bladder
Tissues:	Tendon	Vessel	Muscle	Skin	Bone
Sense organs:	Eye	Tongue	Mouth	Nose	Ear
Manifestations:	Nails	Face	Lips	Body hair	Hair
Voices:	Shouting	Laughing	Singing	Crying	Moaning
Emotions:	Anger	Joy	Worry	Grief	Fear

Adapted from Liu G, Hyodo A, eds. *Fundamentals of Acupuncture and Moxibustion.* Tianjin: Tianjin Science and Technology Translation and Publishing Corporation, 1994, p 20.

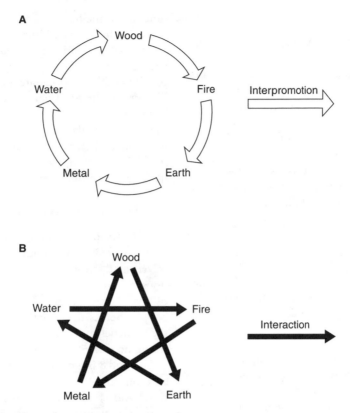

Figure 12.2. Interpromotion and interaction relationships among the five elements. (Reprinted with permission from Liu G, Hyodo A, eds. *Fundamentals of Acupuncture and Moxibustion*. Tianjin: Tianjin Science and Technology Translation and Publishing Corporation, 1994:21.)

erates fire; fire promotes or generates earth. *Interaction* (see Fig. 12.2B) means that one element acts on or controls another in a different order. For example, wood acts on or controls earth; earth acts on or controls water (see Fig. 12.2). Each element represents an internal organ in the body. For example, the liver is associated with wood, the heart with fire, the spleen with earth, the lung with metal, and the kidneys with water. Clinically, pathological changes occur if these dynamic balances are interrupted or destroyed.

Major Components of TCM

Major components of the TCM system include *Qi*, blood, body fluid, the *Zang-Fu* (internal organs), and the *Jing-Luo* (meridian and collateral systems, or pathways, within which *Qi* and blood are circulated through the entire body to maintain equilibrium). These theories explain how the human body maintains its vitality and health physiologicalally.

Qi

Qi denotes vital energy and is an essential substance for maintaining the activities of life. The origins of *Qi* include congenital *Qi*, which is inherited from the parents, and acquired *Qi*, which is obtained from the food eaten and air inhaled. According to the location and functional characteristics of *Qi*, it has different names: primary *Qi*, pectoral *Qi*, nutrient *Qi*, and defensive *Qi*. In general, *Qi* has five functions:

1. Promoting
2. Warming
3. Defending
4. Governing
5. *Qihua* (transforming)

BLOOD

Blood originates from the food essence developed in the spleen and stomach. Blood is dominated by the heart, stored in the liver, and controlled by the spleen. Blood has the function of nourishing the organs and tissues of the body.

Both *Qi* and blood serve as the material basis for life activities. *Qi* is classified as *yang* and blood as *yin* because *Qi* mainly promotes and warms, whereas blood nourishes and moistens. The relationship between *Qi* and blood can briefly be summarized as follows:

- *Qi* generates blood
- *Qi* is the driving force of blood
- *Qi* keeps blood flowing within the vessels
- Blood is the "mother" of *Qi* (i.e., *Qi* originates from and is carried by the blood)

BODY FLUID

Body fluid refers to all normal liquids of the body, such as saliva, tears, nasal discharge, sweat, semen, and urine. Body fluid can reach the skin and hair exteriorly, and the internal organs interiorly to moisten these organs and tissues. The formation, distribution, and excretion of body fluid is a complicated process involving many organs. The key organs in this process are the lung (regulates the water passage), spleen (transports and transforms water), and kidney (dominates water metabolism and the reproductive system).

ZANG-FU (INTERNAL ORGANS)

The theory of the *Zang-Fu* explains the physiological functions and pathological changes of the internal organs through the observation of the outward manifestations of the body. The five *zang* are the solid organs, considered *yin* organs, which are the heart, liver, spleen, lung, and kidney. The six *fu* are the hollow organs, which belong to the *yang* category, consisting of the gallbladder, stomach, small intestine, large intestine, urinary bladder, and *Sanjiao* (triple warmer, which are three compartments—above the diaphragm, the abdomen, and the lower abdomen). The physiological functions of the *zang* organs are to manufacture and store essential substances (e.g., vital essence, which is a function of the health of the kidney; *Qi*; blood; and body fluid). The functions of the *fu* organs are to receive and digest food, and transmit and excrete the wastes. Although some of these physiological functions are similar to those in Western medicine, others are very different. For instance, the heart is said not only to control the blood circulation, but also to take charge of mind activities; the main function of the spleen is digestion, which is very different from its function in Western medicine.

JING (MERIDIANS) AND LUO (COLLATERALS)

The theory of the *Jing* and *Luo* describes the energy system of the body that deals with the travel and distribution of the *Qi*. The meridians, or pathways, are the main trunks that run longitudinally and interiorly-exteriorly within the body, whereas the collaterals, or networks, are the branches running vertically and horizontally throughout the body. There are 12 regular meridians and 8 irregular meridians. The meridians and collaterals relate to the *Zang-Fu* organs interiorly and connect to the extremities and acupuncture points exteriorly, integrating the *Zang-Fu*, tissues, and other organs into a whole. *Qi* flows through the meridians and participates in the homeostatic regulation of various body functions; 361 points are distributed along the meridians and serve as both pathognomic signs of disorder and as loci for acupuncture treatments. Thus, the *Jing-Luo* regulate *Qi* and blood, balance *yin* and *yang*, and keep the functions and activities of all parts of the body in harmony. One of the meridians of the *Jing-Luo* system, as illustrated in a classic textbook from the seventeenth century, is shown in Figure 12.3.

PROVIDER–PATIENT INTERACTION

Patient Assessment

The pathogenic factors of TCM can be classified into three categories: external, internal, and other (neither internal nor external). The six external factors are wind, cold, summer-heat, dampness, dryness, and fire. Normally, they are natural environmental factors and are not harm-

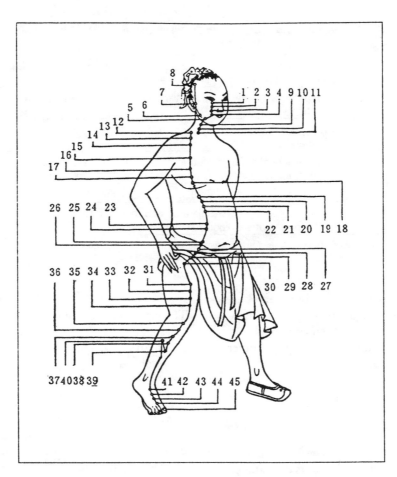

1. ST 1 Chengqi	13. ST 13 Qihu	25. ST 25 Tianshu	37. ST 37 Shangjuxu
2. ST 2 Sibai	14. ST 14 Kufang	26. ST 26 Wailing	38. ST 38 Tiaokou
3. ST 3 Juliao	15. ST 15 Wuyi	27. ST 27 Daju	39. ST 39 Xiajuxu
4. ST 4 Dicang	16. ST 16 Yingchuang	28. ST 28 Shuidao	40. ST 40 Fenglong
5. ST 5 Daying	17. ST 17 Ruzhong	29. ST 29 Guilai	41. ST 41 Jiexi
6. ST 6 Jiache	18. ST 18 Rugen	30. ST 30 Qichong	42. ST 42 Chongyang
7. ST 7 Xiaguan	19. ST 19 Burong	31. ST 31 Biguan	43. ST 43 Xiangu
8. ST 8 Touwei	20. ST 20 Chengman	32. ST 32 Futu	44. ST 44 Neiting
9. ST 9 Renying	21. ST 21 Liangmen	33. ST 33 Yinshi	45. ST 45 Lidui
10. ST 10 Shuitu	22. ST 22 Guanmen	34. ST 34 Liangqui	
11. ST 11 Qishe	23. ST 23 Taiyi	35. ST 35 Dubi	
12. ST 12 Quepen	24. ST 24 Huaroumen	36. ST 36 Zusanli	

FIGURE 12.3. An example of the meridian system: the stomach meridian. It starts from the head and face descending through the anterior part of the trunk and the leg, and ends at the toes. This meridian also connects internally with the organs of the stomach and spleen. The acupuncture points on this meridian can be used for treating the systems of gastrointestinal and oral facial disorders. (Reprinted with permission from Liu G, Hyodo A, eds. Fundamentals of Acupuncture and Moxibustion. Tianjin: Tianjin Science and Technology Translation and Publishing Corporation, 1994:83.)

ful to the human body. However, when they are excessive, or when the defensive *Qi* of the human body declines, these six factors may cause diseases and symptoms. The characteristics of each external factor are listed in Table 12.4. The internal factors refer to the seven emotions: joy, anger, melancholy, worry, grief, fear, and fright. Any of these emotions expressed too strongly or frequently can disturb body processes and cause disease. The other factors in-

Table 12.4. The Properties and Pathogenic Characteristics of the Six Exogenous Factors

EXOGENOUS FACTORS	PROPERTIES AND CHARACTERISTICS
Wind	*Yang* pathogen, tends to invade the upper part of the body, changeable and movable, leading cause among the six factors
Cold	*Yin* pathogen, tends to impair *Yang Qi*, obstructive and coagulative to cause constriction
Summer-heat	*Yang* pathogen, scorching, tends to rise and disperse, apt to impair the body fluid and *Qi*
Dampness	*Yin* pathogen, tends to obstruct *Qi* activities and impairs spleen *yang*, heavy and turbid, viscous and lingering, apt to attack the lower part of the body
Dryness	Tends to exhaust the body fluid and attack the lung
Fire	*Yang* pathogen, tends to flare up and to impair *Qi* and body fluid, apt to disturb the liver and affect blood

Adapted from Liu G, Hyodo A, eds. *Fundamentals of Acupuncture and Moxibustion.* Tianjin: Tianjin Science and Technology Translation and Publishing Corporation, 1994, p 122.

clude dietary irregularities, obsessive sexual activity, taxation fatigue, trauma, and parasites.

The *Si Zhen* (four diagnostic methods) are the examination approaches for TCM differentiation of syndromes:

1. Inspection
2. Auscultation and olfaction
3. Inquiry
4. Palpation.

The aim of the approaches is to collect and analyze information that reflects the status of the body conditions and to determine the pattern of syndromes.

INSPECTION

Inspection refers to the visual assessment of the patient's *Shen* (vitality or spirit), complexion, facial expression, posture, color, and nature of the secretions and excretions. The observation of the *Shen* is important in assessing the prognosis; good spirit suggests a favorable prognosis. Another major component of inspection is the observation of the tongue, in particular the shape, color, markings, and coating. For instance, a pale white tongue with a white coating indicates a cold syndrome and deficiency of *yang* or blood, whereas a deep red tongue with a yellow coating is the sign of a heat syndrome.

AUSCULTATION

Auscultation is the act of listening to the patient's voice for loudness, strength, clearness,

stuffiness, slowness, or rapidity during speaking. The practitioner should be aware of any abnormal sounds, such as hiccups, eructation, asthma, cough, dyspnea, and sighing to differentiate the status of a disease.

OLFACTION

Olfaction is evaluating the odors of breath, body, and excreta. For example, a sour odor in the mouth is often associated with a digestive disorder of the stomach. Foul urine is primarily caused by dampness and heat in the body.

INQUIRING

Inquiring is the act of interviewing the patient to obtain related information about the patient's illness, including the time of onset, the cause and the course of the illness, the location of symptoms, and past history. Inquiring also involves a broad scope of information about the patient's quality of life, including appetite and diet, bowel movement, thirst, urination, sleep, dreams, body temperature (chill/fever), perspiration, conditions of the head, eyes, nose, ears, and throat, status of the trunk (chest/abdomen/back) and limbs, spirit/emotions, pain, menstruation (cycle, duration, amount, color, quality, cramps, and leukorrhea), and pregnancy.

PALPATION

Palpation is a diagnostic method in which the practitioner learns the condition of the patient by palpating the body and the pulse. Body palpation includes using tactile sensation to survey for local coldness, heat, softness, hardness, tenderness, abdominal masses or other abnormal situations in the skin, hands, feet, and abdomen. In pulse palpation, the practitioner typically uses three fingers (i.e., index, middle, and ring fingers), which are placed on the radial arteries of the wrists. The pulse is divided into three sections known as *Cun*, *Guan*, and *Chi*. The region corresponding to the styloid process of the radius at the wrist is *Guan*, with *Cun* just distal and *Chi* just proximal to it. Each hand has three pulse locations corresponding to particular internal organs: the left hand pulses represent the condition of the heart (*Cun*), liver (*Guan*), and kidney (*Chi*), and the right hand pulses represent the condition of the lung (*Cun*), spleen (*Guan*), and kidney (*Chi*). The pulse is assessed in seven aspects: speed, depth, strength, fluency, size/shape, tension, and rhythm. A normal pulse is smooth, even, and forceful, with a frequency of four beats per breath. Classically, 28 types of abnormal pulse have been identified. For example, a superficial pulse means that it is easily felt with gentle, but not with a firmer, touch. This often indicates an exterior syndrome, such as the early stages of a common cold. A surging pulse is broad, large, and forceful, like a roaring wave that comes on powerfully and then fades away. This often indicates excessive heat (e.g., high fever). A tense pulse feels tight and forceful like a stretched rope. It might be indicative of pain.

Differential Diagnosis

BIAN ZHENG (DIFFERENTIATION OF SYNDROMES)

The information collected through the four diagnostic methods (i.e., inspection, auscultation and olfaction, inquiring, and palpation) reflects the pathological changes of the internal organs and the condition of an illness. The differential diagnosis is based on a comprehensive analysis of this information. Several methods of differentiation of syndromes have been developed over the course of the history of TCM clinical practice (Table 12.5). Among them, the differentiation of syndromes according to the eight principles (i.e., *yin* and *yang*, exterior and interior, cold and heat, excess and deficiency) can be used for diagnosis in all clinical situations. The differentiation of syndromes can also be done according to the theories of the *Qi*, blood and body fluids, the *Zang-Fu* organs, the six *Jing* (meridians), and the *Wei*, *Qi*, and *Ying* (see Table 12.5).

An example helps to illustrate the TCM diagnostic approach. A patient presents with a chief complaint of insomnia. In TCM, there are multiple pathologies that can cause insomnia. By using the four diagnostic methods, this patient with insomnia is also found to have mental restlessness, palpitations, dryness of the throat, backache, nocturnal emission, hot flashes, and night sweats. A red tongue with little coating is observed, and a thin, thread-like and rapid

Table 12.5. Traditional Chinese Medicine: Major Types of Differentiation of Syndromes	
TYPES OF DIFFERENTIATION	DESCRIPTION
The Eight Principles	Syndromes of *yin* and *yang*, exterior and interior, cold and heat, deficiency and excess
Qi, Blood, and Fluids	Disorders of *Qi*, blood, and fluids
Zang-Fu Organs	Pathological manifestations of *Zang-Fu* organs
Meridians and Collaterals	Disorders of meridians and their relevant organs
The Six Meridians	Pathological manifestations of six levels of pathogenic factors invasion
Wei, *Qi*, *ying*, and Blood	Syndromes of the four stages of epidemic febrile disease
Sanjiao	Pathological manifestations of acute febrile disease due to the damp-heat in three compartments (upper, middle, and lower *jiao*)

pulse is felt. According to the TCM differentiation described previously, this syndrome is identified as "disharmony between the heart and kidney." Insomnia, mental restlessness, palpitations, dryness of the throat, red tongue, and rapid pulse are the manifestations of hyperactivity of the heart. According to TCM theory, the normal functioning of the heart includes controlling mental activities and housing the mind. Backache, nocturnal emission, hot flashes, night sweats, and thready pulse indicate kidney *yin* deficiency. According to the concept of the five elements, the heart is the organ of fire belonging to *yang*, and the kidney is the organ of water belonging to *yin* (see Table 12.3). Normally, heart fire (i.e., the warm nature of the organ) descends to warm kidney water, and kidney water (i.e., the cool and moist nature of the organ) ascends to nourish heart fire; the equilibrium of these is known as the "harmony of heart and kidney." When this physiological relationship is disrupted by pathogenic factors such as strain, stress, prolonged illness, congenital deficiency, or obsessive sexual activity, disharmony occurs. In the case just described, kidney water has failed to balance heart fire. After the differentiation of syndromes is made, a principle of treatment can be determined to rebalance the disharmony between the heart and the kidney (discussed later in this chapter).

THERAPY AND OUTCOMES

Treatment Options

Since ancient times, the first and most important principle of TCM has been the prevention of illness through proper lifestyle. The *Yellow Emperor's Inner Classic* states that people in the earliest times in China were able to remain healthy because they had a balanced diet, slept and awakened at regular hours, and remained active while avoiding excessive stress. They refrained from overindulging in wine and sex, exercised regularly, and protected the body during harsh weather and seasonal changes. They were thus able to maintain their health against pathogenic factors (9).

Practitioners of TCM carefully observe their patients for signs and symptoms of disease, which can be corrected with lifestyle changes and therapy before the disease can fully develop. As Huang Di, the author of the *Yellow Emperor's Inner Classic*, said:

> In the old days, sages treated disease by preventing illness before it began, just as a good government or emperor was able to take the necessary steps to avert war. Treating illness after it has begun is like suppressing revolt after it has broken out. If someone digs a well when thirsty, or forges weapons after becoming engaged in battle, one cannot help but ask 'Are not these actions too late?'(9).

There are several basic principles of treatment under the TCM system.

CONTROLLING THE INCIDENTAL SYMPTOM (BRANCH) OF A DISEASE WHILE TREATING THE FUNDAMENTAL CAUSE (ROOT)

In urgent situations, one treats the incidental symptom; in chronic conditions, one treats the fundamental cause; and, in complicated cases, one treats both at the same time. For example, easing a patient's breathing during an asthma attack would be considered treating the incidental condition. When the patient's symptoms have subsided, the fundamental cause of the disease is treated by addressing the deficiency of the internal organ, to enhance and thereby prevent or decrease further asthma attacks.

REGULATING YIN AND YANG

Conditions are balanced with appropriate measures (e.g., applying heat for the cold condition, applying cold for the heat condition, reinforcing the deficiency, and reducing the excess). For example, the patient who has excess heat accompanied by constipation may be treated with herbs that clear the bowel, eliminating the constipation and excess heat.

REINFORCING ANTIPATHOGENIC *QI* AND ELIMINATING PATHOGENIC FACTORS

When a person is frequently ill with a common cold, for example, the TCM practitioner focuses on preventing the onset of illness with certain Chinese herbs, appropriate diet, and exercise to enhance antipathogenic *Qi*. If the person currently has a cold, the practitioner provides Chinese herbs in conjunction with acupuncture treatment to eliminate pathogenic factors through sweat.

Description of Treatments

After the principle of the treatment is decided, one or more of the following modalities is then selected: Chinese herbal medicine, acupuncture/moxibustion, *Tui Na* (Chinese massage and acupressure), mind/body exercise (e.g., *Qi Gong, Tai Ji Quan, Gong Fu*) and Chinese dietary therapy.

ZHONG YAO (CHINESE HERBAL MEDICINE)

Zhong Yao has been an integral part of Chinese culture and medical practice for nearly 1600 years. The source of the Chinese *materia medica* includes plants, minerals, and animal parts. Each of the Chinese medicines (or herbs) possesses four natures (i.e., cold, cool, hot, warm) and five flavors (i.e., pungent, sweet, sour, bitter, salty). Chinese herbal medicines are classified based on their function, such as heat-clearing, expectorants and antitussive, dampness-eliminating, and interior-warming (1, 10).

Although each herb has its individual functions and indications, classic Chinese herbal medicine uses a combination of various herbs in a formula. The earliest herbal formulas can be traced back to the end of the third century BC, when approximately 280 formulas for 52 ailments were recorded in the *Ma Wang Tui* tomb document (11). By the time of the Ming dynasty (1368–1644), more than 60,000 formulas had been recorded in the 1406 book *Formulas of Universal Benefit (Pu Ji Fang)* (2, 8, 12). A typical Chinese herbal formula usually includes four components:

1. The **chief (principal) ingredient,** which treats the principal pattern or disease.
2. The **deputy (associate) ingredient,** which assists the chief ingredient in treating the major syndrome or serves as the main ingredient against a coexisting symptom.
3. The **assistant (adjutant) ingredient,** which enhances the effect of the chief ingredient,

moderates or eliminates the toxicity of the chief or deputy ingredients, or can have the opposite function of the chief ingredient to produce supplementing effects.
4. The **envoy (guide) ingredient,** which focuses the actions of the formula on a certain meridian or area of the body or harmonizes and integrates the actions of the other ingredients.

For example, Four-Gentleman Decoction (*Si Jun Zi Tang*) is a Chinese herbal formula used for fatigue, reduced appetite, loose stools, pale tongue, and weak pulse, which occur because of the deficiency of spleen and stomach *Qi* and dampness in the digestive system (11). The formula consists of four ingredients: radix ginseng (*Ren Shen*), rhizona atiactylodis macrocephalae (*Bai Zhu*), sclerotium poriae cocos (*Fu Ling*), and radix glycyrrhizae uralensis (*Zhi Gan Cao*). Among these, radix ginseng is the chief herb. Sweet and warm, it enhances the spleen *Qi*. Rhizona atiactylodis macrocephalae is the deputy herb, bitter and warm, which can strengthen the spleen and dry dampness. Sclerotium poriae cocos is the assistant herb, sweet and bland, which can assist the chief and deputy herbs in strengthening the spleen and leaching out dampness. Radix glycyrrhizae uralensis is the envoy herb, sweet and mild, which can harmonize the other three herbs and regulate the spleen *Qi*. These herbs are formulated to enhance, or tonify, the functioning of the internal organs (in this case, spleen and stomach). This tonification is one of the eight common methods used in Chinese herbal therapy. The other seven methods include diaphoresis, emesis, purging, mediation, warming, cooling, and elimination (11).

ZHEN JIU (ACUPUNCTURE/MOXIBUSTION)

Although acupuncture and moxibustion refer to two different methods, in the history of Chinese medicine, the two, *Zhen* (acupuncture) and *Jiu* (moxibustion), are so interrelated that they are seen as one concept. *Zhen Jiu* has been practiced in China for more than 4000 years (13–15). The earliest acupuncture "needles" unearthed by archaeologists in China dated from 1700 BC. They were made of stone and were named *Bian*. According to acupuncture theory, when the normal flow of energy over a meridian is obstructed (e.g., as a result of tissue injury), pain or symptoms result. The purpose of acupuncture therapy is to use certain devices to stimulate the acupuncture points on the meridians to reopen the normal energy flow, thereby relieving the symptoms.

Classic techniques of acupuncture include needling, moxibustion, and cupping. The needling technique involves inserting a stainless steel filiform needle, usually 0.22–0.25 mm in diameter and 1–1.5 inches in length, into one or more of these specific points to restore the vital flow of energy through the affected meridians. As mentioned, the selection of a formula of acupuncture points is determined by TCM differentiation. For the patient with symptoms of insomnia, which is diagnosed as disharmony of the heart and kidney, the practitioner will select acupuncture points on the heart and kidney meridians, along with needling techniques, to reduce the heart fire and enhance the kidney water. Needles are typically left in place for 20–30 minutes after insertion, and their effects may be augmented with manual or electrical stimulation and/or heat.

Moxibustion is a method in which a moxa herb (*Artemisia vulgaris*) is burned above the skin or on the acupuncture points for the purpose of applying heat to the acupuncture points to alleviate symptoms. It can be used in the form of a cone, stick, loose herb, or can be applied at the end of acupuncture needles.

Cupping promotes blood circulation and stimulates acupuncture points by creating a vacuum or negative pressure on the surface of the skin. Cupping was known as the "*horn method*" because the original cups were made out of the horns of animals. Various materials have been used for cupping, such as bamboo, glass, and ceramic.

TUI NA (CHINESE MASSAGE)

Tui Na, or Chinese massage, is a part of the TCM system, and has been practiced as a therapeutic and health care method in China for at least 2000 years. It was called *Dao Ying* in *Zhuang Zi* (third century BC) and *An Qiao* in the *Yellow Emperor's Inner Classic*. *Tui Na* uses hand manipulation—such as pushing, rolling, kneading, rubbing, and grasping—on specific points and other parts of the body. Like acupuncture, *Tui Na* can be used to balance *yin* and *yang* and to regulate the functions of *Qi*, blood, and *Zang-Fu* organs by stimulating acupuncture points and body tissue. In addition, *Tui Na* can restore the physiological functions through loosening joints, relaxing muscles and tendons, and separating adhesions. For example, a frozen shoulder with a limited range of motion and pain can be treated effectively by *Tui Na* to increase the range of motion and to decrease the pain.

QIGONG (MIND-BODY EXERCISE)

Mind-body exercise is another treatment modality in the TCM system. *Qigong*, which was mentioned in the ancient literature as early as 2000 years ago, has been defined as "energy work," "energy exercise," or "breathing exercise." It is a meditative method that can be combined with body movement to achieve a normal balance of energy in the TCM meridian system. (A detailed description of *Qigong* is delineated in Chapter 23.) *Tai Ji Quan*, also known as Tai Chi, created in the fourteenth century as a martial art, is practiced widely in China. The term itself (*Tai Ji*) refers to the balance of *yin* and *yang*. It consists of sequences of smooth, slow, and flowing movements, which are inspired by the form and movements of animals, as reflected in names for the individual movements such as "white stork spreading wings" and "grasping birds tail." When done correctly, it can be beneficial to the body, mind, and spirit. Recent studies suggest that *Tai Ji Quan* significantly improves balance (16) and reduces mental and emotional stress (17).

TRADITIONAL CHINESE DIETARY THERAPY

As part of Chinese herbal therapy, traditional Chinese dietary therapy is often incorporated into the practitioner's prescription for a specific condition. In fact, the traditional Chinese dietary therapies are deeply ingrained in Chinese culture. Many housewives in China are knowledgeable enough about dietary therapy that they are able to prepare special meals for certain ailments without consulting the practitioner. Examples of dietary therapy include using kelp for a patient with a goiter and, for a postpartum woman with excessive bleeding, serving soup prepared from the herb radix angelicae sinensis (*Dang Gui*), along with an entire hen to enrich the blood.

For the patient with insomnia mentioned earlier, whom TCM diagnostic differentiation determined to have a disharmony of heart and kidney, the classic herbal formula coptis and ass-hide gelatin decoction (*Huang Lian E Jiao Tang*) would be appropriate (3, 11). There are two chief herbs in the formula: coptis (*Huang Lian*) is used to clear fire from the heart and calm the spirit, and gelatinum corii asini (*E Jiao*) nourishes the kidney *yin*. The other ingredients serve deputy, assistant, and envoy roles in the formula. The patient can also be treated by acupuncture in the points of the heart and kidney meridians, such as *Shenmen* (H7—point 7 on the heart meridian) and *Taixi* (K3—point 3 on the Kidney meridian) (Fig. 12.4). The patient is instructed to change his lifestyle by reducing stress, avoiding obsessive sexual activity, and practicing *Tai Ji Quan* or *Qigong* to tranquilize the mind and spirit of the heart and preserve the essence of the kidney (i.e., improve the function of the kidney). In addition, the patient is advised to make a soup of *Lian Xin* (lotus plumule), which nourishes the heart, or include the fruit of *Sang Shen* (morus fruit) to enhance kidney essence.

Treatment Evaluation

The length of treatment in TCM varies according to the method used and the condition being treated. In Chinese herbal therapy, the patient is usually followed up every week or every other week. The herbal formula may be modified at each follow-up evaluation, depending on the condition of the patient. In general, expected changes occur within 1 to 2 months. A longer follow-up treatment may be needed for certain chronic conditions.

Two to three acupuncture treatment sessions per week are usually required for the first couple of weeks. Expected changes may occur within

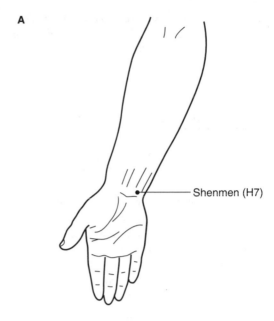

A

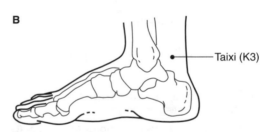

B

FIGURE 12.4. **A.** Point of Heart Meridian Number 7. Located at the ulnar end of the transverse crease of the wrist, in the depression on the radial side of the tendon of m. flexor carpi ulnaris. **B.** Point of Kidney Meridian Number 3. Located in the depression between the medial malleolus and tendo calcaneus, at the level with the tip of the medial malleolus.

5 to 10 treatments. Acupuncture point selection may vary at each treatment depending on the patient's reaction to the treatment. Usually, 10 to 12 treatment sessions constitute one course of treatment. Two or three courses of treatment are required for most chronic conditions. The termination of the treatment is based on the progressed condition of the patient. For example, if the patient with insomnia experiences significantly improved sleep quality after two or three months of treatment, the patient may be discharged. However, the patient will be instructed to maintain a healthy diet, exercise regi-

men, and appropriate stress management. Follow-up evaluations and treatments may be necessary periodically (e.g., once a month or every few months).

USE OF TCM FOR TREATMENT

As an extensive and established medical system, TCM is used by billions of people around the world for every condition known to humankind. It is difficult, therefore, to identify specific Western disease classifications in which TCM is indicated and where it is not. It is clear that modern Western medicine has distinct advantages to other forms of medicine for many problems, especially acute illness and the management of infection and trauma. This advantage has been recognized in China, and Western medicine has been adopted extensively and is officially on "equal footing" with TCM. Western and Chinese medicine are gradually integrating in China, and the use of both approaches to health and disease is emerging.

Major Indications

For the Western physician and health care practitioner, the most useful approach is to consider TCM in circumstances in which Western medicine is not proving adequate, in which good research has identified simple TCM approaches that can be delivered in an uncomplicated fashion, and in which the more complex TCM treatments can be delivered in the context of good medical care. The safety and monitoring of patients are always paramount, and competent TCM practitioners who are able to work with the Western practitioner should be available. Because TCM is largely clinically oriented, the integration of Western medicine and TCM—in which Western medicine provides methods to eliminate or control physical causes and manifestations of disease and TCM provides methods to reduce side effects and improve quality of life and function—is a reasonable approach. In these situations, TCM can be considered a complementary approach.

TCM can be particularly useful as an alternative approach when the Western diagnosis does not help much in the management of the disease. For example, chronic pain syndromes, chronic recurrent infections without overt immunodeficiency, chronic inflammatory conditions and some autoimmune diseases requiring constant suppression, debility of unknown cause, and functional syndromes should all be considered for management with TCM. The more complex, multifactorial, and refractory the condition is to Western management, the more the practitioner may want to consider TCM to provide an alternative assessment. If the TCM diagnosis is clear, the patient is likely to benefit. If the TCM diagnosis is unclear, the less likely TCM will help. For example, a patient with chronic idiopathic nocturnal urticaria was evaluated by an allergist, dermatologist, psychiatrist, and others and was using daily antihistamines, antidepressants, and corticosteroids for several years. No cause for the patient's condition was found. TCM evaluation revealed a clear energy imbalance along both kidney and lung systems. Correction of this imbalance with a combination of dietary changes, short-term herbal use, and acupuncture produced elimination of the urticaria, reduction in medication use, and improvement in mood and energy. Had the TCM diagnosis been unclear, this favorable prognosis would not have been expected.

Although modern research on TCM is still in its infancy, a number of studies have indicated areas in which TCM may be useful as both primary and adjunctive therapy. The Western practitioner may want to consider TCM in the treatment of addictions (18), back pain (19, 20), muscle spasms and neck pain (21–24), eczema (25), osteoarthritis (26), and to improve well-being (14). As an adjunctive therapy, TCM has been demonstrated to be useful in such conditions as cancer pain and nausea and vomiting (27), fibromyalgia (28), ischemic heart disease (29), migraine headache (30), and stroke rehabilitation (31, 32). The World Health Organization has listed over 40 conditions for which acupuncture is indicated as primary or adjunctive therapy, and an NIH consensus conference listed nausea and vomiting (chemotherapy-associated, postoperative, or pregnancy-induced) and postoperative dental pain treatments as especially demonstrated. This panel also found evidence for utility of acupuncture in asthma, carpal tunnel syndrome and contractures, chronic pain (arthritis, low back pain), stroke, addictions, and several other conditions. (The reader is referred to Chapter 19 for more details on the use and precautions of this particular modality.)

Adverse Effects and Contraindications

In China and many other countries, it is generally accepted that most Chinese herbs have few side effects when used properly (33, 25). When marketed as dietary supplements in the United States, Chinese herbs are not subject to regulation by the Food and Drug Administration (FDA) in the same manner as drugs. Although some Chinese herbs are known to have direct toxicity and the majority are safe in the doses recommended in Chinese herbal textbooks (10), casual use and use by those untrained in proper dosing and application can result in serious adverse effects. In addition, data on drug-herb interactions are scarce, and there are contraindications to specific herbs in certain populations, such as pregnant women. For the Western physician who is working with a patient in which extensive Chinese herbal preparations are being taken, it is best to work closely with a well-trained TCM practitioner, monitor the patient for potential adverse effects (e.g., liver function tests), and consult texts on potential adverse effects of these preparations. (Part II of this book catalogues some known adverse effects for many TCM products.) It should also be noted that contaminated products, Western drug adulterants, and erroneous substitutes of patented herb products by commercial manufacturers have been reported as well as the inappropriate use of herbs, all of which can produce toxicity (34, 35).

Serious side effects from acupuncture are uncommon and tend to be associated with violations of sterile procedures or negligence on the part of the practitioner. The few acupuncture complications that have been reported include infectious transmissions (e.g., hepatitis B), tissue infections, and organ and tissue injuries (e.g.,

pneumothorax) (36). Since the introduction of disposable acupuncture needles in the late 1980s, there have been significantly fewer reports associated with infectious disease transmission (36). In addition, certain acupuncture points should not be used under certain conditions, such as during the third trimester of pregnancy and over some skin lesions. Precautions against fainting should also be taken.

Preventive Value

As effective as it is in treating disease, it is thought that TCM's strongest aspect is its prevention of illness. Although the prevention of long-term overt disease is difficult to document, TCM excels in treating early symptomatic and functional symptoms that Western medicine often does not address well. It is thought that by treating early signs of disease, more serious manifestation are averted. Even in cases in which TCM does not completely eliminate the disease, it has been documented that patients often have improved well being and less difficulty managing their illness. According to TCM concepts, wellness and prevention are closely linked. As *The Yellow Emperor's Inner Classic* states (37):

> In peaceful calm,
> Void and emptiness,
> The authentic *Qi*
> Flows easily.
> Essences and spirits
> Are kept within.
> How could illnesses arise?

ORGANIZATION

Training

In ancient China, official schools for TCM existed during many dynasties. However, most TCM practitioners learned their trade through apprenticeship or through their family. Since the 1950s, government-sponsored colleges and universities of TCM have been gradually established in each province in China. The curriculum typically consists of approximately 50% Western medicine and 50% TCM. Individual departments of acupuncture, Chinese herbal medicine, *Tui Na*, and Chinese herbal pharmacology focus on the different aspects of TCM. Most of the Western medical schools in China also offer a few courses in TCM. Additionally, there are postgraduate TCM programs that train Western medical doctors how to use Chinese medicine in their practice.

In the United States, there are now more than 50 schools and colleges of acupuncture and Oriental medicine, many of which are approved by or in candidacy status with the National Accreditation Commission for Schools and Colleges of Acupuncture and Oriental Medicine (NACSCAOM) (38). NACSCAOM standards for a master's degree require a three-year program for acupuncture (approximately 1700 hours) and a four-year program for Oriental medicine (approximately 2100 hours), which includes acupuncture and herbal therapy (24). Some Western medical knowledge, including anatomy and physiology and a clean needle technique (CNT) course are part of the curriculum in most of these schools. There are also at least two postgraduate training programs in

medical acupuncture for physicians, which require approximately 400 hours of study (39).

Quality Assurance

Most states allow MDs to practice acupuncture with little to no training. Non-MD acupuncturists can also practice in more than half of these states and in the District of Columbia, and laws have been passed to regulate their practice (40). The scope of practice in each state may include acupuncture therapy only or may include Chinese herbal therapy. At least six national organizations have been established to promote acupuncture practice in this country. They help to standardize training and licensing requirements, and they also provide the national certification examinations for TCM practitioners. These organizations and their contact information are listed in Table 12.6 (38, 40).

Reimbursement Status

Third-party reimbursements vary by state. In most states, TCM service is not covered by

Table 12.6. National Organizations Associated with Acupuncture and TCM

NAME	YEAR OF ESTABLISHMENT	ADDRESS
American Association of Oriental Medicine (AAOM)*	1981	433 Front Street Catasauque, PA 18032 (610) 266-1433
Council of Colleges of Acupuncture and Oriental Medicine (CCAOM)	1982	8403 Colesville Road, Suite 370 Silver Spring, MD 20910 (301) 608-9175
National Accreditation Commission for Schools and Colleges of Acupuncture and Oriental Medicine (NACSCAOM)	1982	1010 Wayne Avenue, Suite 1270 Silver Spring, MD 20910 (301) 608-9680
National Certification Commission for Acupuncture and Oriental Medicine	1984	P.O. Box 97075 Washington, DC 20090-7075 (202) 232-1404
American Academy of Medical Acupuncturists (AAMA)	1987	5820 Wilshire Blvd., Suite 500 Los Angeles, CA 90036 (213) 937-5514
National Acupuncture and Oriental Medicine Alliance (NAOMA)	1993	P.O. Box 77511 Seattle, WA 98177 (206) 524-3511

* Formerly known as the American Association of Acupuncture and Oriental Medicine (AAAOM).

health insurance companies. Some insurance companies cover acupuncture treatment but not Chinese herbal therapy. Federal payers, such as Medicaid and Medicare, do not generally reimburse for any of the TCM therapies.

FUTURE PROSPECTS

TCM served as the main health care system for people in China for thousands of years before the introduction of modern medicine. It has been disseminated throughout the world, including the United States, Australia, and Europe, and is now gaining acceptance throughout society in general, the medical community, and federal governments. Many Westerners use alternative or complementary medicine, including TCM (41). In 1995, a regional survey in the United States showed that more than 50% of physicians consider acupuncture to be legitimate medical treatment, and 70 to 80% are interested in training in acupuncture and traditional oriental medicine (42). The National Institutes of Health (NIH) established an Office of Alternative Medicine in 1992 that has funded studies of the efficacy, safety, and mechanisms of TCM (1). The FDA recently approved the use of the acupuncture needle as a medical device. From the dramatic increase in the use of TCM in recent years, it is likely that Western medicine will incorporate TCM even more in the future.

SUGGESTED READINGS

Beinfield H, Korngold E. Between heaven and earth: a guide to Chinese medicine. New York: Ballantine Books, 1991.

Kaptchuk TJ. The web that has no weaver. New York: Congdon & Weed, Inc., 1983.

Liu J, Gordon P. Chinese dietary therapy. New York: Churchill Livingstone, 1995.

Stux G, Pomeranz B. Acupuncture: textbook and atlas. New York: Springer-Verlag, 1987.

REFERENCES

1. Ergil KV. China's traditional medicine. In: Micozzi MS, ed. Fundamentals of complementary and alternative medicine. New York: Churchill Livingstone, 1996:185–223.
2. Li JW, Cheng ZF, eds. China's encyclopedia of the medicine, history of medicine (Zhong Guo Yi Xue Bai Ke Quan Shu, Yi Xue Shi). Shanghai: Science and Technology Publishers, 1987. (Chinese).
3. Zhang ZJ. Discussion of cold-induced disorders (Shang Han Lun). Eastern Han Dynasty, 196–204 A.D. Chongqing: Chongqing People's Publishers, 1955. (Chinese).
4. Huang F. A-B classic of acupuncture and moxibustion (Zhen Jiu Jia Yi Jing). 259 A.D. Beijing: People's Health Publishers, 1956. (Chinese).
5. Qin Y. Classic of difficult issues (Nan Jing). Written before Eastern Han Dynasty (25–220 A.D.) Beijing: People's Health Publishers, 1979. (Chinese).
6. Yang J. Great compendium of acupuncture and moxibustion (Zhen Jiu Da Cheng). 1601 A.D. Beijing: People's Health Publishers, 1980. (Chinese).
7. Jiangsu College of New Medicine. Encyclopedia of the traditional Chinese materia medica (Zhong Yao Da Ci Dian). Shanghai: People's Press, 1977. (Chinese).
8. Zhen ZY, Fu WK, eds. History of traditional Chinese medicine (Textbook in Chinese), 4th ed. Shanghai: Science and Technology Publishers, 1987.
9. Ni MS. The Yellow Emperor's classic of medicine: a new translation of the Neijing Suwen with commentary. Boston: Shambhala, 1995:1–7.
10. Bensky D, Gamble A, compiled and translated. Chinese herbal medicine: materia medica. Seattle: Eastland Press, 1993.
11. Bensky D, Barolet R, eds. Chinese herbal medicine: formulas and strategies. Seattle: Eastland Press, 1990:4, 236, 9, 382.
12. Zhu X, Teng S, eds. Formulas of universal benefit (Pu Ji Fang). 1406 A.D. Beijing: People's Health Publishers, 1959. (Chinese).
13. Liu G, Hyodo A, eds. Fundamentals of acupuncture and moxibustion. Tianjin: Tianjin Science and Technology Translation and Publishing Corporation, 1994.
14. Cheng X, ed. Chinese acupuncture and moxibustion. 1st ed. Beijing: Foreign Languages Press, 1987.

15. O'Connor J, Bensky D, eds. Acupuncture: a comprehensive text. Chicago: Eastland Press, 1981.

16. Province MA, Hadley EC, Hornbrook MC, et al. The effects of exercise on falls in elderly patients: a preplanned meta-analysis of the FICSIT trials. JAMA 1995;273:17.

17. Jin P. Efficacy of Tai Chi, brisk walking, meditation, and reading in reducing mental and emotional stress. J Psychosom Res 1992;36(4):361–370.

18. Smith MO, Squires R, Aponte A, et al. Acupuncture treatment of drug addiction and alcohol abuse. Am J Acup 1982;10(2):161–3.

19. Thomas M, Lundberg T. Importance of modes of acupuncture in the treatment of chronic nociceptive low back pain. Acta Anaesthesiol Scand 1994;38:63–69.

20. MacDonald AJR, Macrae KD, Master BR, Rubin AP. Superficial acupuncture in relief of chronic low back pain. Ann Roy Coll Surge Eng 1983; 65:44–46.

21. Zhu C. Use of point Yinmen (UB 37) for treatment of acute lumbar sprain. Shanghai J Acup- Moxi 1984;2:17. (Chinese)

22. Hu XM, ed. Chinese medicine secret recipe. Shanghai: Wenhui Publishers, 1989:2:903–906. (Chinese)

23. Coan R, Wong G, Coan PL. The acupuncture treatment of neck pain: a randomized controlled study. Am J Chin Med 1981;9(4):326–332.

24. Loy TT. Treatment of cervical spondylosis-electroacupuncture versus physiotherapy. Med J Australia 1983;2:32–34.

25. Sheehan MP, Rustin MHA, Atherton DJ, et al. Efficacy of traditional Chinese herbal therapy in adult atopic dermatitis. Lancet 1992;340:13–17.

26. Christenson BV, Iuhl IV, Vilbeck H, et al. Acupuncture treatment of severe knee osteoarthritis: a long term study. Acta Anaesthes Scand 1992; 36:519–525.

27. Dundee JW, McMillan CM. The role of transcutaneous electrical stimulation of Neiguan anti-emetic acupuncture point in controlling sickness after cancer chemotherapy. Physiotherapy 1991;77(7): 499–502.

28. Shoukang L. Treating arthralgia with acupuncture. Internat J Clin Acup 1991;2(1):71–76.

29. Richter A, Herlitz J, Hjalmarson A. Effect of acupuncture in patients with angina pectoris. Eur Heart J 1991;12:175–178.

30. Vincent CA. A controlled trial of the treatment of migraine by acupuncture. Clin J Pain 1989; 5:305–312.

31. Naeser MA, Alexander MP, Stiassny-Eder D, et al. Real versus sham acupuncture in the treatment of paralysis in acute stroke patients: a CT scan lesion site study. J Neuro Rehab 1992;6:163–173.

32. Johanson K, Lindgren I, Widner H, et al. Can sensory stimulation improve the functional outcome in stroke patients? Neurology 1993;43: 2189–2192.

33. Kong XT, Fang HT, Jiang GQ, et al. Treatment of acute bronchiolitis with Chinese herbs. Arch Dis Child 1993;68:468–471.

34. Gertner E, Marshall PS, Filandrinos D, et al. Complications resulting from the use of Chinese herbal medications containing undeclared prescription drugs. Arthritis Rheum 1995;38(5):614–617.

35. Chan TYK, Critchley JAJH, Chan MTV, Yu CM. Drug overdose and other poisoning in Hong Kong—the Prince of Wales hospital (Shatin) experience. Hum Exp Toxicol 1993;13:512–515.

36. Lao L. Safety issues in acupuncture. Journal of Alternative and Complementary Medicine 1996; 2(1):27–31.

37. Claude Larre SJ. The way of heaven: Neijing Suwen Chapters 1 and 2. Cambridge: Monkey Press, 1994:55.

38. Mitchell BB. Legislative handbook for the practice of acupuncture and oriental medicine. Washington, DC: National Acupuncture Foundation, 1995: 59,14,61.

39. Kaplan G. The status of acupuncture legislation in the United States: a comprehensive review. AAMA Review 1991;3(1):7–14.

40. Mitchell BB. Acupuncture and oriental medicine laws. 1995 ed. Washington, DC: National Acupuncture Foundation, 1995:114,137.

41. Eisenberg DM, Kessler RC, Foster C, et al. Unconventional medicine in the United States: prevalence, costs, and patterns of use. N Engl J Med 1993;328(4):246–252.

42. Berman BM, Singh BK, Lao L, et al. Physicians' attitudes toward complementary or alternative medicine: a regional survey. J Am Board Fam Pract 1995;8:361–366.

CHAPTER 13

NATIVE AMERICAN MEDICINE

Ken "Bear Hawk" Cohen

Now! Long Person [a river or stream], I have just come to pray to You.
Wahya hi:nadu! [Wolf thunder]
Now! You will "remake" my soul.
It will become longer.
I will rise again.
Wahya hi:nadu!
I will be greeting You with my soul!

—CHEROKEE HEALING CHANT (1)

BACKGROUND

Definitions: Who is Native American?

Native American medicine is based on widely held beliefs about healthy living, the repercussions of disease-causing activity or behavior, and the spiritual principles that restore balance. These beliefs cross tribal boundaries. However, the particular methods of diagnosis and treatment are as diverse as the languages, landscapes, and customs of the approximately 500 Nations that constitute the indigenous people of Turtle Island, one of the original names of North America.

Therefore it is important to state, from the outset, that there are problems inherent in the term *Native American*, because it implies a uniform culture and healing system. The indigenous people of North America identify themselves by Nation (commonly called tribe[1]), band or community, clan, and family. The term *Native American*[2] became a political necessity—a way for similarly oppressed people to identify their unity in a fight for common rights in the face of the encroachment of white military, religious, and educational imperialism. In pre-contact times (i.e., prior to the arrival of the Europeans), a Native American might identify himself as *Yonah Usdi* (Little Bear), an *Ani Wa-*

---

[1] To preserve brevity, in this essay I will reference Native nations by labels commonly used in EuroAmerican literature. However, the reader should be aware that these labels are generally not the way that Native people refer to themselves. For instance, the "Iroquois," a French adaptation of an Algonquin term meaning enemy, call themselves Haudenosaunee, the People of the Long House. I hope that proper terms for Native nations will gradually be adopted in world literature.
[2] Other commonly used terms include American Indian and First Nations. Although indigenous Americans usually refer to themselves as "Indians," there is no universally acceptable designation in the literature.

hya (Wolf Clan) *Ani Yunwiya* (Cherokee) from the town of Kituhwa (near present-day Bryson City, North Carolina). Today, he might add the name of his reservation.

The healing traditions of the Native Americans have been practiced on this continent since the Clovis Culture at least 12,000 years ago (2), and possibly for more than 40,000 years (3). Esteemed scholar Vine Deloria, Jr. points out serious loopholes in the commonly accepted theory that Native Americans migrated from an original homeland in Siberia over ancient glacial passes in the Bering Straits (4). Native American traditions were probably influenced by migrating peoples, as they were by waves of ocean-faring Asians (5) and, perhaps, Vikings, Celts, or other Europeans (6). However, cultural influences and parallels do not confirm cultural diffusion any more than the presence of animals in the cave paintings at Lascaux and at Newspaper Rock, Utah, prove that the artists at the American petroglyph site were French Neanderthals. According to one school of Native American oral history, Native Americans crossed the Bering Straits *from* North America, and being unappreciative of the lack of civilization in that New World, crossed back again to return home. To Native Americans, the fact that no pre-*Homo sapien* hominid skeletons have been discovered in North America merely confirms their own stories of creation and emergence; to declare otherwise would be as much an assumption of cosmological and theological truth as scientific.

Antiquity is not the only reason for the wealth of Native American healing traditions. Other explanations for healing diversity include:

- The migration of tribes and cultural and intellectual exchange among tribes along established trade routes (7)
- The lack of either precontact literature or churches to rigidify the forms of healing
- The acceptance of personal innovation by visionaries and healers (8)
- Adaptive postcontact strategies of healing (e.g., Native American Church [9], Indian Shaker Church [10], and various synergies of allopathic and traditional Native American healing [11, 12]). Native American healing

is open ended and still evolving. Complementary medicine is a well-accepted principle among Native Americans. White man's diseases—"the diseases of civilization"—often require white man's medicine. Native Americans are pragmatic and down-to-earth in more ways than one.

Transcribing the Ineffable

Many aspects of Native American healing have never been put to paper and never will. At some healing ceremonies, individuals are appointed to protect the grounds from cameras, recorders, notebooks, and uninvited guests. Seneca elder Twylah Nitsch remembers that during her childhood, when anthropologists were spotted nearby, her grandfather, a respected medicine man, would tell the family, "Hide the sacred things, the Bigheads are coming!" (personal communication, 1984). Many aspects of Native American healing are still closely guarded oral tradition. Specific techniques of healing, sacred songs, and healing rituals are received directly from elder healers, from spirits encountered during vision quest, and as a result of initiation into secret societies. To share healing knowledge indiscriminately is to weaken the spiritual power of the medicine (13). There is also a real danger that a medicine person, succumbing to the curiosity of anthropologists, social scientists, or others whom the community defines as "outsiders," will be ostracized by his or her own community. He or she may be perceived as contributing to the exploitation of Native culture.

Yet after five centuries of Red-White interaction, a tremendous amount has been and will continue to be written in books. Native Americans recognize that transcribing healing beliefs and practices may preserve tradition for their own future generations. Today, many Native American healers are willing to engage in dialogue with physicians, other health care professionals, or interested students outside of their culture if these individuals approach them respectfully and unpretentiously, motivated by a common concern to relieve human suffering and recognizing that no culture has a monopoly on healing. Increasing numbers of Native American physicians and nurses are stimulating important cross-cultural insights and prospects for collaboration (14, 15).

Many Native American healers believe that sharing healing ways may be a matter of survival. Indigenous healing traditions and ecology-based values may help people prevent the widely prophesied "Purification" of warfare and "earth changes"—i.e., natural catastrophes as divine retribution for environmental destruction (16).

Review of Literature

Because of the interface between Native healing, spirituality, and culture, the volume of published works about Native American healing is immense. Vogel's *American Indian Medicine* (17) and Beck and Walters' *The Sacred* (18) are important surveys of various Native healing traditions. The "dark side of the force"— malevolent sources of misfortune—are covered in Walker's *Witchcraft and Sorcery of the American Native Peoples* (19). Eliade (20), Kalweit (21), and Krippner and Welch (22) offer cross-cultural perspectives on the relationship between Native American culture and shamanism. The latter work is especially valuable for its discussion of contemporary practitioners and strategies for integrating spiritual healing into psychotherapy, nursing, and medicine. The role of dream and vision seeking—a major source of empowerment and innovation among healers— is carefully analyzed in Irwin's *The Dream Seekers: Native American Visionary Traditions of the Great Plains* (8). Healing is a central theme of the approximately 250,000 member Native American Church (9, 23) and other intertribal spiritual traditions, such as the Indian Shaker Church (10, 24).

Interpretive studies of the healing traditions of particular Native nations can be found in Bahr (25), Hines (26), Jilek (27), Lewis (28), Miller (29), Mooney (30), Powers (31), and Sander (32). Native American botanical medicine is surveyed in Vogel (17) and Moerman (33). Herbal traditions of specific nations are discussed in many works, notably Cochran (34),

Croom (35), Curtin (36), Densmore (37), Herrick (38), Gunther (39), Gilmore (40), Hamel (41), Hungry Wolf (42), and Tantaquidgeon (43). Indigenous herbalism has also influenced popular EuroAmerican writers on herbal medicine; among the most useful for the clinician are those by Moore (44, 45). A great deal can be gleaned from the biographies, autobiographies, or works about Native American healers: Bear Heart (46), Black Elk and Lyon (47), Boyd (48, 49), Horse Capture (50), Jones (51), Lake (52), Lame Deer and Erdoes (53), Mails (54, 55), and Yellowtail (56). Indigenous healing is also explored in *Shaman's Drum: A Journal of Experiential Shamanism* (57). *Winds of Change* magazine (58), published by the American Indian Science and Engineering Society, provides an excellent forum for discussion of Native American views of science, education, and culture. Readers are also directed to the journals *Akwesasne Notes* (59), *News from Indian Country* (60), and the publications of individual Native nations for a broader understanding of the concerns of Native people today.

From the Western scientific perspective, Native American healing is documented only in scattered anecdotes and observations. Native healing methods have not been tested in controlled experiments, nor is this likely to change in the near future. It is impossible to administer "standard doses" in practices that may change from healer to healer and from case to case. Therapeutic methodology and outcome are generally not written down and are known only to individual healers or their close associates. In any case, unmeasurable and nonspecific factors so often outweigh the measurable and specific that it may be impossible to draw accurate conclusions about the efficacy of Native healing from the perspective of Western empirical science. Additionally, many Native Americans are suspicious of the motives of scientists. The results of research may serve political and economic ends that are not in the best interests of the Native American people. Physicist F. David Peat (61) and a former director of the Indian Health Services, Everett R. Rhoades, M.D. (62), offer stimulating overviews of the possibilities for dialogue between indigenous and Western science.

ETIOLOGY OF HEALTH AND DISEASE

Health and Wholeness

According to Native American medicine, a healthy person has a sense of purpose and follows the "original instructions"—i.e., the guidance written in the heart by the Great Spirit. He or she is committed to walking a path of beauty, balance, and harmony, keeping a Good Mind (Iroquois concept), good thoughts towards Creation. The essence of a healthy life— the Good Red Road, as some Native Americans call it—is gratefulness, respect, and generosity.

A basic principle of Native American culture is *wholeness*. According to the Native American spiritual leaders gathered at the University of Lethbridge, Alberta, in 1982, "All things are interrelated. This connectedness derives from the reality that everything is part of a single whole which is greater than the sum of its parts. Hence any given phenomenon can only be understood in terms of the wholeness out of which it comes" (63). The ultimate source of this wholeness is known by many names: *Kitchi Manitou* ("the Great Mystery," Ojibway), *Wakan Tanka* ("the Great Sacred" or "Great Spirit," Lakota), *Acbadadea* ("Maker of All Things Above," Crow), *Shongwàyad¥hs:on* ("the Creator," Iroquois), or simply, God. The manifestation of divine spirit in living beings is life force, or divine breath; known as *ni* in Lakota (64), *nilch'i* in Navajo (65), this concept is common to virtually all indigenous cultures. In 1896, Long Knife, a Lakota holy man, told physician James R. Walker, "A man's *ni* is his life. It is the same as his breath" (66).

Health "can only be understood in terms of the wholeness out of which it comes" (63). Thus, health and disease always have both physical and spiritual components. Speaking of Iroquois notions of disease etiology, Herrick writes, "Because each causal agent is thought to be influencing the balanced, yet constantly fluctuating life force of the individual, there is necessarily the element of spirituality involved in the treatment and diagnosis of *all* illness" (13). Health means restoring the body, mind, and spirit to balance and wholeness: the balance of life energy in the body; the balance of ethical, reasonable, and just behavior; balanced relations within family and community; and harmonious relationships with nature.

Untreatable Conditions

Native American medicine, unlike Western medicine, tends to consider disease in terms of morality, balance, and the action of spiritual power rather than specific, measurable causes. Native American medicine is based on a spiritual, rather than a materialistic or Cartesian, view of life.

Native Americans believe that inherited conditions, such as birth deformities or retardation (including fetal alcohol syndrome), may be caused by the parents' unhealthy or immoral behavior and are not easily treatable. Native healers believe that, among adults, some diseases are the patient's responsibility and the natural consequence of his or her behavior; to treat these conditions may be to interfere with important life lessons. Similar to all health care providers, Native American healers encounter patients who, unfortunately, are unwilling to ask for help when needed. Native healers are bound by their professional ethics not to "missionize" healing, advertise their healing abilities, or in other ways coerce a patient to accept their services. In a certain sense, the *cause* of a patient's ongoing disease may be his or her own stubbornness. However, if the patient is incapable of asking for help—a child, a person with Alzheimer's or mental incapacity, a coma patient— then the healer must ask his or her own intuitive sources of guidance whether he or she should help; this permission may be granted by *Spirit*, a concept that embraces the human spirit, the spirits of the natural world, and the Great Spirit.

Some illnesses are not treated because they are considered "callings," or diseases of initiation: physical and spiritual crises engendered by the breakdown of previous ways of being or by the acquisition of guardian-spirit power. Seneca elder Twylah Nitsch remembers "dying" as a young child. She suddenly and inexplicably stopped breathing. She was revived when her grandfather, the medicine man Moses Shongo, breathed on her to infuse her with healing power (personal communication, 1984). Similarly, Native healer Medicine Grizzlybear Lake (52), who offers one of the few detailed first-person accounts of medicine initiation and training, describes two death experiences, one from illness (rheumatic fever, polio, and pneumonia) and one from drowning, which occurred at ages four and nine. In both cases, he was healed when elderly Native spirits "doctored" him with songs, dance, smoke, and healing power represented by the bear. Lake explains, "The calling comes in the form of a dream, accident, sickness, injury, disease, near-death experience, or even actual death" (67). In the Pacific Northwest "power sickness" is caused when a spirit power pities someone who is sick, sorrowing, or in need of initiation (68). The spirit possesses the person and manifests in symptoms of "restlessness, fainting spells, uncontrollable crying, heavy breathing, sighing and moaning" (69). The illness is resolved when a shaman initiates the person in the winter spirit dance tradition, teaching him or her how to "bring out" the power through song and dance.

Many Native healers believe that people learn to heal best the conditions that they have experienced. When Cherokee elder Keetoowah Christie was questioned about becoming a medicine man, he replied, "I wouldn't wish that curse on anyone" (personal communication, 1978). He explained that during his life he had suffered from typhoid fever, emphysema, prostate cancer, heart disease, and spinal injuries.

Disease Labels: What's in a Name?

Many Native disease labels can only be understood within the context of their originating culture. For instance, in the Piman healing system (25), noxious substances, such as germs, heat, or pus, wander through the body and cause "wandering sickness" which is observed in symptoms such as skin sores, fever, and hemorrhoids. Wandering sickness generally is treated with herbs. The other major disease category among the Pimans is *ka:cim*, or "staying sickness." Staying sickness is the consequence of behaving improperly towards dignified, powerful, and potentially dangerous objects (e.g., hunting or killing an animal in a cruel or thoughtless manner, or using wood from a lightning struck tree). *Ka:cim* "stays" in the body because the person has broken the established order, the sacred laws given to Pimans by the Creator. A patient afflicted with *ka:cim* may demonstrate erratic, lethargic, or disturbed behavior and is returned to wholeness by appealing to the dignity and power of the object or animal offended. The shaman-healer sings and uses the mouth to literally blow in spiritual power or suck out pathogenic forces. He or she may also administer herbs.

Internal and External Causes of Disease

Disease etiology and diagnostic labels vary from tribe to tribe. However, it is possible to analyze many diseases in terms of two broad and interrelated categories: internal and external causes (Table 13.1).

INTERNAL CAUSES

According to the Cherokee medicine man Rolling Thunder, the major internal cause of disease is negative thinking:

- Negative thoughts about oneself: shame, despair, worry, and depression
- Negative thoughts about others: blame, jealousy, anger

According to Nootka healer Johnny Moses, "No evil sorcerer can do as much harm to you as you can do to yourself" (personal communication, 1991). Seneca elder Twylah Nitsch emphasizes the dangers of self-doubt. When personal gifts—"medicine" in Native terminology—are not used, they rot inside, causing sickness. "Healing," says Mrs. Nitsch, "is sometimes not a matter of taking something in—an herb or other medication, but of letting something out, having the confidence to express yourself" (personal communication, 1985). Na-

Table 13.1. Causes of Disease

Internal Causes

Negative thinking (e.g., low self-esteem, anger, jealousy, greed, self-centeredness)

Disturbances in flow of life energy and healing power within the individual or to/from the environment

External Causes

Pathogenic forces, objects (including microbes), people (sorcerers), and/or spirits

Environmental poisons, pollution, and contaminants, including alcoholic drinks and unhealthy food

Traumatic events: physical, emotional, and/or spiritual

Breach of taboo:
- Imbalanced living and inconsiderate behavior
- Not demonstrating proper respect towards an animal, person, place, object, event, or spirit
- Improper performance of ritual or care of ritual objects

tive American healers frequently practice dream interpretation to help a patient discover repressed feelings; unfulfilled needs; or messages from spiritual helpers (*totems,* an Algonquin term) that suggest new, healthier ways of behaving. Early Jesuit missionaries were so impressed by the Iroquois devotion to dreams that they said, "The Iroquois have, properly speaking, only a single divinity—the dream" (70). Native healers, like their colleagues in conventional Western medical practice, believe that psychological distress can cause or make one more susceptible to disease.

Negative thinking is a form of self-centeredness. "People get wrapped up in the past and in their thoughts about the past," says Cherokee healer Hawk LittleJohn, "like a squirrel with a very long tail running through the woods and getting caught in the brambles" (personal communication, 1996). Rigid, obsessive thinking is frequently a sign of prioritizing one's own needs over those of the family, community, or natural world. Self-centeredness creates greed, stinginess, and wastefulness. The self-centered person hoards possessions instead of sharing or giving them away. Interestingly, in Native American communities, a person has a higher status if he or she has given more. An important life event—a birth, a naming, a healing, a good dream—is honored by the "Giveaway" ritual and feast, in which possessions are redistributed in the community. The honored healer often has the least and lives the simplest, most frugal life. In essence, self-centeredness is a definitive

sign that one is negligent in following the original instructions.

External Causes

External causes of disease are pathogenic forces that invade the body, mind, spirit, or all of them. Native American medicine does not reject the theory that microbes can cause disease (71). "Germs are also spirits," says a Lakota colleague Shabari Bird (personal communication, 1986). Like "harmful intrusions," the subtle spiritual pathogens popularized in anthropological literature, germs take hold if the patient is susceptible because of the interplay of imbalanced living, negative thinking, and a feeble constitution. Native healers also recognize that in today's world, physical, environmental, and emotional stress also increase susceptibility to disease-causing agents. Thus the category *external cause* is relative and not absolutely distinguished from internal causes.

Negative Thoughts by Others

A loving, supportive family can greatly aid a person in recovery from disease. Loving thoughts and prayers have healing power, whether or not a patient is consciously aware of their existence. Conversely, negative thoughts of others, expressed or unexpressed, can cause disease. As Larry Dossey, M.D., implies, a physician who labels his patient *terminal* may be creating a self-fulfilling prophecy, which is the essence of a hex (72). In Native tradition, the hex is considered more than a nocebo effect (i.e., the power of negative expectation). It is transcendent power used for evil purposes, transpersonal imagery[3] that harms rather than heals. Hawaiian tradition recognizes both *kahuna lapa'au*, healers who use methods such as herbs, prayer, touch, and love (*alo-ha*) to heal, and *kahuna ana'ana*, who pray people to death (73). In traditional Cherokee culture, healers, called *dida:hnvwi:sg(i)*, "curer of them, he," have the ability to "conjure," that is, pray, a person into a state of health with the aid of invocation and tobacco[4] rituals. His antithesis, the sorcerer who uses knowledge and prayer for personal, unethical ends, is the *dida:hnese:sg(i)*, "putter-in and drawer-out of them, he." The *dida:hnese:sg(i)* projects negative forces (perhaps disease-causing spirits that personify negative thoughts) or removes life energy from the victim (74). In many native societies, it is believed that sorcerers use physical objects to cast spells: stones; herbs; charms; or pieces of clothing, hair, or nails from the intended victim. Sorcery practices have been carefully documented in anthropological literature (19).

However, not all malevolent, pathogenic forces are products of human intent; some are encountered capriciously. Sorcerers, diseases, storms, the dead, certain charms, objects, events, or places may radiate evil influences, called *utgo*[n] in Seneca. Merely being in the presence of these pathogenic forces can cause discomfort, pain, or disease.

Environmental Poisons

Environmental poisons cause disease by clouding the mind, weakening the spirit, and polluting the breath (the energy of life). Environmental poisons include impure air, water, and food. Unnatural foods (e.g., processed, contaminated, or not grown locally) have affected Native American health since the advent of government food rations and the loss of traditional fishing, hunting, foraging, and farming grounds. There is evidence that both Native Americans and European-Americans are genetically ill-adapted to assimilate the macronutrient ratios presented by the modern diet, particularly the increase in fat and refined carbohydrates (75). Alcohol has had a dramatic and devastating effect on the Native population. "Spirits" are antagonistic to Native American spirituality and, according to the elders, drive totems away, causing the mind to become disturbed and delusional. The most successful programs to treat this problem in Native communities are combinations of Western counseling, social work, and traditional Native American healing (76, 77).

Physical and Emotional Trauma

Physical and emotional trauma or shock cause illness by engendering psychological distress, loss of spiritual power, loss of soul, or all of them. For example, the psychological confusion and disorientation commonly experienced by head-injury patients, especially after a car accident, is a sign that identity is shattered, or the spirit is no longer whole. In accord with the metaphysics of Western psychotherapy, dissociated or repressed aspects of the self are believed to be hidden in the unconscious. In both Native American tradition and shamanism in general, these soul-fragments are commonly believed to be lost in inaccessible dimensions of a larger, alternate reality, a "lower world" that may include ancestors or spiritual beings (78, 79). Insight "talk-therapy" may be ineffective, because the healer is only talking to a conscious fragment of the original self, not to the part in need of integration. The Native healer must use ritual (29), physical gestures (e.g., blowing breath [80] or tobacco smoke [81] on the diseased area), or

---

[3] Transpersonal imagery is defined as "imagery that is not confined to a single person's bodymind. It serves as a mode of communication from one person to another, through an unknown, invisible pathway" (120).
[4] Native American moderate and circumspect use of wild tobacco (primarily *Nicotiana Rustica*) as a ceremonial aid and healing agent is sharply contrasted with the EuroAmerican custom of recreational smoking of cultivated varieties of the same genus (primarily *Nicotiana Tabacum*). Several methods of ceremonial tobacco use have a wide distribution among Native nations, including burning tobacco in an open fire, smoking tobacco in a sacred pipe (Lakota: *cannunpa*), blowing tobacco smoke over a patient, using tobacco as an offering of gratitude to a healer or healing powers, or praying while holding tobacco in the hand. Tobacco smoke carries thoughts and prayers to the Great Spirit and when ingested induces a psychological state of heightened awareness, alertness, and intuition. The mind-altering effects can be partially explained by the structural similarity of nicotine to acetylcholine and nicotine's ability to bond to cholinergic receptor sites. Nicotine also triggers the release of norepinephrine, epinephrine, serotonin, dopamine, and other compounds. The pharmacology, traditional use, and lore of tobacco are explored in Wilbert (121).

laying on of hands (82, 83) to physically return soul and power to the patient.

A shocking experience can cause the sudden loss of spiritual and personal power (including sense of control over one's life). Conversely, loss of power, perhaps resulting from negative thinking or childhood trauma, can make one more prone to accidents and misfortune. A balanced and harmonious lifestyle attracts the presence of guardian spirits that ensure improved decision making and transpersonal protection from injury.

Breach of Taboo

Breach of taboo, a frequently cited Native American category of disease etiology, has a much broader meaning than the violation of cultural mores. According to the Yup'ik people of southwestern Alaska, "People brought on disease by transgressing the rules for living, and only through correcting or confessing their offenses could they hope to heal their bodies" (80). These transgressions include neglecting to demonstrate proper respect towards an animal, person, place, event, object, or spirit. For instance, Native Hawaiians believe that certain *heiaus* ("power places") are *kapu*, or forbidden, to non-Hawaiians; these places are guarded by ancient spirits that can cause disease or misfortune to transgressors. Some tribes believe that powerful animals, such as the bear, must be addressed by special names, lest their spirits be offended (84). Totems are offended when their advice is not heeded or when a person is indiscreet in sharing the guidance they offer in sleeping or waking dreams (85). *Discretion* means not boasting or showing off and, sometimes, not revealing the identity of a dream helper.

Cruel words, abusive behavior, and violence are also taboo violations, causing disease in the person, community, and Nation. According to the Code of Handsome Lake, a major religion among the Iroquois, the Creator's law is broken when married people do not love and care for each other and their children or when they desert one another (86, 87). Ignoring the taboo against being in proximity to or eating food prepared by a menstruating woman can cause discomfort, weakness, pain, or disease; this re-

sult is not because menstruating women exude evil *utgo*[n], as some anthropologists believe (88). Instead, the taboo, widely accepted by Native men and women, is a recognition that women are more powerful during their "moon time"— engaged in their own cyclic ceremonies of purification as preparation for childbirth. The isolation of menstruating women and, in many tribes, their period of retreat and meditation in separate "moon lodges," is a custom established by women to improve the physical, mental, and spiritual health of themselves and their communities (Lakota elder Grace Spotted Eagle, personal communication, 1984).

Healers have even more rules of conduct to follow than patients and can become ill because of improper care of ceremonial objects or errors in the performance of ritual. Because healers work with strong healing powers, small mistakes can have serious health consequences.

DIAGNOSIS AND DIVINATION: THE REALM OF SPIRIT

Diagnosis

There are numerous methods of diagnosing disease. Diagnostic ability depends more on the intuition, sensitivity, and spiritual power of the healer than on the precision of a particular diagnostic technique. Therefore, diagnostic methods may vary not only from tribe to tribe, but also from healer to healer. Healers may create new diagnostic methods or find creative adaptations of practiced techniques in any particular healing session.

As in Western medicine, the Native healer observes presenting symptoms and frequently asks the patient to describe them. The healer pays attention to the age and gender of the patient, the history and duration of the problem, and nonverbal cues, such as posture, breathing, tone of voice, and general deportment. The Lakota holy man, Fools Crow, would talk to the patient about his philosophy of healing (54). He would also discuss the possible causes of the disease, the patient's lifestyle and relationships, and how the patient's disease was affecting his family. The purpose of this lengthy discussion was not merely diagnostic, but also "to draw the people completely into the curing process, to engage their total persons, to get them communing fully with *Wakan-Tanka* [the Great Spirit] and the Helpers, and to enhance their own curing abilities and those of the 'hollow bones' [clear-minded healers] who treated them" (89). Fools Crow would enter the sweat lodge or practice other rituals of purification and communion to ask his helping spirits, the Great Spirit, or both for further information about diagnosis and treatment.

Among the Navajo, if the medicine man is unsure about diagnosis, diagnostic specialists may be consulted: "They are able to place themselves in a state of trance at will, and diagnose illness by divination—hand trembling, star gazing, crystal gazing, or 'listening'" (90). These Navajo diagnosticians practice techniques in common with healers of many other Native traditions. Wintu shaman Flora Jones enters an altered state of consciousness by smoking wild tobacco, drinking clear acorn water—an offering to her helping spirits— and singing sacred songs, accompanied by an assistant (or "interpreter"), the patient, and various friends and family members. According to author P.N. Knudtson's observations, "With the diagnostic powers of the spirit-helpers acting through her hands, she begins to move her fingers carefully across the patient's body sensing unseen, internal injuries or abnormalities" (91). Flora Jones feels the patient's disease or pain in her own body: "I become a part of their body."

Divination

Medical divination is the attempt to elicit medical information from divine or spiritual forces. It is commonly practiced by interpreting dreams, waking visions, or omens seen in such apparently random events as a toss of coins, a pattern in flowing water, or the crackling of a fire. Medical divination has a world-wide distribution. It was practiced by the Chinese more than three thousand years ago. African Zulu shamans cast "the bones," seeing the diagnosis and prognosis of disease in a prayerful toss of ivory and other

personally meaningful objects. Native Americans employ water, fire, smoke, stones, crystals, or other objects as projective fields in which they can "see" the reason and course of a disease. Sometimes, the patient is asked to read the markings on a stone in a type of free association to help both the patient and the healer discover relevant information from the *realm of Spirit*— what we might call the *unconscious*, both personal and collective. This realm of Spirit may also be accessed in the pan-Indian Sweat Lodge Ceremony (92), during the Lakota Yuwipi (31) or Cree *Kosāpahcikéwin,* "Shaking Tent" (93), during which helping and diagnostic spirits speak to the holy person in the darkness. Spirits also supply diagnoses during the darkness of dream-time. Before sleep, the healer cleanses herself with the smoke of a sacred plant, such as sage or cedar, and prays that the dream spirits inform her of diagnosis, treatment, and prognosis.

Divination plays a prominent role in Cherokee diagnostics (94). The healer holds a pebble in each fist and recites a prayer formula. When the healer opens his or her hands, if the pebble in the right hand moves, the answer to the diagnostic question is favorable; if the pebble in the left hand moves, the answer is unfavorable. In a similar way, a silver coin may be immersed in water and its movements interpreted. In another Cherokee divination, a freshly cut stick is partially immersed in a stream at daybreak. The healer recites his or her own name and the name of the patient, and while circling the stick in a prescribed manner recites the formula, "Now! Long Person. . .," quoted at the opening of this chapter. The healer must then interpret the clarity of the water, the presence of floating debris, or the omens presented by passing fish or birds flying overhead.

It must be emphasized, again, that the essence of Native American diagnostics is not the technique, but the ability of the healer to see the patient with the inner eye of spirit, to sense disturbances of energy with the hands and heart, and to commune with higher sources of knowledge. For this reason, the diagnostic procedures are ineffective if merely imitated and cannot be easily taught to those who do not participate in Native tradition.

Table 13.2. Common Therapeutic Methods*

METHOD	PURPOSE
Prayer and chant	Prepare and focus the mind; induce altered state of consciousness; commune with, invoke, empower, and express gratitude to sacred healing forces; attend gathering and administration of herbs or other medicines

Music
  Voice
  Drum
  Rattle
	Same as prayer and chant; entrain consciousness of healer, patient, and helpers; accompaniment to dance and ceremony

Smudge
  Sage
  Cedar
  Sweetgrass
	Cleanse space, healer, patient, helpers, and ritual objects; induce altered state of consciousness and increased sensitivity

Herbs	Establish physical, mental, and spiritual balance; combat specific physical or spiritual pathogens

Laying on of hands
  Massage
  Non-contact treatment
	Aid healing of body, mind, and spirit; relieve pain; transmit healing energy and/or spiritual power

Counseling
  Talking things out
  Advice of elder/advisor
  Dream and vision interpretation
  "Native American Rorschach":
  stones, fire, water, and other
  projective fields
  Healing imagery
  Humor
	Discover emotional/psychological correlate of problem; help patient find new sources of inner strength and understanding; strengthen family and community relations

Ceremony	Support and context for any methods above; commune with natural and spiritual forces, the Great Spirit, and/or the spirit of the disease; induce altered consciousness; affirm cultural identity and values

* *Nature, social support,* and *sacrifice* are common elements that may increase the efficacy of therapy. The patient may expose him or herself to the healing power of nature or the healer may invoke their presence. Family and community are frequently asked to join healer and patient in administering any of the therapeutic methods. Patient and healer may practice fasting or other forms of personal sacrifice as purging or purification and to demonstrate courage, commitment, and dedication to Spirit.

SACRED TECHNOLOGY: HOW MEDICINE PEOPLE PRACTICE HEALING

Methods of treatment are as varied as methods of diagnosis. The most common methods include prayer, chanting, music, smudging—purification with the smoke of sacred herbs—herbalism, laying on of hands, counseling, and ceremony (Table 13.2).

Prayer and Chanting

Healing always begins with prayer. The healer prays each day to prepare himself or herself for the work ahead. The healer may also pray with and for the patient. In addition to the invoca-

tion of transcendent powers and presence, prayers serve a very practical purpose for the patient. They focus his or her mind on the problem at hand. Among northern plains nations, the patient wraps pinches of tobacco in small pouches of cloth ("tobacco ties") while praying for health and divine help. The patient's prayerful preparation for healing is, of itself, healing.

Prayers are directed towards the highest good and generally closed with the traditional expression, "All My Relations." This expression is far more than a Native American version of Christianity's "Amen." "All My Relations" is a statement of the basic Native American philosophy that we should always dedicate prayers to the health, harmony, and balance of all natural and spiritual relations: the Stones, Plants, Animals, Two-leggeds, Earth, Sky, Sun, Moon, Ancestors, Spirit Helpers, and, most importantly, the Great Spirit.

Chants, like prayers, may be spontaneous or culture-specific formulas, such as the complex Night Chant of the Navajo or the "remaking" chants of the Cherokee. Some chants, such as those used in *Si.si.wiss* ("Sacred Breath"), an intertribal healing tradition from the Puget Sound region of Washington State, use specific breathing techniques along with sacred words to drive noxious forces out of the body or to attract healing power.[5]

Music

Many prayers are sung. There are songs to express gratitude, to celebrate, or to invoke the power and blessings of every aspect of nature; there are songs to willow trees, thunder spirits, snow flakes, salmon, bear, the winds of the Four Directions, water, fire, and to healing and guardian spirits. Songs may attend the gathering and preparation of herbal medicines. In *Si.si.-wiss* tradition, songs empower the healer and provide a continuous background during the laying on of hands. Some songs *are* healing power: they enter the patient to seek out and remove pathogenic forces or invading spirits. Songs are received in dreams or visions, or are learned from elders and medicine people.

Most songs are accompanied by a regular drum-beat. Sometimes, the drum itself is an agent of healing; its rhythm entrains the minds of both healer and patient and leads them to an expanded awareness of self and spirit. Many healers substitute or add the rattle to their healing sessions, using the sound and movement of the rattle to shake away disease. In the Indian Shaker Church, bells, a new "medicine" borrowed from Christianity, accompany the healing songs and evoke God's healing power. The Indian flute, although rarely used in healing others, can be an important instrument of self-healing. Patients play the flute to empty the

mind of worries and preoccupations while meditating with Nature and attuning to Her healing power.

Smudging

Native healing sessions frequently begin with smudging, which is a ritual cleansing of place, healer, helpers, patient, and ritual objects with the smoke of a sacred plant, typically sage (*salvia apiana*, other salvia subspecies; or referring to the wormwoods: *artemisia vulgaris, a. tridentata, a. frigida,* etc.), cedar (*libocedrus descurrens* or *juniperus spp.*), or sweetgrass (*hierochloe odarata*). Some healing ceremonies consist of nothing more than smudging the patient while praying. Smudging induces an altered state of consciousness, heightened emotions[6], and increased sensitivity. Because the tools of the Native healers are hands, heart, and spirit, sensitivity to energetic or spiritual imbalance is a necessity for diagnosis and therapy.

Herbalism

Native Americans generally believe that, in ancient times, there was a local plant cure for every disease. Today, because of drastic changes in the environment and population and the scourge of new diseases, these remedies are not as effective. Most of my Native relations do not hesitate to see a conventional medical doctor for any condition that generally requires antibiotics or surgery. Native Americans use herbs *and* Western medications, realizing that each has its strengths and weaknesses.

Native American herbal medicine, like the gifts of Native agricultural technology, saved the lives of early colonists and continues to save lives today. According to Virgil J. Vogel's classic *American Indian Medicine,* "about 170 drugs which have been or still are official in the *Pharmacopeia of the United States of America* or the *National Formulary* were used by North American Indians north of Mexico, and about 50 more were used by Indians of the West Indies, Mexico, and Central and South America" (95).

---

[5] The author is an initiate and practitioner of this tradition.
[6] A result of the olfactory-limbic connection. Altered awareness may be explained, in part, by sensory stimulation on many levels: olfactory from smudging; auditory from drumming and singing; visual from masks, candlelight, and sacred objects; and kinesthetic from healing dances.

Jacques Cartier (1491–1557) was cured of scurvy by a Huron decoction of pine needles, which are high in vitamin C. Native Americans taught Europeans to cure malaria with quinine, to expel toxins with ipecac, and to treat constipation with the most commonly used laxative in the world today, cascara sagrada (*rhamnus purshiana*).

Herbal remedies can reduce fevers, inflammation, and pain and, when applied topically, prevent infection. Weatherford (96) has an unsurpassed narrative account of the gifts of Native American medicine to Western pharmacology. Some herbs, such as "Grandfather Peyote," are considered medicines for the body and soul and are ingested in a spiritually charged atmosphere of drumming, singing, prayer, and cedar smoke. Peyote has been attributed with cures of leukemia, tuberculosis, pneumonia, stroke, and other disorders (97).

Native herbalists may have a repertoire of 300 or more herbs (98, 99), used singly or in various combinations. Some herbalists use only the plants that appear to them in dreams, which is often a result of praying for a particular patient. In the 1920s, a Lakota healer told Frances Densmore, "A medicine man would not try to dream of all herbs and treat all diseases, for then he could not expect to succeed in all nor to fulfill properly the dream of any one herb or animal" (100). It may be futile to look for distinct chemical agents in Native American medicine as explanations for efficacy, because much of an herb's effect may be due to ritual methods of gathering and usage. At St. Regis, Mohawk Nation, there are approximately 200 ways of gathering plant medicines (101). In the Navajo Night Chant, some plants are gathered only when the lightning flashes or used only during specific chants (32).

Laying on of Hands

Massage, healing touch, and non-contact healing are practiced by Native healers throughout North and South America. Native Americans find it amusing that therapeutic touch, a similar modality, is being tested in modern medical and nursing research. Yet few nurses have sought pointers from America's senior practitioners! In Native practice, the intent of massage is not merely physical. Often the hands are used to sweep away or remove spiritual intrusions or to brush in healing powers.

Cherokees warm their hands over coals and circle their palms either on or above an affected area (102; and personal communication, Cherokee medicine man Keetoowah[7], 1978). Some healers hold their hands to the front and back of an affected area, creating what they now call "electrodes within the body" (103). The healer imagines that electricity is moving from one hand to the other. Sometimes the muscles are rubbed in a manner similar to Western massage. The Cherokee use massage to relieve tension, sprains, and pain. Massage oils made of buffalo fat, bear grease, or sea algae may also be applied. To increase the healing effect, the medicine person massages specific therapeutic points (104) or practices an ancient indigenous form of acupuncture and moxibustion (the application of heat or burning herbs to the body) (105). For example, Eagle Plume, a renowned Blackfoot medicine man, treated his son's knee injury by inserting rose thorns into the skin and burning them down to the bottom (106).

Counseling

Because Native healers recognize that *all* health problems affect the mind and spirit, counseling is frequently a major part of the intervention. Clan mothers, respected female elders, are especially known for their ability to offer kind, wise, yet strong advice during times of emotional difficulty. Native counseling emphasizes health rather than pathology. The counselor generally seeks to augment a person's strengths rather than analyze or focus on weaknesses. Humor is frequently used to help break obsessive and overly serious thinking or behavior. The goal is not to return a person to an average or "normal" state; instead, the goal is to help the patient actualize his or her fullest potential by dis-

---

[7] The author was principal apprentice to Cherokee medicine man Keetoowah from 1976 until his death in 1987.

covering the gifts of Spirit—"the original in-structions."

Counseling may take the form of talking things out or listening to the insight of an elder or medicine person. The counselor may help the patient create or discover an image of improved health, perhaps by interpreting patterns seen in projective fields (e.g., fire, smoke, stones). Or, the healer may help the patient access healing guidance by interpreting his or her dreams or visions. The counselor may also use his or her own visualization of healing powers to affect a proximal or distant patient. The healer's "of-fice" is often the sacred sweat lodge, hogan, or other ceremonial lodge, where both healer and patient can more easily discard avoidance, de-nial, or hindrance to the truth.

Ceremony

Ceremonial healing includes both healer and patient. The most basic form of ceremony is communicating with the spirit of a disease through prayer and ritual. Although the goal of the ceremony is to gather information, leading to the release of pathogenic forces, sometimes the patient must first make an offering to these forces—a symbolic gift of words or gesture—to demonstrate acknowledgment and respect.

In Duran's (77) effective adaptation of tradi-tion in the treatment of Native American alco-holism, the patient speaks to the spirit in the bottle. When a patient was offered an alcoholic drink at a social event, this approach "allowed for the psyche of the client to become aware as to the risk involved as well as to activate the unconscious process of the group. . ." (107). According to Duran, the patient has "taken the offensive 'warrior' stance as opposed to the victim stance."

Healing power is present in the ubiquitous Sweat Lodge (also called the Purification Lodge or Stone People Lodge). The Sweat Lodge is a dome of willow branches covered by blankets in which the patient, healer, and helpers pray and counsel together while ladling water onto red-hot stones. The lodge, pitch black but for the glow of the rocks, is a symbolic womb, a return to primal wisdom. Traditionally, separate

ceremonies are conducted by and for women and men. In some ceremonies, the sacred pipe is smoked to further open the mind to healing guidance (108, 109).

Healing ceremonies received during dreams and visions belong only to an individual healer. Other ceremonies are culture specific and are powerful affirmations of cultural identity and values. There are an extraordinary number of these unique healing ceremonies. The following are just a few:

* Navajo "sings" and sand-painting
* The Green Corn and Midwinter rites of the Seneca "faces": *gagosa*, which are masks that personify spiritual beings and powers and are often made to fulfill a dream
* The Lakota Yuwipi
* Native American Church ceremonies
* Healing rites of the Ojibway Midewewin and other medicine societies
* Shamanic exorcisms of the Inuit
* Winter "spirit dances" of the Salish

Other Healing Sources

All Native Americans recognize the source of healing in Nature and Spirit. For example, natu-ral elements, such as earth, water, mountain, and sun, are considered *elder healers;* by harmo-nizing with them, patients may experience spon-taneous healing or find intuitive solutions to their problems. Native Americans also recognize the healing power of fasting and inner silence as ways to become more receptive to any healing influence. Family and community are also im-portant facets of many healing sessions. "Help-ers" are often essential to add healing power and to reintegrate the person into the commu-nity. As all human beings can attest, illness cre-ates a feeling of alienation both from one's own normal self and from normal relations with one's community.

Duration of Therapy

Disease can have a slow or sudden onset. Simi-larly, healing can occur quickly or over a long period of time. However, even in serious or chronic disease, long-term therapy may not be required. The intensity of therapy is generally considered more important than the duration (110). Research in dissociative identity disorder (111–113) suggests that sudden changes in consciousness may result in sudden changes in physiology. One alter (i.e., a disassociated identity) may suffer from diabetes or allergies, whereas another alter may be asymptomatic and apparently healthy.

In Native American healing, the change of consciousness is not from one pathological adaptive state to another, but rather from an unhealthy condition of mind and body to a healthier state. The healing ritual shocks the patient into a new awareness of self and Creation. Healing may not be a gradual process but rather a quantum leap. However, Native healers recognize that patients must make lifestyle and behavioral changes that reinforce and maintain the improved condition. Although healing may occur quickly, way of life makes healing last.

ORGANIZATION

Lifelong Training

Healing power can be inherited from ancestors, transmitted from another healer, or developed through training and initiation (Johnny Moses, personal communication, 1988). However, the best way to develop, strengthen, and maintain healing power is through rigorous personal training. Among the Snohomish, "individuals sometimes inherit a power from a grandmother, grandfather, aunt, or uncle. . . . If they want that power to be strong, they have to fast and go through a lot of sacrifice" (114). The only prerequisite is patience.

Native healers generally train under one principal mentor, often a family or clan member. As anthropologist William S. Lyon notes, "It is really the function of the teacher to train the novice how to be trained directly by the spirits" (115). However, today, with the greater ease of travel and intertribal communication, many healers have several mentors. Wallace Black Elk (47) had 11 "grandfathers." Medicine Griz-

zlybear Lake (52) had 16. Whis.stem.men.knee (Johnny Moses) was asked to carry on his family's medicine at age 13, after being shamanically cured of cancer. He studied northern Nootka and Saanich traditions with his grandparents and later with several other medicine people (116). Among the Yakima, a boy or girl might prepare for spiritual training at age 6, when he or she was brought by an elder to secluded places in nature (26). Following the practice of many Native nations, the child leaves for his or her first vision quest at puberty. After years of continued training and power seeking, sometimes lasting into middle age, the Yakima novice would participate in the "Shaman's Inaugural Dance."

The English word *medicine man* implies a uniform role and gender, which is incorrect. As we have already seen, some medicine people are ritual experts; others specialize in curing snake bites, setting bones, countering sorcery, divining, prescribing herbs, and so on. The Lakota distinguish the *pejuta wicasa*, herbalist, from the *wicasa wakan*, the "holy person" who communicates directly with the healing powers.

OJIBWAY MEDICINE TRAINING

Medicine training is sometimes the domain of specific medicine societies. Among the Ojibway, this "university" is called the *Midewewin* (117), a word meaning "the sounding [of sacred instruments: drum or rattle]" or perhaps a contraction of *Mino* (good) and *daewaewin* (hearted). A member-sponsor recommends a male or female candidate, who is invited to join only after a long period of character assessment. A new member must generally pass through four Orders, or Degrees, before being fully accredited as a medicine person. In each Order, a new tutor is assigned.

In the first Order, the candidate is instructed once or twice weekly for one year in the sacred knowledge of plants, songs, and prayers. After initiation rites and testing, he proceeds to the second Order; in this Order, the novice learns the history of his people and how to keep the spiritual senses open. In the third Order, the member learns to commune with and summon spiritual powers and generate healing energy in the ill. In the fourth Order, the initiate is further purified, tested, and initiated to assure that he or she can resist malevolent forces. On completion of the fourth Order, the member can test candidates and confer and confirm power in others. Although now fully accredited, his education is not finished. The member continues to learn and train and to abide by the moral code of the Midewewin.

NAVAJO MEDICINE TRAINING

Among the Navajo, medicine training is extremely long, requiring the exact memorization of complex chants, sand paintings, and rituals. Some begin learning in their teens, others not until their 50s, generally learning from a relative, clan member, or friend. Medicine man Denet Tsosi recounted that it took six years to learn one of the chants from his brother (32). In the 1970s, the National Institutes of Mental Health began funding a program in Rough Rock, Arizona, to train Navajo medicine men to teach apprentices (11, 118). The program began with 6 medicine men training 12 students. The average age of the students was 50, and the average age of the faculty was 85. Students also learned complementary interventions from Western psychiatrists. The program indicates a growing recognition by psychiatrists that culture and cultural expectations can affect treatment outcome.

Payment for Services

The exorbitant fees charged by Western medical practitioners are, from the Native American point of view, a sign of contemptible professional ethics. Because healing is a gift from the Great Spirit, it is beyond price and should never be equated with a specified bundle of "frog skins." Although many healers accept monetary or material offerings, most do not charge a set fee. Illness is a time for generosity by a caring community. One should not take advantage of someone when he or she is down.

Frequently, the only required gift is a pouch of tobacco. In some traditions, acceptance of the tobacco offering seals a contract between patient and healer. Giving tobacco is a way of saying, "I respect your ways, and I offer prayers of smoke to the Great Spirit." In Cherokee tradition, payment for services is called *ugista'ti*, probably derived from the verb *tsi'giû*, meaning "I take" or "I eat." On a practical level, gifts may help the healer to eat. This is not payment in the common sense of the word, but rather a necessity for "the removal and banishment of the disease spirit" (119). The offering ensures success of treatment because healing spirits appreciate generosity. Value is placed on the source of healing, not primarily on the healer. Hundreds of years ago, the gift was commonly a deer skin or pair of moccasins. Today, cloth, groceries, money, and/or other personal expressions of respect and gratitude are offered.

To consider a healing, the Comanche medicine woman Sanapia (51) required a ritual offering of dark green cloth, a 5/8-ounce bag of Bull Durham tobacco, and four corn shuck "cigarettes papers." The patient would roll a cigarette, take four puffs, and offer the cigarette to Sanapia. Her acceptance of the cigarette was a contract between them, signifying her willingness to help. As a final payment at the conclusion of her services, Sanapia would accept whatever was offered. In 1972, her average payment was about $30, groceries, and enough cloth to make several dresses. She treated an average of 20–30 patients per year.

Flexible, sliding scale fees or barter may, nevertheless, place a demand on the resources of an impoverished patient. The patient is responsible for providing food and sometimes accommodations for the medicine person, his or her helpers, and others, including community members, who assist in healing ceremonies that may last several days. The patient, if he or she is educated in traditional protocol, will probably also wish to make a "sacrifice" of money or material goods to demonstrate sincerity and respect towards the healing powers. I have personally met a man who gave away his printing press—his only source of income—to a medicine man in gratitude for curing him of psychotic behavior caused by substance abuse. On the other hand, I have seen this same medicine man gratefully accept a pouch of tobacco and a twenty-dollar bill from a poor Indian patient who genuinely gave all he had. The medicine person, in turn, gives freely to those in need. He eschews greed and acquisitiveness.

PROSPECTS FOR THE FUTURE

Native American healing has made a comeback. More and more Native youth are learning to appreciate their tradition and to realize its strengths. Americans and Europeans are also demonstrating an extraordinary interest. This is a mixed blessing, because many non-Natives pursue a romanticized form of "Indian healing" as a way of rebelling against the dominant society's values and without learning the wisdom of their own ethnicity. The misrepresentation of Indian teachings by the New Age Movement and the stereotyping of Indian behavior present a threat to Indian identity.[8]

The passing of the Indian Religious Freedom Act in 1978 was a significant step in restoring the right of Native Americans to practice their spiritual and healing traditions. Although this law does not yet have sufficient "teeth," it is a step in the right direction. Much more needs to be done to restore sovereignty, to return illegally appropriated lands, and to preserve the biodiversity necessary for a sustainable and evolving Native herbal tradition. Without their original land base—the source and training ground of Native American healing—this most ancient form of holistic medicine can only be a fragment of what it was.

References

1. Kilpatrick JF, Kilpatrick AG. Run toward the nightland: magic of the Oklahoma Cherokee. Dallas: Southern Methodist University Press, 1967:118.
2. Bryan L. The buffalo people: prehistoric archaeology on the Canadian plains. Edmonton, Alberta: University of Alberta Press, 1991.
3. Jennings F. The founders of America. NY: W. W. Norton, 1993.
4. Deloria V Jr. Red earth, white lies. NY: Scribner, 1995.
5. Needham J, Lu GD. Trans-Pacific echoes and resonances: listening once again. Unpublished Manuscript, 1977.
6. Fell B. America B.C. New York: Simon & Schuster, 1989.
7. Terrell JU. Traders of the western morning: aboriginal commerce in precolumbian North America. Los Angeles, CA: Southwest Museum, 1967.
8. Irwin L. The dream seekers: Native American visionary traditions of the great plains. Norman, OK: University of Oklahoma Press, 1994
9. Smith H, Snake R. One nation under God: the triumph of the Native American Church. Santa Fe, NM: Clear Light Publishers, 1996.
10. Ruby RH, Brown JA. John Slocum and the Indian Shaker Church. Norman, OK: University of Oklahoma Press, 1996.
11. Bergman RL. A school for medicine-men. Am J Psychiatry 1973;130(6):663–666.
12. Swinomish Tribal Community. A gathering of wisdoms, tribal mental health: a cultural perspective. La Conner, WA: Swinomish Tribal Mental Health Project, 1991.
13. Herrick, JW, Snow DR, eds. Iroquois medical botany. Syracuse, NY: Syracuse University Press, 1995:35.
14. Mehl-Madrona L. Coyote medicine. New York: Scribners, 1997.
15. Plumbo, MA. Living in two different worlds or living in the world differently: a qualitative study with American Indian nurses. Journal of Holistic Nursing 1995;13(2):155–173.
16. Hill D, Monture R. Cry of the eagle: prophecies and preparation. Akwesasne Notes 1995;1(3/4):100–108.
17. Vogel VJ. American Indian medicine. Norman, OK: University of Oklahoma Press, 1970.
18. Beck PV, Walters AL. The sacred. Tsaile (Navajo Nation), AZ: Navajo Community College Press, 1977.
19. Walker DE Jr. Witchcraft and sorcery. Moscow, ID: University of Idaho Press, 1989.
20. Eliade M. Shamanism: archaic techniques of ecstasy. Princeton, NJ: Princeton University Press, 1964.

---

[8] The locus of control over how Native American tradition is expressed should be in the hands of Native people. The National Museum of the American Indian is helping to correct some of these problems by presenting the public with a more authentic view of Native tradition, as understood by Native Americans themselves. It is hoped that this trend will continue and that various national and multinational organizations, such as the United States Office of Alternative Medicine and the World Health Organization, will include indigenous healers and scholars in health care planning and delivery. The World Health Organization and the Global Initiative for Traditional Systems (GIFTS) of Health have, so far, focused only on traditional health systems in developing countries (122). Although universal and affordable health care is certainly an admirable and necessary goal, it seems to me that no country can "afford" to ignore the accumulated wisdom of indigenous science.

21. Kalweit H. Shamans, healers, and medicine men. Boston: Shambala Publications, 1992.

22. Krippner S, Welch P. Spiritual dimensions of healing. New York: Irvington Publishers, 1992.

23. Stewart OC. Peyote religion: a history. Norman, OK: University of Oklahoma Press, 1987.

24. Ruby RH, Brown JA. Dreamer-prophets of the Columbia Plateau. Norman, OK: The University of Oklahoma Press, 1989.

25. Bahr DM, Gregorio J, Lopez DI, Alvarez A. Piman shamanism and staying sickness. Tucson: University of Arizona Press, 1974.

26. Hines DM. Magic in the mountains, the Yakima shaman: power & practice. Issaquah, WA: Great Eagle Publishing, Inc., 1993.

27. Jilek WG. Indian healing: shamanic ceremonialism in the Pacific Northwest today. Blaine, WA: Hancock House, 1982.

28. Lewis TH. The medicine men. Lincoln: University of Nebraska Press, 1990.

29. Miller J. Shamanic odyssey. Menlo Park, CA: Ballena Press, 1988.

30. Mooney J. Myths of the Cherokee and sacred formulas of the Cherokees. Nashville, TN: Charles and Randy Elder—Booksellers Publishers, reproduced 1982.

31. Powers WK. Yuwipi. Lincoln: University of Nebraska Press, 1982.

32. Sander D. Navaho symbols of healing. Rochester, VT: Healing Arts Press, 1991.

33. Moerman DE. Medicinal plants of Native America, 2 vols. Ann Arbor, MI: University of Michigan Museum of Anthropology, 1986.

34. Cochran W. A guide to gathering and using Cherokee medicinal herbs. Park Hill, OK: Cross Cultural Education Center, 1984.

35. Croom EM Jr. Herbal medicine among the Lumbee Indians. In: Kirkland J, Mathews HF, Sullivan III CW, Baldwin K, eds. Herbal and magical medicine: traditional healing today. Durham, NC: Duke University Press, 1992:137–169.

36. Curtin LSM. By the prophet of the earth: ethnobotany of the Pima. Tucson, AZ: University of Arizona Press, 1984.

37. Densmore F. How Indians use wild plants for food, medicine & crafts. New York: Dell Publications, 1974.

38. Herrick, op. cit.

39. Gunther E. Ethnobotany of western Washington. Seattle: University of Washington Press, 1981.

40. Gilmore MR. Uses of plants by the Indians of the Missouri River region. Lincoln: University of Nebraska Press, 1977.

41. Hamel PB, Chiltoskey MU. Cherokee plants. Sylva, NC: Herald Publishing Co., 1975.

42. Hungry Wolf A. Teachings of nature. Invermere, British Columbia: Good Medicine Books, 1975.

43. Tantaquidgeon G. Folk medicine of the Delaware and related Algonkian Indians. Harrisburg, PA: Pennsylvania Historical and Museum Commission, 1977.

44. Moore M. Los remedios: traditional herbal remedies of the southwest. Santa Fe, NM: Red Crane Books, 1990.

45. Moore M. Medicinal plants of the mountain west. Santa Fe, NM: Museum of New Mexico Press, 1979.

46. Bear Heart, Larkin M. The wind is my mother: the life and teachings of a Native American shaman. New York: Clarkson N. Potter, 1996.

47. Black Elk W, Lyon WS. Black Elk: the sacred way of a Lakota. San Francisco: Harper & Row, 1990.

48. Boyd D. Mad Bear. New York: Simon & Schuster, 1994.

49. Boyd D. Rolling Thunder. New York: Dell Publishing, 1974.

50. Horse Capture G, ed. The seven visions of Bull Lodge. Ann Arbor, MI: Bear Claw Press, 1980.

51. Jones DE. Sanapia: Comanche medicine woman. Prospect Heights, IL: Waveland Press, 1984.

52. Lake MG. Native healer. Wheaton, IL: Quest Books, 1991.

53. Lame Deer JF, Erdoes R. Lame Deer seeker of visions. NY: Simon & Schuster, 1972.

54. Mails TE. Fools Crow. Garden City, NY: Doubleday & Co, 1979.

55. Mails TE. Fools Crow: wisdom and power. Tulsa, OK: Council Oak Books, 1991.

56. Yellowtail, Fitzgerald MO. Yellowtail, Crow medicine man and sun dance chief. Norman, OK: University of Oklahoma Press, 1991.

57. Shaman's drum: a journal of experiential shamanism. Willits, CA: the Cross-Cultural Shamanism Network.

58. Winds of change. (quarterly) Boulder, CO: American Indian Science & Engineering Society.

59. Akwesasne notes. (quarterly) Kahniakehaka Nation Territory, Rooseveltown, NY: Akwesasne Notes Publishing.

60. News from Indian Country: the native nations journal. (twice monthly) Hayward, WI: Indian Country Communications, Inc.

61. Peat DF. Lighting the seventh fire: the spiritual ways, healing, and science of the Native American. New York: Birch Lane Press, 1994.

62. Rhoades ER. Two paths to healing: can traditional and western scientific medicine work together? Winds of Change 1996;11(3):48–51.

63. The Four Worlds Development Project. Over-

view: the Four Worlds Development Project. Lethbridge, Alberta: University of Lethbridge, No date.

64. Walker JR. Lakota belief and ritual. Lincoln: University of Nebraska Press, 1980.

65. McNeley JK. Holy wind in Navajo philosophy. Tucson: University of Arizona Press, 1982.

66. Walker, op. cit.:83.

67. Lake, op. cit.:17.

68. Amoss P. Coast Salish spirit dancing: the survival of an ancestral religion. Seattle: University of Washington Press, 1978:54.

69. Jilek, op. cit.:42.

70. Wallace AFC. Dreams and the wishes of the soul: a type of psychoanalytic theory among the seventeenth century Iroquois. American Anthropologist 1958;60:235.

71. Krippner, op. cit.:44.

72. Dossey, L. Meaning & medicine. New York: Bantam Books, 1991:60.

73. Pukui MK, Haertig EW, Lee CA. Nana i ke kumu (Look to the source), 2 Vols. Honolulu, HI: Queen Lili'uokalani Children's Center, 1972.

74. Kilpatrick JF, Kilpatrick AG. Walk in your soul: love incantations of the Oklahoma Cherokees. Dallas, TX: Southern Methodist University Press, 1965:9.

75. Eaton SB, Shostak M, Konner M. The paleolithic prescription. New York: Harper & Row, 1988.

76. Bopp M, ed. Developing healthy communities: fundamental strategies for health promotion. Lethbridge, Alberta: Four Worlds Development Project, University of Lethbridge, 1985.

77. Duran E, Duran B. Native American postcolonial psychology. Albany: State University of New York Press, 1995.

78. Ingerman S. Soul retrieval: mending the fragmented self. San Francisco: HarperSanFrancisco, 1991.

79. Harner M. The way of the shaman. San Francisco: Harper & Row, 1980.

80. Fienup-Riordan A. The living tradition of Yup'ik masks. Seattle: University of Washington Press, 1996:191.

81. Horse Capture, op. cit.:46.

82. Vogel, op. cit.:187.

83. Miller, op. cit.:45.

84. Nelson RK. Make prayers to the raven: A Koyukon view of the northern forest. Chicago: University of Chicago Press, 1983:174.

85. Applegate RB. Atishwin: the dream helper in south-central California. Socorro, NM: Ballena Press, 1978.

86. Chief Thomas J, Boyle T. Teachings from the longhouse. Toronto, Canada: Stoddart Publishing Co., 1994.

87. Wallace AFC. The death and rebirth of the Seneca. NY: Vintage Books, 1969.

88. Herrick, op. cit.:37.

89. Mails (1991), op. cit.:155.

90. Sander, op. cit.:30.

91. Knudtson PM. The Wintun Indians of California and their neighbors. Happy Camp, CA: Naturegraph Publishers, 1977:64.

92. Bruchac J. The Native American sweat lodge history and legend. Freedom, CA: The Crossing Press, 1993.

93. Brown JSH, Brightman R. "The orders of the dreamed": George Nelson on Cree and northern Ojibwa religion and myth, 1823. St. Paul: Minnesota Historical Society Press, 1988.

94. Kilpatrick (1967), op. cit.

95. Vogel, op. cit.:267.

96. Weatherford J. Indian givers: how Indians of the Americas transformed the world. NY: Fawcett Columbine, 1988.

97. Smith, op. cit.:57–64.

98. Green J. Kwi-tsi-tsa-las: portrait of an herbalist. In: Tierra M, ed. American herbalism: essays on herbs & herbalism by members of the American Herbalist Guild. Freedom, CA: The Crossing Press, 1992:69–84.

99. Winston D. Nvwote: Cherokee medicine and ethnobotany. In: Tierra M, ed. American herbalism: essays on herbs & herbalism by members of the American Herbalist Guild. Freedom, CA: The Crossing Press, 1992:86–99.

100. Densmore, op. cit.:323.

101. Herrick, op. cit.:69.

102. Vogel, op. cit.:187.

103. Bear Heart, op. cit.:96.

104. Mails TE. Secret Native American pathways: a guide to inner peace. Tulsa, OK: Council Oak Books, 1988:296–297.

105. Vogel, op. cit.:183.

106. Hungry Wolf, op. cit.:16.

107. Duran, op. cit.:146.

108. Brown JE, ed. The sacred pipe: Black Elk's account of the seven rites of the Oglala Sioux. NY: Penguin, 1971.

109. Paper J. Offering smoke: the sacred pipe and Native American religion. Moscow, ID: University of Idaho Press, 1988.

110. Duran, op. cit.:16.

111. O'Regan B. Multiplicity and the mind-body problem: new windows to natural plasticity. In: Noetic sciences collection. Sausalito, CA: Institute of Noetic Sciences, 1991:20–23.

112. Braun BG. Psychophysiologic phenomena in multiple personality and hypnosis. Am J Clin Hypn 1983a;26:124–137.

113. Braun BG. Neurophysiological changes in multiple personality due to integration: a preliminary report. Am J Clin Hypn 1983b;26:84–92.

114. White T. Northwest coast medicine teachings: an interview with Johnny Moses. Shaman's Drum 1991;23(Spring):40.

115. Black Elk, op. cit.:xix.

116. White, op. cit.:36–43.

117. Johnston B. Ojibway heritage. New York: Columbia University Press, 1976.

118. Steiger B. Indian medicine power. Gloucester, MA: Para Research, 1984:47–53.

119. Mooney, op. cit.:337.

120. Achterberg J, Dossey B, Kolkmeier L. Rituals of healing: using imagery for health and wellness. New York: Bantam Books, 1994:51.

121. Wilbert J. Tobacco and shamanism in South America. New Haven: Yale University Press, 1987.

122. J Altern Complement Med 1996;2(3).

CHAPTER 14

TIBETAN MEDICINE

Vladimir Badmaev

BACKGROUND

Definition and Description

Tibetan medicine is rooted in several ancient traditions. Its first written document is approximately 1,300 years old (1, 2). The consensus among Tibetologists is that this medical system developed under the influence of Buddhist philosophy and Ayurvedic medicine, which were brought to Tibet from India (3–5). Tibetan medicine was also molded by Western (6) (i.e., Greek) and Chinese influences (5). According to some accounts, Tibetan medicine originated in the pre-Buddhist religion Bon (also known as Bonpo), a unique tradition of Tibetan origin (7, 8). Tibetan medicine is also practiced in Mongolia (5, 9), the Buryat Republic of Russia, St. Petersburg (5, 10–13), Northern India (3, 4, 7, 8), various European countries (10, 14), and the United States (15–17).

History

The origins of Tibetan medicine, based on accounts of the Bonpo tradition, can be traced to the teacher sTon-pa gShen-rab, who lived approximately 500 years before Buddha Shakya-muni (7, 8). The first king of Tibet, Nya-khri bTsan-po, who ruled around 150 BC, had a prominent physician, Dung-gi Thor-cog, who most likely practiced an indigenous Tibetan medical art. The Bonpo traditions have been misunderstood and undervalued, particularly after Tibetan culture was influenced by Buddhism in the seventh and eighth centuries AD.

KEY FIGURES AND LITERATURE

The historical period of the Tibetan Empire shaped the body of knowledge known as Tibetan medicine (1). The Tibetan Empire lasted from the seventh to the ninth centuries AD and extended south to the plain of the Ganges, north to Samarkanda, and included part of China. The vast and culturally varied territory of that empire effected development of Tibetan medicine, mostly because of special interest that the three consecutive rulers of that empire had in acquiring and nourishing knowledge of other cultures (1, 2).

The three kings who ruled the Tibetan Empire were, in chronological order, Song-tsen Gam-po, Ti-song De-tsen, and Rolpa-chon. They are regarded as the most prominent figures in Tibetan history (1, 2). In the eighth century AD, one of the three rulers, king Ti-song De-tsen, invited Padma-Sambhava, a famous Buddhist teacher, to Tibet. Since then, Buddhist philosophy has been essential in the medical education of Tibetan culture (1, 2). Symbolically, Buddha occupies an important position in the medical hierarchy of Tibet. One of his titles is Supreme Physician, and he is often thought of as the Tibetan Aesculapius. The Tibetan Empire was also highlighted by a medical convention that took place between 755 and 797 AD at Samye (5, 10). During that meeting, renowned physicians from Persia, Greece, India, China, Afghanistan, Nepal, East Turkestan, and

Kashmir translated their medical works into the Tibetan language.

The eighth and ninth centuries are also noted for the work of a physician known as the Elder gYu-thogYon-tan mGon-po, or the Excellent Protector (18). He is credited with writing a first document on Tibetan techniques of diagnosis and treatment. He and one of his descendants contributed to the final form of the *yGyud-bzhi* (pronounced Zud-shi, meaning "Four Roots"), a canon textbook in Tibetan medicine (2). The nucleus document of the *yGyud-bzhi* was probably written in Sanskrit in the fourth century AD and was brought to Tibet from India during the active period of the Empire (19). Most likely, the translation into the Tibetan language was accomplished in the eighth century by the Buddhist scholar Vairochana, with the assistance of the Tibetan physician Zla-ba mNon-dgha (2). In the late nineteenth and early twentieth centuries, that ancient work was translated from Tibetan and Mongolian into Russian by the present author's great grand-uncles Alexander Badmaev, MD (known by his Buddhist name as Sul-Tim-Badma) and Peter Badmaev, MD (known by his Buddhist name as Zhamsaran-Badma) (20).

EARLY TIBETAN MEDICAL EDUCATION

Historically, medical education in Tibet has been based on a highly structured system, with Buddhist monasteries functioning as medical schools (2). The first medical college in Tibet, Kong-po-menlung, was built in the eighth century at Lhasa. Among medical schools established since then, the best known are the Chagpori Medical College, built in the seventeenth century, and Mentsi Khang, built in 1915. Since 1959, the Tibetan Medical Institute at Dharamsala, India, has been the center that upholds both the medical tradition and the Tibetan culture under the guidance of His Holiness Dalai Lama (5, 9).

Partly because of the vast cultural influence of the Tibetan empire, Tibetan medicine has also been practiced in Mongolia (5, 9, 10). According to some accounts, Tibetan medicine was particularly welcomed in that country because of a Tibetan physician named Sakaja (first half of the thirteenth century) who cured Godon, the ruler of that country, of a form of paralysis (9). In recognition of the Tibetan and Buddhist contributions to their medical knowledge, the Mongolian people awarded the ruling priest-prince of Tibet in 1547 the Mongolian title of Dalai-Lama, meaning Ocean Priest (5). In the twentieth century, Tibetan medicine was brought from Mongolia to the Asiatic part of Russia, and the principles of both that medicine and Buddhism have flourished in the Buryat Russian Republic, where it has been taught in the Aga monastery, which is in the vicinity of Lake Baikal (5, 10–13).

TIBETAN TRADITIONS AND LINEAGES

Although all Tibetan medicine teachings have central texts and core concepts, the actual practice of Tibetan medicine has developed variations from different lineages or traditions. These lineages usually follow the special practices of one teacher or family tradition. In addition, these lineages will take on certain characteristics of the local medicine traditions where they are practiced. It would be beyond the scope of this chapter to describe all these lineages and their practices. The author is trained in one of these traditions that came to the West via Russia and was taught by his ancestor, Buryat physician Dr. Sul-Tim-Badma, who settled in St. Petersburg in the late 1800s and changed his name to Dr. Alexander Badmaev (11–13, 22, 23). Descendants of Alexander and his brother Peter continue to practice in St. Petersburg (22–24). The examples of specific herbal treatments described in this chapter come out of this lineage and are not used by all Tibetan physicians. They do, however, serve to illustrate basic principles of Tibetan plant use and similar formulae are used in Tibetan practices around the world.

Unlike Chinese and Ayurveda medicine, Tibetan medicine has only recently come to the attention of the West. Probably the greatest pioneer of Tibetan medicine for the West was Alexander Csoma de Koros, called the Hungarian "hero of learning," who spent years in seclusion in Tibetan monasteries studying Tibetan medical treatises and translating them for the

West (21). The Badmaev family also brought Tibetan medical practices to the West. After Alexander and Peter Badmaev, Valdimir N. Badmaev, MD, Sr. (Buryat name Jamayan Badma) established a Tibetan pharmacy and practice in Warsaw in the 1930s. Later, his son (Peter Badmaev, MD, Jr.) and Mr. Karl Lutz helped to establish the commercial manufacture and clinical testing of herbal and mineral treatments based on the Badmaev tradition (14). In 1985, the present author established the Laboratory of Applied Pharmacology in New York to carry on the development and testing of these formulae for the Western market (17). The PADMA company in Switzerland is another company that has developed and tested Tibetan formulae for Western use.

More recently, and under the guidance of His Holiness the Dalai Lama, other Tibetan traditions have been introduced to the West. Tibetan physicians trained at the Tibetan Medical Institute in Dharamsala and elsewhere have come to the West to give demonstrations and open practices in conjunction with conventional Western clinics. In addition, organizations like the Dharma Hinduja Indic Research Center at Columbia University; Pro-Cultura, Inc.; the Alternative Medicine Foundation, Inc., and the Smithsonian Institute have stimulated increased understanding and exchange of information on Tibetan medicine traditions and lineages in the West. In recent years, a number of institutes for the practice of Tibetan medicine have opened in Western countries.

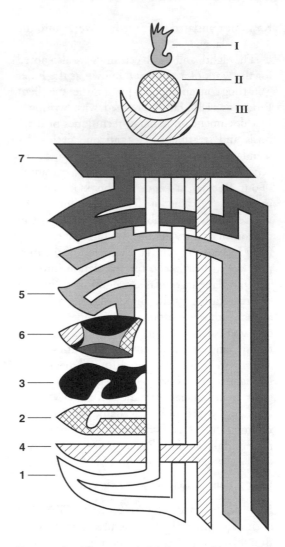

FIGURE 14.1. The ten essential elements of humans (all forms and processes of universal existence): I, awareness; II, willpower; III, compassion; 1, element of structure and temperature; 2, element of gaseous, aqueous, and solid substances; 3, element of plants; 4, element of gender; 5, element of animals; 6, element of man; 7, element of mind.

PRINCIPAL CONCEPTS

The three elements, or the *triadic theory,* is the distinguishing medical theory in Tibetan medicine. This theory is a Tibetan doctor's basis for the determination of psychosomatic types of humans, as well as for the prevention, diagnosis, and treatment of a disease.

The triadic theory evolved from the philosophical perception that every form of existence depends on other factors and requires the three essential elements: *Chi* (different meaning than the Chinese *chi*), *Schara*, and *Badahan* (25). At the level of the macrocosm (the universe), *Chi* can be illustrated by the element of space. *Schara* is the element of energy, and *Badahan* is the material element. According to the triadic theory, these elements can exist by depending on each other; according to Tibetan theory, in reality there cannot be an absolute space without the elements of energy and the matter contained therein. Subsequently, it is the dominance of either *Chi, Schara,* or *Badahan* that determines the nature of a perceived phenomenon or form of existence.

The interdependence of the three elements and the dynamic balance among them are manifested by the transition of one quality into the other—analogous to the known paradigm in physics where energy (equal to *Schara*), matter (equal to *Badahan*), and light (medium of transition in space equal to *Chi*) are interdependent and interchangeable. As part of the macrocosm, earthly life is permeated by the infinite number of examples of the three elements at work.

The human is seen as one of the expressions of *Chi, Schara,* and *Badahan* elements, and as such it incorporates all forms and processes of the universal existence (Fig. 14.1) (26). The concept of 10 essential elements points to the links among the anatomical forms, physiological and psychological function in humans, and any conceivable elements of the larger Universe, including animate and inanimate matter as well as psychic existence. Subsequently, the *Chi, Schara,* and *Badahan* elements in the human are approximated to the universal forms of those elements.

For example, the space (*Chi*) is perceived as a supportive element in the Universe to facilitate transition of energy (*Schara*) to matter (*Badahan*) and matter to energy. At the level of the human body, a form of Universe in miniature, the *Chi* element can be exemplified by the skeleton, which supports body tissues, organs, and systems, and facilitates the physiological functions. In principle, the *Chi* element represents the tissues, organs, systems, and physiological functions that provide the body with structure and integrity (e.g., cell membranes, connective tissue, skeleton, skin); basic support of life by introducing and carrying nutrients to the mind and body (i.e., sensory stimuli as nutrients), oxygen supply as nutrient, and the food-derived nutrients (e.g., receptacles of sensory nerves, receptors of autonomic nervous system, nasopharynx, bronchial tree, upper digestive tract); and basic support of life through elimination of metabolic waste from the body (e.g., large intestine, urinary tract, excretory functions). Element *Chi* therefore *initiates* and makes possible the process of life.

In the universe, *Schara* represents the element of energy. In humans, *Schara* is associated with the digestive processes (applicable to the three categories of nutrients mentioned) and the distribution of the absorbed nutrients. Therefore, *Schara* is primarily located in the relevant tissues, organs, and systems, and is expressed by corresponding physiological functions (e.g., muscles, upper gastrointestinal tract, liver, pancreas, energy channels [subtle body], nervous and cardiovascular systems).

The matter, or the element, of *Badahan* is understood in the triadic theory as an outcome of interaction between *Chi* and *Schara*—an element of energy being realized within the space. Thus, *Badahan* is listed as a third essential element, after the space (*Chi*) and energy (*Schara*), which in a way secures and justifies the existence of space and energy. Consequently, the *Badahan* element is represented by the tissues, organs, systems, and physiological functions that secure and protect the functioning of the other two elements in the body. In this capacity, the *Badahan* element dominates and regulates the nutrients' absorption and processing (e.g., converting sensory perception into intellectual process, such as hearing verbal commands and coordinating the reaction and response to them), diffusion of oxygen and its use by the tissues, and absorption and integration (bioavailability) of absorbed food nutrients within the tissues. *Badahan* element predominates, for example, in the adipose tissue, the upper gastrointestinal tract (absorptive functions), the lungs, the brain, and the immune system. *Badahan* is the outcome of the process initiated by *Chi* and implemented by *Schara*.

The processes that govern state of health, transition to a disease, and determination of disease origin represent the dynamic interactions taking place among the *Chi, Schara,* and *Badahan* elements in the body. The balance among those elements corresponds to the state of well-functioning homeostasis and health; disruption of these elements corresponds to the disease condition. It should be noted that it is not the absence of any physical ailment that defines health solely. For example, a physically healthy person may be unfulfilled spiritually and emotionally. Therefore, it is the spiritual, mental, and physical (balance) well-being along with the absence of the physical ailment that characterize optimal health in Tibetan practice.

The Human as a Psychic Phenomenon

THE EMPIRIC SOUL

Knowledge of human psychology dominates the theory and practice of Tibetan medicine and stresses a practical approach to the human psyche, which is comparable with the approach that a physician takes in examining the physical body. The *empiric soul,* which is distinct from the nonmaterial and clinically inaccessible absolute soul, is a key to understanding the structure and clinical relevance of the human psyche in Tibetan medicine. The classic ancient text in Indian medicine by Caraka Samhita describes the concept of the empiric soul. The empiric soul is comprised of the mind, the mind's attributes (i.e., intellect, ego, memory, emotions), and the senses (i.e., sound, touch, vision, taste, smell). Although the empiric soul is an autonomous entity in relation to the absolute soul, its function depends on the absolute soul; these two entities communicate through spirituality. It is believed that a properly functioning empiric soul is conductive to spirituality.

The mind is the most important element of the empiric soul. Because it receives, records, and analyzes information from the other five sense organs, the intellect, the ego, and so forth, the mind is regarded as a separate sixth sense. The mind has the ability to process the information provided, which leads to understanding.

Emotions such as happiness, sorrow, misery, love, and one particularly important emotional state—compassion—originate in the mind. Memory also originates in the mind. The senses provide critical information about the outside world; they are a source of external information for the functioning of the mind. The five senses and their attributes are traditionally listed in a specific order—sound, touch, vision, taste, and smell—based on the increasing quantity of attributes that are believed to be inherent to a particular sense.

The intellect and ego are considered inseparable in Tibetan understanding. Intellect is the executive branch of the empiric soul, which implements the understanding provided by the mind. At the same time, it also reports the implementation and results of the understanding by continuing feedback to the mind.

Ego is perceived as being derived from the intellect. Ego is seen as a result of the ongoing self-evaluation and validation process that is a direct outcome of the feedback provided by the intellectual process. Ego may indeed frequently play a negative role in human psychology. For example, when there is too much preoccupation with the personal image, then there is, paradoxically, little energy left for self-improvement, which is exactly what is needed to become perceived by others in a better light.

Maintaining Health and Disease Prevention: General Rules

Maintaining health, disease prevention, or both are, according to Tibetan medicine, primarily the individual's responsibility. The important aspects of that responsibility involve proper nutrition, good lifestyle habits, proper adjustment to the seasons of the year, and self-awareness of one's physical and psychological predisposition. To fulfill these four conditions, besides devoting time and effort to the task, a person has to be at peace with oneself and understand one's place within the family, community, society, and universe. Being at peace with the self is understood in triadic philosophy as the state of objectivity or adequacy in a given reality. This state is often referred to and measured by Tibetan practitioners as a feeling of *compassion.* It should be noted, however, that although compassion is commonly understood to be an emotional feeling, it is used here to mean *feeling emotionless,* which should *not* be confused with the state of emotional exhaustion. And compassion should also not be mistaken for the feeling of being "in love." Objectivity or compassion can also be defined as the state of mind devoid of ignorance, attachment, anger, jealousy, and pride. The embodiment of this state conductive to health is known in Tibetan medicine as the high levels of "living warmth," or vitality.

WISDOM

In traditional Tibetan understanding, the state of objectivity in the universe is achieved by certain laws of nature. To comprehend, learn, and follow these laws are separate tasks for every living creature. The animal upholds these laws by instinct. Humans, however, have been provided with a far greater skill than the animal, and that skill originates with a special kind of wisdom. This wisdom is derived from an individual's faith in God. Tibetan medicine stresses the vital need for each of us to seek out and cultivate our relationship with God to strengthen our faith in the divine authority of God.

Failure to obtain this wisdom disconnects a person from reality, compromises the overall well-being, and may initiate the transition from optimal health to an overt disease. This failure is not simply a lack of intelligence, but a lack of faith in life and the creative approach to life, which, as just explained, is equated to lack of faith in the divine authority of God.

SPIRITUALITY

This health-sustaining wisdom can actually be cultivated by our spirituality, or harmonious communication between the empiric and absolute souls, as exercised by awareness, willpower, and compassion; these are three important functions of the mind and the intellectual process that correspond to the *Chi, Schara,* and *Badahan* elements, respectively. The function of awareness, willpower, and compassion in developing spirituality can be described as follows: *awareness,* or the inspiring force of *Chi,* provides a direction or framework for the individual's actions yet to be fulfilled; the fulfilling act of *willpower* then follows due to the energy of *Schara.* As a result of this interaction between *Chi* and *Schara,* a person can accomplish the state of objectivity measured by the feelings of *compassion.* The state of objectivity or compassion embodies *Badahan,* which facilitates the healthy functioning of *Chi* and *Schara* by making them "worthwhile." Conversely, if awareness and willpower have not been used properly in the first place (e.g., the wrong action for the wrong reason, or the right action for the wrong reason, such as self-pleasing or merely pleasing others), then the effort has not been made "worthwhile," and the state of objectivity has not been accomplished.

Exercising spirituality is important and, if left unfulfilled, can make an individual vulnerable to a host of health-compromising conditions and disease vectors.

Maintaining Health and Disease Prevention: Nutrition and Its Adjustment to the Seasons of the Year

According to the triadic theory, food is considered a form of the three elements—*Chi, Schara,* and *Badahan*—which, as such, are transformed into every aspect of the living and well-functioning organism. A singular cell, tissue, organ, or system of the body is composed of particular proportions of these three basic elements. Those proportions change due to seasonal variations of atmospheric conditions that are both responsive to and designed to meet the natural challenge of the environment. These seasonal differences in the three elements' proportions require appropriate nutrient delivery, which reflects the changing needs of the organism to maintain both short-term and long-term well-being. Balancing the dynamic processes in the body depends on timely (i.e., hourly, daily, and seasonal) delivery of the proper combination of supporting nutrients.

DELIVERY OF NUTRIENTS

According to Tibetan medicine, one of the most important factors in sustaining health is timely delivery of nutrients. Lack of timely nutrition results in states leading to illness. This condition may not put people in the hospital, prevent them from working, or alienate them from family, but it can restrict their full potential, eventually exhausting their lifespan prematurely. Therefore, delivery of nutrients unsynchronized with daily and seasonal requirements amounts to poor nutrition. According to Tibetan tradition, the optimal diet is calculated partly on the basis of carbohydrate, fat, and protein content, but primarily on the taste value of the food.

Taste

The taste of food is a practical and important guide to adjust nutrition with changing seasons. Three kinds of basic, supplementary tastes are recognized:

1. Pungent-sweet.
2. Bitter-salty.
3. Sour-astringent.

These three basic tastes promote or modify specific functions done by those organs and systems in which elements of *Chi, Schara,* and *Badahan* predominate, respectively. The three complementary tastes moderate or modify the *Chi, Schara,* and *Badahan* action of the corresponding basic tastes.

Pungent taste stimulates organs and systems with a predominance of *Chi,* those of which participate in excretion of metabolites from the organism and improve alertness and awareness. Bitter taste stimulates the functions of organs and systems with a predominance of *Schara,* those of which are related to the digestion of food and absorption of nutrients and promote willpower and self-control.

Sour taste promotes the functions of organs and systems that have a predominance of *Badahan,* that is, those organs and systems that carry nutrients into the organism (e.g., upper gastrointestinal tract, lungs [oxygen nutrient]). Sour taste promotes the storage of nutrients, which induces feelings of satiety, calmness, and tranquility.

SEASONAL FOOD ADJUSTMENTS

Just as we have to adjust to the physical environment that we live in, proper nutrition is a logical step when we adjust to changes of weather. A monodiet throughout the year, no matter how well fitted to calorie and essential nutrient requirements, will likely result in too little or too much, too rich or too restricted, nutrition for a given season. Traditionally, the season is not determined exactly according to the calendar, but is based on the atmospheric conditions characteristic of a particular season.

Winter Nutrition

In a healthy individual, when the cold weather arrives, the digestive (*Schara, Badahan*) and absorptive (*Badahan, Schara*) functions are well balanced and ready for the heavy seasonal demands of providing energy from the caloric value of food. The excretory *Chi* functions of the body are diminished to further save energy. The nutritional mission in the winter is to eat a variety of foods, with no particular food-taste admonition. Meals should be frequent and in small quantities to continuously sustain the di-

gestive capacities and nutritional demands of the body. It is particularly important to eat regularly and not go hungry during the winter season. A disproportion between increased demand and diminished food supply may, in the short term, cause indigestion; it may also have a far-reaching detrimental effect on health and disease prevention.

Spring Nutrition

Between the winter and summer solstices, the digestive functions of the gastrointestinal tract are gradually diminishing in comparison to their activity in the winter. The changing atmospheric conditions, as measured by increased solar energy, decrease the need for energy supplied by digestion and absorption. Thus, the functions of *Schara* and *Badahan* become progressively weaker and are prone to be upset by dietary errors. The spring menu is recommended to prevent an upset of *Schara* and *Badahan* functions, particularly until unstable atmospheric conditions yield to the more stable conditions of summer. The menu should be based on the rough, bitter, astringent, and pungent tastes characteristic of spring vegetables and fruits. Of all the seasons, spring is the most plausible time to eat sparingly or even fast (if needed) to provide the least burden to body homeostasis.

Summer Nutrition

The peak solar energy operating during the summer puts little stress on digestion to extract energy for the body. The digestive tract exercises the option of economy: it does not work to its full potential because it does not have to. That dormant state of the gastrointestinal tract makes it nevertheless vulnerable to strong-tasting foods that may stimulate and upset the unprepared functions of *Schara.* During the summer, food should be light and cool, with a predominantly sweet taste. Bitter, pungent, and astringent foods should be avoided. Greasy, heavy, and canned food should also be avoided. By avoiding the bitter taste, functions of *Schara* will not be upset; also, salty taste will moderate an undesired stimulation of *Schara* with bitter-tasting foods.

It is preferable to quench a summer thirst

with warm tea and lemon rather than a cold drink. This is recommended to avoid upsetting thermoregulation, a *Schara*-dependent process, which is particularly vulnerable during the summer. For example, the common cold or cold sores are often experienced during summer because of the poor response of the body's thermoregulatory mechanism to challenging conditions, such as drafts, swimming after a prolonged sunbath, ice-cold drinks, and alcoholic beverages.

Autumn Nutrition

As summer advances toward autumn, the menu gradually becomes limited. Traditionally, it is believed that energy from the sun is decreased and the digestive functions, particularly related to *Schara* and *Badahan,* undergo transition in preparation for their peak activity during the winter. Because the digestive functions are again in transition, from low to high activity, they are prone to be upset by dietary errors. The autumn menu should consist of light food with predominantly sour, salty, astringent, and sweet tastes (in that order). The main purpose of the autumn diet is to avoid strong, stimulating tastes and heavy food while a gradual increase in overall gastrointestinal performance is accomplished.

Meals should be frequent and small to keep digestive functions moderately busy, but not overwhelmed. Although meals should always be enjoyed, it is particularly important to have a specially designated time and place for daily meals during the autumn.

TRADITIONAL BOTANIC FORMULAE

Not only has the Tibetan medical tradition recognized the importance of nutrition in maintaining health, but, more importantly, it has recognized the *fallibility* of humans to maintain a proper nutritional regimen. Therefore, the Tibetan medical art is particularly abundant in the use of herbs and minerals as well as compound formulae used to assist the digestive process, particularly the process disrupted by nutritional errors. Although seasonal adjustment of the menu is the first step in nutritional intervention, the traditional botanic formulae have often been used to assist nutritional intervention.

Mental and Emotional Digestion

In Tibetan medicine, central nervous system functioning is often likened to the functioning of the digestive tract, which transforms food into the elemental nutrients that can sustain metabolism and life. Therefore, reference to the "mental and emotional digestion" of an individual is made. The "food" for the empiric soul is the complex source of sensory stimuli and information that is transformed into the mental energy that makes life possible. The concept of mental and emotional digestion is a clinically useful way to approach some of the most difficult aspects of human life and existence (i.e., psychological phenomena in health and disease).

Attaining harmonious mental digestion depends on an individual's day-to-day life. An important aspect of the digestive process is recognition and knowledge of what constitutes proper nutrition and digestion. A healthy empiric soul has all the necessary potential to recognize the importance of proper mental and emotional digestion and is fully equipped to seek the solution that realizes an individual's mental and emotional well-being. No one is born with the solution, and seeking it is a task for each individual. This continuous search is gradually rewarded by peace of mind. Peace of mind is traditionally defined as the state of joyful *but* purposeful existence and should not be mistaken for the feeling of an unconditional serenity.

Recognizing the importance of seeking true peace of mind has a cost: suffering and fear. A person can then understand that whatever causes the misery, and the misery itself, is totally foreign to and runs against the individual's deepest nature. This understanding is linked to the faculties of mind and memory. A person cannot truly be healthy without a sense of identity, which memory provides. Memory pervades all that we do, who we are, our personalities, and how we interact with other people; it literally creates our internal and external worlds.

Mind and Memory

Understanding mind and memory is indispensable for understanding the process that causes

Table 14.1. Attitudes and Actions that Cause Emotional, Mental, and Physical Harm

ATTITUDE OR ACTION	EXAMPLES
Engaging in risky behaviors	Sexual promiscuity, substance abuse
Forcible suppression of natural urges and needs	Need for emotional expression
Fear	Fear of success or failure
Untimely action and reaction	Outbursts of anger, impatience, bewilderment; rushing through life
Complacency	Not standing up to challenges; vanity, greed
Disrespect	Showing disrespect and envy for someone's accomplishment
Unfit friendships	Friendship with a person who is unable or unwilling to relate emotionally, or who dominates or is dominated
Avoidance of healthy activities	Avoiding healthy physical activity or relaxation (or inability to relax); workaholism
Negligence of treatment	Avoiding a visit to a doctor for fear of "bad news"

suffering and fear; it is also indispensable for finding practical solutions and peace of mind. Memory impairment leads an individual towards hurtful circumstances as well as those that cause ill effects and a never-ending sequence of self-inflicted suffering and fear. An individual will continue to revisit the *hurtful* past for as long as he or she is ignorant of his or her innermost nature and/or does not remember and understand that certain actions and situations cause emotional, mental, and physical harm. Examples of these attitudes and actions are covered in Table 14.1.

Proper memory functioning, therefore, can be viewed as a necessary element to maintain or restore mental and emotional digestion, which results in peace of mind.

Another important consideration of mental and emotional digestion is the perception of ego. Ego is often viewed as a culprit that causes misery. A selfish ego is blamed for unhappiness, for the inability to draw mental strength from intellect and patience, and for failing to take a proper "history" lesson from memory. In Western culture, a healthy, integrated, and rationally functioning personality is strengthened by the loss of what Tibetan medicine calls the selfish ego, which is characterized by infantile craving, attachment, and anxiety. Ego should be limited to a useful, not a disturbed, function. The French philosopher and mathematician René Descartes said, *"Cogito ergo sum"*—"I think, therefore I am." This statement may be

an appropriate definition of a useful function of ego: awareness of existence, but only awareness. According to Tibetan medicine, care for an individual's deep nature—not his or her image—should be the priority.

Realization of the inevitability of decay and death as well as the ephemeral nature of life (e.g., relationships, interests, professional and personal positions and possessions) provides additional understanding of misery and self-inflicted fear; why fear something that is unavoidable in the course of life?

As mentioned, attaining harmonious mental and emotional digestion is a continuous process that, according to Tibetan medicine, depends primarily on an individual effort. Having had a glimpse of true peace of mind allows a person to more peacefully reconcile with the common experience of the occasional "mental and emotional" indigestion. This measure is the Tibetan way to attain first-hand knowledge of good mental and emotional nutrition, digestion, and health.

PATIENCE

According to traditional Tibetan understanding, patience is the most important factor in sustaining peace of mind. Patience alone pacifies ego and sustains a harmonious intellectual process. Patience in this context is understood primarily not as a "patient waiting," but as an acquired ability to contain emotions and desires in favor of mental and emotional discipline. Patience is praised in Western culture as a great virtue, but it is not fully recognized that patience can be used therapeutically. In Tibetan medical tradition, the true peace of mind is equated with unquestioning recognition of the divine authority of God. Also, the true peace of mind signifies a special kind of wisdom that is a guide to a total and sustained health.

PRACTITIONER–PATIENT INTERACTION

Diagnosis of Health, the Transition to Disease, and Disease

According to Tibetan tradition, the first visit to a doctor should be scheduled in the morning, when the patient is well rested and fasting. Obtaining relevant information includes noting the patient's appearance (e.g., psychosomatic, or triadic, type; facial expression; expression of eyes); obtaining information on the patient's complaints (e.g., eating habits, behavior, mental state, sexual activity, personal and social life); and physical examination and additional tests (e.g., pulse reading, evaluation of patient's urine).

DETERMINATION OF THE PSYCHOSOMATIC TYPE

Determining a person's triadic type is an important step toward the diagnosis and self-diagnosis of individual health. In Tibetan medicine, the three basic psychosomatic types are *Chi, Schara,* and *Badahan.*

Chi

A person of *Chi* type has the following somatic characteristics: a tall, lean physique; poor muscle tone; long, thin neck; narrow chest; long extremities with small, thin hands and feet, and relatively long fingers and toes; thin, dry nails; and dry skin, with prominent veins and dull complexion. The head, covered with scanty and soft hair, is small and elongated with a narrow forehead, thin eyebrows, and small eyelashes. The eyes are small, unfocused, and usually blue. The nose is small, thin, sharp, and crooked; the ears are projecting; the shoulders are narrow and dropping; and the abdomen is small and flat.

On the mental and emotional level, a *Chi* type may be anxious, with nervous behavior (similar to the stereotype of an artist's personality). The *Chi* person has an everchanging, chimerical, and adaptable mind in search of new ideas. New ideas come easily to the *Chi* type, but often are not followed through, mostly because of lack of perseverance and courage to implement. The *Chi* type is intelligent but impractical, and creates a mental picture of an ideal world. These individuals do not have good paternal or maternal instincts and are often troubled by parental duties.

The sexual life of a *Chi* type is characterized by strong desire but low energy and multiple partners. The favorite foods are sweet, hot, and light in nature.

A *Chi* type is very susceptible to disease, but at the same time shows good resistance and adaptability to disease. These individuals are prone to nervous disorders (e.g., psychoneurosis, schizophrenia, insomnia) and neurological disorders (e.g., epilepsy, neurodegenerative disorders, neuralgia, herpes zoster, optic neuritis, and neurological conditions affecting urogenital and rectal regions). This psychosomatic type often suffers from rheumatoid arthritis and osteoarthritis. *Chi*-type disorders tend to break out or be aggravated in the fall and winter, and they tend to afflict the elderly.

Schara

A person of the *Schara* type is characterized by a well-proportioned physique; medium height; strong muscles; strong, medium-size neck; well-developed chest; strong arms and legs; medium-size hands and feet; medium-size soft, square pink nails; and skin with a pink complexion that is often covered with moles, freckles, or acne. The head is short and covered with moderate, early graying and balding hair; the forehead is wide and has folds. The eyebrows and eyelashes are fine; the eyes are medium-size, often congested (bloodshot), and attentive; the nose is medium- size; and the ears are proportionate and well-formed. The shoulders are medium-size and straight, and the abdomen is small and muscular.

The psychological features of *Schara* are similar to the stereotype of a strong-willed political or corporate leader. The *Schara* type has an intelligent, penetrating, and critical mind. This person implements well-defined ideas with bold, reckless determination. The *Schara* type can be ruthless, caring more about ideas than about people.

The sexual life of this type is passionate and dominating. As a parent, *Schara* represents a demanding, unsentimental, authoritarian individual. The *Schara* type is fond of sweet and bitter foods (which also can be described as dense and cool foods).

The *Schara* type has low resistance to disease but good endurance against psychological and physical suffering. A *Schara* type is prone to infectious diseases, venereal diseases, and resulting infectious psychoses. The *Schara* type is also prone to neoplastic diseases. *Schara* types often complain of digestive disorders manifested by hyperacidity, gastrointestinal ulcers, infectious diseases of the liver, and diseases of the pancreas. Allergic and infectious skin disorders, rashes, and boils often afflict persons with the *Schara* constitution. These *Schara* conditions tend to flare up in late spring and summer and are more likely to affect young and middle-aged adults.

Badahan

A person of the *Badahan* type is characterized by a heavy physique that tends to be overweight; a short, beefy neck; a broad, overdeveloped chest; inappropriately short extremities compared with the trunk; large hands and feet; large, thick, white nails; pale, thick, moist, and smooth skin. The person's head is large and oval and covered with abundant, thick, lustrous hair. The forehead is large, with thick and bushy eyebrows; the eyelashes are large and firm; and the eyes are wide, prominent, and expressive. The nose is thick, big, and firm; the ears and earlobes are large. The shoulders are broad and firm, and the abdomen is large.

The *Badahan* type is similar to the stereotype of a caring figure of the community: he or she provides a sense of stability, love, and compassion, but not necessarily leadership. This type of person has a pleasant personality, is a good listener, but is slow to react, is not talkative, and is not imaginative. The sexual life of *Badahan* is characterized by good sexual energy and devotion to one partner. *Badahan* values comfort and peaceful surroundings of the home. *Badahan*-type males are family-oriented men; *Badahan*-type females are good wives and mothers, with strong maternal instincts. *Badahan* types are particularly fond of foods with sour and strong flavors.

Badahan types have high resistance to disease. However, once this resistance is broken, the person shows low endurance. These people are prone to states of emotional deprivation and abnormal metabolism, which results in metabolic intoxications (e.g., diabetes, cardiovascular disease, tumors, skin diseases, asthma, bronchitis, and emphysema). They also tend to have decreased acuity of taste and smell. *Badahan* disorders are aggravated in late winter and early spring; children and young people (up to 16 years of age) are more prone to the disorders of *Badahan* than are other age groups.

It should be noted that the clear-cut *Chi, Schara,* and *Badahan* types are rarely, if ever, encountered in practice. Usually a person has a combination of the three factors, with the predominance of one or two types. Often there may be no match-up between the physical and psychological characteristics described for the particular psychosomatic type. For example, a *Badahan* steadfast mind may not necessarily be in the *Badahan* body frame, but can be present in either the lean *Chi* physique or well-built *Schara* types.

APPEARANCE OF THE PATIENT

A patient's general appearance, which is affected by thoughts, desires, actions, and overall physical and mental condition, can provide an important clue for the examining physician. A person who has *Chi* disorder has worried, fearful, and examining eyes in the absence of a direct reason for this display of emotions. In *Chi* disorders, a carefully interviewed patient may report premonitions, sentimentalism, telepathy, and telekinesis. A person who has *Schara* disorder appears aggressive and tense, which may be underscored by blood-shot eyes; this appearance often brings to mind a "human machine." Upon careful interview, a picture emerges of an arrogant, contemptuous mind, with constant scheming and plotting activities, as well as workaholic and perfectionist behaviors. A person who has *Badahan* disorder appears with hollow eyes and an emotionless facial expression. The appearance often brings to mind a "mask face." The careful interview may reveal a wandering, blunt mind and feelings of persecution, prejudice, self-pity, greediness, and lack of general direction and purpose in life. These examples provide *extreme* facial and bodily expressions, which in clinical practice can be less easily distinguishable.

PRESENTING TRIADIC DISORDERS

In *Chi* disorders, the patient usually complains of feeling tired, uneasy, and giddy, and of experiencing aches and pain, shivering, and stiffness. The patient may appear hyperactive, with disorganized speech and poorly coordinated body movements. The patient may have an acidlike, rancid body odor, and the breath may be unnatural, sharp, and rusty smelling. In *Chi* disorders, the patient's tongue tends to turn red or dark brown, have irregular cracks, and be rough; the mouth may feel dry and taste bitter. The pulse feels hollow and spurts up and down.

In *Schara* disorders, the patient may report feelings of warmth, excessive sweating, thirst, frequent urination, purging, and nausea. The patient's body language exhibits impatience, and the speech is rushed, with an angry and arrogant-sounding tone. The body odor may be strong and pungent, and the breath may have a putrid smell (as in liver disorder, hyperacidity, or tooth decay), or it may smell like stomach acid. The tongue is often covered with a furry yellow to yellow-green coat. The patient may report that the mouth tastes bitter-sour. The pulse feels hard and pulsates fast.

In *Badahan* disorders, patients complain of tiredness, mental depression, and desire for sleep. They often report generalized skin itching and stiffness of extremities and joints. The patient's speech may be slow and slurred, and body reactions and movements tend to be subdued. The body odor may be rancid, and the breath may impart a "bad breath" odor (e.g., as in periodontal disease or tooth decay). The patient may report that his or her breath often *acquires* the smell of the environment. The tongue is typically covered with a white coat, and taste sensation may be diminished. The pulse feels low and beats at a slow pace.

Pulse Reading

Pulse reading is an important and complex diagnostic technique used by Tibetan physicians. Pulse reading provides information not only about the cardiovascular system, but also about other major systems and organs. The accuracy of the pulse readings depends on the patient, who should be well rested and on a light diet at least 1 day before examination; accuracy also depends on the physician's experience and ability to concentrate.

The pulse is read at the radial artery at each wrist (1 inch from the wrist joint), and the index, middle, and ring fingers are used for this purpose. The varying pressures of the three fingers are applied to determine the pulse (i.e., the ring finger is applied with more pressure than the middle finger, and the middle finger is applied with more pressure than the index finger). The three examining fingers should not touch each other. For a male patient, the physician first reads the left wrist using the right hand fingers; in a female patient, the physician first reads the right wrist using the left hand fingers. Gender differences in pulse readings are due to different anatomies of the energy channels for the lungs and heart.

Each finger feels two beats, with the radial and ulnar side of the tip. An examiner will feel heart–large intestine beats on the left wrist index finger; spleen–stomach beats on the middle finger; and left kidney–genital beats on the ring finger. Also, the examiner will feel lungs–small intestine beats on the right wrist index finger; liver–gallbladder beats on the middle finger; and kidney–bladder beats on the ring finger. In the female patient, the heart readings are taken on the right wrist, and the lung readings are taken on the left wrist. Because of the close proximity of the heart and lungs, pulse readings should not be taken on the vessels of the neck; also, pulse readings should not be taken on leg vessels because they are too far away from the vital organs.

The pulse rate is evaluated in beats per breathing cycle (i.e., inhalation and exhalation). A healthy person has 5 beats per respiratory cycle; a person with a feverish condition will have more than 5 beats; and a person with below-normal body temperature will have less than 5 beats per respiratory cycle. The pulse rate and qualitative change in the pulse beats help the physician in final diagnosis.

Evaluation of the Urine

Urine sample evaluation (i.e., odor, color, steam, bubble formation, and sedimentation) provides the physician with an important diagnostic clue. Urine evaluation, however, requires compliance and cooperation from a patient. On the evening before the examination, the patient must eat a simple diet, avoiding food rich in fats, protein, and simple carbohydrates. The patient's thirst should be quenched satisfactorily, preferably with spring water. After a good night's rest, the midstream urine passed at dawn should be collected in a clean, transparent vessel.

The urine of a healthy person should be straw-colored, form a moderate quantity of bubbles, give a typical uremic smell, and have a light vapor with moderate sediment. When the urine cools, it should have a clear appearance and whitish yellow color. The urine of those suffering from *Chi* disorder (and often elderly people) is bluish, forms big bubbles, and has a rusty smell; steam disappears quickly, and the sediment has a sprinkled appearance. Upon standing and cooling, the color of this urine remains bluish.

The urine of those affected by *Schara* disorder is dark yellow, forms few bubbles that disappear quickly, and smells like burnt butter; the steam is dense, and the sediment is plentiful. In cases of indigestion afflicting *Schara*, the urine has a food smell. Upon standing and cooling, the color of this urine remains yellow.

The urine of those suffering from *Badahan* disorder is colorless (but may be dark brown in cases of metabolic intoxication), forms small bubbles, and has a stale odor; steam disappears quickly, and the sediment is scant. Upon standing and cooling, the color of this urine becomes brown to dark brown.

THERAPY

Physician as Healer

In addition to technical knowledge, a good physician in the Tibetan tradition has to have certain qualities, including wisdom in implementing the knowledge and equal compassion for all patients. The art of healing is a result of combining those qualities. The qualities of a healer can in part be inherited but, above all, must be acquired and sustained by continuous training and contact with patients. The relationship between physician and patient should not be casual, and the mind of a physician should operate in absolute concentration (or in a *zone*) when dealing with a particular patient. The ability for absolute concentration requires continuous training of the concentrating ability of the mind on present time. As a result of the training, a physician is able to isolate his or her mind from past and anticipated future events, and instead focus on the patient. Working in the zone translates to gaining the patient's confidence, which is of paramount importance to a physician.

In the Tibetan tradition, initial eye contact is critical in establishing the physician–patient relationship. With good eye contact, a physician can convey a message of assurance to the patient and also learn about the patient's emotional and physical condition by skillfully reading the patient's eye expressions.

A proper physician–patient relationship, leading to an open-minded and positive attitude from a patient, is important for a physician, whose role is to educate patients about the nature of the disease and eventually gain full support and patient compliance with the treatment regimen. An important step in this interactive process is helping the patient realize that none of the techniques devised by humans against any disease can be as helpful as the body's own means of fighting the disease. Thus, it is important to educate patients about individual predispositions and how to take advantage of this knowledge; specifically, to increase strengths and diminish weaknesses for optimal functioning and recovery from a disease.

This physician-mediated awakening to one's abilities is particularly important in the sphere of spirituality, psychology, and emotional life. According to Tibetan medicine, our individual triadic makeup can operate at different potentials, contributing to either healing process, an intermediate state, or disease—that is, the optimal, the middle, and the lowest states. Each of these states can be recognized by a psychological and emotional profile of an individual. The optimal state is characterized by a great ability to love, compassion for everybody, poise, steadfastness, and confidentiality in relationships. The middle state is characterized by disturbed qualities of the optimal state (e.g., the inability to share one's good nature with everybody, but rather with a particular person). The lowest state does not have any good qualities, but rather certain faults (e.g., being prone to anger, inability to have gratitude and to forgive, lack of patience, inability to speak well about others, being unreliable). The role of a good physician in recognizing a patient's good qualities and faults can help enhance the patient's spirituality and bring out full potential in the healing process.

Finally, a physician's healing qualities and services should not be confused with those provided by a spiritual teacher. This confusion should be avoided, particularly in view of Tibetan tradition in which the titles *lama* or *priest* are often held by physicians. Spiritual teaching, as typically provided by a lama, should be received by a person who is healthy and ready to receive that teaching. Persons who have unresolved personal conflicts and psychological or psychiatric problems should receive professional help from a physician who is also trained as a lama. Spiritual teaching cannot be a substitute for help from a properly trained physician. Also, a healing process that is facilitated by enhanced spirituality should be augmented, in addition to the medical intervention, by living a proper life style, maintaining proper nutrition, and

meeting specific personal needs in various seasons of the year.

The State of Disease

In the practice of Tibetan medicine, disease is defined as an unphysiological increase in *Chi, Schara,* or *Badahan.* Treatment is aimed primarily at alleviating the out-of-range function. As a secondary aim, treatment adjusts the remaining two elements, which tend to be particularly afflicted in chronic conditions.

Food as Medicine

Both foods and medicines are prepared in Tibetan tradition based on specific taste combinations. There are three basic tastes groups—sweet, bitter, and sour—and their respective moderating tastes are pungent, salty, and astringent. These pairs of tastes are used to prepare meals appropriate for a specific season of the year. Also, because these tastes directly affect the psychosomatic elements of *Chi, Schara,* and *Badahan,* they may be used in regulating the corresponding taste elements. A correlation between eating habits/patterns and foods/flavors that either bring on symptoms of a disease or produce relief from symptoms is important in determining the diet for a given disease.

As a rule, *Chi* diseases are alleviated by smooth and heavy foods that taste sweet, sour, or astringent; *Chi* diseases are aggravated by rough and cool foods that taste bitter and acrid. For example, a recommended menu for *Chi* diseases includes dried meat, sour cream, butter, sesame seed oil, fresh milk, and raw sugar.

Schara diseases are treated with cool and soft foods that taste bitter and astringent; *Schara* diseases are aggravated by warm, sharp, and smooth foods that taste sour, salty, and acrid. For example, a recommended menu for *Schara* diseases includes goat and game meat, raw barley, black tea, and spring water.

Badahan diseases are treated with light, rough, and sharp foods that taste sour, salty, or astringent; *Badahan* diseases are aggravated by heavy, smooth, and cool foods that taste sweet and bitter. For example, a recommended menu in *Badahan* diseases includes mutton, fish, honey, sour milk, yogurt, and boiled water.

There are exceptions to these food rules that can be recognized by a trained practitioner. For example, some foods, although astringent, are not effective against *Chi* or *Badahan* diseases. Garlic and long pepper, although acrid, do not aggravate the diseases of *Badahan*. The cited exceptions are caused by secondary food qualities of these acrids, rendering potentially deleterious primary qualities of the food harmless (i.e., the acrid qualities of garlic or long pepper are modified by these herbs' other components, making them harmless against functions of *Badahan*). The distinction between deleterious versus harmless can often be made only by understanding the inner nature of the food stuff acquired through the ability to meditate.

Botanic Treatment

According to the tradition carried by the Badmaev family lineage, there is a regimen for herbal treatments based on the concept of proper nutrition (18). The treatment usually starts with a digestive formulation because, in Tibetan medicine, disease is considered primarily a derangement of nutrition and the nutrient delivery process. There are three kind of nutrients: nutrients derived from "mental and emotional" (sensory) food, oxygen as nu-

Table 14.2. Partial List of Products Used in Clinical Practice in Badmaev Family Tradition

FORMULA NO.	USE[c]
2[a]	Osteoarthritis, rheumatoid arthritis, gout; combined with formulae 179, 28, 162, 96, 173, 269
8[b]	Degenerative kidney disorders, pyelonephritis, nephrolithiasis, cystitis, prevention and treatment in UTI, BPH; combined with formulae 149, 179, 28, 96, 162, 173
13[b]	PMS, menopause, female infertility due to PID, endometritis, vaginitis; combined with formulae 269, 173, 137, 96, 179, 151, 155
28[a]	Peripheral vascular disease
34[a]	Chronic liver disorders, outcome of viral heptitis; prevention and treatment of cholelithiasis; maldigestion secondary to insufficient secretion of bile; combined with formulae 147, 28
85[a]	Upper respiratory tract infection, inflammation, congestion; sore throat, laryngitis; respiratory tract care, and prevention of lung disease due to indoor and outdoor pollution; combined with formulae 179, 147, 96, 173, 269
96[b]	Biological response modifier and adaptogen of thermoregulation and "living warmth"; flu, common cold; depurative in metabolic diseases, goiter; lymphoproliferative diseases; arthritis, fibromyalgia, sciatica; neuropathies; anxiety neurosis, depressive illness; combined with formulae 179, 28, 151, 162, 155, 173, 147
115[b]	Psychosomatic illness affecting gastrointestinal tract, manifesting with dyspepsia, hyperacidity, increased fermentation, irritable bowel syndrome, and peptic ulcer; combined with formulae 137, 151, 96, 269
137[a]	Psychosomatic illnesss affecting primarily stomach and small intestine, inflammatory bowel diseases, gastritis, peptic ulcer; combined with formulae 115, 28, 151, 96, 269
147[b]	Emphysema, chronic bronchitis, bronchial asthma; combined with formulae 28, 173, 96
149[a]	Male andropause; BPH; combined with formulae 151, 155, 8, 28, 179
151[a]	Depressive illness; obsessive-compulsive disorder; substance abuse, alcoholism, drug abuse; psychosomatic diseases, psychological stress; combined with formulae 179, 155, 28, 96, 173, 269, 115, 137
155[a]	Pain relief, muscle tension relief, tension headaches, migraines; poor short-term memory; combined with formulae 2, 28, 179, 34, 151, 96, 173, 269

continued

Table 14.2. Partial List of Products Used in Clinical Practice in Badmaev Family Tradition

FORMULA NO.	USE[c]
162[b]	Depurative properties, used in metabolic and chronic disorders causing retention of metabolites and toxins; lymphoproliferative disorders, biological (bacterial, viral, parasitic) and chemical intoxications (diabetes); inflammation, degenerative conditions, hepatitis, nephritis, prostatitis, venereal diseases, skin diseases (psoriasis), arthritis, atherosclerosis; combined with formulae 269, 173, 96, 179, 28, 2, 8
173[a]	Biological response modifier similar to No. 96; lowers blood pressure, slows pulse rate; decreases swelling of lymph nodes, size of enlarged spleen (lymphoproliferative diseases); decreases enlarged thyroid in cases of goiter; combined with formulae 28, 162, 96, 269
178[a]	Disorders of the veins; varicose veins, spider veins; hemorrhoids; combined with formulae 96, 28, 13, 149, 179, 173, 269
179[a]	The basic care of the digestive tract and principal formula in preventing disease; indigestion, gas, constipation, obesity, psychosomatic disorders, prevention of gastrointestinal cancer; combined with all of the formulae as needed
194[a]	Solid tumors of the GI tract; combined with formulae 269, 173, 96, 162
201[a]	Smoking deterrent providing a true sensory incompatibility with cigarette smoke, protects lungs from cigarette smoke, second-hand smoke and air pollution; combined with formulae 151, 85, 147
269[a]	Prevention of environmental and occupational conditions affecting the immune system. Biological response modifier similar to Nos. 96 and 173; combined with formulae 28, 162, 179, 96, 173

[a] Tablets, taken with sufficient water.
[b] Decoctions, prepared according to directions.
[c] Combined treatments are listed in order from most to least used.

trient, and the food-derived nutrients. Herbal and mineral formulae, as passed down in the family tradition, have been referred to as *condensed food* for specific disease conditions. Along with the treatment of the suspected nutritional pathology, the appropriate treatment of any secondary disease is instituted.

The herbal formulations are composed of several herbal and/or mineral ingredients. These formulations have been arranged based on triadic philosophy into three therapeutic groups of ingredients:

1. The main-acting ingredients.
2. The ingredients that support the main action.
3. The ingredients that prevent any untoward effects of the first two groups and increase gastrointestinal absorption of the active principles.

Table 14.2 shows a *partial* list of herbal and mineral formulae developed and used for more than 100 years in the Badmaev family tradition. Each formula is known by its numerical designa-

tion. The cited list is partial, including only the most commonly used formulae that have been made available to patients and health practitioners in Russia, Europe, and the United States.

Tibetan Massage

This form of physiotherapy is performed on the abdomen, spine, head, and neck. The massage regulates the pressure between the organs in the abdomen, improves digestion, increases the lymphatic circulation, increases the blood supply, increases peristalsis, lowers blood pressure, and improves respiration. Massage also has a stimulating effect on a patient's mental condition; in the course of therapy, the patient's psychological status changes from passive to active. Towards the end of the massage session, the majority of patients feel relaxed, and some of them even fall asleep; patients who have respiratory difficulties (e.g., asthma) start to breathe more normally during massage.

The technique of massage can be exemplified by the abdominal massage: The massage should be performed after a complete examination of the patient and exclusion of all contraindications. The patient should have an empty stomach. The hands of the physician should be warm and soft. The first contact with the abdomen must be very gentle to produce relaxation of the muscles. Massage is usually started from the right lower quadrant. The classical physiological narrowings, such as the ileocecal valve, the hepatic flexure, the splenic flexure, and the sigmoid, should be massaged longer. The right hand performs vibratory movements in the direction of peristalsis. The left hand presses slightly on the epigastrium to divert the patient's attention from the action of the right hand. The massage is carried on along the large bowel, particularly over all intumescences, until they disappear. After massage of the large bowel is complete, the epigastrium and hypogastrium along the middle line is the next area. Contraindications for this massage include all acute diseases of the abdomen, internal hemorrhage, patients receiving anticoagulant therapy, and abdominal aortic aneurysm. The massage can

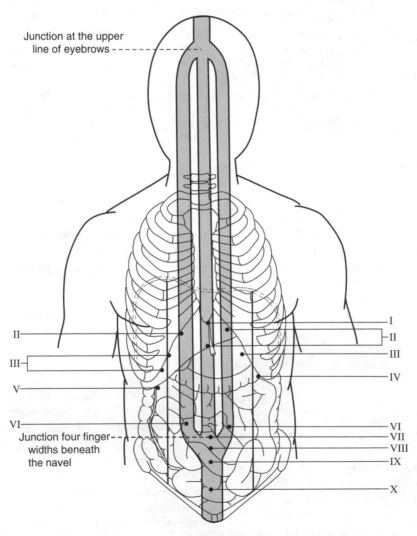

FIGURE 14.2. The massage points of the abdominal area; outline of the main energy channels (central, left, and right): I, heart; II, stomach; III, liver; IV, spleen; V, gallbladder; VI, large intestine; VII, triple caloripher; VIII, kidneys; IX, small intestine; X, urinary bladder.

concentrate on particular areas corresponding to the internal organs, as depicted in Figure 14.2.

Subtle Body and Energy Channels in Therapeutic Intervention

In many cases, Tibetan medical therapy is based on the concept of the *subtle body*, which is described as a network of channel structures carrying energy in the transformed form from the three categories of physical nutrients—that is, sensory-, oxygen-, and food-derived nutrients. In the transformed form, this energy is called *psychic energy,* which pervades the body and has a controlling and overriding role over the body's somatic functions. The subtle body is not an anatomic entity like the nervous or cardiovascular system. According to Tibetans, the subtle body can be discovered through visualization and imagination, as is done in the process of meditation. That is, this network runs parallel to the body's nerves and blood vessels, facilitating and coordinating the conductivity of neural impulses and the blood flow. The physiological processes are regarded as functions of the psychic energy.

Although the energy channels form a network maze in the body, the three main channels are most commonly described and used in Tibetan medicine therapy—that is, the central, left, and right channels, or columns. The central channel runs from the top of the head (the "Gate of Brahma," Brahma being a mythic figure of creation in Indian culture) to an area located approximately four finger widths beneath the navel called the triple caloripher, because it is formed by the merging of the three energy channels (Fig. 14.2). This central channel is visualized as hollow and blue, representing the philosophical emptiness, which is an absolute aspect of wisdom (wisdom being used interchangeably with psychic energy). The left and right columns are born out of the main channel immediately above the eyebrows, run parallel approximately 1 inch to the central channel, and rejoin it just below the navel. The left channel (visualized as white) and the right channel (visualized as red) are filled with a physical nutrient-like atmospheric air to be transformed into psychic energy.

ENERGY TRANSFORMATION

There is an exercise that leads to energy transformation best explained in conjunction with the respiratory process. During inspiration, the left and right columns are inflated with the physical air brought in through the left and right nostrils. This physical air has to be held skillfully in the area where the three channels merge. With proper mental exercise, this allows the person to visualize the transformation of the ephemeral and imperfect aspects of the physical air into the psychic air (conversion of ignorance into wisdom). Although the psychic air, or "air of wisdom," supplies the central column—providing psychic energy to the subtle body network—the remnants of physical air are exhaled. The simple way to visualize this transformation is to see the red and white color of the right and left channels, respectively, being gradually changed at the merging point with the central channel into the translucent blue color (i.e., color symbolizing the central channel).

This described exercise creates a vital energy called the "living warmth." This energy also arises when a person is experiencing the feeling of compassion. In Tibetan medicine, the living warmth is an all-important concept: It is a measure of the state of health, the ability to withstand adverse conditions, and the ability to recover from a disease. The levels of living warmth can be evaluated by a skilled practitioner by analyzing the overall appearance of the patient; the way he or she listens, speaks, and behaves; and pulse reading.

Preventive and therapeutic interventions are aimed at securing the physiological flow of energy in the subtle body. For example, the *moxa* technique uses both mechanical and thermal stimuli to influence the subtle body. In this technique, a needle slightly covered with a vegetable tinder is placed at the *moxa*-point on the skin, and then the tinder is lit at the upper end of the needle. The needle is removed at the moment the smoldering tinder touches the skin. This treatment aims to remove the energy blockage and redirect the flow of energy to the deprived sections of the subtle body. A similar purpose is served by yogic breathing exercise, massage, and Tibetan pharmacological treatments.

USE OF TIBETAN MEDICAL PRACTICE IN THE CONTEMPORARY HEALTH CARE SYSTEM

Integration of Tibetan medicine into contemporary health care requires properly trained medical professionals in the United States and other countries. Training activities are needed to provide ready-to-use information for the accredited programs in medical schools and to develop new diagnostic and therapeutic methods derived from ancient, time-proven traditions.

Major Indications/Preventive Value

In addition to the discussion of Tibetan medicine's approaches as a means to attain health, the concepts of synthesis medicine and Tibetan pharmacology are inspirations for a better health care delivery system.

SYNTHESIS MEDICINE

The terms *medycyna syntetyczna* and *syntetische medizin,* corresponding to the English term *synthesis medicine,* was first used in 1930s Tibetan medicine literature (27). The term refers to a specific reasoning in diagnostic and therapeutic approach. Practicing synthesis medicine is based on a physician's ability to deal effectively with a medical condition with relatively simple means of diagnosis and treatment at his or her disposal. For example, with a single measurement of the radial pulse, a well-trained Tibetan practitioner can obtain an in-depth reading from the patient's organs and body systems. By comparison, Western medicine uses a sum of analytic findings taken separately that results in a *synthetic* picture and diagnosis of a disease. According to synthesis medicine, a patient is not a compilation (a sum) of parts working together, but an outcome of a psychosomatic fusion, or *synthesis,* occurring within the mind and body. In synthesis medicine, the patient, rather the cell, is seen as the elementary unit on which the diagnostic and therapeutic efforts are focused.

The concept of the subtle body provides important insight into the theoretical precepts of synthesis medicine. The subtle body and its energy channels run parallel to the cardiovascular and nervous systems of the body. Whereas the cardiovascular and nervous systems are the anatomical entities, the energy channels can be perceived only through meditation and visualization techniques. This comparison may illustrate a distinguishing feature of synthesis medicine: Because the subtle body can be accessed by visualization, it cannot and does not need to be analyzed to be *perceived.* However, the anatomical cardiovascular and nervous systems need to be dissected and analyzed; based on these analyses, the structure and functioning of the systems emerge.

In general, practicing synthesis medicine brings a physician closer to a patient. The synthesis approach allows the physician to grasp the "big picture" in the process of diagnosis, treatment, and follow-up, effectively minimizing diagnostic and therapeutic errors. Practicing synthesis medicine leads to diagnosis and treatment primarily because of the physician's ability to relate to the patient at both personal and psychological levels.

The synthesis approach does not diminish the importance of analytical thinking. In fact, Tibetan medical texts provide plenty of examples of analytical approaches (e.g., anatomy and physiology charts, distinguishing types and subtypes of a particular disease, and the causative and symptom-oriented treatments). Therefore, synthesis medicine complements the analytical approach by maintaining focus on a patient and the totality of that patient's well-being.

The theory of synthesis medicine is best represented by the triadic concept. Understanding the interaction among the *Chi, Schara,* and *Badahan* is helpful in developing skills of synthesis thinking. For example, understanding that element *Chi* leads to *Schara* and subsequently results in *Badahan* provides a model for the synthesis.

TIBETAN PHARMACOLOGY

The design of Tibetan pharmacological therapies was the result of synthesis medicine. These therapies are based on a *uniform three-group design* for each pharmacological preparation (i.e., providing active ingredients, ingredients to modify gastrointestinal absorption, and ingredients to offset the potential adverse effects of the active ingredients). The broad range of therapeutic activity secured by this design has provided a basis for a recent discussion of the newly defined bioprotectant mechanism of Ayurveda- and Tibetan-based formulae; that is, pharmacological action operating through *prevention* and *intervention* on the disease pathology (28). This approach leads to very complex combinations of herbs (Table 14.3).

Table 14.3. Ingredients of Formula 28*

Aegle sepiar fructus (L. Raffin) 0.02
Amomum medicinalis fructus (L. Merril) 0.025
Aquilegiaviridifolia foliae (Linn.) 0.015
Calendula officinalis flores (Linn.) 0.005
Camphora japonicum (Nees.) 0.02
Costus amarum radix (Dcne. Clarke) 0.04
Calcium sulfate 0.02
Elettaria cardamomum fructus (Maton) 0.03
Eugeniacaryophyllata fructus (Spreng. Thunb.) 0.012
Glycyrrhiza glabra radix (Linn.) 0.015
Hedychium spicatum rhizoma (Ham. ex. Smith) 0.01
Lactuca sativafoliae (Linn.) 0.006
Lichen islandicus (Ach.) 0.04
Melia toosend fructus (Linn.) 0.035
Plantaginis lanceolata herba (L.) 0.015
Polygonum aviculareherba (Linn.) 0.015
Potentilla aurea herb (L.) 0.015
Prunus spinosus flores (L.) 0.005
Pterocarpus santalinus lignum (Linn.) 0.03
Andropogon muriaticus (L.) 0.01
Santalum album lignum (Linn.) 0.03
Sida cordifolia radix (Linn.) 0.01
Terminalia chebulae fructus (Retz.) 0.03
Valeriana officinalis radix (Linn.) 0.01
Aconitum nepellus radix (Linn.) 0.001

* = in 500-mg tablets.

Research: Comparison to Western Pharmaceuticals

The following formulations and a description of related research are examples of how treatment modalities derived from Tibetan medicine can gradually be introduced into contemporary health care through continuous research. Continuous research to validate and improve those therapeutic herbal methods is important. For example, a Tibetan treatment successfully implemented through a research program led to the standardization of 25 herbal and mineral ingredient nutraceuticals with clinically proven efficacy in 5 double-blind studies in the treatment of peripheral vascular disease (PVD) (29–33). This formula is referred to here as Formula 28. Ingredients of the formula are listed in Table 14.3.

According to a literature data comparison, Formula 28 appears to provide more therapeutic benefit than most cited pharmaceutical drugs in improving PVD conditions (Table 14.4). Based on these findings and indications from Tibetan medical theory, the results of an open field study in improving mental performance in elderly patients (44), the effectiveness of the formula in treating CNS inflammatory vascular condition in experimental animals (28), and plans for a clinical study of Formula 28 in patients with the memory loss due to cerebrovascular insufficiency are in process.

THE FUTURE

Based on past and recent history, the development of botanic treatments derived from Tibetan medicine will continue and complement the development of synthetic drugs. As illustrated in Figure 14.3, both developmental processes from the different pharmacological concepts are complementary in that they provide different approaches for research and improvement of pharmacological treatments.

Integration of Tibetan medicine with Western medical practice can improve existing health care systems considerably. But it is not only a matter of advanced technology that allows people to become and feel healthier. Despite tre-

Table 14.4. Comparison of Badmaev Formula 28 Therapeutic Results with Those of Synthetic Pharmaceutical Drugs in Improving PVD

COMPOUND NAME	DURATION OF TREATMENT	PERCENT INCREASE OF MAXIMAL WALKING DISTANCE	REFERENCE
Formula 28	12 weeks	54%*	29
	16 weeks	98%	30
	16 weeks	93%	31
	16 weeks	97%	32
	16 weeks	112%	33
Pentoxifylline [Trental]	24 weeks	58%	34
	4 weeks	40%	35
	24 weeks	33%	36
	8 weeks	47%	37
	24 weeks	50%	38
	90 days	25%	39
Neftidrofuryl [Praxilenel]	24 weeks	70%	40
	12 weeks	54%	41
Buflomedil [Loftyll]	12 weeks	97%	42
	90 days	28%	39
Bencyclan [Fludilat]	6 weeks	34%	43
Nifedipine	90 days	21%	39

* Hurlimann study assessed pain-free walking distance.

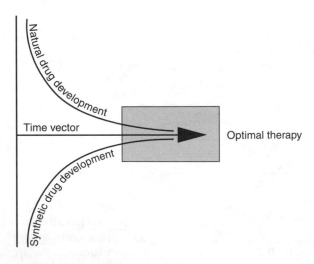

FIGURE 14.3. Coexistence of the development of natural and synthetic drugs.

mendous advancement in medical technology, we, as a modern society, are still plagued with chronic disease. We need, therefore, to learn more, and in different ways. To learn and understand more, we may have to set aside preconceptions and follow the advice of the European philosopher and Tibetan scholar, Cyrill von Korvin-Krasinski: ". . . theoretical medical science cannot be separated from its practical application, nor the teaching from life in community, nor the finished doctrine be acquired without personal experience of its truth." To experience and perceive Tibetan medicine firsthand is the best way to understand it.

DEDICATIONS

To the work of my predecessors, my wife Eulalia Badmaev, MD, and son Michael.

ACKNOWLEDGMENTS

Thanks and appreciation go to Dr. Muhammed Majeed, Todd Norton, Thomas & Dee Mower, William S. Coury, Curtis Jacquot, Dr. Maja Nowakowski, Dr. Henry M. Wisniewski, Dr. Georgia Schuller-Levis, Dr. Peter B. Kozlowski, Dr. George Weissmann, Ms. Janette Carlucci, Ms. Jackie Woottan, and Dr. Herbert Schwabl.

REFERENCES

1. Sarton G. The time of Jabir Ibn Haiyan. In: Sarton G, ed. Introduction to the history of science. Baltimore: Williams & Wilkins, 1927:520–542.
2. Kunzang J. History of Tibetan medicine. In: Kunzang J, ed. Tibetan medicine. Berkeley and Los Angeles: University of California Press, 1973:8–28.
3. Clifford T. Tibetan Buddhist medicine and psychiatry. The diamond healing. The medicine of dharma. York Beach, ME: Samuel Weiser, Inc., 1984:13–33.
4. Clifford T. Tibetan Buddhist medicine and psychiatry. The diamond healing. The medicine of dharma. York Beach, ME: Samuel Weiser, Inc., 1984:35–45.
5. Dhonden LY. Tibetan medicine a short history. Tibetan Rev 1974;17:13–14.
6. Beckwith ChI. The introduction of Greek medicine into Tibet in the seventh and eighth centuries. J Am Oriental Soc 1979;99:297–313.
7. Clifford T. Tibetan Buddhist medicine and psychiatry. The diamond healing. The medicine of dharma. York Beach, ME: Samuel Weiser, Inc., 47–63.
8. Tenzin Wangyal. Wonders of the natural mind. The essence of Dzogchen in the native bon tradition of Tibet. Tarrytown, NY: Station Hill Press, 1993:218.
9. Olschak BC. The art of healing in ancient Tibet. CIBA Symposium 1973;12:129–134.
10. Clifford T. Tibetan Buddhist medicine and psychiatry. The diamond healing. Introduction by Dr. Lokesh Chandra. York Beach, ME: Samuel Weiser, Inc., 1984:XV–XX.
11. Berthenson LB. O russkich buddistah I ob tibetskoj medicinie. St. Petersburg: Ruskii Vrach 1906; 5:418–421.
12. Berthenson LB. Uber russische Buddistah und die sogenannte tibetanische Medzin. Med Wochenschr 1906;24:248–257.
13. Semicov BV. Die tibetische Medizin bei den Burjaten. Janus 1935;39:1–2.
14. Kowalewski K. Wladimir Badmajeff, Tibetan doctor in Europe. J Res Indian Med 1973;8:101–109.
15. Editorial in Med Tribune. Father-son MD team have Tibetan legacy. Med Tribune (USA) 1983; July 13:13.
16. Rockwood M. Tibetan cure. OMNI 1985;6:24, 148.
17. Ross M. Tibet: ancient remedies gain new acceptance as research explore "mysterious" medicines. The Medical Post (Canada) 1990;July 10:14.
18. Kunzang J. The life of the great physician-saint g Yu-thog Yan-tan mGon-po. In: Kunzang J, ed. Tibetan medicine. Berkeley and Los Angeles: University of California Press, 1973:147–319.
19. Winder M. Introduction. In: Kunzang J, ed. Tibetan medicine. Berkeley and Los Angeles: University of California Press, 1973:1–7.
20. Badmaev PA. O sistemie vrachebnoi nauki Tibeta (On the Tibetan medical system). Contains translation and commentaries on the first two books of the yGyud-Bzhi, St. Petersburg:1898:234.
21. Csoma de Koros A. Tibetan studies (a reprint of the articles contributed to the Journal of the Asiatic Society of Bengal). J Asiatic Soc Beng 1911; 7:1–172.
22. Badmajew P, Badmajew V, Park L. Healing herbs. Berkeley: Lotus Press, 1982:80.
23. Glatfelter RE. Peter Badmaev. In: Wieczynski JL, ed. The modern encyclopedia of Russian and Soviet

history. Vol. 2. London: Academic International Press, 1976:234–237.

24. Grekova T. Tibetska Medicina vy Rossii (Tibetan medicine in Russia). Nauka Religia 1988;August 8;10–15.

25. Badmajeff W. CHI SCHARA BADAHAN Grundzuge der tibetanische Medzin (Autorisierte Uebersetzung von Dr. Anna Koffler-Harth). Johannes Baum Verlag: Pfulligen in Wurtt 1933:47.

26. Korvin-Krasinski C von. Die Tibetische Medizinphilosophie. Zurich: Origo-Verlag, 1953:339.

27. Kunzang J. Bibliography of European works on Tibetan medicine. In: Kunzang J, ed. Tibetan medicine. Berkeley and Los Angeles: University of California Press, 1973:98–102.

28. Badmaev V, Kozlowski PB, Schuller-Levis GB, Wisniewski H. The therapeutic effect of an herbal formula Badmaev 28 (Padma 28) on experimental allergic encephalomyelitis (EAE) in SJL/J mice. Phytother Res. In Press, 1998.

29. Hurlimann F. Eine lamaistische Rezeptformel zur Behandlungderperipherenarteriellen Verschlusskrankheit [A lamaistic formula for the treatment of peripheral arterial occlusive disease]. Schweiz Rundsch Med 1979;67:1407–1409.

30. Schrader R, Nachbur B, Mahler F. Die Wirkung des tibetanischen Krauterpraparates Padma 28 auf die Claudicatio intermittens [The effect of the Tibetan herbal preparation Padma 28 on intermittent claudication]. Schweiz MedWochenschr 1985; 115:752–756.

31. Samochowiec L, Wojcicki H, Kosmider K, et al. Wirksamkeitsprufung von Padma 28 bei der Behandlung von Patienten mit chronischen arteriellen Durchblutungsstorungen [Potency test of Padma 28 in the treatment of patients with chronic arterial circulatory disturbances]. Polbiopharm Rep 1985; 21:3–40.

32. Drabaek H, Mehlsen J, Himmelstrup H, Winther K. A botanical compound, Padma 28, increases walking distance in stable intermittent claudication. Angiology 1993;44:863–867.

33. Smulski HS, Wojcicki J. Placebo-controlled, double-blind trial to determine the efficacy of the Tibetan plant preparation Padma 28 for intermittent

claudication. Alternat Therap Heath Med 1995; 1(3):44–49.

34. Porter JM, Baur GM. Pentoxifylline: pharmacologic treatment of intermittent claudication. Surgery 1982;92:966.

35. Volker D. Behandlung von Arteriopathien mit Trental 400. Ergebnisse einer Doppleblindstudie. Med Welt 1979;29:1244.

36. Porter JM, Cutler BS, Le BY, et al. Pentoxifylline efficacy in the treatment of intermittent claudication. Am Heart J 1982;104(2):66–72.

37. Bojan A. Beneficial hemorheologic therapy of chronic peripheral arterial disorders with pentoxifylline: results of double-blind study versus vasodilator-nylidrin. Am Heart J 1982;103:864.

38. Lindgarde F, Jelnes R, Bjorkman H, et al. Conservative drug treatment in patients with moderately severe chronic occlusive peripheral arterial disease. Circulation 1989;80(6):1549–1556.

39. Chacon-Quevedo A, Eguaras MG, Calleja F, et al. Comparative evaluation of pentoxifylline, buflomedil and nifedipine in the treatment of intermittent claudication of the lower limbs. Angiology 1994;45(7):647–653.

40. Phole W, Hirche H, Barmeyer G, et al. Doppelblindstudie mit Naftidrofuryl-Hydrogenoxalat bei Patienten mit peripherer artereller Verschlusskrankheit. Med Welt 1979;30:269–272.

41. Maass U, Cachovan M, Alexander K. Einfluss eines kontrollierten Intervall trainings auf die Gehstrecke bei Patienten mit Claudicatio intermittens. VASA 1983;12:326–332.

42. Trubestein G, Balzer K, Bisler H, et al. Buflomedil bei arterieller Verschlusskrankheit. Ergebnisse einer kontrollierten Studie. Dtsch Med Wschr 1982; 107:1957–1981.

43. Holle W, Schneider B. Bencyclan, Pentoxifylline und Placebo bei peripheren Durchblutungsstoerungen. Mod Medizin (Germany, West) 1980; 8(4):167–177.

44. Panjwani HK, Priestley J, Lewis AE. Clinical evaluation of Padma 28 in treatment of senility and other geriatric circulatory disorders: a pilot study. Alt Med 1987;2(1):11–17.

CHAPTER 15

CHIROPRACTIC MEDICINE

Dana J. Lawrence

BACKGROUND

Definition and Descriptions

Chiropractic is one of the major branches of Western medicine. The major difference between chiropractic and other forms of Western medicine, such as osteopathy and allopathic medicine, is that chiropractic focuses on the spine as integrally involved in maintaining health, providing primacy to the nervous system as the primary coordinator for function, and thus health, in the body. The approach of chiropractic is the maintenance of optimal neurophysiological balance in the body, which is accomplished by correcting structural or biomechanical abnormalities or disrelationships. The primary method for accomplishing this balance is spinal manipulation, known as the chiropractic adjustment.

FOUNDER AND KEY FIGURES

The following are the key figures from chiropractic's history:

Daniel David Palmer (1845–1913) was the founder of the profession. His interest in healing grew from his initial forays into spiritualism and magnetic healing. His adjustment of Harvey Lillard led to the creation of the chiropractic profession. He founded the first chiropractic school in 1898.

Bartlett Joshua Palmer (1882–1961) was the son of Daniel Palmer. Bartlett voraciously promoted the profession and helped keep its flame alive during years of trial and tribulations.

Solon Langworthy (dates unknown) was a student of David Palmer. He founded his own school and introduced the use of traction tables and naturopathic remedies to the fledgling profession.

Oakley Smith (1880–1967) was another early Palmer graduate. He felt that the true cause of interference to the nervous system came from cramping in the connective tissue, which he called a *ligatite*. He later founded the naprapathic profession, and he was coauthor with Langworthy and Minor Paxon of the first chiropractic text, *A Textbook of Modernized Chiropractic* (1).

John A. Howard (1876–1954) was the founder of today's National College of Chiropractic (then the National School of Chiropractic). He had left Palmer's college with the blessing of David Palmer after disagreeing with the direction that Bartlett had chosen for the Palmer School. Howard emphasized a scientific approach to training chiropractors, referred to today as *rational chiropractic*.

William Schulze (1870–1936) purchased the National School of Chiropractic from John Howard and maintained the emphasis on training in basic science.

Willard Carver (1866–1943) was a tremendously influential early chiropractor who developed a systems approach to subluxation that emphasized compensatory adaptations to preexisting subluxations elsewhere in the spine. He also influenced early legislative and licensing laws for the profession.

Tullius Ratledge (1881–1967) helped pass

the first licensing regulation in the nation and went to jail rather than accept a license as a drugless healer. He founded Ratledge College, which is known today as Cleveland Chiropractic College in Los Angeles.

John Nugent (1891–1971) was to chiropractic education what Abraham Flexner was to medical education—the man who almost single-handedly revamped its educational system. Under his direction as Director of Education for the National Chiropractic Association (known today as the American Chiropractic Association), he led reforms to standardize the chiropractic curriculum and to move the chiropractic institutions to become nonprofit and professionally owned.

Leo Spears (1884–1956) was the founder of the first chiropractic hospital, the Spears Hospital and Free Clinic for Poor Children.

Joseph Janse (1909–1985) was a man of formidable intellect and perseverance who led the National College of Chiropractic for 38 years (Fig. 15.1). Under his stewardship, the college made a number of important advances for the profession. He helped found the Council on Chiropractic Education, the National Board of Chiropractic Examiners, the Federation of Chiropractic Licensing Boards, scientific councils, and the residency program in chiropractic radiology. His college was first to receive regional accreditation and the first to found a journal (the *Journal of Manipulative and Physiological Therapeutics*) that became internationally indexed; it remains the only chiropractic journal indexed in *Index Medicus*.

Carl Cleveland (1896–1982) led two chiropractic colleges for 60 years. His sons, Carl, Jr., and Carl III, also led chiropractic colleges. Carl III is currently the president of Cleveland Chiropractic College.

There are many significant historical figures not mentioned in this list. A more comprehensive list would also include Sylvia Ashworth, Homer Beatty, William Budden, Andrew Davis, James Drain, James Firth, Arthur Forster, Henri Gillet, Almeda Haldeman, George Hariman, George Haynes, Arthur Hendricks, A. Earl Homewood, Fred Illi, Craig Kightlinger, Lyndon Lee, Joy Loban, Hugh and Vinton Logan, Ernest Napolitano, Earl Rich, Leo Steinbach, Harry Vedder, Claude Watkins, and Clarence Weiant as just some of those who played a significant role in chiropractic's historical development. Even a comprehensive list does not account for many of the "movers and shakers" helping the profession in modern times.

KEY PUBLISHED WORKS AND REFERENCES

Important texts of the early and middle period of chiropractic are listed in Table 15.1 (1–11). Also, one of the most complete lists of early chiropractic texts can be found in the reference list to Gaucher-Peslherbe's text *Chiropractic: Early Concepts in Their Historical Setting* (12).

The modern era of chiropractic texts was ushered in by the 1975 publication of *The Research Status of Spinal Manipulative Therapy* (13), edited by Murray Goldstein. This text grew out of a critically important workshop held under the auspices of the National Institute of Neurological and Communicative Disease and Stroke. Since then, a large number of texts have

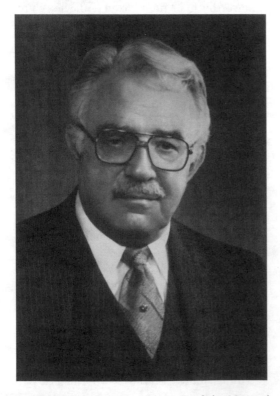

FIGURE 15.1. Joseph Janse (courtesy of the National College of Chiropractic).

Table 15.1. Important Texts of the Early and Middle Chiropractic Era

Early Texts (1906 to 1917)

A Textbook of Modernized Chiropractic (1)

The Chiropractor's Adjuster: A Textbook of Science, Art and Philosophy of Chiropractic for Students and Practitioners (2)

The Chiropractor (3)

The Science of Chiropractic: Its Principles and Philosophies (4)

Carver's Chiropractic Analysis of Chiropractic Principles as Applied to Pathology, Relatology, Symptomatology, and Diagnosis (5)

Principles and Practice of Spinal Adjustment: For the Use of Students and Practitioners (6)

Encyclopedia of Chiropractic (the Howard System) (7)

Midperiod Texts (1947 to 1962)

Fundamentals of Chiropractic from the Standpoint of a Medical Doctor (8)

The Vertebral Column: Life Line of the Body (9)

Neurodynamics of the Vertebral Subluxation (10)

Chiropractic Principles and Technic (11)

been published. In part, this growth of texts is due to market forces; there are more students in chiropractic college, and more practitioners scattered around the country, so there is an obvious market waiting to be tapped. Also, many chiropractic texts have been published because of the growth of chiropractic research and education; more faculty and researchers means a greater critical mass of potential writers. Some of the best texts of the past two decades are listed in Table 15.2, although this list should not slight any of the many other texts or authors who made important contributions to the chiropractic biomedical literature during the past 20 years.

History and Development

Although manipulation has been used as a medical therapy since ancient times, the chiropractic profession itself only celebrated its centennial in 1995. The profession was founded when Daniel David Palmer (Fig. 15.2), an itinerant scholar,

Table 15.2. Important Texts of the Modern Chiropractic Era

Modern Developments in the Principles and Practice of Chiropractic (1980) (14)

Chiropractic: History and Evolution of a New Profession (1992) (15)

Essentials of Skeletal Radiology (1987) (16)

The Chiropractic Theories (1995) (17)

Low Back Pain: Mechanism, Diagnosis and Treatment (1990) (18)

Fundamentals of Chiropractic Diagnosis and Management (1987) (19)

Whiplash Injuries (1995) (20)

Foundations of Chiropractic: Subluxation (1996) (21)

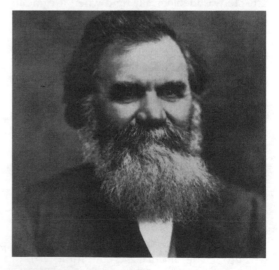

FIGURE 15.2. D. D. Palmer (courtesy of the National College of Chiropractic).

grocer, and magnetic healer, was able to restore the hearing of Harvey Lillard, who had suffered from deafness for some time. Lillard had noted that his hearing loss began after he felt something "snap" in his neck. Palmer palpated for the spinous process, found it abnormally positioned, and reasoned that this abnormal position, or *subluxation*, could be involved in the etiology of the hearing loss. Palmer thus was involved in two "firsts"—the use of the spinous process as a lever for manual adjusting of the spine, and the application of then current medical knowledge to create a new approach to healing, based on his contention that illness is effectively functional and becomes organic only as an end process (22).

From this inauspicious beginning, within two years Palmer had founded his first Chiropractic School and Cure; at the same time, he expanded on the concept of the subluxation as a factor in creating, contributing to, or perpetuating disease. For his efforts, Daniel Palmer is now known as "The Founder."

Daniel's son, Bartlett Joshua (Fig. 15.3), took over his father's college when he was only 25 years of age. Within 10 years, Bartlett had developed one of the nation's largest nonmedical institutions, and thus was later known as "The Developer" of chiropractic. A truly controversial figure, Bartlett's entrepreneurial spirit helped protect and expand the fledgling healing art. He was ideologically rigid when it came to his healing art, and it was under his stewardship that a schism that still exists within the chiropractic profession began. Bartlett was essentially a fundamentalist concerning chiropractic, practicing what came to be known as *straight* chiropractic. It was Bartlett's unyielding beliefs that ultimately led John A. Howard to found the National School of Chiropractic, seen today as the leading institution following the *mixer* approach to chiropractic. The split between Bartlett Palmer and John Howard started over the former's refusal to obtain cadavers for anatomical study, which Howard felt was essential for proper anatomical study. Howard, with the help of William Schulze, created a rational alternative to chiropractic practice and education (23).

Those early days of chiropractic were fraught with trouble, both with education and licensure (or lack thereof). Many chiropractors were sent

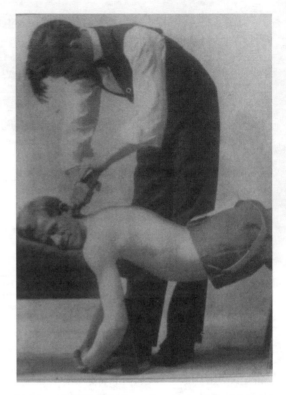

FIGURE 15.3. B. J. Palmer (courtesy of the National College of Chiropractic).

to jail for practicing without a license, even after being offered the opportunity to pay a fine in lieu of jail (24). At the same time, the educational institutions had many of the same problems that beset their medical counterparts and which led to the famous Flexner Report (25). Some institutions were quite good, but many were poorly equipped and managed. The Flexner Report spurred the development of the modern day Council on Chiropractic Education, which was initiated under the early leader of John Nugent.

PRINCIPAL CONCEPTS

There are four general areas that chiropractic philosophy and practice emphasize:

1. **Nervous system.** In the human being, the nervous system is highly evolved and developed and influences all other body systems. It therefore plays important roles in health and disease.

2. *Vis medicatrix naturae.* The human body has an innate ability to heal itself and seeks to maintain that health via homeostatic mechanisms.

3. **Effect of subluxation or joint dysfunction.** When subluxation or joint dysfunction is present in the body, it may interfere with the ability of the neuromuscular system to act in an optimal fashion, and may therefore lead or contribute to the presence of disease.

4. **Diagnosing and treating subluxation.** One primary goal of chiropractic diagnosis and treatment is to identify, via appropriate medical and chiropractic procedures, subluxations and dysfunctions and to correct or eliminate them. This will then optimize the healing process in the human body.

Because an assessment of the spine is paramount in determining the presence of subluxation or joint dysfunction, the chiropractic physician relies more heavily on manual palpation of the body than other health care practitioners. This palpation and its associated procedures are performed alongside other standard medical diagnostic procedures.

Chiropractic is a holistic form of health care that recognizes that function cannot be separated from structure. This belief is not only from a macroscopic point of view but also from a cellular, microscopic view.

The National College of Chiropractic, in its "Profile of the Practice of Chiropractic" (26), provides a comprehensive statement regarding modern-day chiropractic practice. This statement admirably summarizes modern chiropractic practice and the principles on which that practice is based:

The National College of Chiropractic holds that the practice of the chiropractic physician embraces the whole person with emphasis upon conservative health care which facilitates the inherent potential of the human organism to develop and maintain a state of self-regulation and to invoke self-healing processes with minimal therapeutic risk at reasonable cost. Chiropractic practice embodies:

- Recognition of a diversity of factors which impact upon human physiology, among which are biomechanical dysfunction, genetics, trauma, hygiene, microorganisms, nutritional status, exercise, motion, posture, environment, stress, emotion and human relationships.

- Primary care of patients based upon diagnostic evaluation, including patient history, physical examination, clinical laboratory data, diagnostic imaging, and other special diagnostic measures, as well as those procedures which are unique to the chiropractic evaluation of human spinal and structural balance and integrity.

- The application of a diversity of spinal and other adjustments and manipulations for the treatment, correction, and prevention of neurologic, skeletal or soft-tissue dysfunction and the production of beneficial neurologic effects.

- The use of other conservative means including, but not limited to, nutritional counseling, physiologic therapeutics, meridian therapy/acupuncture, trigger point therapy, life-style counseling, emotional support and stress management.

- The chiropractic doctor is a primary-care, first-contact physician who practices within the legal scope of licensure, emphasizes the importance of the doctor/patient relationship, recognizes the need for other kinds of treatment when indicated, and who, therefore, interacts fully with other members of the health care delivery team, always in the best interest of the patient (26).

There is a continuing intraprofessional debate about the role of modern chiropractic. One faction feels that chiropractic is a primary health care profession that should have full "gate-keeper" status for managing the health concerns of its patients, whereas the second faction feels that chiropractic should take pride in its ability to act as a strict musculoskeletal specialty, given that low back pain is ubiquitous and pervasive in modern culture. This debate is ongoing, and no consensus has yet developed, although it appears that the chiropractic colleges have for the most part hewed to the primary care approach.

PROVIDER-PATIENT INTERACTION

Patient Assessment Procedures

The chiropractic physician uses the same standard diagnostic approach as that of the medical or osteopathic physician, but adds a number of special procedures unique to the chiropractic profession as described.

HISTORY-TAKING AND PHYSICAL DIAGNOSIS

A visit to the chiropractor starts with a history (anamnesis) and a standard physical examination, the latter driven by the specific presentation of the patient. A standard systems review (e.g., cardiovascular system, genitourinary system, gastrointestinal system) is part of the examination, as is neurological examination, orthopedic examination, radiological examination, and so on as required by the specific nature of the patient's case.

OTHER DIAGNOSTIC METHODS: SPINAL EXAMINATION

Bergmann has succinctly noted that the chiropractor views the human body as a dynamic, integrated, and complex living system which, having innate intelligence, therefore has a re-

markable capacity for self-healing (27). Chiropractors can serve as a gatekeeper for entry into the health care system and as a potential primary care practitioner. (Chiropractors are primary care practitioners in the eyes of many, but not in the eyes of some.) The chiropractic physician must by necessity be able to use the findings from a standard physical examination, integrate them with the findings from chiropractic procedures, and then use the combined information to fashion both an appropriate diagnosis and management plan for the patient.

Given that spinal adjustment is the primary therapeutic tool used by a chiropractor, spinal examination becomes a paramount part of the patient evaluation process. Spinal examination allows the chiropractor to determine the nature of the lesion, whether subluxation or spinal dysfunction. There are a number of procedures used to evaluate the spine. Bergmann has coined the term *PARTS* to help define the diagnostic criteria for identifying spinal dysfunction (Table 15.3) (28). Within the parameters formed by these components are a number of specific procedures, including postural analysis (via plumb line examination or via more sophisticated computer systems), gait analysis, static articular palpation, motion palpation, muscle strength testing, spinal percussion, and motion analysis.

Palpation, in general terms, is the art of feel-

Table 15.3. PARTS: Diagnostic Criteria for Identifying Spinal Dysfunction (28)

P: Pain/Tenderness
Pain and tenderness should be defined in terms of their location, quality, and intensity. Pain is typically seen in most musculoskeletal conditions. Pain and tenderness may be identified using the procedures of observation, palpation, and percussion.

A: Asymmetry
This may occur at the gross level, the sectional level or the spinal segmental level, and can be identified via observation (i.e., of gait or posture), palpation, and radiographic analysis.

R: Range of Motion Abnormalities
There should be assessment of active motion, passive motion, and motion into the paraphysiological space (joint play, or accessory motion). There may be elements of increased, decreased, or aberrant motion. The most common manner in which range of motion is examined is by motion palpation, although stress radiographs may be helpful.

T: Tissue, Tone, Texture, and Temperature Abnormality
These may accompany structural or functional changes affecting the spine. They can be identified via observation, palpation, heat sensing devices, algometers, and tests for strength and stretch.

S: Special Tests
A variety of special tests (e.g., electromyography, diagnostic ultrasound) might be considered, where appropriate, to provide more comprehensive information.

ing by hand to determine a variety of parameters governing the health and mobility of the tissues on or near the surface of the body. Static palpation is used to help analyze the bony or soft tissue structures of the body in a fixed position (e.g., palpation of the location of the spinous process). Motion palpation, which was originally developed by the Belgian chiropractor Henri Gillet (29), is designed to help assess the dynamic motion of the vertebrae and extravertebral joints. Specifically, it assesses the presence or absence of joint play, an accessory joint motion not under direct control of the voluntary muscles. Postural analysis helps determine the presence of gross (i.e., directly observable) physical abnormalities. This may be accomplished through visual observation using a plumb line or through computerized systems such as the Metrecom device.

Differential Diagnosis

DISEASE CLASSIFICATION AND TAXONOMY

Chiropractors use standard medical diagnostic and disease classifications, but differ in the manner in which they assess involvement of the human nervous system in disease processes. The key concept undergirding the chiropractic profession is that of *subluxation*, which should not be interpreted in the medical sense of "less than a luxation." The concept of subluxation has undergone continual evolution and controversy. There is no single, agreed-on definition, although a recent consensus panel defined subluxation as "a motion segment in which alignment, movement integrity, and/or physiologic function are altered although contact between joint surfaces remains intact" (30) The role of subluxation in health and disease is considered a significant area for chiropractic research. The presence of subluxation, however defined, and its related neurological sequelae are seen as important concomitants of disease states or other conditions.

DETERMINING TREATMENT

Treatment is determined by combining the results of the standard physical examination with the results of specialized chiropractic examination procedures. For example, a patient who has suffered a bout of back pain will undergo a standard physical examination, which might determine that the problem is essentially an uncomplicated strain. The chiropractic examination will then determine which specific areas of the spine are involved as well as which areas are to be adjusted and how they are to be adjusted.

THERAPY AND OUTCOMES

Treatment Options

The basic therapeutic tool used by a chiropractic physician is the chiropractic adjustment, which is applied to the articulations of the body, particularly to those located in the spine. Chiropractors also use a host of other interventions, including physiotherapeutic tools and devices, exercise, nutrition, and orthotics. In addition, when the patient's condition warrants, the best tool may be referral to a medical practitioner.

The chiropractic adjustment helps restore proper motion between articular surfaces, which then has potentially beneficial effects on the nervous system. Within the chiropractic profession, many schools exist, each with a specified body of technique to offer. Included in these are the Activator technique, diversified technique, Cox flexion/extension technique, sacro-occipital technique, Gonstead technique, Thompson terminal point technique, Logan basic technique, and upper cervical technique.

Description of Treatments

The chiropractic adjustment is delivered to joints in the spine or extraspinal regions of the body. The adjustment entails placement of the doctor's hands onto contact points on the body, followed by positioning of the joint and, most often, a high-velocity short-amplitude thrust to that joint. Force is introduced by the doctor for that to occur, although the actual maneuver is gentle.

For example, a patient with a mild strain

of the low back musculature may receive the following approach to therapy (obviously there is some variability in the approach selected by any individual doctor): Assuming that the patient's problem is uncomplicated low back pain, the course of therapy may begin with the use of hot moist packs followed by gentle soft tissue massage, such as a petrissage procedure. Some chiropractors may follow this with trigger point therapy to deactivate any active trigger points, followed perhaps by an electrical modality, such as high-volt galvanism or interferential current; other chiropractors might not use these procedures at all. Finally, the patient will receive the adjustment.

Before the adjustment, the doctor would have already assessed the patient's spine, likely using a palpatory procedure, such as motion palpation. Areas of decreased mobility or static malposition would be noted, and adjustments would then be directed to those regions. For purposes of example, assume that there is a rotational restriction noted at the fourth lumbar vertebra on the right. The patient would then be placed on his or her side, with the side of restriction placed up. The patient's lower arm would be placed under the head; the upper arm would be placed on the side of the body. The up leg would be bent so that the foot can be placed near the knee of the lower leg. The doctor would then position him or herself so that the cephalad arm is placed on the patient's arm, and his or her body would be placed so that it comes over the patient's body. The caudal hand would have its pisiform placed on the spinous process of the fourth lumbar vertebra. After removing tissue tension by rotating the patient gently, the thrust is gently but quickly delivered in a posterior to anterior direction.

The profession has designed a multitude of such procedures for all areas of the human body.

Treatment Evaluation

A number of outcomes may be used to monitor patient progress:

- Changes in scales, such as the visual analogue scale or the Oswestry instrument
- Changes in function, as may be assessed by a

variety of parameters: EMG, Oswestry scale, Roland-Morris scale, neck disability index, headache diary
- Changes in spinal mobility, as may be assessed by motion palpation
- Patient response to therapy

Thus, it is possible to look for either decreases in pain (or other symptomatology) or increases in function (e.g., muscle strength, spinal mobility).

Pain may be assessed through visual analogue scales or pain drawings. Function may also be assessed through manual palpation of the spine to determine mobility of individual spinal motion segments.

Research has indicated that spinal manipulation is most useful in the short term for patients suffering a variety of low back and cervical problems (31). Thus, such improvements in pain and function occur within a relatively short period of time (i.e., within about two weeks). However, there is a growing body of evidence to show that these improvements may extend over longer amounts of time (32, 33).

As in most forms of medical care, treatment is altered when care fails to provide expected results, the patient does not respond, or the situation worsens.

USE OF THE SYSTEM FOR TREATMENT

Major Indications

CHIROPRACTIC AS A PRIMARY APPROACH

Most people associate chiropractic with treatment for low back pain, and indeed that is where the greatest amount of scientific support exists. There is strength of evidence for the use of manipulation in patients suffering from low back pain without radiculopathy when used in the first month of problems (34).

In general, chiropractic finds its greatest usefulness in managing conditions affecting the neuromusculoskeletal system, such as strains, sprains, disk disease or herniation, tendinitis, bursitis, headache, spondylolisthesis, whiplash injury, osteoarthritis, myofascial pain, disorders of the cervical, thoracic, and lumbar spine and pelvis, and so forth. These conditions comprise the so-called Type M disorders. There are also visceral conditions that have spinal overlays and that are managed by chiropractors (e.g., hypertension [35]). Bergmann, Peterson, and Lawrence provide a more complete discussion of this topic (28).

CHIROPRACTIC AS A COMPLEMENTARY APPROACH

The use of chiropractic care in specific visceral conditions, such as hypertension or ulcer, is complementary rather than primary. The chiropractic physician works alongside another medical or osteopathic physician in managing the musculoskeletal manifestations that accompany the disease process.

Contraindications

Chiropractic management is less useful or not recommended in managing infectious disease and other Type O conditions. Risks for complications caused by manipulation, though, are quite low (36). Manipulation is contraindicated in situations in which vertebral artery narrowing is present, when aneurysm is present, and with tumor, bone infection, and fracture. Gatterman lists these conditions as absolute contraindications (37). This list is not comprehensive; common sense should rule.

Preventive Value

Hawk and Dusio (38) surveyed 753 randomly selected chiropractors to assess their attitudes towards prevention-related training, especially those that pertain to primary care practice. Although this study did not assess actual knowledge or training in prevention-related topics, it did provide an overview of the attitudes that drive these issues. Of the 65% who did respond, the majority (greater than 90%) considered themselves primary care practitioners, although less than 80% thought they had received adequate training in primary care during their chiropractic education. The more recent graduates reported greater amounts of such training.

Hawk and Dusio concluded that there is an apparent need for greater training in matters pertaining to preventive and primary care.

Scope of Practice

Scope of practice is dictated by state law, and therefore varies from state to state. Some states are more liberal in what they allow, whereas others are restrictive (the so-called 10 finger states). Lamm (39) has shown that greater than 50% of those state licensing boards that responded to a questionnaire (90% response rate; 54 of 60 questionnaires returned) allow the following procedures:

- Ordering or performing clinical laboratory procedures
- Routine physical examination
- Female pelvic examination
- Rectal examination
- Electromyography
- Nerve conduction velocity studies

Greater than 80% of the states that answered the questionnaire allow x-ray examination, Doppler studies, and either computed tomography or magnetic resonance imaging. And greater than 90% allow chiropractors to employ physiotherapy, adjust soft tissue or extremities, provide vitamin supplements, and perform impairment ratings (39). A full state-by-state breakdown of allowable procedures can be found in Lamm's article.

ORGANIZATION

Training

GENERAL REQUIREMENTS

In general, chiropractic colleges in the United States require the following criteria for matriculation (40):

- High school diploma
- A minimum of 2 years of 60 semester credit hours (90 quarter hours) leading to a bachelor's degree in the arts or sciences

–Those credits must be earned in an accredited institution (as listed in the United States Office of Education's Directory of Colleges and Universities)

–Those courses must be from appropriate areas of study, such as the biological sciences, general or inorganic chemistry, organic chemistry, physics, psychology, English, humanities, social sciences, or communication skills

• The College Level Examination Program (CLEP) is accepted

For people from foreign countries who desire entry into United States chiropractic colleges, the entry requirements are the same as those for a native citizen. Transcripts from foreign countries may be evaluated by outside agencies, depending upon the country of origin. Recently, several chiropractic colleges have announced efforts to raise entry requirements, so that both higher grade-point averages and more college course work are necessary. Advanced standing credit may be awarded if previous college course work matches that of the specific curriculum, although no credit can be awarded for clinical course work.

BASIC CURRICULUM OF CHIROPRACTIC EDUCATION

There are three basic components to chiropractic education: basic science course work, clinical science course work, and clinical internship.

Basic science course work tends to fall in the earlier semesters of the curriculum. Topics covered in detail include anatomy, biochemistry, histology, microbiology, physiology, genetics, embryology, and so on. The mid to latter semesters, before the final internship, are generally composed of the clinical science courses. These include general diagnosis, biomechanics, all chiropractic technique classes, radiological diagnosis, orthopedic diagnosis, neuromusculoskeletal diagnosis, neurology, cardiology, nutrition, rehabilitation and exercise, physiological therapeutics, and so on. These courses combine standard medical diagnostic and therapeutic procedures (excluding invasive procedures, pharmacology, and surgery) with specific chiropractic diagnostic and therapeutic procedures,

such as motion palpation, radiographic mensuration, and various types of chiropractic manipulative procedures. The final internship involves application of the didactic portion of the program in a controlled clinical setting and under the supervision of licensed chiropractic physicians.

The typical course of study is 5 academic years; this can be completed, if a student takes summer courses, in a little less than four complete years. Basic science course work generally occurs during the first 4 (of 10) semesters of the curriculum. Clinical science courses are then taken in the next 4 semesters, and the full internship program then takes place in the final 2 semesters. A semester lasts approximately 4 months. The total number of hours over the entire course is approximately 5000.

A movement within the chiropractic educational community toward problem-based education is introducing students to clinical matters far earlier in the chiropractic program than was traditional. It has also allowed for a potentially more effective integration of basic and clinical science courses than in the past. This is rather new, with only two colleges (National and Los Angeles) moving toward full problem-based learning programs, although many others have initiated smaller changes in their curriculum.

Most colleges, and some state and professional organizations, also offer full postgraduate and continuing education programs, some of which offer a variety of specialty certifications.

Quality Assurance

LICENSURE AND CERTIFICATION

In the United States, licensure requires the student to have (1) passed all courses in the chiropractic curriculum with a passing grade average per department, (2) pass all elements of the National Board of Chiropractic Examiners examinations, and (3) pass the licensure test for the specific state in which the chiropractor desires to practice. All applicants for licensure must also have attended a chiropractic college accredited by the Council on Chiropractic Education (CCE), or one that meets equivalent standards. The CCE has developed educational standards for chiropractic education. This specialized accrediting body focuses its attention on the particular program that the chiropractic college uses. There is also institutional accreditation within chiropractic, such as might be conferred by the North Central Association of Schools and Colleges or the Western Association of Schools and Colleges; this examines the entire institution rather than just its program.

McNamee notes that "the accreditation of an institution by an institutional accrediting body certifies to the general public that the institution: (a) has appropriate purposes; (b) has the resources needed to accomplish its purposes; (c) can demonstrate that it is accomplishing its purposes; and (d) gives reason to believe that it will continue to accomplish its purposes" (39). Other countries have their own accreditation process: for example, the Australasian Council on Chiropractic Education, the Council on Chiropractic Education (Canada), and the European Council on Chiropractic Education.

All 50 states and the District of Columbia have their own chiropractic licensing boards, as do the provinces of Canada. There are also licensing boards in other countries, including Australia, Belgium, Denmark, France, Great Britain, Italy, Japan, Netherlands, Norway, Puerto Rico, South Africa, Sweden, Switzerland, and other European and Asian countries.

PROFESSIONAL SOCIETIES

The profession is served by a multitude of professional societies, ranging from American national organizations, such as the American Chiropractic Association (the largest association in the profession) and the International Chiropractic Association, to national foreign organizations (e.g., the Japanese Chiropractic Association or the Canadian Chiropractic Association), to state and provincial organizations, and to research organizations such as the Foundation for Chiropractic Education and Research. In the United States, each state is served by at least one chiropractic organization, and some have more than one (including Pennsylvania, Illinois, and Michigan). States in which there are more than one organization reflect the different philosophies regarding the practice of chiropractic.

CONTINUING EDUCATION

Postgraduate and continuing education is regulated by statute and differs from state to state or from country to country. In general, each state requires a certain number of continuing education hours yearly; these hours may be earned by attending postgraduate classes offered by the colleges or state and professional organizations. These courses may cover the gamut from orthopedics to nutrition, from chiropractic technique to neurology, to sports therapy and radiology. Some hours may be earned by reading professional scientific publications. In addition, the majority of chiropractic colleges offer residency postgraduate programs. Current residency programs include orthopedics, radiology, neurology, family practice, research, rehabilitation, sports and recreational injuries, ergonomics, physiological therapeutics, meridian therapy/acupuncture, and pediatrics. These programs require 2 years of on-campus training beyond initial degree status.

Reimbursement Status

Chiropractic is covered under most insurance policies and is involved in managed care networks.

Relations with Conventional Medicine

Although the two professions have a history characterized by rancor and ill will, this has changed substantially in the last decade as chiropractic research and practice has grown. The Wilk trial (41) may have been the impetus for some of this change in that it finally made organized medicine take stock of the positions it had held for so long. Wilk and some other chiropractors brought suit against the AMA, AOA, and 10 other medical organizations, charging that they had conspired to unreasonably restrain the practice of chiropractic; a permanent injunction against the AMA was entered in 1987. Today, chiropractors can be found on staff at many hospitals, chiropractic research is respected and important, and chiropractors are playing significant roles in both legislative and research matters. As a result, the cooperation between the two professions is growing, and the traditional opposition to chiropractors has decreased. It is not, however, absent.

Most medical professionals recognize that chiropractors refer patients when appropriate, and good working relationships between the two professions exist everywhere. Referrals are also made from medical physicians to chiropractors. This is perhaps the best recognition of the diagnostic and therapeutic acumen that chiropractors possess. Indeed, perhaps the greatest challenge for the profession today comes not from medical opposition, but from within the profession itself as it tries to communicate to policy makers charged with reforming health care. The profession's move toward evidence-based practice will be of significant aid in this regard.

PROSPECTS FOR THE FUTURE

The chiropractic profession has undergone an unprecedented growth in its public and professional acceptance. Today, the United States has over 55,000 chiropractors, and nearly another 12,000 are enrolled in the nation's chiropractic colleges. Chiropractic research has contributed significantly to basic understanding of low back pain, cervical pain, and headache, and is involved in examining several other major health problems, including dysmenorrhea, carpal tunnel syndrome, and otitis media. Chiropractors have begun to enjoy staff privileges in hospital settings, and some colleges are again offering rotations through participating hospitals. Chiropractors participate on federal panels and organizations, such as the Office of Alternative Medicine of the National Institutes of Health. They have also been involved in programs, such as merit review for the Interdisciplinary Training Grants for Rural Health Care program run under the auspices of the Health Resources and Services Administration (HRSA) (M. Brand, personal communication, May 1995).

An area of great potential is in the growth of the chiropractic profession outside the United

States. The World Federation of Chiropractic (WFC) has been invited to join the World Health Organization (DA. Chapman-Smith, personal communication, January 1997). The WFC represents the interests of chiropractic associations and chiropractors from a multitude of locations, including Ireland, Great Britain, France, Italy, Mexico, Japan, Taiwan, Norway, Sweden, Switzerland, and Finland, and this is by no means a complete list. Chiropractic has a growing presence outside its traditional stronghold in the United States. An example is the new RMIT:Japan Unit, a college based in Japan and coordinated through the Royal Melbourne Institute of Technology. The latter institute has its own chiropractic college.

Most chiropractic colleges are private, nonprofit institutions. Of the chiropractic colleges in the United States, only the University of Bridgeport College of Chiropractic has an institutional affiliation. The Canadian Memorial Chiropractic College is now investigating university affiliation. Two chiropractic colleges are becoming universities: Palmer University (through combining its Palmer and Palmer West colleges) and Life University (which now offers programs in addition to the chiropractic program). National College is investigating implementing master's degree programs (D. Wickes, personal communication, March 1997). Whether there will be a greater movement towards university affiliation remains to be seen, but it would be a welcome development.

Managed care offers its own set of challenges. The chiropractic profession would like to see the adoption of an "any willing provider" provision of health care reform, fearing that many gains might be lost if it is deprived of playing a role in the managed care networks under development, especially those that require a medical gatekeeper. This situation is in tremendous flux, and it remains to be seen how this will evolve. It is interesting to note that chiropractic-specific reimbursement codes have been developed.

Curriculum revision is occurring within the chiropractic institutions. Programs such as Los Angeles College of Chiropractic's *Advantage* curriculum and National College of Chiropractic's *Guided Discovery* curriculum are exploring full-blown problem-based education. Other programs have made their own in-roads into curriculum revision, although not to the scale that these two institutions have.

The issue of whether chiropractic is primary care must be debated further. The vast majority of chiropractic practices involve spinal manipulation for musculoskeletal issues. In many situations, however, it is incontestable that chiropractors do render primary care. This is especially true in the rural setting, where the chiropractor may be the sole deliverer of health care for the community. Efforts are currently underway to develop collaborations between chiropractic physicians and Area Health Education Centers (AHECs). HRSA made special effort to include chiropractors as merit reviewers in the Interdisciplinary Training Grant for Rural Health Care program. The thinking was that because chiropractors now represent a significant force in health care, it would be smart to consider them in terms of answering shortages that exist in delivery of health care to medically underserved areas. There now stands a chance that approximately every 4 years another 10,000 chiropractors will enter the work force; efforts must be made to do long-term planning to address national needs and trends.

A growing number of people within the chiropractic profession would argue that chiropractic medicine is no longer complementary and alternative medicine but now mainstream.

REFERENCES

1. Langworthy SM, Smith OG, Paxson MC. A textbook of modernized chiropractic. Cedar Rapids, IA: American School of Chiropractic, 1906.
2. Palmer DD. The chiropractor's adjuster: a textbook of the science, art and philosophy of chiropractic for students and practitioners. Portland, OR: Portland Printing House, 1910.
3. Palmer DD. The chiropractor. Los Angeles: Beacon Light Publishing Co., 1914.
4. Palmer BJ. The science of chiropractic: its principles and philosophies. Davenport, IA: Palmer School of Chiropractic, 1917.
5. Carver W. Carver's chiropractic analysis of chiropractic principles as applied to pathology, relatology, symptomatology, and diagnosis. Oklahoma City, OK: Warden-Elbright Printing Co., 1909.
6. Forster AL. Principles and practice of spinal adjustment: For the use of students and practitioners. Chicago: National College of Chiropractic, 1915.
7. Howard JF. Encyclopedia of chiropractic (the Howard system). Chicago: National College of Chiropractic, 1912.
8. Beiderman F. Fundamentals of chiropractic from the standpoint of a medical doctor. Germany: Haug Verlag, 1959.
9. Illi FWH. The vertebral column: life line of the body. Chicago: National College of Chiropractic, 1951.
10. Homewood AE. Neurodynamics of the vertebral subluxation. Thornhill, Ontario: self-published, 1962.
11. Janse J, Hauser H, Wells BF. Chiropractic principles and technic, 2nd ed. Chicago: National College of Chiropractic, 1947.
12. Gaucher-Peslherbe PL. Chiropractic: early concepts in their historical setting. Lombard, IL: National College of Chiropractic, 1993:228–261.
13. Goldstein M, ed. The research status of spinal manipulative therapy. Workshop held at the National Institutes of Health, February 2–4, 1975. National Institutes of Neurological and Communicative Disorders and Stroke (NINCDS). Bethesda, MD: DHEW Pub. No. (NIH76–998).
14. Haldeman S. Modern developments in the principles and practice of chiropractic. New York: Appleton-Century-Croft, 1980.
15. Wardwell W. Chiropractic. History and evolution of a new profession. St. Louis: Mosby Year Book, 1992.
16. Yochum TR, Rowe L. Essentials of skeletal radiology. Baltimore: Williams & Wilkins, 1987.
17. Leach R. The chiropractic theories, 3rd ed. Baltimore: Williams & Wilkins, 1995.
18. Cox JM. Low back pain: Mechanism, diagnosis and treatment. 5th ed. Baltimore: Williams & Wilkins, 1990.
19. Lawrence DJ, ed. Fundamentals of chiropractic diagnosis and management. Baltimore: Williams & Wilkins, 1987.
20. Foreman S, Croft A. Whiplash injuries, 3rd ed. Baltimore: Williams & Wilkins, 1995.
21. Gatterman M. Foundations of chiropractic: subluxation. St. Louis: Mosby Year Book, 1996.
22. Gibbons R. Evolution of chiropractic. In: Haldeman S. Modern developments in the principles and practice of chiropractic. New York: Appleton-Century-Croft, 1980.
23. Beideman RP. Seeking the rationale alternative: the National College of Chiropractic 1906 to 1982. Arch J Assoc Hist Chiropr 1983;3:17–23.

24. Gibbons RW. Go to jail for Chiro. J Chiropr Humanities 1994;4:61–71.
25. Flexner A. Medical education in the United States and Canada. New York: Carnegie Foundation for the Advancement of Teaching, 1910.
26. National College of Chiropractic. Profile of the Practice of Chiropractic. Lombard, IL: National College of Chiropractic, 1989.
27. Bergmann TF. Chiropractic technique. In: McNamee KP, ed. The chiropractic college directory: 1994–95. Los Angeles: KM Enterprises, 1994.
28. Bergmann TF, Peterson D, Lawrence DJ. Chiropractic technique. New York: Churchill Livingstone, 1993.
29. Gillet H, Liekens M. Belgium chiropractic research notes. Davenport, IA: Palmer College of Chiropractic, 1951.
30. Gatterman MI, Vernon H. Development of chiropractic nomenclature through consensus. J Manipulative Physiol Ther 1994;17:302–309.
31. Shekelle PG, Adams AH, Chassin MR, et al. The appropriateness of spinal manipulation for low back pain. Santa Monica: RAND, 1991.
32. Koes BW, Bouter LM, Mameran van H, et al. Randomized clinical trial of manual therapy and physiotherapy for persistent back and neck complaints: results of one year follow up. Br Med J 1992;304:601–605.
33. Meade TW, Dyer S, Browne W, et al. Low back pain of mechanical origin: randomised comparison of chiropractic and hospital outpatient treatment. Br Med J 1990;300:1431–1437.
34. Bigos S, Bowyer O, Braen G, et al. Acute low back problems in adults. Clinical practice guideline No. 14. AHCPR Publication No. 95-0642. Rockville, MD: Agency for Health Care Policy and Research, Public Health Service, U.S. Department of Health and Human Services. December, 1994.
35. Crawford J, Hickson G, Wiles M. The management of hypertensive disease: a review of spinal manipulation and the efficacy of conservative therapeusis. J Manipulative Physiol Ther 1986;9:27–31.
36. Gatterman M. Contraindications and complications of spinal manipulative therapy. ACA J Chiro 1981;18:S75–S86.
37. Gatterman M. Chapter 4: Complications of and contraindications to spinal manipulative therapy. In: Gatterman M, ed. Chiropractic management of spine-related disorders. Baltimore: Williams & Wilkins, 1990:55–69.
38. Hawk C, Dusio ME. A survey of 492 U.S. chiropractors on primary care and prevention-related issues. J Manipulative Physiol Ther 1995;18:57–64.
39. Lamm LC, Wegner E, Collord D. Chiropractic scope of practice: what the law allows—update 1993. J Manipulative Physiol Ther 1995;18:16–20.
40. McNamee KP, ed. The chiropractic college directory: 1994–95. Los Angeles: KM Enterprises, 1994.
41. Wilk CA et al. vs. AMA et al. Complaint 76C3777 filed October 12 in the United States District Court for the Northern District of Illinois, Eastern Division.

CHAPTER 16

OSTEOPATHY

Harold Goodman

BACKGROUND

Definition

Osteopathy, or osteopathic medicine, may be defined as a complete system of health care that teaches and practices according to the following tenets (1):

1. The body is a unit.
2. The body has its own self-protecting and self-regulating mechanisms.
3. Structure and function are reciprocally interrelated.
4. Treatment proceeds from the first three principles.

As a primary care practitioner, the osteopathic physician uses any and all therapeutic and diagnostic approaches that best support these principles and most effectively, gently, and functionally promote local and systemic homeostasis.

Founder

Andrew Taylor Still, MD (1828–1917), the father of osteopathy, was an allopathic physician and Civil War surgeon who practiced in the midwestern United States during the nineteenth century. After many years of practice and clinical observation, he concluded that what was called health care was mostly fixated on disease and that medicine per se consisted of the suppression of symptoms and little else. He was galvanized into action by the death of several of his children to spinal meningitis. He thought that the enlightened mind of humans could certainly come up with something better than what passed for medicine. He believed that by diligently observing nature and, specifically, the living anatomy and physiology of humans, some guidance might be gleaned. Over the years he evolved a system of diagnosis and treatment, which he announced to the world in 1874 as osteopathy. *Osteo*, the Greek word for bone, emphasized the new approach to physical and nonphysical structure.

History and Development

Dr. Still saw his work as a reformation of medicine, surgery, and midwifery (obstetrics) and as an expansion of the traditional medical–surgical model (2). It was never his intention to start a new profession. He believed that over time logical, rational men and women would accept his contributions for the overall betterment of society. Instead he was hounded by the medical community, driven out of Kansas where he practiced, and ended up in Kirksville, Missouri. In 1892 in Kirksville, he founded the first school of osteopathy, the American School of Osteopathy. This school, which was empowered by the state to award the MD degree, instead issued a new degree, the doctor of osteopathy (DO), which distinguished its graduates from the medical profession and insured professional and legal autonomy. A major emphasis in the osteopathic curriculum was a mastery of the basic sciences, especially anatomy (which he called the alpha and omega of osteopathy), as well as applied physiology. Dr. Still also emphasized the mastery of osteopathic philosophy, which he believed was his major contribution to the discipline. Specific manipulative technique was not initially taught. Dr. Still believed that, based on a thorough background in applied basic science, a well-supported diagnosis, and reasonable skill, any osteopathic physician could devise a treatment for any specific condition. However, within a few years, *technique*, as osteopathic treatment was termed, became an established part of the nascent curriculum. Dr. Still saw osteopathy and medicine as diametrically opposed and loudly denounced attempts to integrate the two approaches. Traditional osteopathy continued to grow (by the time of Dr. Still's death in 1917, there were 5000 DOs). But by the 1940s, when early antibiotics were introduced, the previously drugless profession of osteopathy began to embrace pharmacology and a symptom-oriented medical model.

Although there has always been a small, active minority embracing and attempting to implement classical osteopathic approaches, the majority of osteopathic graduates and the professional osteopathic colleges have adopted the allopathic model with little training in traditional osteopathic principles. However, within the last few years the trend has begun to reverse; more and more younger osteopaths show interest in Dr. Still's original teachings and observations. For example, the Undergraduate American Academy of Osteopathy, which was almost moribund in the early 1980s, is quite vibrant today. Most of these practitioners participate in the American Academy of Osteopathy and its subsections, such as the Cranial Academy. Over the years, entirely new territories have been developed in the art and science of osteopathy. Some examples are the cranial concept (3); the embryological approach (best exemplified by the work of James Jealous, DO, of the New England College of Osteopathic Medicine); the use of the percussion hammer (as exemplified by the teachings of Robert Fulford, DO, for over 15 years); and fluid- and energetic-based approaches to osteopathy.

Key Published Works and References

The history of the profession is chronicled in two books. The first book, by E. R. Booth (2), covers the profession up to the 1920s, whereas the second book, by Norman Gevitz (4), covers the profession up to the 1970s. The Gevitz book is written by someone outside the profession and is thought by some osteopaths to contain historical inaccuracies and major omissions of key aspects of osteopathic history.

The literature of osteopathy is available in both monographic and journal form. Unfortunately, much of the classical literature is out of print. However, many of the classics in osteopathy are being republished by the American Academy of Osteopathy and by Health Resources Press. Dr. Still published four books, including *The Autobiography of A. T. Still*, *Philosophy of Osteopathy*, and his final work, *Osteopathy: Research and Practice* (1910). From a clinical perspective, his most valuable work is *The Philosophy and Mechanical Principles of Osteopathy* (1902). Arthur Hildreth, a friend and student of Dr. Still, wrote and published an excellent biography, *The Lengthening Shadow of Dr. Andrew Taylor Still*. Other outstanding authors and leading figures in the profession include:

- William Garner Sutherland, who discovered the cranial concept
- Beryl Arbuckle, one of the most creative developers of the cranial concept and the leading authority on osteopathic pediatrics
- Carl McConnell, a skilled, prolific writer on core concepts in osteopathy
- F. P. Millard, the leading developer of the osteopathic approach to lymphatics
- Rollin E. Becker, a student of Dr. Sutherland
- Robert Fulford, a student of Drs. Sutherland and Arbuckle and developer of the percussion hammer

Some of these authors have only published in journals. In addition, there are a number of other recent authors, such as Kuchera, Greenman, Mitchell, Jones, and others represented in the bibliography.

The *Journal of the American Osteopathic Association* (*JAOA*, 1901 to present) has an excellent index up to the mid-1950s, after which much of the journal's index can be found in the *Index Medicus*. Two other excellent but unfortunately defunct journals are the *Journal of Osteopathy* and *Osteopathic Profession*; the former ran from 1892 to around 1967, was founded by Dr. Still, and contained articles by him and his original students. Several anthologies based on these and other osteopathic journals are available from Health Resources Press.

Overall, the best representation of osteopathic thought outside of the pre-1950 years of the *JAOA* and the writings of Dr. Still can be found in the *Yearbooks of the American Academy of Osteopathy*, a monograph that ran from 1938 to the late 1970s, after which issues have been released only sporadically.

PRINCIPAL CONCEPTS

Dr. Still often said that his major contribution to osteopathy was in the realm of ideas, principally in the elaboration of osteopathic philosophy, which he believed was an accurate reflection of the essential laws of nature applied to the human being.

The first principle of osteopathy is that the body is a unit and functions as such. Reductionistic attempts to view the body as a collection of disparate parts ignore the reality that this is not how the system actually functions. The next principle is that structure and function are reciprocally interrelated. This is a central underlying theme of all osteopathic work, which, in diagnosis and practice, distinguishes it from other health care systems. The form or structure (from the macroscopic to the microscopic level) of each living creature is a perfect reflection of its function. Osteopathic physicians believe that nature is deliberate in its evolutionary development. Dr. Still would often study human structures and ask, "Why, in order to best accomplish its function, *must* this bone take the form that it does?" In this manner, the osteopathic physician can intimately understand the human biosystem. And, just as structure absolutely governs function, abnormal structure governs dysfunction.

Other basic principles of osteopathy are (5):

- The body possesses self-regulatory mechanisms.
- The body has the inherent capacity to defend and repair itself.
- When normal adaptability is disrupted or when environmental changes overcome the body's capacity for self-maintenance, disease may ensue.
- Movement of body fluids is essential to health.
- The nervous system plays a crucial role in controlling the fluids of the body.
- There are somatic components to disease that are not only manifestations of disease, but also are factors that contribute to maintenance of the diseased state.

These basic principles are, as applicable, elaborated on many levels because humans are viewed as simultaneously experiencing physical, emotional, mental, and spiritual realities. Dr. Still alluded to this in part when he presented his discovery of what he called the Law of Mind, Motion, and Matter. In this sense, motion in the patient is seen as a material manifestation of the effects of the underlying forces in the universe.

A consistent theme in osteopathy is to constantly support the system in its quest for homeostasis and normalized function. Osteopathy concentrates on health and not on the eradication of disease; it is a system that views the body as an ally and teacher, not as the enemy or simply a mass of tissues; and it is a system that embraces life and all of its manifestations as part of a greater, intelligent, self-generating, self-healing Unity.

PROVIDER-PATIENT ASSESSMENT

The purpose of osteopathic evaluation and patient assessment is to provide sufficient interaction with the patient to initiate the treatment phase.

The physician begins by observing the patient. This observation includes but is not limited to body habitus, dress, emotional state, posture, and anything else that may reflect the essential, underlying patterns of the patient as a unique individual. As the patient walks into the examination room (assuming he or she is ambulatory), the physician pays close attention to how he or she moves through space.

The history and physical examination are of crucial importance in osteopathy. They form the foundation for future clinical work and must be undertaken in a careful and thorough manner. The history covers the major medical parameters; specific information about prenatal, labor, and delivery history; and neonatal, pediatric, and adolescent physical and psychosocial history. Significant traumas and illnesses must also be elicited. The physician also must determine if the patient is right- or left-handed and if this was ever consciously or otherwise changed.

In eliciting the chief complaint as well as other complaints, the practitioner must accurately establish the onset of symptoms and specific history of any pathological development. It is especially important to understand the personal factors (e.g., family or personal crises, emotional traumas) that occurred in the patient's life within six months preceding and up to the complaint. This information may change the physician's understanding of the situation. Previous therapies of any nature must be elicited.

THE STRUCTURAL EXAMINATION

General Considerations

As in any approach to medicine, the physician must develop certain clinical skills to gather sufficient data. There are many exercises that assist the clinician or student in further developing palpatory abilities (6). For example, some of my teachers had us practice placing our hand on the center of a long table which had a coin tucked under one of its legs. Our job was to identify the location of the coin by palpating the center of the table. Another exercise involved placing a hair under successive sheets of paper and then to accurately identify its location under the many sheets. An elderly clinician who graduated from an osteopathic college in the early 1940s told me that he was asked to identify

bones placed in a bag. Normally this would not be difficult; however, all of the bones has been disfigured, with many of the major landmarks removed, and the remainder of the bones were cut into small pieces. From this point, the physician graduates to palpating the living system in all of its subtlety and dynamic manifestation.

Just as someone who lives in a foreign country is under a tremendous handicap if he or she fails to comprehend the local language, so too will the physician be extremely limited in his or her work with the living system if he or she fails to learn the language of the living body. The system is *alive*. The living body has the ability to communicate to the physician in the most incredible manner, but only if the physician is open to receiving the information being offered. Many clinicians view the body as a thing to be experienced via the lens of laboratory tests, radiography, and other static interactions with a living, dynamic system. From the osteopathic perspective, the overreliance on static information is one of the greatest shortcomings of medicine, especially when it becomes the main arbiter of how one approaches the patient.

RESPIRATION

In observing the patient, the physician should note the full extent of respiration. Subtle respiration may be sensed all the way from the clavicles to the pubes in a healthy patient; anything less than this is dysfunctional and is later addressed in treatment. The osteopathic approach to functional anatomy identifies several diaphragms, including, but not limited to, the tentorium cerebri, tentorium cerebelli, fascial-muscular aspect of the thoracic inlet, the diaphragm proper at the thoracic outlet, and the pelvic diaphragm. Any asynchronous functioning of these structures is noted.

POSTURE

Posture in both the static and dynamic state is a major source of clinical data. Because osteopathy is particularly concerned with the structure–function relationship in the living system, osteopaths are especially interested in understanding the ways the musculoskeletal system homeostatically adapts to various physical (e.g., gravity) and nonphysical (e.g., emotional) stressors. On one level, this is referred to as postural compensation and takes in all structures from the base of the skull to the feet. Because of gravity, osteopaths are especially interested in the more caudad structures like the lower extremities, sacrum, and pelvis and their relationship relative to more cephalad regions. This perspective enables the practitioner to readily identify structural compensation for somatic dysfunction in other areas. These patterns manifest underlying tendencies on the part of a system that is constantly seeking homeostatic balance on all levels.

Several factors lead to postural compensation, including traumatic, personal conditions (e.g., emotional state), and abnormal gait. Other patterns, including various forms of scoliosis, kyphosis, and lordosis, of both anatomic and functional nature, are noted.

LEG LENGTH

Apparent leg length discrepancies are important to identify because they adversely affect the structure–function of anything cephalad. In general, osteopathic physicians have noted that actual anatomic leg length discrepancies are rare compared with functional states secondary to sacral base dysfunction and lumbar rotoscoliosis.

Observation and Palpation

Observation is conducted on numerous levels, ranging from the gross to the subtle. Gross observation may reveal relative asymmetry of the body in general (e.g., left versus right), as well as of specific regions or structures relative one to the other (e.g., scapulae, levels of the iliac crests, levels of the mastoid processes).

Palpation may also be conducted on numerous levels, ranging from the gross to the subtle. Certain osteopathic practitioners have reputations for their skills in palpation on very subtle levels. Major factors that greatly influence palpation results include personal intention when undertaking the task as well as where or on what level the physician's attention or focus is placed.

The practitioner must learn to distinguish

normally functioning tissue from any variation from the anatomico-physiological norm. Because most medical curricula focus on disease, recognition of normal function requires additional study on the part of the physician.

Basic palpatory skills may help confirm the acuteness or chronicity of a complaint. Much of this is related to the action of the sympathetic nervous system over time on the musculoskeletal realm. Another vital component noted during palpation is *skin drag*. Skin drag represents relative resiliency of the superficial tissues and fascia. For example, with the patient in the supine position, the physician places the palm of his or her hand on the sternum and with slight posterior pressure makes contact and then slowly rotates the hand to the right and then to the left. In a dysfunctional state, the hand rotates better in one direction compared with the other. Variations of this maneuver may be performed all over the body and can provide valuable information regarding the functional state of the fascias.

Tissue findings during palpation, including tone, temperature, relative resistance to pressure, texture, and moisture, also provide information regarding the sympathetic nervous function in the region. In addition, segmental muscle and visceral function may be evaluated both directly and indirectly using palpation.

Informed muscular palpation may yield extremely valuable information. For example, one of the most commonly found causes of sciatica is secondary to contraction of the piriformis muscle. Evaluation takes approximately 5 to 10 seconds and, besides providing instant feedback, may save much needless and costly traditional workup. Other important muscles commonly implicated in major symptomatic complaints include the scalenes (so-called thoracic outlet syndrome); various intraoral muscles, especially the masseter (temporomandibular joint pain); and the psoas (incapacitating low back pain). The writings of Janet Travell, MD, are most helpful for students of such palpation (7).

Evaluation of fascial function is key to the osteopathic evaluation. The main dysfunctions found in the fascia, which is ubiquitous, being continuous from the most macroscopic to the microscopic levels (it actually ensheathes individual muscle fibers), involve sprains and various strain patterns. These are secondary to a variety of sources, including postural, emotional, traumatic, and others. Some of these patterns may be recent, whereas others may be traced back to early traumas. One aspect of such palpation actually allows the clinician to approximately date the onset of the dysfunction. Regardless of the origin, these fascial dysfunctions all inevitably contribute to functional impairment, resulting in disease and pathology on many levels. Dr. Still said, "I know of no part of the body that equals the fascia as a hunting ground"(8).

EVALUATION OF JOINT FUNCTION

Evaluation of joint function is a mainstay of the osteopathic examination. The major function of the joint, regardless of its size or location, is motion. Therefore, this aspect must be evaluated thoroughly because any decrease in joint function leads to compensation and dysfunction on other levels as a simple concomitant of the homeostatic process. Range of motion exists and may be palpated in any joint of the body, whether on a gross level (e.g., the hip joint), a less gross level (e.g., the individual vertebral facets), or a subtle level (e.g., the relatively microscopic motion documented in the cranial sutures). A clinician's failure to palpate this motion should not be interpreted as lack of motion in the system.

On a gross level, the patient is examined for joint motion in standing, sitting, and supine/prone positions. The axial skeleton is evaluated for motion range using side bending, rotation, and anteroposterior movement (forward-to-backward bending), as is the sacrum and sacrococcygeal joint. The same evaluation is done for the ribs, clavicles, scapulae, bones of the pelvis, lower and upper extremities, and cranium. In addition, bones without joints (e.g., the hyoid) may be evaluated. The form in which this range of motion is expressed follows specifically defined osteopathic terminology, which is addressed later in this chapter.

Because of the intimate link between structure and function, the body's motion preferences (i.e., the way the tissues move with least resistance) may lead to a deeper understanding of the state of the autonomic nervous system. Many clinicians are unaware that much of the autonomic innervation is directed to the musculoskeletal system, which comprises 60% of the body. When this is evaluated during examination, findings may lead a physician to suspect changes in the internal milieu of the patient merely from examining the musculoskeletal system. The further a physician journeys in the realm of osteopathy, the more he or she will encounter this method of clinical reasoning. This method, which is based on basic applied anatomy and neurophysiology, has been substantiated in the laboratory by researchers such as Denslow, Korr, and others (9).

LYMPHATIC SYSTEM

The lymphatic system is found in all regions of the body and instantly responds to homeostatic changes. By carefully examining the regional lymphatics, a physician can receive valuable feedback as to where to hunt for dysfunction on many levels. A number of osteopathic physicians, most notably F.P. Millard, DO, author of the text *Applied Anatomy of the Lymphatics*, and one of his students, Gordon Zink, DO, have contributed to our clinical understanding in this field. Dr. Millard developed a quick total-body lymphatic screen that the experienced clinician may complete in 2 to 3 minutes (10).

CONNECTIVE TISSUE

The connective tissue system, particularly the fascia, provides another fruitful avenue of clinical exploration. Because fascial continuity is uninterrupted from the cranium to the feet, skilled assessment provides a total-body picture of major areas of somatic dysfunction. From this, regional, transregional, and interregional sprains and strain patterns can provide invaluable information about the body's functioning, especially when considering that all the vasculature, nervous structures, and lymphatics must pass through the various layers of fascia and will be adversely affected by fascial dysfunction. These fascial patterns underlie the essential motion patterns found in our muscles, bones, and organs. Our habitual postural patterns may only be addressed adequately by working on the level of the fascias as the students of Ida Rolf, PhD, (founder of *rolfing*, an approach to structural realignment that focuses mainly on the fascias, and a student-patient of an osteopathic physician over many years) will attest. You may thus understand why Dr. Still wrote, "We see in the fascia the framework of life, the dwelling place in which life sojourns" (8).

Additional Approaches to the Structural Examination

Frank Chapman, DO, an early twentieth century osteopathic practitioner, discovered a large number of reflex points throughout the body. He noted that these reflex points had a direct correspondence with visceral dysfunction and, when stimulated and diminished, brought about a corresponding decrease in the visceral dysfunction. These points, which feel like small BBs or lumps, are chiefly found on both sides of the torso and are generally uncomfortable when palpated. Chapman believed that these gangliform contractures were neurolymphatic reflexes. One of the most famous of the Chapman reflex points is found on the tip of the right twelfth rib. It is tender in appendicitis and reverts to a nontender state after the problem is corrected. This is one of many useful osteopathic clinical pearls (11).

Lawrence Jones, DO, an osteopathic physician who lived and practiced most of his life in a small town in Oregon, discovered another well-known system of diagnosis used in the osteopathic exam. Dr. Jones found a correspondence between certain well-delineated tender points and specific joint dysfunctions. After many years of clinical observation and experimentation, he described points for virtually the entire panoply of somatic dysfunction. The treatment of these points referred to as "Jones tenderpoints" in the literature actually leads to correction of these joint dysfunctions, as determined by subsequent range of motion retesting of the joints. He called his approach Strain/Counterstrain, and he taught it widely both in classes and in written form until his recent death (12). This approach is now a standard part of the curriculum in osteopathic colleges in the United States.

The work of William Garner Sutherland, DO, of Mankato, Minnesota, has revolutionized our understanding of the system in ways which we are still just beginning to comprehend. A student at the American School of Osteopathy in Kirksville, Missouri, in the late nineteenth century, Dr. Sutherland noticed that the beveling of the temporal bone was similar in form to the gills of a fish. Understanding that structure and function are intimately interrelated, he later spent many years experimenting on himself in a lengthy series of trials. He determined that there was small but definitely palpable movement in the dural membranes surrounding the central nervous system. These membranes are continuous in nature with the inner plane of the cranial bone, the bone itself once having been membrane in its development. In the living person, these sutures always have some movement which, as in any joint, may be palpated. Unfortunately, research on cadavers did not detect this until recent research at Michigan State University in East Lansing corroborated Dr. Sutherland's findings in a laboratory setting (13–18). Today the examination and treatment of the cranial-sacral system is a standard part of all American osteopathic curricula. Postgraduate courses in this field are also offered to licensed physicians and medical students (contact the Cranial Academy, 3500 Depauw Blvd., Indianapolis, IN 46268). Cranial diagnosis and treatment is a subdivision of the wider osteopathic approach and is not intended to be used in an isolated fashion.

Fred Mitchell, Jr., DO, at the Michigan State University College of Osteopathic Medicine, has elaborated a 10-step screening examination. This examination is highly recommended to any physician wishing guidance in learning the gross osteopathic evaluation (19).

DISEASE CLASSIFICATION: TAXONOMY IN OSTEOPATHY

The manner in which dysfunction is classified in osteopathy reflects the profession's understanding of the relationship of structure and function. Although standard medical and surgical terminology is fully used, uniquely osteopathic descriptors are also used. Essentially, much of the terminology describes findings in terms of either restrictions or allowances in range of motion. One approach is based on the work of Harrison Fryette, DO. In 1918, Dr. Fryette first described what he called the "physiologic movement" of the spine (20, 21).

Guidelines for discriminating different types of dysfunction in the axial skeleton are known as Fryette's Laws. There are three types of patterns described, the first two of which exclusively apply to the thoracic and lumbar spines and the third to any part of the spine. Thus, the reader of osteopathic literature may encounter references to Type I or Type II dysfunctions.

The general term for osteopathic musculoskeletal dysfunction is *somatic dysfunction*. Somatic dysfunction is currently defined as "impaired or altered function of related components of the somatic system: skeletal, arthrodial, and myofascial structures, and related vascular, lymphatic and neural elements" (22). The American Osteopathic Association annually publishes a yearbook that is widely available and that contains the complete "Glossary of Osteopathic Terminology," which is an excellent resource for anyone seeking information relating to osteopathic terminology (22).

International Classification of Disease (ICD-9) codes for somatic dysfunction exist and are widely used by practitioners and third-party payers specifically to code osteopathic findings. They are qualified by body region to be more specific. All of the specialized approaches to osteopathic evaluation previously mentioned (e.g., cranial, fascial, Jones tenderpoints) have also developed specialized vocabulary depending on their unique orientation.

DETERMINANTS OF TREATMENT

Treatment is specifically determined by body feedback that is gained from the physical evaluation, while accounting for the key elements of the patient's history. In considering the restrictions and dysfunctions enumerated, an osteopathic physician tries to understand conditions from the system's viewpoint, why it was that the system developed this symptomatic manifestation, and how it was accomplished. These factors, as well as the acuteness or chronicity of the condition, compensatory nature of the findings, age of the patient, previous experience with osteopathic treatment, and sensitivity to treatment, play a role in determining treatment. Treatment is based on specific findings of an anatomicofunctional nature and *not*, as in allopathic practice, a disease label. There is no protocol, for example, for the treatment of otitis media. An osteopathic physician will treat the *patient* who may carry such a diagnostic label but he or she will never provide routine treatment for the diagnostic label itself. Osteopathic physicians diagnose specific deviations from normal function and work solely towards the restoration of normalized function.

THERAPY AND OUTCOMES

When considering osteopathic therapeutic intervention, most people immediately think of manipulation. However, manipulation may not always be used. Because the practitioner is a licensed physician and surgeon, there is a vast array of treatment possibilities. The founders of osteopathy considered the unique osteopathic philosophy, not manipulation, to be the profession's key contribution to the world. Manipulation is one of a number of tools used by the physician to implement osteopathic philosophical goals, the result of which is the restoration of homeostasis and functional normalcy in the system.

Other means to achieve treatment goals include (but are not limited to) nutrition, psychotherapy, various types of pharmacology, surgery, physical therapy, occupational therapy, speech therapy, exercise, orthotic and prosthetic devices, biofeedback, and spiritual support. These tools are frequently combined with manipulation, which is one "spoke" on the therapeutic "wheel." To insist on the exclusive use of manipulation to treat all conditions is as medically unwarranted as to believe that pharmacological therapy, for example, is a panacea. The osteopathic physician is a complete physician and uses a variety of tools.

Osteopathic Manipulative Treatment

Osteopathic manipulative treatment (OMT) is often used to support the homeostatic forces of the body, promote healing, combat the effects of compensation and decompensation, and help relieve underlying dysfunctional patterns.

Some research on the basic mechanisms by which OMT promotes homeostasis has been done. Michael Patterson, PhD, a reflex neurophysiologist, has demonstrated that all disease is characterized by a hypersympathetic component to one degree or another, that facilitated spinal cord segments are perpetuated by somatic dysfunction, and that osteopathic manipulation specifically works to reduce this hypersympathetic activity locally and systemically (24). Dr. Patterson has also demonstrated how somatic dysfunction specifically promotes visceral dysfunction via somatovisceral reflex arcs and may be a harbinger of chronic disease. Clearly, more research on OMT mechanisms and effects is needed.

Basic Treatment Approaches

Many of the basic approaches for diagnosis and assessment previously discussed equally apply to treatment. As in diagnosis, the physician is constantly receiving feedback from the system regarding the treatment effect. This feedback, in turn, helps guide the treatment, similarly to how a skilled navigator uses data and feedback during his or her journey. In addition, the physician's intention and focus of attention are critical determinants in any treatment. Always the ultimate goal of treatment is not the removal of symptoms but rather the restoration of homeostasis and normalized function.

A manipulative prescription based on diagnostic findings is used to plan treatment. It accounts for goals, method of application of treatment, dosing (how long to treat), and frequency of treatment. The degree of dysfunction in the patient must also be understood. For example, purely structural dysfunction (e.g., patient falls and sprains ankle) is approached in one way. However, a condition involving both structural and related functional–structural dys-

Table 16.1. Classification of Osteopathic Manipulative Treatment

Direct	Indirect
High-velocity, low-amplitude	Functional
Muscle energy	Ligamentous, articular balancing
	Counterstrain
	Fascial unwinding

function (e.g., patient falls but the pain disappears on its own in a few days, then after a while the patient develops a persistent headache related to compensation for the first injury) or a condition involving structural and visceral dysfunction of the entire system must be treated differently.

Other determinants of treatment involve, but are not limited to, acuteness or chronicity of the problem, structural or bodily responses, age, sex, other dysfunction, size of patient, responses to similar treatments, and metastatic, surgical, or arthrodial joint restriction (23).

In general, OMT may be classified into two categories—direct and indirect (Table 16.1). In direct techniques, the dysfunctional unit is placed into at least one of several barriers to motion and force is applied against the barrier. Indirect treatment takes the dysfunctional unit away from the restricted motion barrier and uses the body's inherent forces via balanced tension to make a correction.

DIRECT TECHNIQUES

Thrust, or high-velocity, low-amplitude (HV LA) technique is an example of direct technique; HVLA technique has been a mainstay of osteopathic treatment since inception of the profession. The patient is placed in a position so that the joint is brought into its physiological restricted barrier to motion. The physician applies a small amount of force quickly, just enough to go beyond the restrictive barrier. Then, motion is reassessed. The expected result is improved function (i.e., motion). This is a passive treatment because the physician provides the force.

An example of thrust technique is a patient

who presents with anterior chest wall pain. The most common etiology of this complaint is somatic dysfunction of the ribs. Assuming this is the diagnosis, the physician determines the barrier to rib head motion and after positioning the patient, gently and swiftly overcomes the barrier to motion. Besides improved motion, one expects immediate alleviation of pain.

Muscle energy technique is another example of direct treatment. This form, unlike thrust, is an active technique in that the patient helps provide the corrective force. An example is a patient who presents with acute lumbar pain. On examination, the practitioner finds that the L-5 vertebra rotates easier to the right than the left (i.e., rotated right) and sidebends easier to the left than the right (i.e., sidebent left). The patient is positioned, and the physician has the patient rotate to the right and sidebend to the left in the lumbar region against resistance applied by the doctor.

Cranial manipulation may also involve direct treatment. For example, if a neonate refuses to suckle, this problem may be caused by suboccipital compression secondary to labor and compressive forces of the birth canal. This in turn puts pressure on the involved cranial nerves, which decompression may relieve. The expected result is immediate improvement in suckling.

INDIRECT TECHNIQUES

Indirect techniques of manipulation involve taking the dysfunctional unit in a direction away from the restricted motion barrier until a state of balanced tension is obtained. Functional and indirect ligamentous balance technique uses these principles. For example, an athlete suffers a sprained ankle on the soccer field. Before any other intervention is done the physician cradles the proximal aspects of the tibia and fibula in one hand and grasps both malleolae in the other. He or she holds them in a state of balanced, ligamentous tension, feeling the release of the strain-sprain take place. When the tissues feel palpably normalized the physician retests motion. The usual result is immediate: alleviation of dysfunctional symptoms. In many cases, depending on severity, the athlete can immediately return to the game.

Strain-counterstrain is another form of indirect manipulation. A tenderpoint related to a specific somatic dysfunction is located. The ends of the muscle or muscles in which it occurs are approximated and held for about 90 seconds, at which point they are slowly released. At this point the muscle contraction and tenderpoint will be gone, and retesting of the joint motion reveals less dysfunction. An example is a patient with acute torticollis. The physician palpates the most tenderpoint along the anterior or posterior articular pillars in the cervical paraspinal musculature. Then the physician presses the point and asks the patient to quantify the pain (e.g., the most pain is equivalent to $1.00) Then he or she repositions the spine so that when he or she presses on the point again the patient tells the physician that 25¢ or less of the pain remains. The physician then holds the patient in this position for 90 seconds and then, without any help from the patient, brings the patient to a neutral position and firmly presses the point. Reevaluation of the specific joint dysfunction will reveal an improved range of motion and the patient will report significantly less pain. This form of manipulation is one of the best for the neophyte to begin with when starting to learn osteopathic manipulation because it involves only the most elementary type of palpation, is easily grasped, and produces excellent, longlasting results.

OTHER TYPES OF OMT

There are many other types of osteopathic manipulation: Chapman's reflex points, fascial unwinding, fluid techniques, such as V-spread, energetic treatments, percussion hammer work of Robert Fulford, DO, embryologically based treatment of James Jealous, DO, indirect forms of cranial manipulation and the work of Rollin Becker, DO, John Upledger, DO, and others, to name but a few options.

TREATMENT EVALUATION

After treatment, the physician would expect to palpate increased range of motion as well as encounter more normalized function locally and systemically. Often the patient will report lessening of symptoms, especially pain, although occasionally things may actually seem worse initially. This initial worsening of symptoms represents a shifting and rebalancing of the system and usually passes without further intervention. Change is assessed using standard methods of evaluation as previously detailed. Patients must understand that the longer they have had the condition, the longer will it take for symptoms to resolve. Osteopathic treatment unleashes a homeostatic process that functions over days, weeks, and months, depending on the amount of dysfunction. The physician may hear from the patient that many more symptoms have resolved between the visits than what was reported immediately after treatment. Acute onset complaints may require relatively few visits for resolution compared to chronic ones. During each visit there is constant, multileveled evaluation going on. Based on this immediate feedback from the system, the various parameters of the ongoing treatment are established, reweighed, and accordingly altered. As always, the essential measurement of progress is normalization of function and improvement in symptoms on all levels.

USES OF OSTEOPATHIC MANIPULATIVE TREATMENT

Because osteopathic treatment promotes homeostatic balancing and normalized function for the entire system, most pathological states may benefit to some degree from this approach. However, certain conditions in particular lend themselves to an osteopathic approach.

Indications

MUSCULOSKELETAL CONDITIONS

Osteopathic manipulation is often the treatment of choice for musculoskeletal conditions, particularly those involving trauma to the soft tissues, sprains and strains, range of motion restrictions, pain, impingement of nerves, and related areas. Most busy osteopathic practices see many patients with complaints of lumbar and cervical pain, both chronic and acute, localized and radiating. Some of this pain is caused by somatic dysfunction and some is secondary to nerve impingement, either discogenic or further along the route of the nerve. Manipulation is indicated in most of these situations with a few exceptions, one being in which extensive surgery has been performed and the effects of massive scar tissue impede osteopathic efforts and in emergencies, such as sudden loss of bowel and bladder function. However, even postsurgical cases often derive benefits arising from improved systemic function. Another key factor as with any approach is that of patient compliance. Reinjury of any kind must strictly be avoided.

Extremity pain, such as thoracic outlet syndrome, certain types of carpal tunnel syndrome in which repetitive motion reinjury can be avoided for a while, frozen shoulders, shoulder pain, and hip, knee, ankle and many types of foot pain seem to respond well.

Headaches of many kinds, with the exception of classical migraines (especially in their full-blown state), lend themselves to osteopathic treatment, as do sinusitis, temporomandibular joint dysfunctions, and closed-head injuries (with proper surgical consultation, of course).

CHILDHOOD CONDITIONS AND PREGNANCY

Although more research is needed, children with otitis media who have undergone many trials of antibiotic treatment with the infections always returning seem to respond well to OMT (24). The infections disappear, and the patients often avoid further antibiotics and tubes. In addition, the author has seen excellent response in patients with acute and chronic vertigo. In both of these conditions, cranial manipulation is useful.

Children diagnosed with attention deficit disorder and hyperactivity often benefit from an osteopathic cranial approach, as do many patients labeled developmentally delayed (25–27).

Pregnant women respond especially well to gentle osteopathic treatment. It provides them with a relatively low pain pregnancy and is excellent physiological and anatomical preparation for delivery (28). Because most neonatal problems (e.g., colic, respiratory and upper respiratory problems, failure to suckle) can be treated in one to two visits, the author usually recommends mothers to bring in their newborn with these conditions. Issues such as plagiocephaly (i.e., misshapen heads) are best dealt with as early as possible and respond to direct cranial molding techniques.

HYPERSYMPATHETIC SYNDROMES, RESPIRATORY DISORDERS, AND OTHER CONDITIONS

One of the most valuable uses of OMT is in dealing with frank hypersympathetic syndromes, such as ileus. Until recently, standing orders were common at most osteopathic hospitals for preoperative and postoperative OMT for many surgical patients to prevent ileus. A clinical study demonstrating the value of such treatment for prevention of ileus was conducted at the osteopathic hospital in Waterville, Maine (29).

Although there are few formal studies conducted, I have found a number of conditions that are frequently helped with OMT. OMT is often helpful, for example, in respiratory disorders, such as asthma, pneumonia, and pulmonary sarcoidosis. Some data were collected on this in the 1918 influenza epidemic, which was in the preantibiotic era. American osteopathic clinics and hospitals reported a mortality rate of 0.25% for flu and 10% for the sequela of pneumonia compared with the allopathic rates of 9.8 to 27% for flu and 26 to 73% for the sequela of pneumonia at that time. Even now with antibiotics, OMT helps respiratory function in these conditions and can be a useful adjunct treatment (30–32).

Other conditions that I have found responsive to osteopathic treatment include radiation fibrosis, hepatitis, mononucleosis, anterior chest wall pain, angina, amblyopia, neuritis, Bell's palsy, epilepsy with an unknown focal source, and whiplash.

There are also many conditions in which OMT may be a useful adjunct. Some of these are dental equilibration, swallowing disorders, tinnitus, stabilization of arrhythmias, infertility of unknown cause, gastroesophageal reflux, coli-tis, and stroke rehabilitation. OMT can also be helpful with the pain of cancer.

Contraindications

OMT is not recommended in certain conditions. Examples are cancer, nutritional problems, emotional problems, continuing repetitive trauma, or conditions of a psychosocial etiology.

With the exception of thrust technique, there are few contraindications (33). Obviously in muscle energy, an active technique, the patient must be able to follow commands adequately. Contraindications to thrust include fractures at the site of thrust, increase of pain or neurological symptoms while positioning the patient, severe rheumatoid arthritis, and metastatic cancer at the site of the thrust. Relative contraindications include carotid bruits in cervical thrust, advanced osteoporosis, acute spasms, and advanced mechanical motion restrictions (e.g., in certain types of arthritis).

ORGANIZATION

Training

American osteopathic physicians follow a parallel track with their allopathic medical colleagues in training. They have identical premedical course and testing requirements. Osteopath applicants must work with the American Association of Colleges of Osteopathic Medicine (AACOM) application service by applying to any of the 19 American osteopathic medical schools. The four-year osteopathic curriculum is equivalent to that of the allopathic medical school, except that the osteopathic student is required to take additional coursework in osteopathic principles and practice. Traditionally there is greater emphasis on understanding certain aspects of the basic sciences, such as anatomy, and later integrating that learning into the clinical setting than is commonly found in conventional allopathic medical schools.

After graduation as a doctor of osteopathy (DO) and before beginning postgraduate specialty training, DOs must do a one-year internship in an approved osteopathic clinical teaching institution. This hospital internship is roughly equivalent to the MD transitional year; the physician spends three months doing surgery and then several months in internal medicine, pediatrics, obstetrics, and so forth. This assures hands-on skills and exposure to all areas of practice in an osteopathic atmosphere. After the internship year, the physician is encouraged to complete a multiyear specialty or subspecialty residency. Presently, DOs are eligible for admission to all residencies in all specialties and subspecialties of medicine and surgery in all American MD and DO teaching hospitals. After this, additional fellowship training is available. Postgraduate training is also available in osteopathic manipulation.

Licensure and Certification

The National Board of Osteopathic Medical Examiners administers a three-part, six-day exam which, except for its specifically osteopathic component, mirrors its MD counterpart exam. These and other exams qualify DO's for licensure as full-practice physicians and surgeons in all 50 states. As a result of their advanced specialty training in residencies and fellowships, DOs are also eligible to sit for all AOA and AMA certifying examinations. They may and do serve on the staff of any allopathic or osteopathic hospital. They are also eligible to serve as fully commissioned medical officers in the armed forces, public health service, and other government programs.

Professional Societies

The central unifying organization in the United States is the American Osteopathic Association. The AOA has numerous component subsections and societies that are concerned with local affairs (e.g., state societies), specialty colleges (e.g.,. anesthesiology), research (e.g., National Osteopathic Foundation), and philanthropic groups. One group that has been around since the 1930s, the American Academy of Osteopa-

thy, is concerned with furthering the teaching and development of osteopathic manipulation and principles. It also has numerous component societies for special interests in this area (e.g., Cranial Academy). There also exists a National Osteopathic Museum in Kirksville, Missouri, home to the first osteopathic school.

Osteopathic physicians are licensed by the states in which they practice. Approximately 17 states have specific boards just for DOs. The rest of the states and territories use composite and MD boards to license DOs (34).

Reimbursement Status and Relations with Conventional Medicine

American DOs are considered identical to MDs as far as third-party and government reimbursement for their services is concerned. There are specific ICD-9 codes for somatic dysfunction as well as the Physician's Current Procedural Terminology (CPT) codes specific for osteopathic manipulation done by a licensed physician (35). As of 1997, there were 129 hospitals accredited by the AOA. Many of these sponsored internship, residency, and fellowship postdoctoral specialty and subspecialty training (36).

The profession's relationship with the medical profession is at present cordial. For most of the profession's history, however, and as recently as the early 1960s, conventional mainstream medicine waged a steady campaign to weaken the osteopathic profession. In 1962, for example, the California affiliate of the AMA in league with the national organization got the legislature to pass a provision outlawing the licensing of DOs in that state. As a result, the osteopathic profession lost over 30 osteopathic hospitals, which were taken over by MDs. The College of Osteopathic Physicians and Surgeons (founded 1901) was also taken over and became the University of California School of Medicine at Irvine. In 1974, the California State Supreme Court declared the 1962 law a violation of the antitrust amendment, but the damage had been done. This example is only one of many ways in which mainstream medicine has treated the osteopathic profession over the years (37, 38).

PROSPECTS FOR THE FUTURE

Ironically, the *AMA News* published an article which noted that as of the last few years it is actually more competitive to get into a DO school than an MD school (39). This may be because of the American trend of people looking for fully licensed physicians with a holistic orientation and good primary care skills, both major aspects of osteopathy today. Currently almost 40,000 DOs, which is 5% of all fully licensed physicians in the United States, serve over 10% of the American population. This trend is increasing daily. Today there are 19 osteopathic schools, compared with the late 1960s when there were only 5. New osteopathic schools are being approved at a time when medical schools are being closed and consolidated. It appears that organizationally, the osteopathic profession is doing well. There also appear to be renewed efforts to recapture the uniquely osteopathic orientation that first distinguished the profession and without which it will in all probability not survive as a distinctive, separate stream in American health care. Thus, despite tremendous pressures to the contrary, Dr. Still's reported final words to "Keep it pure" are being adopted by an small but increasing minority within the American osteopathic profession.

REFERENCES

1. Kuchera W, Kuchera M. Osteopathic principles in practice. 2nd ed. Kirksville, MO: Kirksville College of Osteopathic Medicine Press, 1991:2.
2. Booth ER. History of osteopathy and twentieth-century medical practice. 2nd ed. Cincinnati, Ohio: The Caxton Press. 1924:80.
3. Di Giovanna E, Schiowitz S. An osteopathic approach to diagnosis and treatment. Philadelphia: JB Lippincott Company, 1991:369.
4. Gevitz N. The D.O.'s: osteopathic medicine in America. Baltimore: The Johns Hopkins University Press, 1982.
5. Sprafka S, Ward R, Ness D. What characterizes an osteopathic principle? J Am Osteopathic Assoc 1981;81(1):29–81.
6. Kuchera.op. cit. 113.
7. Travell JG, Simons DG. Myofascial pain and dysfunction: the trigger point manual. Baltimore: Williams & Wilkins, 1983.
8. Truhlar R. Dr. A.T. Still in the living. Cleveland: Private printing, 1950.
9. Dowling DJ. Neurophysiologic mechanisms related to osteopathic diagnosis and treatment. In: Di Giovanna, Schiowitz S. An osteopathic approach to diagnosis and treatment. Philadelphia: JB Lippincott, 1991:12–19.
10. Millard FP. Applied anatomy of the lymphatics. Kirksville, Mo: Journal Printing Co., 1922:22–27.
11. Owens C. An endocrine interpretation of Chapman's reflexes. Chatanooga, TN: Private, 1937.
12. Jones L. Strain and counterstrain. Newark, OH: American Academy of Osteopathy, 1981.
13. Upledger J. The reproducibility of craniosacral examination findings: a statistical analysis. J Am Osteopath Assoc 1977;76:890–899.
14. Upledger J, Karni Z. Mechano-electric patterns during craniosacral osteopathic diagnosis and treatment. J Am Osteopath Assoc 1979;78:782–791.
15. Greenman P. Roentgen findings in the craniosacral mechanism. J Am Osteopath Assoc 1970; 70:24–35.
16. Michael DK, Retzlaff EW. A preliminary study of cranial bone movement in the squirrel monkey. J Am Osteopath Assoc 1975;74:866–869.
17. Retzlaff EW, et al. Cranial bone mobility. J Am Osteopath Assoc 1975;74:869–873.
18. Dunbar HS, et al. A study of the cerebrospinal fluid pulse wave. Arch Neurol 1966;14:624–630.
19. Mitchell F Jr. The muscle energy manual. Vol 1. East Lansing, MI: MET Press, 1995.
20. Fryette HH. Physiologic movements of the spine. J Am Osteopath Assoc 1918;18:1.
21. Fryette HH. Principles of osteopathic technic. Kirksville, MO: Academy of Applied Osteopathy, 1954.
22. American Osteopathic Association, Publications Dept., 142 E. Ontario St.,Chicago,Ill. 60611.
23. Dowling DJ. Neurophysiologic mechanisms related to osteopathic diagnosis and treatment. In: Di Giovanna, Schiowitz S. An osteopathic approach to diagnosis and treatment. Philadelphia: JB Lippincott, 1991:12–19.
24. Gintis B. AAO case study. Recurrent otitis media. AAOJ 1996;6:2:16.
25. Agresti LM. Attention deficit disorder. The hyperactive child. Osteopathic Annals 1989;14:6–16.
26. Frymann V, et al. Effect of osteopathic medical management on neurologic development in children.J Am Osteopath Assoc 1992;92:729–744.
27. Frymann V. Learning difficulties of children viewed in the light of the osteopathic concept. J Am Osteopath Assoc 1976;76:46–61.
28. Johnson K. An integrated approach for treating the

OB patient: treating the five diaphragms of the body. Part I. AAOJ 1991;1:4:6.

29. Stiles, E.G. Osteopathic manipulation in a hospital environment. J Am Osteopath Assoc 1976;76: 243–258.

30. Magoun H Sr. Practical osteopathic procedures. Belen, NM/Kirksville, MO: Journal Printing Co, 72–73.

31. Anonymous. Osteopathy's epidemic record. Osteopathic Physician 1919;36:1.

32. Smith RK. Influenza mortality, one hundred thousand cases; with death rate of one-fortieth of that officially reported under conventional medical treatment. J Am Osteopath Assoc 1920;19: 172–175.

33. Kuchera. op. cit. 295–296.

34. Citation 23 for address of AOA which publishes directory.

35. AOA directory contains latest guideline. Address citation 23.

36. Yearbook and directory of osteopathic physicians. 87th ed. Chicago, IL: American Osteopathic Association, 1996:665–669.

37. Gevitz N. The D.O's. Baltmore: The Johns Hopkins University Press, 1982.99–136.

38. Bartosh L. The history of osteopathy in California. Journal of the Osteopathic Physicians and Surgeons of California 1978;5:30–33.

39. AMA News. May 10, 1993.

CHAPTER 17

NATUROPATHIC MEDICINE

Michael T. Murray and Joseph E. Pizzorno

Nature is doing her best each moment to make us well. She exists for no other end. Do not resist. With the least inclination to be well, we should not be sick.

Henry David Thoreau

The doctor of the future will give no medicine, but will interest his patient in the care of the human frame, in diet and in the cause and prevention of disease.

Thomas Edison

BACKGROUND

Naturopathic medicine, also known as "nature cure," is more than a health care system—it is a philosophy and, for many, a way of life. It is based on the belief in the ability of the body to heal itself—the *vis medicatrix naturae* (the healing power of nature). The expectation that the body can heal, if given the proper opportunity, is fundamental to the practice of naturopathic medicine. This opportunity involves living within the laws of nature and using therapies that support normal body function, instead of using drugs that supplant body function. Naturopathy also involves a strong commitment to improving the quality of the environment.

Naturopathic physicians believe that most disease is the direct result of the ignorance and violation of Natural Living Laws. Healing will result from the following:

- Consumption of natural, unrefined, organically grown foods
- Ensuring adequate amounts of exercise and rest
- Living a moderately paced lifestyle
- Having constructive and creative thoughts and emotions
- Avoiding environmental toxins
- Maintaining proper elimination

The typical naturopathic practice is characterized by maintenance of health, prevention of disease, patient education and self-responsibility, as well as diagnosis and the use of natural therapies that support regeneration of the body's systems.

Although the term *naturopathy* was coined in the late nineteenth century, its philosophical roots date back thousands of years, drawing on the healing wisdom of many cultures, such as those of India (Ayurvedic), China (Taoist), Greece (Hippocratic), Germany (homeopathy, hydrotherapy, nature cure), the Roman Empire (hydrotherapy), England (botanical medicine), Native America (botanical medicine, spiritual guidance), and early America (natural hygiene, detoxification, spinal manipulation). Unlike many other health care systems, naturopathy is not identified with any particular therapy, but rather with a philosophy of health promotion rather than simply disease treatment or symptom alleviation.

This philosophical approach necessitates a broad range of diagnostic and therapeutic skills and accounts for the eclectic interests of the naturopathic profession. Because the goal of the naturopathic physician is to restore normal body function (rather than the application of a particular therapy), virtually every natural medicine therapy is used. In addition, virtually every disease is in the realm of naturopathic treatment because strengthening the body's own healing systems always benefits the patient regardless of the pathologic diagnosis. However, not every disease process can be reversed and, in keeping with their role as primary care physicians, naturopaths also employ office surgery, acute prescription drugs, and referral to specialists when it is in the patient's best interests.

In addition to providing recommendations on lifestyle, diet, and exercise, naturopathic physicians use a variety of therapeutic modalities to promote health. Some naturopathic physicians emphasize a particular therapeutic modality, whereas others use a number of modalities. Some naturopaths focus on a particular medical field, such as pediatrics, natural childbirth, or physical medicine, whereas others are generalists.

Today's naturopathic doctor (ND) is an extensively trained and state-licensed physician equipped with a broad range of conventional and unconventional diagnostic and therapeutic skills. The modern ND considers herself (66% of naturopaths are women) or himself an integral part of the health care system and takes full responsibility for the common public health issues.

Historical Perspective

Enriched by its philosophical links to many cultures, naturopathic medicine as a distinct profession in America grew out of natural healing systems of the eighteenth and nineteenth centuries. Naturopathy began with the teachings and concepts of Benedict Lust (1870–1945). In 1892, at the age of 23, Lust came from Germany as a disciple of Father Kneipp to bring hydrotherapy practices to America. Exposure in the United States to a wide range of practitioners and practices of natural healing arts broadened Lust's perspective. After a decade of study, he purchased the term *naturopathy* from Scheel of New York City in 1902 (who coined the term in 1895) to describe the eclectic compilation of doctrines of natural healing that he envisioned as the future of natural medicine. Naturopathy, or "nature cure," was defined by Lust as both a way of life and a concept of healing, employing various natural means of treating human infirmities and disease states (1). In 1902, Lust also opened the first health food store.

In a January, 1902, editorial in the first issue of *The Naturopathic and Herald of Health*, Lust began promoting a new way of thinking of health care with the following:

We believe in strong, pure, beautiful bodies . . . of radiating health. We want every man, woman and child in this great land to know and embody and feel the truths of right living that mean conscious mastery. We plead for the renouncing of poisons from the coffee, white flour, glucose, lard, and like venom of the American table to patent medicines, tobacco, liquor and the other inevitable recourse of perverted appetite. We long for the time when an eight-hour day may enable every worker to stop existing long enough to live; when the spirit of universal brotherhood shall animate business and society and the church; when every American may have a little cottage of his own . . . when people may stop doing and thinking and being for others and be for themselves; when true love and divine marriage and pre-natal culture and controlled parenthood may fill this world with germ-gods instead of humanized animals.

In a word, Naturopathy stands for the reconciling, harmonizing and unifying of nature, humanity and God.

Fundamentally therapeutic because men need healing; elementary educational because men need teaching; ultimately inspirational because men need empowering . . . . (2)

Although the terminology is almost 100 years old, Lust's concepts provided a powerful foundation that has endured despite almost a century of active political suppression by the dominant school of medicine. The wisdom he garnered from the insights of many natural healers is now well documented. For example, in the modern textbook, *Natural Medicine*, there are 10,000 citations to the peer-reviewed scientific literature.

During the past century, the profession has progressed through several fairly distinct phases (Table 17.1) . Because of its eclectic nature, the history of naturopathic medicine is as complex as any healing art.

The Halcyon Years of Naturopathy

Naturopathy was most popular from the 1920s until 1937. The success of the early naturopaths, in the face of the relative inadequacy of conventional medicine of this era, initiated a health fad movement that cause great public awareness, interest, and concern. Many famous people and politicians of the day proclaimed the benefits of naturopathic cures.

The naturopathic journals of the 1920s and 1930s provide insight into the prevention of disease and the promotion of health. Much of the dietary advice focused on correcting poor eating habits, including the lack of fiber in the diet and an over-reliance on red meat as a protein source. Although scientific data were lacking in the 1930s, the pronouncements of the National Institutes of Health and the National Cancer Institute in the 1990s confirmed many of the early assertions of naturopaths that these dietary habits would lead to degenerative diseases, including cancers associated with the digestive tract and the colon.

The December 1928 volume of *Nature's Path* was the first American publication of the works of Herman J. DeWolff, a Dutch epidemiologist who was one of the earliest researchers to assert, based on studies of the incidence of cancer in the Netherlands, that there was an association between exposure to petrochemicals and various types of cancerous conditions. He saw a connection between chemical fertilizers and their usage in some soils, which led to the fertilizer remaining in vegetables after they had arrived at the market and were purchased for consumption. This was almost 50 years before orthodox medicine confirmed such assertions.

Suppression and Decline

In 1937, the popularity of naturopathy began to decline. Conventional medicine had developed effective therapies and the public became enamored by technology. Benedict Lust died in September of 1945 in residence at the Yungborn facility in Butler, New Jersey, preparing to attend the 49th Annual Congress of his American Naturopathic Association. Right before his death, he noted his concerns for the future, especially his frustration with the success of the medical profession in blocking the naturopaths' efforts to establish state licensing laws. These

---

Table 17.1. Historical Overview of Naturopathic Medicine

Latter part of the Nineteenth century: *The Founding by Benedict Lust.* Origin in the Germanic hydrotherapy and nature cure traditions

1900–1917: *The Formative Years.* Convergence of American dietetic, hygienic, physical culture, spinal manipulation, mental and emotional healing, Thompsonian/eclectic herbalism, and homeopathic systems

1918–1937: *The Halcyon Years.* During a period of great public interest and support, the philosophical basis and scope of therapies diversified to encompass botanical, homeopathic, and environmental medicine

1938–1970: *Suppression and Decline.* Growing political and social dominance of the AMA, America's desire for technology, and the emergence of "miracle" drugs and effective modern surgical techniques resulted in legal and economic suppression

1971–Present: *Naturopathic Medicine Reemerges.* Reawakened awareness in the American public of the importance of health promotion, prevention of disease, and concern for the environment; establishment of modern, accredited, physician-level training reestablished public interest in naturopathic medicine, resulting in rapid regrowth

laws would not only establish appropriate practice rights for NDs, but also protect the public from the pretenders—that is, those who would call themselves naturopaths without attaining formal training—a problem that continues to plague the profession today. His concerns were part of the official program for the Annual Congress of the American Naturopathic Association in October 1945. Just before his death, he wrote:

> Now let us see the type of men and women who are the Naturopaths of today. Many of them are fine, upstanding individuals, believing fully in the effectiveness of their chosen profession—willing to give their all for the sake of alleviating human suffering and ready to fight for their rights to the last ditch. More power to them! But there are others who claim to be Naturopaths who are woeful misfits. Yes, and there are outright fakers and cheats masking as Naturopaths. That is the fate of any science—any profession—which the unjust laws have placed beyond the pale. Where there is no official recognition and regulation, you will find the plotters, the thieves, the charlatans operating on the same basis as the conscientious practitioners. And these riff-raff opportunists bring the whole art into disrepute. Frankly such conditions cannot be remedied until suitable safeguards are erected by law, or by the profession itself, around the practice of Naturopathy. That will come in time.

The public infatuation with technology, introduction of "miracle medicine," the second World War's stimulation of the development of surgery, the Flexner Report, growing political sophistication of the American Medical Association, the growth in numbers of the "pretenders," and the death of Benedict Lust in 1945 combined to cause the decline of naturopathic medicine and natural healing in the United States.

Lack of insurance coverage, public confusion over educational standards, lost court battles, and a hostile legislative perspective progressively restricted practice until the core naturopathic therapies became essentially illegal and practices financially nonviable.

Naturopathic Medicine Reemerges

The combination of the counterculture years of the late 1960s, the public's reawakening interest in nutrition and the environment, and America's disenchantment with organized institutional medicine (when it became apparent that orthodox medicine has its limitations and is expensive), resulted in newfound respect for alternative medicine in general and the rejuvenation of naturopathic medicine. At this time, a new wave of students were attracted to the philosophical precepts of the profession. They brought with them a new appreciation for the appropriate use of science, modern college education, and matching expectations. In addition, the emergence of Bastyr University (founded in 1978), with its focus on teaching and researching science-based natural medicine, played a major role.

PRINCIPAL CONCEPTS

Naturopathic medicine is vitalistic in its approach—that is, life is more than the sum of biochemical processes, and the body is believed to have an innate intelligence that strives for health. The role of the physician is to understand and aid the body's efforts, and to help the patient understand why he or she is sick and how to become (and stay) healthy.

In this context, health is more than the absence of disease. Health is a vital dynamic state that enables a person to function well in a wide range of environments and stresses. Health and disease are points on a continuum, with death at one end and optimal function at the other. The naturopath believes that a person who engages in an unhealthy lifestyle will more rapidly progress to greater dysfunction.

The profession's efforts to codify this philosophy of health promotion and work in concert with nature has led to a series of principles to guide patient care:

Principle 1: The healing power of nature
(*vis medicatrix naturae*)
    Naturopathic physicians believe that the body has considerable power to heal itself.

It is the physician's role to facilitate and enhance this process with the aid of natural, nontoxic therapies.

Principle 2: Identify and treat the cause (*tolle causam*)

The naturopathic physician is trained to seek the underlying causes of a disease rather than simply suppress the symptoms. Symptoms are viewed as expressions of the body's attempt to heal, and the causes may spring from the patient's physical, mental–emotional, and spiritual levels.

Principle 3: First do no harm (*primum no nocere*)

The naturopathic physician seeks to do no harm with medical treatment by employing safe and effective natural therapies.

Principle 4: Treat the whole person

Naturopathic physicians are trained to view an individual as a whole entity composed of a complex interaction of physical, mental–emotional, spiritual, social, and other factors.

Principle 5: The physician as teacher

The naturopathic physician is foremost a teacher educating, empowering, and motivating the patient to assume more personal responsibility for his or her health by adopting a healthy attitude, lifestyle, and diet.

Principle 6: Prevention is the best cure

Naturopathic physicians are preventive medicine specialists. Prevention of disease is accomplished through education and lifestyle habits that support health and prevent disease.

Principle 7: Establish health and wellness

Establishing and maintaining optimum health and promoting wellness are the primary goals of the naturopathic physician. Although health is defined as the state of optimal physical, mental, emotional, and spiritual well-being, wellness is defined as a state of health characterized by a positive emotional state.

The naturopathic physician strives to increase the level of wellness regardless of the disease or level of health. Even in cases of severe disease, a high level of wellness can be achieved.

Naturopathic Principles in Clinical Practice: Case Analysis

Applying these principles to clinical practice takes extensive training, careful insight, and years of practice. When evaluating a patient, the well-trained naturopathic doctor asks the following questions:

- What is the first cause of the disease or symptom?
- How is the body trying to heal itself?
- What is the minimum level of intervention needed to facilitate the self-healing process?
- What are the patient's underlying functional weaknesses?
- What education does the patient need to understand why he or she is sick and how to become healthier?
- How does the patient's physical disease relate to his or her psychological and spiritual health?

Table 17.2 lists more questions the naturopathic students is taught to consider. Although the practice of naturopathic medicine is grounded in *vis medicatrix naturae*, it also recognizes that intervention in the disease process may sometimes be efficacious or absolutely necessary. Naturopathic physicians have a long-standing tradition of integrating aspects of traditional, alternative, and conventional medicine in the interest of the patient. As appropriate, patients are referred to specialists and other health care practitioners. Whenever possible, every effort is made to use all treatment techniques in a manner that is harmonious with the naturopathic philosophy.

PROVIDER–PATIENT INTERACTIONS

The modern naturopathic physician provides all phases of primary health care. Clinical assessment involves a medical history, physical exami-

Table 17.2. Naturopathic Case Analysis

Principle 1. The Healing Power of Nature (*vis medicatrix naturae*)
How is the healing power of Nature supported in the case?
Is the person in balance with Nature?
What is being in balance with Nature?
Is this person in balance with his/her environment?
How are you assessing the healing powers of this individual?
What is the prognosis for this individual?

Principle 2. Find the Cause (*tolle causam*)
What level of healing are you aiming for? (i.e. suppression, palliation, cure)
Where and/or what are the limiting factors in this person's life? (concept: health is freedom from limitations)
Where is the center of this person's disease? (i.e., physical, mental, emotional)
What are the causative factors contributing to disease in this individual? Of these causative factors, which are avoidable or preventable?

Principle 3. First Do No Harm (*primum non nocere*)
What is the potential for harm with this particular treatment plan?
Are you doing no harm? How?
What is the appropriate course of action?

Principle 4. Treat the Whole Person
How are you working holistically?
Can you see the person beyond the disease?
What aspects of the person are you addressing?
What aspects of the person are you not addressing?
Would a referral to another health care practitioner assist you in working holistically? When? To whom?
What are the patient's goals and expectations in relationship to their health and treatments?
What are your goals and expectations for the patient? What are the differences between yours and the patient's? How are they similar?
How will the treatment plan help the patient take more responsibility for his/her health and healing?
Are you empowering the patient? How?
What is the vitality level of this patient?

Principle 5. Doctor as Teacher (*Docere*)
What type of patient education are you providing?
How can you determine the level of a patient's responsibility?
In what ways do you cultivate and enhance your role as teacher?

Principle 6. Prevention is the Best Cure
What is being done or planned in regard to prevention?
Doctor means teacher: What are you teaching this person about his/her health?
Have you done a risk factor assessment for this patient?
Does this patient do regular health screening self-exams?

Principle 7. Establish Health and Wellness
What is being done to cultivate wellness?
How are you contributing to optimal health in this individual?
How can you contribute to optimal health in this individual?
What are the patient's goals and expectations in relationship to his or her own wellness (e.g., creativity, energy, enjoyment, health, balance)?
How can these goals be achieved? Are the expectations realistic?
How can achievement of these goals be measured?
Once achieved, how can the patient maintain an optimal level of wellness?
Are you stimulating wellness or treating disease, or both?
Is the patient demonstrating positive emotion, thought, and action? If not, why?
Can the patient recall or imagine a state of wellness?
Is the patient able to participate in his/her own process toward a state of wellness?

nation, radiological and laboratory evaluation, and other well-accepted conventional diagnostic procedures that are supplemented with nonconventional diagnostic techniques. For example, naturopathic physicians use extensive laboratory methodologies to assess nutritional status, toxin load, detoxification function, food intolerance, intestinal bioses, digestive function, and other functional aspects.

A typical first office visit with a naturopathic physician lasts for one hour. Because teaching a patient how to live healthfully is a primary goal of naturopathy, the physician devotes time to discussing and explaining principles of health maintenance. This approach sets naturopaths apart from many other health care providers.

The physician–patient relationship begins with a thorough medical history and interview process designed to review all aspects of a patient's lifestyle. As appropriate, the physician performs diagnostic procedures, such as physical examination; blood, urine, and stool analysis; and various laboratory procedures to assess physiological function. When the patient's health and disease status is established and understood (making a diagnosis of a disease is only one part of this process), the doctor and patient together establish a treatment and health-promoting program. Proper assessment of outcomes using conventional assessment tools (e.g., patient interview, physical examination, laboratory tests, radiologic imaging) is an important part of patient follow-up.

Therapeutic Modalities

Naturopathy incorporates a variety of healing techniques. Naturopathic physicians are trained in a large scope of treatments: clinical nutrition, botanical medicine, homeopathy, Chinese medicine and acupuncture, hydrotherapy, physical medicine including massage and therapeutic manipulation, counseling and other psychotherapies, and minor surgery. In certain states (most notably Oregon and Washington), licensed naturopathic physicians are granted prescription privileges for naturally derived prescription substances, including vitamins, minerals, hormones

(e.g., corticosteroids, estrogen, thyroxine), pancreatin, bile acids, antibiotics, and plant-based drugs (e.g., belladonna, scopolamine).

Naturopathic medicine uses natural medicines and intervention therapies as needed. When properly used, natural medicine and therapies generally have low invasiveness and rarely cause suppression of symptoms or side effects. These medicines and therapies generally support the body's healing mechanisms rather than take over or inhibit the body's processes.

CLINICAL NUTRITION

Clinical nutrition, or the use of diet as a therapy, serves as the foundation of naturopathic medicine. There is an ever-increasing body of knowledge that supports the use of whole foods and nutritional supplements in the maintenance of health and treatment of disease. The recognition of unique nutritional requirements due to biochemical individuality has provided a strong theoretical and practical basis for the appropriate use of megavitamin therapy. Controlled fasting is also used therapeutically.

BOTANICAL MEDICINE

Plants have always been used as medicines. Naturopathic physicians are professionally trained herbalists, and they know both the historical uses and modern pharmacological mechanisms of plants. Although many botanical medicines can be used (or misused) as replacement for conventional drugs, the naturopathic physician prefers to use them to support the body's healing processes.

HOMEOPATHY

Homeopathy is a system of medicine that treats a disease with a dilute, potentized agent, or drug, that will produce the same symptoms as the disease when given to a healthy individual. The fundamental principle of this system is that *like cures like*. Homeopathic medicines are derived from a variety of plant, mineral, and chemical substances.

TRADITIONAL CHINESE MEDICINE AND ACUPUNCTURE

Traditional Chinese medicine and acupuncture are part of an ancient system of medicine that enhances the flow of vital energy (*Chi*). Acupuncture involves the stimulation of specific points on the body along *Chi* pathways (termed *meridians*). Acupuncture points can be stimulated by inserting and withdrawing needles, applying heat (moxibustion), massage, laser therapy, electrical stimulation, or a combination of these methods.

HYDROTHERAPY

Hydrotherapy is the use of water in any form (e.g., hot or cold; ice, steam) and methods of application (e.g., sitz bath, douche, spa and hot tub, whirlpool, sauna, shower, immersion bath, pack, poultice, foot bath, fomentation, wrap, colonic irrigations). Hydrotherapy is an ancient method that has been used to treat disease and injury by many different cultures, including the Egyptians, Assyrians, Persians, Greeks, Hebrews, Hindus, and Chinese. Its most sophisticated applications were developed in eighteenth-century Germany.

PHYSICAL MEDICINE

Physical medicine refers to the use of physical measures in the treatment of an individual. It involves the use of physiotherapy equipment (e.g., ultrasound, diathermy, other electromagnetic devices), therapeutic exercise, massage, joint mobilization (manipulative) and immobilization techniques, and hydrotherapy.

DETOXIFICATION

Recognition and correction of endogenous and exogenous toxicity is an important theme in naturopathy. Liver and bowel detoxification, elimination of environmental toxins, correcting the metabolic dysfunction that causes the buildup of non-end-product metabolites are important ways of decreasing toxic load.

COUNSELING AND LIFESTYLE MODIFICATION

A naturopath is formally trained in mental, emotional, and family counseling. A naturopath typically implements the following:

1. Interviewing and responding skills, active listening, assessing body language, and other contact skills necessary for the therapeutic relationship.
2. Recognizing and understanding prevalent psychological issues, including developmental problems, abnormal behavior, addictions, stress, and sexuality.
3. Various psychological treatment measures, including hypnosis and guided imagery, counseling techniques, correcting underlying organic factors, and family therapy.

THERAPEUTIC APPROACH

Use of Naturopathic Medicine for Treatment

Because naturopathic medicine encompasses numerous therapies, the naturopathic physician must select the best treatment option based on the patient and his or her condition and health status. The discussions of individual modalities throughout this book highlight their appropriateness, strengths, limitations, and contraindications for various health conditions. In general, naturopathic medicine is best suited for the typical problems seen in a general practice, with particular applicability in the prevention and treatment of chronic diseases, such as atherosclerosis-related vascular disease; hypertension; diabetes; osteoarthritis; osteoporosis; Alzheimer's disease; kidney stones; inflammatory bowel disease; psoriasis; eczema; benign prostatic hyperplasia; and autoimmune diseases, including rheumatoid arthritis, multiple sclerosis, and lupus. It is also well suited for helping patients enhance normal physiological processes and deal with stress, or for those with low immune function, chronic infections, digestive disturbances, liver disorders, allergies, hormonal disturbances, premenstrual syndrome, and fatigue.

Scientific literature supports many (although not all) of the modalities naturopathic physicians commonly use in the treatment of these conditions, especially nutritional and botanical therapies (2).

Often, natural pharmacological agents, such as botanical preparations and nutritional supplements, are used as direct substitutes for conventional drugs. However, an important distinction must be made: the best use of these natural pharmacological agents involves promoting the healing process rather than simply alleviating symptoms. The use of glucosamine sulfate instead of nonsteroidal antiinflammatory drugs (NSAIDs) in the treatment of osteoarthritis illustrates this point.

Clinical and experimental research indicates that many NSAIDs used in the treatment of osteoarthritis may produce short-term benefit, but may accelerate the progression of the joint destruction by inhibiting the manufacture of glycosaminoglycans (GAGs), which are key components of the cartilage matrix (3–9). In contrast, glucosamine sulfate has shown equal to or better results for improving pain scores and Lequesne's index scores in double-blind studies versus placebo or NSAID in patients with osteoarthritis. These results are accomplished primarily through enhancing GAG synthesis rather than analgesic or pain relieving effects (3–6). Although NSAIDs offer symptomatic relief, glucosamine sulfate appears to address an underlying causative factor of osteoarthritis—that is, reduced manufacture of GAGs. Glucosamine sulfate not only improves the symptoms, including pain, but may also help the body repair damaged joints. This effect is unique and consistent with naturopathic goals, especially when glucosamine's safety and apparent lack of side effects are considered.

Complementary Aspects of Naturopathic Medicine

In addition to being used as primary therapy, naturopathic medicine is useful as a complementary approach to conventional medicine, especially in more severe illnesses requiring pharmacological and/or surgical intervention,

such as cancer, angina, congestive heart failure, Parkinson's disease, and trauma. For example, a patient with severe congestive heart failure requiring drugs (e.g., digoxin, furosemide) may benefit from the appropriate use of thiamin, carnitine, and coenzyme Q_{10} (CoQ_{10}) supplementation (10–16). Although there are double-blind studies demonstrating the value of these agents as complementary therapies in congestive heart failure, they are rarely prescribed by conventional medical physicians in the United States.

Using Naturopathic Medicine as Prevention

Ultimately, the greatest value of naturopathic medicine is disease prevention. Naturopathic physicians are trained to teach patients the importance of adhering to a health-promoting lifestyle, diet, and attitude in a family practice setting. True primary prevention involves addressing a patient's risk for disease (especially for heart disease, cancer, stroke, diabetes, and osteoporosis) and instituting a course of action designed to reduce controllable risk factors.

The health benefits and cost-effectiveness of disease prevention programs have been clearly demonstrated. Studies have consistently found that participants in wellness-oriented programs reduced their number of days of disability (43% in one study), number of days spent in a hospital (54% in one study), and amount spent on health care (up to 76% in one study) (17).

The therapeutic approach of the naturopathic doctor is basically twofold: to help patients heal themselves, and to use the opportunity to guide and educate the patient in developing a more healthy lifestyle. Many supposedly incurable conditions, such as osteoarthritis, respond very well to naturopathic approaches.

Clinical Application of Naturopathic Principles

Although every effort is made to treat the whole person (not just a disease), this chapter is limited to a description of only typical naturopathic therapies of specific conditions in a simplified, disease-oriented manner. The following are a few examples of how the person's health can be improved, resulting in alleviation of the disease.

MIGRAINE HEADACHE

Although the pathophysiology of migraine headaches entails vasomotor dysfunction, from the naturopathic perspective the underlying cause is maldigestion and a damaged intestinal mucosa that leads to food intolerance and nutritional deficiencies.

Double-blind, placebo-controlled studies have demonstrated that the detection and removal of allergic or intolerant foods eliminates or greatly reduces migraine symptoms in the majority of patients. Depending on the detection methodology, success ranges from 30 to 93% (18–23). When not carefully selected for food allergy, only about 30% of patients respond (18). However, when food intolerance is included, response rate increases to 84% (19–23). The key intolerant foods are cow's milk, wheat, chocolate, eggs, and the food additive benzoic acid.

Although maldigestion can result in nutritional deficiencies, only a few deficiencies have been studied in relationship to migraine headache. For example, several researchers have found a substantial link between low magnesium levels and both migraine and tension headaches (24–27). A magnesium deficiency increases vasomotor instability, setting the stage for the migraine attack. However, magnesium supplementation is only effective in migraine sufferers who are magnesium deficient (28, 29). Low tissue levels of magnesium are common in patients with migraine, but most cases go unnoticed because most physicians rely on serum magnesium levels to indicate magnesium levels; this serum measure is unreliable because most of the body's store of magnesium lies within cells, not in the serum. A low magnesium level in the serum reflects end-stage deficiency. More sensitive tests of magnesium status for migraine patients are the level of magnesium within the red blood cell (erythrocyte magnesium level) and the level of ionized magnesium (the most biologically active form) in serum.

Another possible benefit of magnesium in migraine sufferers may be its ability to improve mitral valve prolapse. Mitral valve prolapse is thought to be linked to migraines because it leads to damage to blood platelets, causing them to release vasoactive substances like histamine, platelet-activating factor, and serotonin. Up to 85% of patients with mitral valve prolapse may have chronic magnesium deficiency, in which case magnesium supplementation is indicated (30). This recommendation is further supported by several studies showing oral magnesium supplementation improving mitral valve prolapse.

Many botanical medicines have a long history of being used as folk cures for migraine headache. The most widely researched of these is *Tanacetum parthenium* (feverfew). A survey and several controlled studies have demonstrated moderately good clinical response with few side effects (31–34). However, from the naturopathic perspective, this is not a curative approach because it only relieves the symptoms without addressing the underlying causes.

BENIGN PROSTATIC HYPERPLASIA (BPH)

Prostatic hyperplasia affects most older men and is, from the naturopathic perspective, not a natural sequelae of aging. Rather, it is associated with a life-long inadequate consumption of zinc and essential fatty acids (EFAs) combined, in some cases, with excessive exposure to several toxins, such as alcohol.

Adequate zinc intake and absorption are paramount to proper function of the prostate. Zinc supplementation has been shown to reduce the size of the prostate—as determined by rectal palpation, x-ray, and cystoscopy—and to reduce symptomatology in the majority of patients (35, 36). The clinical efficacy of zinc is probably caused by its critical involvement in many aspects of androgen metabolism. In addition, zinc has been shown to inhibit the activity of 5-alpha-reductase, the enzyme that irreversibly converts testosterone to dehydrotestosterone (DHT) (37–41).

The administration of an EFA complex containing linoleic, linolenic, and arachidonic acids can result in significant improvement for many of these patients (42). In an uncontrolled study, all 19 subjects showed diminution of residual urine, with 12 of the subjects having no residual urine by the end of several weeks of treatment. These effects appear to be caused by the correction of an underlying EFA deficiency because these patients' prostatic and seminal lipid levels and ratios are often abnormal (43, 44).

Higher alcohol intake is associated with BPH. For example, a 17-year study of 6,581 men in Hawaii found that an alcohol intake of at least 25 oz/month was associated with the diagnosis of benign prostatic hyperplasia (45). Environmental toxins from pesticides and other contaminants (e.g., dioxin, polyhalogenated biphenyls, hexachlorobenzene, dibenzofurans) may increase 5-alpha reduction of steroids.

In addition to correcting the underling nutritional deficiencies and toxin exposure, the naturopathic physician helps facilitate the healing process with specific foods and botanical medicines. For example, soybeans, rich in phytosterols (especially beta-sitosterol) and the isoflavonoids genistein and daidzein, which have also been shown to improve BPH, may be recommended. In a recent double-blind study consisting of 200 men receiving beta-sitosterol (20 mg) or placebo three times daily (46), the beta-sitosterol produced an increase in maximum urine flow rate from a baseline of 9.9 mL/second to 15.2 mL/second and a decrease in mean residual urinary volume of 30.4 mL from 65.8. No changes were observed in the placebo group. An increased consumption of soy and soyfoods is also associated with a decrease in the risk of prostate cancer (47).

The liposterolic extract of the fruit of the palm tree *Serenoa repens* (Saw palmetto, also known as *Sabal serrulata*), native to Florida, has been shown to significantly improve the signs and symptoms of BPH in numerous clinical studies. The mechanism of action is related to inhibition of DHT binding to both the cytosolic and nuclear androgen receptors, inhibition of 5-alpha-reductase, and interfering with intraprostatic estrogen receptors. Roughly 90% of men with mild-to-moderate BPH experience improvement in symptoms, especially nocturia, during the first 4 to 6 weeks of therapy, with the condition continuing to improve with longer use (48–54).

CARDIAC FAILURE

The naturopathic approach to cardiac failure is to reverse the underlying causes: cardiac muscle degeneration secondary to poor blood supply and chronic nutritional deficiencies. Treatment focuses on improving myocardial energy production, because cardiac failure is characterized by an energy depletion status. This impaired energy production is often related to a nutrient or coenzyme deficiency, such as magnesium, thiamin, coenzyme Q_{10} (CoQ_{10}), and carnitine.

Low magnesium levels (particularly white blood cell magnesium) are common findings in patients with cardiac failure. This association is particularly significant because magnesium levels have been shown to correlate directly with survival rates. In one study, patients with normal levels of magnesium had 1- and 2-year survival rates of 71% and 61%, respectively, compared with rates of 45% and 42% for patients with lower magnesium levels (55). These results are not surprising considering that magnesium deficiency is associated with cardiac arrhythmias, reduced cardiovascular function, worsened ischemia, and increased mortality in acute myocardial infarction. Magnesium deficiency in these patients is probably due to a combination of inadequate intake and increased wasting secondary to overactivation of the renin-angiotensin-aldosterone system.

In addition to providing benefits of its own in congestive heart failure (CHF), magnesium supplementation also prevents the magnesium depletion caused by the conventional drug therapy for CHF (i.e., digitalis, diuretics, and vasodilators such as beta-blockers and calcium channel blockers). Magnesium supplementation has even been shown to produce positive effect in CHF patients receiving conventional drug therapy, even if serum magnesium levels are normal (56). Finally, magnesium is a critical nutrient for the production of adenosine triphosphate (ATP).

The frank thiamin deficiency of "wet beriberi" is known to result in cardiovascular dysfunction (i.e., sodium retention, peripheral vasodilation, heart failure). Although severe thiamin deficiency is relatively uncommon (except in alcoholics), many Americans do not consume even the RDA of 1.5 mg, especially elderly patients in hospitals or nursing homes. Depending on the thiamin measurement, plasma versus red blood cell thiamin, low levels (defined as a level below the lowest reference range for younger aged groups) were found in 57% and 33%, respectively, in one study (57). Interestingly, furosemide (Lasix), the most widely prescribed diuretic, has been shown to cause thiamin deficiency in animals and patients with cardiac failure.

Although the first study to look at thiamin as a potential adjunct in the treatment of cardiac failure showed only modest benefits, several subsequent studies have shown that daily doses of 80 to 240 mg of thiamin daily improved left ventricular ejection fraction by 13 to 22% (58).

Normal heart function is critically dependent on adequate concentrations of carnitine and CoQ_{10}. These compounds are essential in the transport of fatty acids into the myocardium and mitochondria for energy production. Although the normal heart stores more carnitine and CoQ_{10} than needed, cardiac ischemia rapidly depletes carnitine and CoQ_{10} levels. Several double-blind clinical studies have shown carnitine supplementation to substantially improve cardiac function in patients with cardiac failure (59–61). In one double-blind study, only one month of treatment (500 mg three times daily) was needed to cause significant improvement in heart function (60). The longer carnitine was used, the more substantial was the improvement. After six months of use, the carnitine group demonstrated an increase in the maximum exercise time of 25.9% and a 13.6% increase in ventricular ejection fraction.

Studies have also shown that CoQ_{10} supplementation is effective in the treatment of cardiac failure, typically as an adjunct to conventional drug therapy. In an early study, 17 patients with mild congestive heart failure received 30 mg/day of CoQ_{10} (62). All 17 patients improved, and 9 of them (53%) became asymptomatic after 4 weeks. In a more recent double-blind Scandinavian study of 80 patients, participants were given either CoQ_{10} (100 mg/day) or placebo for 3 months and then crossed over. The improvements noted with CoQ_{10} were greater than those obtained from conventional drug therapy alone (63).

Preparations of *Crataegus spp.* (Hawthorne) appear to be useful in correcting one of the underlying problems of cardiac failure: poor blood supply and ischemic damage. *Crataegus* is especially useful in the early stages as a sole agent and in the latter stages in combination with digitalis cardioglycosides. The effectiveness of *Crataegus* has been demonstrated in double-blind studies (64–66). In a recent study, 30 patients with congestive heart failure (NYHA Stage II) were assessed in a randomized double-blind study (66). The group receiving the *Crataegus* extract showed a statistically significant advantage over placebo in terms of changes in heart function as determined by standard testing procedures. Systolic and diastolic blood pressure were also mildly reduced. No adverse reactions occurred.

RESEARCH

Until the last decade, original research at naturopathic institutions has been limited. The profession has relied on its clinical traditions and the worldwide published health care research. The most comprehensive compilation of the scientific documentation of naturopathic philosophy and therapies can be found in *Natural Medicine* (Churchill-Livingstone, 1998) coauthored and edited by this chapter's authors. First published in 1985, the textbook now comprises over 200 chapters and references over 10,000 studies from the peer-reviewed scientific literature. The profession publishes the peer-reviewed *Journal of Naturopathic Medicine*.

The most current study of the efficacy of naturopathic practices evaluated 135 consecutive patients seen by naturopathic physicians in five clinics (Table 17.3). Patients in this survey showed a 53% decrease in those persistent health problems that were *not* the primary focus of treatment. This result is an indication of the nonspecific effects of the naturopathic approach to comprehensive patient treatment and education—that is, improved health and well-being.

Another promising study was the evaluation of an innovative health insurance program using

Table 17.3. Results of 135 Consecutive Patients Seen by Naturopathic Physicians in Five Clinics

Lowered or discontinued conventional treatment	49%
Self-care education (excellent or good)	96%
Effect on lifestyle (excellent or good)	92%
Successful treatment	68%
Persistent problems, other than primary complaint, improved as side effect of therapy	53%

naturopathic physicians as both wellness-educators and primary care providers. After one year, overall health care costs were decreased 30% (67).

There are a few studies that have directly compared patient satisfaction using natural medicines with patient satisfaction using conventional medicines. The largest study was done in the Netherlands, where natural medicine practitioners are an integral part of the health care system (68). This observational study compared satisfaction in 3,782 patients seeing either a conventional physician or a "complementary practitioner." As shown in Table 17.4, the patients seeing the natural medicine practitioner reported better results for most conditions. In this series, the patients seeing the complementary practitioners were somewhat sicker at the start of therapy; in 4 of the 23 conditions the conventional medical patients reported better results.

An in-depth review of evidence of safety, effectiveness, and cost-effectiveness of modern naturopathic medicine using government re-

Table 17.4. Patient Satisfaction with Complementary Practitioners Compared With Medical Specialists

SYMPTOM	COMPLEMENTARY PRACTITIONER PATIENTS (% IMPROVED)	CONVENTIONAL MEDICAL PATIENTS (% IMPROVED)
Palpitations	63	59
Stiffness	67	54
Feeling very ill	75	78
Itching or burning	71	50
Tiredness or lethargy	70	60
Fever	86	100
Pain	70	58
Tension or depression	69	65
Coughing	76	50
Blood loss	100	100
Tingling, numbness	59	40
Shortness of breath	77	53
Nausea and vomiting	71	67
Diarrhea and constipation	67	50
Poor vision or hearing	31	47
Paralysis	80	67
Insomnia	58	45
Dizziness and fainting	80	53
Anxiety	65	64
Skin rash	58	50
Emotional instability	56	63
Sexual problems	57	57
Other	75	56

views and audits, insurance company statistics, clinical trials, and other studies demonstrated that naturopathic medicine can contribute to the improvement of several common health problems affecting Americans (69). These studies need cautious interpretation, however, because they did not involve actual case studies, the 125 consecutive patients were not controlled, and the Netherlands' study is not entirely relevant to naturopathic medicine in the United States. More carefully conducted outcomes studies are needed to fully show the effectiveness of naturopathic medicine.

In the past decade, Bastyr University, National College of Naturopathic Medicine, and Southwest College of Naturopathic Medicine have all developed active research departments. This has resulted in the publication of original research in several peer-reviewed journals, both alternative and mainstream. In October, 1994, Bastyr University was awarded a three-year, $840,000 grant by the United States National Institutes of Health's Office of Alternative Medicine to establish a research center to study alternative therapies for patients with HIV/AIDS.

ORGANIZATION

Training

The education of the naturopathic physician is extensive and incorporates the diversity that typifies the natural health care movement. The training program is similar to conventional medical education, but the primary differences are in the therapeutic sciences. To be eligible to enroll, prospective students must first successfully complete a conventional premedicine program, which typically requires a college degree in a biological science.

The naturopathic curriculum is a four-year program. The first two years concentrate on the human biological sciences, basic diagnostic sciences, and introduction to the various treatment modalities. The conventional basic medical sciences include anatomy, human dissection, histology, physiology, biochemistry, pathology, microbiology, public health, pharmacology, biostatistics, and so on. The development of

diagnostic skills is initiated with courses in physical diagnosis, laboratory diagnosis, and clinical assessment. Finally, introductory natural medicine subjects, such as environmental health, pharmacognosy (pharmacology of herbal medicines), naturopathic philosophy, Chinese medicine, Ayurvedic medicine, homeopathy, counseling, spinal manipulation, nutrition, and hydrotherapy, are covered.

The last 2 years are oriented towards the clinical sciences of diagnosis and treatment. Not only are the standard diagnostic techniques of physical, laboratory, and radiological examination taught, but there is a special emphasis on preventive diagnosis, such as diet analysis, recognition of the early physical signs of nutritional deficiencies, laboratory methods for assessing physiological dysfunction before it progresses to cellular pathology and end-stage disease, and methods of assessing toxic load and liver detoxification efficacy. The natural therapies, such as nutrition, botanical medicines, homeopathy, acupuncture, natural childbirth, hydrotherapy, fasting, physical therapy, exercise therapy, counseling, and lifestyle modification, are also studied extensively.

During the last 2 years, students also work in clinical settings seeing patients, first as observers and later as primary care providers under the supervision of licensed NDs. Unlike MD and DO schools, most naturopaths do not go on to internship or residency training, although a limited number of optional residencies are available. Naturopaths do not do inpatient training or care; therefore, they generally do not deal with seriously ill patients who require hospitalization. These patients are referred for conventional treatment.

Professional Organizations

Three national organizations define and ensure the standards of naturopathic medicine: the Council on Naturopathic Medical Education (CNME), American Association of Naturopathic Physicians (AANP), and the Naturopathic Physicians Licensing Examination (NPLEx). The CNME is recognized by the United States Department of Education as the accrediting agency for schools and programs of naturopathic medicine. The AANP is the national professional association and counts the majority of licensed NDs in the United States as members of the associations. NPLEx provides nationally recognized standardized tests for licensing.

Licensing

Naturopathic physicians (NDs or NMDs) are currently licensed as primary health care providers in Alaska, Arizona, Connecticut, Hawaii, Maine, Montana, New Hampshire, Oregon, Puerto Rico, Utah, Vermont, and Washington. Legal provisions allow the practice of naturopathic medicine in several other states. There are currently efforts to gain licensure in other states. Naturopathic physicians are also recognized in most of the provinces in Canada. Naturopaths also practice in other states without government approval; however, without licensing standards, individuals with little or no formal education can proclaim themselves naturopaths.

All states and provinces with licensure laws require a resident course of at least 4 years and at least 4,100 hours of study from a college or university recognized by the State Examining Board. To qualify for a license, the applicant must satisfactorily pass the Naturopathic Physicians Licensing Exam, which includes basic sciences, diagnostic and therapeutic subjects, and clinical sciences. An applicant must satisfy all licensing requirements for the individual state or province to which he or she has applied as well. This requirement in most states licensing naturopathic physicians is a comprehensive written state board exam divided into main areas of focus and given over a 2- to 3-day period.

Unlicensed, self-proclaimed naturopaths are a serious problem for both the public and the naturopathic profession. With either no education or only correspondence school study, their health care credentials are, at best, problematic. In unlicensed states, the best criteria to determine if a naturopathic physician is legitimate is if he or she is a graduate from one of the three schools listed previously or a member of the AANP.

Reimbursement Status

Similar to licensure, insurance reimbursement differs from state to state. Insurance reimbursement ranges from government-mandated reimbursement, as occurs in Connecticut and Washington, to no reimbursement. Reimbursement standards for naturopathic physicians are of growing interest for insurance groups in many states.

Relations with Conventional Medicine

Because naturopathic physicians are primary care providers, it is essential they interact with conventional medical doctors. Naturopathic physicians, out of necessity for good patient care, develop a good working relationship with the various medical specialists to whom their patients must be referred when needed. Referral is required when more interventionist therapy or hospitalization is required. Examples of cases in which referrals are appropriate include life-threatening situations (e.g., acute myocardial infarction, stroke, sepsis, appendicitis, ruptured spleen), conditions in which the disease process has become advanced to a stage that is organ- or life-threatening (e.g., severe angina, very high blood pressure, advanced osteoporosis, nephrotic syndrome, brittle diabetes), and any condition outside the scope of practice for the individual naturopathic physician (e.g., broken bones, traumatic injuries requiring surgery).

The difficulty many naturopathic physicians experience in attempting to interact with conventional medical doctors stems from misconceptions the medical doctor may have about naturopathic medicine or from fraudulent naturopathic practitioners. These issues are usually displaced when conventional medical doctors interact with a well-trained modern naturopathic physician.

PROSPECTS FOR THE FUTURE

To some, naturopathic medicine, as well as the entire concept of natural medicine, appears to be a fad that will soon pass away. However, naturopathic physicians believe they are at the forefront of a better health care system.

One of the myths about naturopathic medicine is that there is no firm scientific evidence for the use of the natural therapies. However, numerous research studies and observations have not only backed the validity of diet, nutritional supplements, herbal medicines, detoxification, and physical medicine, but also have lent some support to more esoteric natural healing treatments, such as acupuncture, biofeedback, meditation, and homeopathy. In some cases, the scientific investigation has not only validated the natural measure, but also led to greater understanding of the pathophysiology and healing processes of the practices. In the past 30 years, there have been advances in understanding about how many natural therapies and compounds work to promote health or treat disease. Research has not lent support to all naturopathic practices. For example, recent studies on the effect of several naturopathic on the progress of HIV disease have shown no benefit from such practices. Undoubtedly, other established naturopathic practices will be shown to be ineffective or possibly even harmful as more and better research is conducted. The naturopathic organizations are committed to conducting those studies and improving naturopathic practices as resources for such research become available.

Scientific tools exist to assess and evaluate the fundamental principles and therapies of naturopathic medicine. It is becoming more common for conventional medicine to adopt and endorse a number of age-old naturopathic techniques, such as lifestyle modification, stress reduction, exercise, consuming a whole foods diet, supplemental nutrients, toxin reduction, and others.

There is a paradigm shift occurring in medicine. What was once scoffed at is now becoming generally accepted as effective. In many cases of common illnesses, the naturopathic alternative offers significant benefit over standard medical practices. In the future, it is likely that many of the concepts, philosophies, and practices of naturopathy will be demonstrated.

The naturopathic profession is growing rapidly. The therapeutic and diagnostic skills of practitioners are becoming more sophisticated; licensing is being established in new states; and public interest is strong. Key to the profession's future is becoming an integral part of the health care system.

REFERENCES

1. Cody G. History of naturopathic medicine. In: Pizzorno JE, Murray MT, eds. A textbook of natural medicine. Seattle, WA: Bastyr University Publications, 1998.
2. Pizzorno JE, Murray MT, eds. A textbook of natural medicine. Seattle, WA: Bastyr College Publications, 1998.
3. Dingle JT. The effect of NSAIDs on human articular cartilage glycosaminoglycan synthesis. Eur J Rheumatol Inflamm 1996;16:47–52.
4. Brandt KD. Effects of nonsteroidal anti-inflammatory drugs on chondrocyte metabolism in vitro and in vivo. Am J Med 1987;83(suppl.5A):29–34.
5. Shield MJ. Anti-inflammatory drugs and their effects on cartilage synthesis and renal function. Eur J Rheumatol Inflamm 1993;13:7–16.
6. Brooks PM, Potter SR, Buchanan WW. NSAID and osteoarthritis—help or hindrance. J Rheumatol 1982;9:3–5.
7. Newman NM, Ling RSM. Acetabular bone destruction related to non-steroidal anti-inflammatory drugs. Lancet 1985;2:11–13.
8. Noack W, Fischer M, Forster KK, et al. Glucosamine sulfate in osteoarthritis of the knee. Osteoarthritis Cartilage 1994;2:51–9.
9. Vaz AL. Double-blind clinical evaluation of the relative efficacy of ibuprofen and glucosamine sulfate in the management of osteoarthrosis of the knee in out-patients. Curr Med Res Opin 1982;8:145–9.
10. Leslie D, Gheorghiade M. Is there a role for thiamine supplementation in the management of heart failure. Am Heart J 1996;131:1248–1250.
11. Goa KL, Brogden RN. L-carnitine—a preliminary review of its pharmacokinetics, and its therapeutic use in ischemic cardiac disease and primary and secondary carnitine deficiencies in relationship to its role in fatty acid metabolism. Drugs 1987; 34:1–24.
12. Mancini M, Rengo F, Lingetti M, et al. Controlled study on the therapeutic efficacy of propionyl-L-carnitine in patients with congestive heart failure. Arzneim Forsch 1992;42:1101–1104.
13. Pucciarelli G. The clinical and hemodynamic effects of propionyl-L-carnitine in the treatment of congestive heart failure. Clin Ter 1992;141: 379–384.

14. Hofman-Bang C, Rehnquist N, Swedberg K. Coenzyme Q10 as an adjunctive treatment of congestive heart failure. J Am Coll Cardiol 1992;19:216A.

15. Morisco C, Trimarco B, Condorelli M. Effect of coenzyme Q10 therapy in patients with congestive heart failure: a long-term multicenter randomized study. Clin Investig 1993;71(Suppl.8):S134–136.

16. Baggio E, Gandini R, Plancher AC, et al. Italian multicenter study on the safety and efficacy of coenzyme Q10 as adjunctive therapy in heart failure. CoQ10 Drug Surveillance Investigators. Mol Aspects Med 1994;15(Suppl.):S287–294.

17. Pelletier KR. A review and analysis of the health and cost-effective outcome of comprehensive health promotion and disease promotion at the worksite: 1991–1993 update. Am J Health Promotion 1993;8:50–61.

18. Mansfield LE, Vaughan TR, Waller ST, et al. Food allergy and adult migraine: double- blind and mediator confirmation of an allergic etiology. Ann Allergy 1985;55:126–129.

19. Carter CM, Egger J, Soothill JF. A dietary management of severe childhood migraine. Hum Nutr: Appl Nutr 1985;39A:294–303.

20. Hughes EC, Gott PS, Weinstein RC, Binggeli R. Migraine: a diagnostic test for etiology of food sensitivity by a nutritionally supported fast and confirmed by long-term report. Ann Allergy 1985;55:28–32.

21. Egger J, Carter CM, Wilson J, et al. Is migraine food allergy? Lancet 1983;2:865–869.

22. Monro J, Brostoff J, Carini C, Zilkha K. Food allergy in migraine. Lancet 1980;2:1–4.

23. Grant ECG. Food allergies and migraine. Lancet 1979;1:966–969.

24. Mazzotta G, et al. Electromyographical ischemic test and intracellular and extracellular magnesium concentration in migraine and tension-type headache patients. Headache 1996;36:357–361.

25. Swanson DR. Migraine and magnesium: eleven neglected connections. Perspect Biol Med 1988; 31:526–557.

26. Ramadan NM, Halvorson H, Vande-Linde A, et al. Low brain magnesium in migraine. Headache 1989;29:590–593.

27. Gallai V, Sarchielli P, Morucci P, et al. Magnesium content of mononuclear blood cells in migraine patients. Headache 1994;34:160–165.

28. Pfaffenrath V, Wessely P, Meyer C, et al. Magnesium in the prophylaxis of migraine—a double-blind placebo-controlled study. Cephalalgia 1996;16:436–440.

29. Peikert A, Wilimzig C, Kohne-Volland R, et al. Prophylaxis of migraine with oral magnesium: results from a prospective, multi-center, placebo-controlled and double-blind randomized study. Cephalalgia 1996;16:257–263.

30. Galland LD, Baker SM, McLellan RK. Magnesium deficiency in the pathogenesis of mitral valve prolapse. Magnesium 1986;5:165–174.

31. Johnson ES, Kadam NP, Hylands DM, et al. Efficacy of feverfew as prophylactic treatment of migraine. Br Med J 1985;291:569–573.

32. Murphy JJ, Heptinstall S, Mitchell JRA. Randomized double-blind placebo-controlled trial of feverfew in migraine prevention. Lancet 1988; 2:189–192.

33. Barsby RWJ, Salan U, Knight BW, Hoult JRS. Feverfew and vascular smooth muscle: extracts from fresh and dried plants show opposing pharmacological profiles, dependent upon sesquiterpene lactone content. Planta Medica 1993;59:20–25.

34. Heptinstall S, Awang DV, Dawson BA, et al. Parthenolide content and bioactivity of feverfew (Tanacetum parthenium (L.) Schultz-Bip.). Estimation of commercial and authenticated feverfew products. J Pharm Pharmacol 1992;44:391–395.

35. Bush IM. Zinc and the prostate. Presented at the annual meeting of the AMA, 1974.

36. Fahim M, Fahim Z, Der R, Harman J. Zinc treatment for the reduction of hyperplasia of the prostate. Fed Proc 1976;35:361.

37. Leake A, Chrisholm GD, Busuttil A, Habib FK. Subcellular distribution of zinc in the benign and malignant human prostate: evidence for a direct zinc androgen interaction. Acta Endocrinol 1984;105:281–288.

38. Zaichick VY, Sviridova TV, Zaickick SV, et al. Zinc concentration in human prostatic fluid: normal, chronic prostatitis, adenoma and cancer. Int Urol Nephrol 1996;28:687–694.

39. Leake A, Chisholm GD, Habib FK. The effect of zinc on the 5-alpha-reduction of testosterone by the hyperplastic human prostate gland. J Steroid Biochem 1984;20:651–655.

40. Wallae AM, Grant JK. Effect of zinc on androgen metabolism in the human hyperplastic prostate. Biochem Soc Trans 1975;3:540–542.

41. Judd AM, MacLeod RM, Login IS. Zinc acutely, selectively and reversibly inhibits pituitary prolactin secretion. Brain Res 1984;294:190–192.

42. Hart JP, Cooper WL. Vitamin F in the treatment of prostatic hyperplasia. Report Number 1, Lee Foundation for Nutritional Research, Milwaukee, WI, 1941.

43. Scott WW. The lipids of the prostatic fluid, seminal plasma and enlarged prostate gland of man. J Urol 1945;53:712–718.

44. Boyd EM, Berry NE. Prostatic hypertrophy as part of a generalized metabolic disease. Evidence of the presence of a lipopenia. J Urol 1939;41:406–411.

45. Chyou PH, Nomura AM, Stemmermann GN, et al. A prospective study of alcohol, diet, and other lifestyle factors in relation to obstructive uropathy. Prostate 1993;22:253–264.

46. Berges RR, Windeler H, Trampisch HJ, et al. Randomized, placebo-controlled, double-blind clinical trial of beta- sitosterol in patients with benign prostatic hyperplasia. Lancet 1995;345:1529–1532.

47. Morton MS, Griffiths K, Blacklock N. The preventive role of diet in prostatic disease. Br J Urol 1996;77:481–493.

48. Boccafoschi S, Annoscia S. Comparison of *Serenoa repens* extract with placebo by controlled clinical trial in patients with prostatic adenomatosis. Urologia 1983;50:1257–1268.

49. Cirillo-Marucco E, Pagliarulo A, Tritto G, et al. Extract of *Serenoa repens* (Permixon[R]) in the early treatment of prostatic hypertrophy. Urologia 1983;5:1269–1277.

50. Tripodi V, Giancaspro M, Pascarella M, et al. Treatment of prostatic hypertrophy with *Serenoa repens* extract. Med Praxis 1983;4:41–46.

51. Champlault G, Patel JC, Bonnard AM. A double-blind trial of an extract of the plant *Serenoa repens* in benign prostatic hyperplasia. Br J Clin Pharmacol 1984;18:461–462.

52. Mattei FM, Capone M, Acconcia A. *Serenoa repens* extract in the medical treatment of benign prostatic hypertrophy. Urologia 1988;55:547–552.

53. Braeckman J. The extract of *Serenoa repens* in the treatment of benign prostatic hyperplasia: a multicenter open study. Curr Ther Res 1994;55: 776–785.

54. Bach D, Ebeling L. Long-term drug treatment of benign prostatic hyperplasia—results of a prospective 3-year multicenter study using Sabal extract IDS89. Phytomed 1996;3:105–111.

55. Gottlieb SS, Baruch L, Kukin ML, et al. Prognostic importance of serum magnesium concentration in patients with congestive heart failure. J Am Coll Cardiol 1990;16:827–831.

56. Gottlieb SS. Importance of magnesium in congestive heart failure. Am J Cardiol 1989;63:39G–42G.

57. Chen MF, Chen LT, Gold M, et al. Plasma and erythrocyte thiamin concentration in geriatric outpatients. J Am Coll Nutr 1996;15:231–236.

58. Leslie D, Gheorghiade M. Is there a role for thiamine supplementation in the management of heart failure. Am Heart J 1996;131:1248–1250.

59. Goa KL, Brogden RN. L-carnitine—a preliminary review of its pharmacokinetics, and its therapeutic use in ischemic cardiac disease and primary and secondary carnitine deficiencies in relationship to its role in fatty acid metabolism. Drugs 1987; 34:1–24.

60. Mancini M, Rengo F, Lingetti M, et al. Controlled study on the therapeutic efficacy of propionyl-L-carnitine in patients with congestive heart failure. Arzneim Forsch 1992;42:1101–1104.

61. Pucciarelli G, Masturi M, Latte S, et al. The clinical and hemodynamic effects of propionyl-L-carnitine in the treatment of congestive heart failure. Clin Ter 1992;141:379–384.

62. Ishiyama T, Morita Y, Toyama S, et al. A clinical study of the effect of coenzyme Q on congestive heart failure. Jpn Heart J 1976;17:32.

63. Hofman-Bang C, Rehnquist N, Swedberg K. Coenzyme Q_{10} as an adjunctive treatment of congestive heart failure. J Am Coll Cardiol 1992;19:216A.

64. O'Conolly VM, Jansen W, Bernhoft G, et al. Treatment of cardiac performance (NYHA stages I to II) in advanced age with standardized crataegus extract. Fortschr Med 1986;104:805–808.

65. Leuchtgens H. Crataegus Special Extract WS 1442 in NYHA II heart failure. A placebo controlled randomized double-blind study. Fortschr Med 1993;111:352–354.

66. Schmidt U, Kuhn U, Ploch M, et al. Efficacy of the hawthorn (Crataegus) preparation LI 132 in 78 patients with chronic congestive heart failure defined as NYHA functional class II. Phytomed 1994;1:17–24.

67. American Western Life Insurance. San Francisco, CA, 1994.

68. Oojendijk WT, Mackenback JP, Limberger HHB. What is better? An investigation into the use and satisfaction with complementary and official medicine in the Netherlands. Netherlands Institute of Preventive Medicine and Technical Industrial Organization, 1980.

69. Bergner P. Safety, effectiveness, and cost effectiveness in naturopathic medicine. Seattle, WA: American Association of Naturopathic Physicians, 1991.

CHAPTER 18

HOLISTIC NURSING

Barbara Dossey

BACKGROUND

Definition and Description

Holistic nursing is a philosophy and a model that integrates concepts of presence, healing, and holism. Although holistic nursing is not a system of nursing practice, it is recognized as an important way to conceptualize and practice professional nursing. The American Holistic Nurses Association (AHNA) defines and describes holistic nursing as follows (1):

Holistic nursing embraces all nursing practice which has healing the whole person as its goal. Holistic nursing recognized that there are two views regarding holism: that holism involves studying and understanding the interrelationships of the bio-psycho-social-spiritual dimensions of the person, recognizing that the whole is greater than the sum of its parts; and that holism involves understanding the individual as an integrated whole interacting with and being acted upon by both internal and external environments. Holistic nursing accepts both views, believing that the goals of nursing can be achieved within either framework.

Holistic practice draws on nursing knowledge, theories, expertise, and intuition to guide nurses in becoming therapeutic partners with clients in strengthening the clients' responses to facilitate the healing process and achieve wholeness.

Practicing holistic nursing requires nurses to integrate self-care in their own lives. Self-responsibility leads the nurse to a greater awareness of the interconnectedness of all individuals and the relationships to the human and global community, and permits nurses to use this awareness to facilitate healing.

The *AHNA Standards of Holistic Nursing Practice* defines and establishes the scope of holistic practice (2). These standards are based on the philosophy that nursing is an art and a science whose primary purpose is to provide services that strengthen individuals so they can achieve the wholeness inherent within them. The concepts of holistic nursing are based on broad and eclectic academic principles. Holistic concepts incorporate a sensitive balance between art and science, analytic and intuitive skills, and the ability and interconnectedness of body, mind, and spirit. Table 18.1 lists the two major parts and nine core values addressed in the *AHNA Standards of Holistic Nursing Practice.*

History and Development

The formation of the AHNA was a driving force behind the holistic nursing movement in the United States. In 1980, founder Charlotte McGuire and 75 founding members began the national organization in Houston, Texas. There are currently 4500 members. The AHNA mission is the renewal of holistic nursing with an

Table 18.1. Standards of Holistic Nursing Practice*

Part I: Discipline of Holistic Nursing Practice

Core Value I: Holistic philosophy

Core Value II: Holistic foundation

Core Value III: Holistic ethics

Core Value IV: Holistic nursing theories

Core Value V: Holistic nursing and related research

Core Value VI: Holistic nursing process

Part II: Caring for the Whole Client and Significant Others

Core Value VII: Meaning and wholeness

Core Value VIII: Client self-care

Core Value IX: Health promotion

* As addressed in the *American Holistic Nurses Association Standards of Holistic Nursing Practice*

emphasis on the discipline of holistic nursing and on caring for the whole client and significant others. Although the concepts in holistic nursing are not new, the AHNA focuses on holistic principles of health, preventive education, and the integration of allopathic medicine with complementary and alternative interventions for healing the whole person.

The key published AHNA works are the *Journal of Holistic Nursing* (3), the *IPAKHN Survey* (*Inventory of Professional Activities and Knowledge Statements of a Holistic Nurse*) (4), and the *American Holistic Nurses' Association Core Curriculum for Holistic Nursing* (5). There are now many nurse clinicians, educators, authors, and researchers who are key figures in holistic nursing at university-based schools of nursing as well as within other professional nursing organizations.

Principal Concepts of the Philosophy and Model of Holistic Nursing

PRESENCE, HEALING, AND HOLISM

Holistic nursing provides both substance and form for the ancient caring–healing practices of nursing. These practices can be used in the modern and demanding health care setting of today and the future. The three principal concepts of holistic nursing are presence, healing, and holism.

The first concept, *presence,* has significant implications in all areas of holistic nursing education, practice, and research. A common definition for presence is "being." As a noun, *being* is commonly defined as "existence" and "actuality." As a synonym, being is defined as "essence." Two components of *presence* have been identified: the physical "being there" and the psychologicalal "being with," which includes the nurse's use of spirituality, individuality, and authentic self. A holistic nurse integrates presence to be an effective guide. The art of guiding clients to tell their personal stories assists individuals in discovering and recognizing new health behaviors and choices, in exploring purpose and meaning in life, and in developing insight on how to cope more effectively. Guiding is a special art and a healing intervention that holistic nurses may use at all times. For example, a patient with pain describes the pain as squeezing, hard, and walled-off in a box. After a holistic assessment, the nurse will determine the most appropriate treatment. Many times pain can be relieved by guiding patients with relaxation and breathing exercises, possibly combined with imagery, music, or massage. Even when pain medication is required, these healing strategies can also be combined for best results.

The second concept, *healing,* is viewed in holistic nursing as a lifelong journey and process for all individuals. Clients often come to holistic nurses in search of healing, but holistic nurses remind these people that they always bring their healing with them. Holistic nurses enter into a state of "healing intention" with a client to bring to the present moment a person's fullest potential (6). It is a state of presence in the moment to care and to facilitate healing, not curing. Holistic nurses are becoming more aware of being an "instrument of healing" (7). For holistic nurses to evolve their own personal process, they reflect on their healing journey and ask the same questions of themselves as they do their clients, such as:

- How do I find meaning in my life?
- How do I define spirituality?
- When I use the words *guiding force, higher power, God,* or *absolute,* what kind of link with a universal wholeness do I experience?

The third concept addressed in holistic nursing, *holism,* explores basic assumptions about humans and humankind. Holism is a way of viewing everything in terms of patterns and processes that combine to form a whole, instead of viewing things as fragments, pieces, or parts. Natural systems theory, derived primarily from the work of von Bertalanffy, provides a way of comprehending the interconnectedness of natural structures in the universe (8). According to this theory, natural structures are composed of vastly different sizes, from the level of subatomic particles to the level of the entire universe. Each structure possesses definite characteristics at each level and is governed by similar principles of organization. Therefore, if any one part of the hierarchy changes, all the other parts are affected. Changes are occurring in the other levels simultaneously, which in turn affects the level to which an individual is attending to at the moment and vice versa. For example, the ripple effect of a pebble thrown in a body of water changes the water surface while simultaneously changing the air surface above and below as well. The analogy of a kaleidoscope is also useful: a slight turn of the kaleidoscope changes the whole configuration. This differs from the traditional Western allopathic view of disease which is usually from the level of the organelle to the level of body system or person.

Integration of Natural Systems Theory in the Holistic Nursing Model

The pathogenesis and etiology of health and illness in the holistic nursing model integrates the natural systems approach into nursing, giving a more complete perspective of disease. Viewed from a holistic perspective, disease can be caused by a disturbance anywhere from the subatomic to the transpersonal level; and disease may be caused by a force that disturbs or disrupts the structure of the natural systems themselves. Health is on a continuum, and the goal is to work with the patient to decrease the disturbances and stressors caused by his or her illness. As the patient and his or her family strive to reweave the social fabric of their lives and move towards achieving more harmonious interaction, these interactions affect all components of the natural systems hierarchy.

A key characteristic of the hierarchy of natural systems is informational flow (9). The result of illness causes chaos in the person's family with a temporary disharmony that further affects a person's work, the community, and up the hierarchy depending on the individual's involvement in society. The death of President John F. Kennedy in the early 1960s is an example of the magnitude of a disturbance at one level affecting the whole hierarchy. The world still reflects on this tragedy over 35 years after his death. Regardless of where the information originates, it spreads up and down the components of the hierarchy. Information flow has a domino effect because the whole system is affected by information originating at any point in the system. Holism and natural systems theory have important implications for providing a holistic perspective of caring and healing for individuals in their health or in all aspects of an illness.

The Bio-Psycho-Social-Spiritual Model

When making a holistic nursing diagnosis, holistic nurses use a bio-psycho-social-spiritual model to understand the whole person or situation. This model provides a complete and holistic understanding of how human beings function (10). This model also guides all of holistic clinical nursing practice, education, and research. In this model, all four components—the biological, psychological, sociological, and spiritual—are interdependent and interrelated. The tenants of this model assert that all of these components must be addressed to achieve optimal therapeutic results. Regardless of the technology, therapy, or treatment used, the human spirit is also included as a major healing force in reversing, stabilizing, and producing remission in all stages of an illness.

The biological dimension of this model includes those basic needs that help individuals maintain their health, such as food, sleep, water, exercise, fresh air, and a healthy environment. The psychologicalal dimension includes language, perceptions, cognition, mood, thoughts, symbolic images, memory, intellect, and the ability to analyze and synthesize data. The sociological dimension includes aspects that are involved in relationships with oneself as well as with family, friends, the community, and the universe.

The spiritual dimension in this model incorporates spirituality in a broad context that encompasses a person's values, meaning, and purpose in life. It reflects the human traits of caring, love, honesty, wisdom, and imagination. It may reflect evidence of a higher power or existence, or a guiding spirit. The concept of *spirit* implies a quality of transcendence, a guiding force, or something outside the self and beyond the individual nurse or patient; this concept may include organized religion, which pertains to an organized group worship experience with other people who have a similar belief system. Spirit may suggest a purely mystical feeling or a flowing dynamic quality of unity that is ineffable. If one could clearly define the spirit, then it would no longer be the spirit. It is undefinable, yet it is a vital force profoundly felt by the individual and capable of affecting life and behavior. The human spirit becomes enfolded in one's being, and one's perceptions of meaning can make the difference between life and death.

Holistic nurses distinguish spiritual elements from psychological elements (11). Spiritual elements are those capacities that enable a human being to rise above or transcend the circumstances at hand. These elements are characterized by the ability to seek purpose and meaning in life, to love, to forgive, to pray, to worship, and to transcend, move, or rise above ordinary circumstances.

It is possible to ignore spiritual concerns, meaning, and purpose or confuse them with religion or religious beliefs. However, spiritual factors are crucial in healing, and the human spirit plays a major role in who lives and dies. Giving attention to the role of the human spirit helps the treatment plan to be complete. Dissecting spirit during the healing process does not interfere with and is not harmful to conventional medical treatment.

Using this model, appropriate traditional, complementary, and alternatives therapies are chosen in a relationship-centered care process (12). The holistic nurse never heals the client, but uses herself or himself as an instrument of healing by guiding and facilitating clients in their healing process. The holistic nurse continues to refine and clarify the use of the most appropriate caring–healing modalities that can heal the human spirit.

PROVIDER–PATIENT/CLIENT INTERACTIONS

Patient Assessment Procedures

The holistic nursing process guides the nurse in all aspects of client interactions. The six parts of the holistic nursing process (13) are as follows:

1. Holistic assessment
2. Holistic nursing diagnosis
3. Client outcomes
4. Plan
5. Implementation
6. Evaluation

HOLISTIC ASSESSMENT

In a holistic assessment, the nurse listens to the client tell his or her story (i.e., history-taking), using both scientific approaches (e.g., physical assessment, noninvasive and invasive data) as well as intuitive approaches (e.g., therapeutic touch, presence, intuition). The client's data are recorded and organized according to the nine human response patterns of the Unitary Person framework, as described in Figure 18.1, a holistic assessment tool (14).

According to the North American Nursing Diagnosis Association (NANDA), a Unitary Person framework focuses on a person as an open system who interacts with the environment (15). After the holistic history data collection, the nurse uses the nine human response patterns of the Unitary Person framework to determine the most appropriate nursing diagnoses. Depending on the clinical situation and the client's needs, the holistic nurse may also perform an energetic (energy field) assessment, such as is used in therapeutic touch, pain assessment, imagery assessment, and with different caring–healing modalities such as touch therapies, movement, exercise, and cognitive therapies. Significant findings are marked on the human figure drawings at the end of the tool.

Another assessment tool, the spiritual assessment tool (Figure 18.2), can also be used in diagnosis (16). There are three defining characteristics of spirituality in this tool: meaning and purpose, inner strengths, and interconnections (17). *Meaning and purpose* refer to one's experience about life's purpose and meaning, mystery, uncertainty, and struggles. *Inner strengths* refer to a sense of awareness, as well as a sense of self, consciousness, inner resources, sacred source, unifying force, inner core, and transcendence. *Interconnections* include relatedness, connectedness, and harmony with oneself, others, a higher power, and the environment.

The spiritual assessment tool provides reflective questions for assessing, evaluating, and increasing spiritual awareness in clients and their significant others. The reflective questions in this tool can facilitate healing because they stimulate spontaneous, independent, meaningful initiatives to improve the client's capacity for recovery and healing. Use of bio-psycho-social-spiritual tools and integration of complementary and alternative therapies also assist nurses in meeting the mandate by the Joint Commission on Accreditation of Healthcare Organizations (JCAHO) to deliver the Patient Bill of Rights and to improve the quality of health care. The Patient Bill of Rights (RI.1.1.2) states that "care of the patient must include consideration of the psychosocial, spiritual, and cultural variables that influence the perception of illness. The provision of client/patient care reflects consideration of the patient as an individual with personal value and belief systems that impact upon his/her attitude and response to the care that is provided by the organization" (18).

HOLISTIC NURSING DIAGNOSIS

A holistic nursing diagnosis can be defined as a clinical judgment about the individual, the family, or the community responses to actual or potential health problems and life processes. These diagnoses provide the basis for selecting nursing interventions to achieve the desired client outcomes for which the nurse is accountable. The *taxonomy* of specific *holistic nursing diagnoses* is described in the nine human response patterns of the Unitary Person framework (see Figure 18.1). Each holistic nursing diagnosis has been or is currently being researched to further refine the etiology and defining characteristics of each holistic nursing diagnosis. When making a holistic nursing diagnosis, the human response patterns are considered basic for the nurse to perceive the meaning inherent with each person and his or her situation.

CLIENT OUTCOMES

After a holistic nursing diagnosis, client outcomes are established, which direct the plan of holistic nursing care. These client outcomes are direct statements of the desired end that the client will reach within a specific time frame. It indicates the maximum level of wellness that is realistically attainable for the client. Each outcome will specify something that should or should not occur, the time at which it should occur, and the expected results. Outcome criteria describe the specific tools, tests, or observations that will be used to determine whether the client outcomes are achieved. To achieve outcomes, they must be established by the client with the assistance of the holistic nurse, the family, and significant others. The client must be motivated and must want to change to establish healthy patterns of behavior.

Holistic Nursing Assessment Tool for Outpatients

Name _____ Date of Birth _____ Sex _____

Address _____ Telephone _____

Significant Other _____ Telephone _____

Date _____ Education _____ Employment _____

Medical Diagnosis _____

Reason for Seeking Holistic Nursing Care _____

_____

Height _____ Weight _____ B/P _____ T _____ P _____ R_____

Nursing Diagnosis
(Altered/High Risk for/
Potential for Enhanced)

Communicating—A pattern involving sending messages

Verbal: _____ [Communication, altered]

Nonverbal: _____   Verbal
                                                             Nonverbal

"Valuing/Transcending"—A pattern involving spiritual growth

Meaning and Purpose in Life: _____ [Spiritual State]

Inner Strengths: _____   Spiritual well-being

Interconnections (self, others, universe, higher power): _____   Spiritual distress
                                                                    Hopelessness
_____   Powerlessness

Relating—A pattern involving establishing bonds

Role (marital status, children, parents): _____ Role performance, altered
                                                                 Parenting, altered
_____   Parental role conflict
                                                                 [Work]
_____   Sexual dysfunction

_____

Occupation: _____ Family process, altered

Sexual Relationships: _____ Sexuality patterns, altered

Socialization: _____ [Socialization, altered]
                                                             Social interaction,
_____   impaired
                                                             Social isolation

FIGURE 18.1. Holistic nursing assessment tool. Developed by Pamela Potter Hughes, RN, BSN, MA, and adapted by Barbara M. Dossey, RN, MS, HNC, FAAN and Noreen Frish, RN, PhD. (Adapted with permission from Guzzetta CE, Bunton SD, Prinkey LA, Sherer AP, Seifert PC. Clinical assessment tools for use with nursing diagnosis. St. Louis: Mosby, 1989.)

PLAN

During planning, the holistic nurse helps the client and family identify methods of instituting new patterns of behavior to achieve a healthier state. The holistic nurse generally chooses an intervention by determining if it will be useful in helping the client reach a desired outcome; determining if the intervention should target etiology, signs, symptoms, or potential problems; evaluating the intervention; determining the feasibility of administering the intervention based on surrounding circumstances (e.g., time, cost, other diagnoses the patient may have) as well as how the client feels about the intervention; and by ensuring the nursing competency

Nursing Diagnosis
(Altered/High Risk for/
Potential for Enhanced)

Knowing—A pattern involving the meaning associated with information
Orientation: _____
_____
_____
_____

Memory: _____
_____
_____

Previous Illnesses/Hospitalizations/Surgeries: _____

Identified Health Problems (Present/History): _____

Current Medications (Medication Allergies): _____

Risk Factors (Smoking, Family History, etc.): _____

Perception/Knowledge of Health/Illness: _____

Expectations of Holistic Health Intervention: _____

Readiness to Learn (Ready, Willing, Able): _____
_____

Thought processes,
altered
[Orientation]
[Confusion]
[Memory]

Knowledge deficit
(Specify)

[Learning]

Feeling—A pattern involving the subjective awareness of information
Comfort: _____
_____
_____
_____

Emotional Integrity States: _____
_____
_____
_____
_____
_____
_____
_____
_____
_____
_____
_____
_____

[Comfort, altered]
Pain, chronic
Pain, acute
[Discomfort, chronic]
[Discomfort, acute]
[Grieving]
Anticipatory
Dysfunctional
Anxiety
Fear
[Anger]
[Guilt]
[Shame]
[Sadness]
Post-Trauma Response

Moving—A pattern involving activity
Activity (Physical Mobility Limitations): _____
_____
_____
_____

Rest: _____
_____
_____
_____

[Activity, altered]
Activity Intolerance
Impaired physical
mobility
Fatigue
Sleep Pattern
disturbance
[Hypersomnia]
[Insomnia]
[Nightmares]

FIGURE 18.1. (*continued*)

Nursing Diagnosis
(Altered/High Risk for/
Potential for Enhanced)

Recreation: _____

Environmental Maintenance: _____

Health Maintenance: _____

Self-Care: _____

Diversional activity
  deficit
Impaired home
  maintenance
  management
    [Safety Hazards]
Health maintenance,
  altered
Bathing/hygiene deficit
Dressing/grooming
  deficit
Feeding deficit
Toileting deficit

Perceiving—A pattern involving the reception of information
Sensory Perception: _____

[Sensory Perception,
  altered]
  Visual
  Auditory
  Kinesthetic
  Gustatory
  Tactile
  Olfactory
  Unilateral Neglect

Self-Concept: _____

[Self-Concept, altered]
  Body image
    disturbance
  Personal identity
    disturbance
  Self-Esteem
    disturbance
    —Chronic low
    —Situational

Choosing—A pattern involving the selection of alternatives
Coping: _____

Judgment/Decisions: _____

Participation: _____

Individual coping,
  ineffective
Adjustment: impaired
Conflict: decisional
Coping: defensive
Denial: impaired
Noncompliance

Family Coping: _____

[Family Coping,
  ineffective]
  Compromised
  Disabled

Figure 18.1. (*continued*)

Exchanging—A pattern involving mutual giving and receiving

Nutrition: _____
_____
_____
_____
_____
_____

Elimination: _____
_____
_____
_____
_____
_____
_____

Renal/Urinary: _____
_____
_____
_____
_____
_____

Physical/Tissue Integrity: _____
_____
_____
_____
_____
_____
_____
_____
_____

Physical Regulation: _____
Immune: _____
_____
_____
_____
_____
_____

Circulation: _____
_____
_____
_____
_____
_____
_____
_____
_____

Nursing Diagnosis
(Altered/High Risk for/
Potential for Enhanced)

[Nutrition, altered]
[Nutritional deficit]
< or > Body
Requirements
Oral mucus membranes,
impaired

[Bowel elimination,
altered]
Bowel incontinence
Constipation: colonic
Constipation:
perceived
Diarrhea
GI tissue perfusion
[Urinary elimination,
altered]
Incontinence (specify)
Retention
[Enuresis]
Renal tissue perfusion
[Tissue integrity,
impaired]
Impaired skin
integrity
[Injury: Risk]
Aspiration
Disuse syndrome
Poisoning
Suffocation
Trauma
[Physical regulation,
altered]
Infection: risk
Altered protection
Thermoregulation,
ineffective
—Hypothermia
—Hyperthermia
Cardiac output,
decreased
[Tissue perfusion, altered]
Cardiopulmonary
Cerebral
Peripheral
[Fluid volume, altered]
Deficit
Deficit: risk
Excess

FIGURE 18.1. (*continued*)

Oxygenation: _____

_____

_____

_____

_____

Hormonal/Metabolic Patterns: _____

_____

_____

_____

Energy Field Patterns

Nursing Diagnosis
(Altered/High Risk for/
Potential for Enhanced)

[Respiration, altered]
   Airway clearance,
      ineffective
   Breathing pattern,
      ineffective
   Gas exchange, impaired
[Menstrual Patterns]
[Premenstrual syndrome]

Energy Field Disturbance

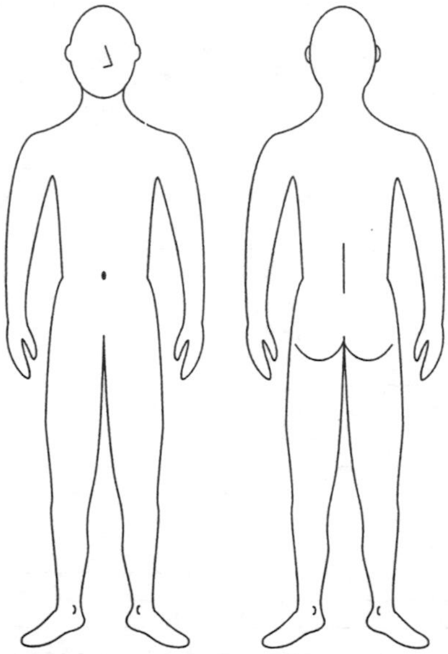

ADDITIONAL COMMENTS:

_____

_____

_____

_____

_____

_____

_____

Goals
  1. _____
  2. _____
  3. _____
  4. _____
  5. _____

FIGURE 18.1. (*continued*)

**Prioritized Nursing Diagnosis/Problem
List/Theory-Based Plan of Care**   Date

1. _____   _____
2. _____   _____
3. _____   _____
4. _____   _____
5. _____   _____

Signature _____ Date _____

Holistic Nursing Care Plan

Name: _____   Client Goals:

Date: _____   1. _____

                                                      2. _____

                                                      3. _____

                                                      4. _____

Nursing Diagnosis and Related Factors	*Client/Patient Outcomes Outcome Criteria*	*Therapeutic Intervention*	*Evaluation*

Client Signature _____

Date _____

Figure 18.1. (continued)

To facilitate the healing process in clients/patients, families, significant others, and yourself, the following reflective questions assist in assessing, evaluating, and increasing awareness of the spiritual process in yourself and others.

MEANING AND PURPOSE These questions assess a person's ability to seek meaning and fulfillment in life, manifest hope, and accept ambiguity and uncertainty.

- What gives your life meaning?
- Do you have a sense of purpose in life?
- Does your illness interfere with your life goals?
- Why do you want to get well?
- How hopeful are you about obtaining a better degree of health?
- Do you feel that you have a responsibility in maintaining your health?
- Will you be able to make changes in your life to maintain your health?
- Are you motivated to get well?
- What is the most important or powerful thing in your life?

INNER STRENGTHS These questions assess a person's ability to manifest joy and recognize strengths, choices, goals, and faith.

- What brings you joy and peace in your life?
- What can you do to feel alive and full of spirit?
- What traits do you like about yourself?
- What are your personal strengths?
- What choices are available to you to enhance your healing?
- What life goals have you set for yourself?
- Do you think that stress in any way caused your illness?
- How aware were you of your body before you became sick?
- What do you believe in?
- Is faith important in your life?
- How has your illness influenced your faith?
- Does faith play a role in regaining your health?

INTERCONNECTIONS These questions assess a person's positive self-concept, self-esteem, and sense of self; sense of belonging in the world with others; capacity to pursue personal interests; and ability to demonstrate love of self and self-forgiveness.

- How do you feel about yourself right now?
- How do you feel when you have a true sense of yourself?
- Do you pursue things of personal interest?
- What do you do to show love for yourself?
- Can you forgive yourself?
- What do you do to heal your spirit?

These questions assess a person's ability to connect in life-giving ways with family, friends, and social groups and to engage in the forgiveness of others.

- Who are the significant people in your life?
- Do you have friends or family in town who are available to help you?
- Who are the people to whom you are closest?
- Do you belong to any groups?
- Can you ask people for help when you need it?
- Can you share your feelings with others?
- What are some of the most loving things that others have done for you?
- What are the loving things that you do for other people?
- Are you able to forgive others?

These questions assess a person's capacity for finding meaning in worship or religious activities and a connectedness with a divinity or universe.

- Is worship important to you?
- What do you consider the most significant act of worship in your life?
- Do you participate in any religious activities?

FIGURE 18.2. Spiritual assessment tool. (Adapted with permission from Burkhardt M. Spirituality: an analysis of the concept. Holistic Nursing Practice 1989;3[3]:69.)

- Do you believe in God or a higher power?
- Do you think that prayer is powerful?
- Have you every tried to empty your mind of all thoughts to see what the experience might be like?
- Do you use relaxation or imagery skills?
- Do you meditate?
- Do you pray?
- What is your prayer?
- How are your prayers answered?
- Do you have a sense of belonging in this world?

These questions assess a person's ability to experience a sense of connection with all of life and nature, an awareness of the effects of the environment on life and well-being, and a capacity or concern for the health of the environment.

- Do you ever feel at some level a connection with the world or universe?
- How does your environment have an impact on your state of well-being?
- What are your environmental stressors at work and at home?
- Do you incorporate strategies to reduce your environmental stressors?
- Do you have any concerns for the state of your immediate environment?
- Are you involved with environmental issues such as recycling environmental resources at home, work, or in your community?
- Are you concerned about the survival of the planet?

FIGURE 18.2. *(continued)*

needed for successful implementation. Compatibility with other treatments and cooperation by the patient and family are essential parts of any comprehensive plan.

IMPLEMENTATION

Awareness is critical when a holistic nurse approaches the implementation of an intervention. The basic framework when implementing care is that the holistic nurse is aware that clients are active participants in their care, that the care must be performed with purposeful and focused intention, and that a client's humanness is an integral factor in implementation.

EVALUATION

Data about the clients' responses to intervention, as well as their bio-psycho-social-spiritual status, are continually collected and reported during the holistic nursing process. In evaluation, the holistic nurse attempts to determine if the client outcomes are successful and to what degree. The evaluation process includes not just the holistic nurse and client, but also the client's family and other members of the health care profession involved with the client.

THERAPY AND OUTCOMES

Treatment Options

After the holistic assessment, holistic nursing diagnosis, client outcomes, and planning, the most appropriate treatment options are determined by using a relationship-centered care approach with the client and significant others. From this coparticipatory perspective, the holistic nurse helps the client and his or her significant others choose the most appropriate therapies that integrate technology when needed along with complementary and alternative therapies. Another nursing taxonomy, the Nursing Interventions Classification (NIC), is also being used with increasing frequency (19). The complementary and alternative therapies listed in Table 18.2 are those most frequently used by holistic nurses in clinical practice (20). These therapies are usually referred to in holistic nursing as caring–healing modalities.

Description of Treatment Interventions and Evaluation

Descriptions of many of the treatments, outcomes, and treatment evaluations used in holistic nursing are developed throughout this book.

Table 18.2. Most Frequent Complementary and Alternative Therapies Used in Holistic Nursing*

Acupressure
Aromatherapy
Addictions counseling
Art therapy
Biofeedback
Cognitive therapy
Death and grief counseling
Environmental counseling
Exercise and movement
Goal setting and contracts
Healing touch
Holistic self-assessments
Humor and laughter
Imagery
Journaling
Massage
Meditation
Music and sound therapy
Nutrition counseling
Therapeutic touch
Play therapy
Prayer
Reflexology
Rituals of healing (combining several caring–healing modalities)
Relationship counseling
Self-reflection
Sexual abuse counseling
Spiritual counseling
Smoking cessation
Violence counseling
Weight management
Wellness counseling

* More frequently referred to as caring–healing modalities in holistic nursing.

The reader is referred to specific chapters within this book which correspond to therapies in Table 18.2 for details.

USE OF THE SYSTEM FOR TREATMENT

Meanings of Health and Illness

Holistic nursing considers the meanings a person attaches to symptoms or illness as integral to practice. These meanings are an important factor and influence the journey of one's life through a crisis (21). Human beings often view illness from one or more of at least eight frames of reference (22). Illness can be viewed as challenge, enemy, punishment, weakness, relief, strategy, irreparable loss or damage, or value.

Holistic nurses explore the meanings of health and illness with each individual and encourage these individuals to explore and share their story (23). Meanings are individual and personal and are congruent with the person's experience, belief systems, rationality, expectations, and context of the event. Context assumes significance in uncovering meaning and involves a person's past and present life story as well as what one believes about future events (24). The holistic nursing assessment explores these meanings with the individual clients looking at wholes, broad relationships, insights, and patterns.

Specific treatments are used depending on the holistic assessment, nursing diagnoses, client outcomes, and plan. These therapies include many mind-oriented therapies to treat physiological as well as psychological and spiritual sequelae of illness. Mind therapies are used as means of activating inner healing, thus augmenting the effects of drugs, surgery, and technological therapies and significantly improving morbidity and mortality rates and the quality of life. Holistic nurses consider complementary and alternative therapies as adjuncts or complements to conventional medical treatments and not necessarily as replacements for them. They advocate a *both/and* instead of *either/or* approach.

Doing and Being Therapies

Both *doing* and *being therapies* are used in holistic nursing. *Doing therapies* involve many forms of modern medicine, such as medications, procedures, dietary manipulations, radiation, acupuncture, and so forth. *Being therapies* do not employ medications or procedures; instead, these therapies use states of consciousness through imagery, prayer, meditation, quiet contemplation, and the use of presence and intention by the holistic nurse. Being therapies are therapeutic because of the psyche's power to affect the body.

These therapies generally are used in either of two ways: directed or nondirected (25, 26). When a patient employs a directed mental strategy, he or she attaches a specific outcome to the imagery, prayer, meditation, and so forth. For example, a patient may imagine coronary artery disease regressing or the blood pressure normalizing. When a nondirected approach is used, the patient does not assign a specific outcome to the strategy. Instead, the patient imagines the best outcome for the particular situation, without trying to steer the situation in any particular direction. The patient relies on the inherent intelligence within him- or herself to come forth and manifest, acknowledging the intrinsic wisdom and self-correcting capacity within nature. Doing therapies are highly directed in their approach. These therapies employ things and actions (e.g., medication, procedures) and they have a specific goal of outcome. The classic body–mind approach, however, employs the use of being therapies that can be directed or nondirected, depending on the mental strategies one decides to use, such as entering a state of relaxation or meditation. The individual moves to a level in which he or she feels a sense of interconnectedness that is beyond ordinary day-to-day involvement. It is actually a "not-doing," to become conscious of releasing, emptying, trusting, and acknowledging that we have done our best, regardless of the outcome.

Ritual

Rituals are an important aspect of holistic nursing. Holistic nurses can help to create a time for rituals that have specific meaning and to assist others in the art of ritual in daily living (27). Although there are no absolute rules that should be followed in creating ritual, a few guidelines are useful. A ritual should have a structure—a beginning, middle, and end. It helps to plan the details of a ritual carefully in advance (e.g., similar to what one does in anticipation of a special house guest). For example, when you are expecting a guest in your home, you give attention to details in a guest room by adding fresh flowers and books of art or poetry at a bedside, so that a sacred space is created. Ritual also happens when we create a sacred space to be alone and reflect on healing awareness.

The first phase of a ritual, the *separation phase*, is a symbolic act of breaking away from life's busy activities. For example, it may involve going to a quiet room for 15 to 20 minutes, taking shoes off, sitting on a pillow on the floor, putting on the answering machine, and honoring the silence. A sacred healing place can be made more personal with a special object, such as a burning candle, mandala or religious symbol, and to focus on that object brings a sense of calmness.

The second phase of ritual, the *transition phase*, helps individuals more easily identify areas in life that need attention. It is a time of facing the shadow, the hero's journey, where one can recognize the dark and the difficult as one searches for self and for what is real and worthy and in need of healing in the deepest sense. It is the time to go into an unknown terrain—the *limen*, or the meaning threshold—in which one leaves one way of being to enter into another way of participating.

The last phase of the ritual, the *return phase*, allows for a formal release. An individual can put aside or leave old fears, anger, or memories that no longer serve in daily living. This phase challenges a person to integrate a new way of acting, choosing, and relating, or to "walk one's talk" of healing awareness. Healing awareness is the ability to be present in the moment and to understand the meaning of the moment. In this state of being present, a noninterfering attention allows natural healing to flow.

The reader is directed to specific chapters in

this book for treatment approaches, recommendations, contraindications, preventive or nondiagnostic values, scope of practice, and evaluations corresponding to some of the complementary and alternative therapies listed in Table 18.2.

ORGANIZATION

Training

Training in holistic nursing first involves the basic nursing curriculum that leads to becoming a registered nurse; some academic nursing curriculums are more holistic than others. A nurse can receive additional training in holistic nursing through graduate education, various continuing education nursing programs, and professional nursing organizations.

The AHNA has established the knowledge and clinical competency in holistic nursing through the AHNA Holistic Nurse Certification Program and the AHNA Holistic Nurse Certification (HNC) Examination. The prerequisites for both routes to certification are that the registered nurse must be in good standing and be registered at a state level. The curriculum components for the AHNA Holistic Nurse Certification Program and the HNC examination are found in the *AHNA Core Curriculum for Holistic Nursing* (28). The *AHNA Standards for Holistic Nursing Practice* serves as the blueprint for both certification processes.

The AHNA Holistic Nurse Certification Program is a four-part program that lasts 18 to 24 months, depending on the nurse's pace. The participant learns about holistic nursing and caring–healing modalities. A nurse who has experience in holistic nursing may go straight to the HNC examination. On successful completion of the HNC examination, an HNC is awarded.

Quality Assurance

Quality assurance in these two certification routes have been established and are maintained

by the AHNA Certification Board. The AHNA completed the *IPAKHN Survey*, a role delineation/job analysis study that defined and validated the professional activities and knowledge requisite for competent holistic nursing practice in various practice environments (29). The *IPAKHN Survey* data analysis ensured the adequate content validity for the HNC examination blueprint as well as the percent of HNC examination questions that should be apportioned for each content area. The *IPAKHN Survey* and the *AHNA Core Curriculum for Holistic Nursing* both use the *AHNA Standards of Holistic Nursing Practice* as the organizational framework.

The successful completion of the AHNA Holistic Nurse Certification Program and the HNC examination are both a personal and a professional mark of achievement. HNC certification recognizes the holistic nurse as having the distinction of excellence in the area of holistic nursing. Nurses who complete either process have the honor to list HNC (holistic nurse certified) after their name. The legal status and regulations for the practice of holistic nursing, as with use of complementary and alternative therapies, are different in each state. Holistic nurses must know which complementary and alternative therapies they are covered to use in their professional practice as specified in their state's nurse practice act.

Emerging organizations and professional societies are increasing the number of offerings for holistic nurses in complementary and alternative therapies. The best references for these organizations are university nursing programs and their continuing nursing education departments.

Reimbursement Status and Relations with Conventional Medicine

The reimbursement status for holistic nurses is different in each state. Holistic nurses must know their nurse practice act and follow their state guidelines and regulations for reimbursement when in independent practice.

Many holistic nurses are joining other allopathic and complementary and alternative practitioners to offer holistic nursing services. Allopathic physicians are beginning to honor the mission and work of holistic nurses and are inviting them to join in collaborative practices to improve the quality of health care for their clients.

PROSPECTS FOR THE FUTURE

The prospects for the future are bright for holistic nurses. By the Year 2000, the majority of nurses will likely be practicing in the community, integrating holistic nursing and complementary and alternative therapies. Two major challenges are emerging in holistic nursing (30). The first is to integrate the concepts of technology, mind, and spirit into nursing practice; the second is to create models for health care that guide the healing of self and others.

Holistic nurses will continue to use, examine, and research complementary and alternative therapies that can facilitate healing, and determine which ones work, for which conditions, and with what results. They will explore further the values that clients and their significant others attach to complementary and alternative therapies and that holistic nurses attach to them. They will also continue to investigate anticipated complications that result from complementary and alternative therapies.

Holistic nurses can reduce the devastating effects of an individual's crisis and illness by using tools for assessing the bio-psycho-social-spiritual human dimensions and integrating complementary and alternative therapies. These tools and therapies are bridges for holistic nurses to better understand the emotions and meaning involved in clients' illnesses, crises, and life events.

RESOURCES

For information on the American Holistic Nurses Association Certificate Program in Holistic Nursing and the Holistic Nursing Certification Examination:

American Holistic Nurses Association
2733 East Lakin Avenue
Flagstaff, AZ 86004
(520) 526–2196
(800) 278-AHNA
(520) 526–2752 FAX

For audio and education video information on holistic nursing:

The Art of Caring: Holistic Healing Using Relaxation, Imagery, Music Therapy, and Touch (1995)
Sounds True Audio Tapes
(817) 773–2337
Boulder, CO

AHNA Video on Holistic Nursing (1996)
American Holistic Nurses Association
(800) 278-AHNA

At the Heart of Healing: Experiencing Holistic Nursing (1994)
Kineholistic Foundation
P.O. Box 719
Woodstock, NY 12498
(800) 255–1914/ext. 277

REFERENCES

1. American Holistic Nurses Association description of holistic nursing. Flagstaff, AZ: American Holistic Nurses' Association, 1993.
2. American Holistic Nurses Association standards of holistic nursing practice. Flagstaff, AZ: American Holistic Nurses' Association, 1994.
3. Journal of Holistic Nursing. Thousand Oaks, CA: Sage Publications, Inc, 1997.
4. IPAKHN SURVEY (The role of a holistic nurse: an inventory of professional activities and knowledge statements). Flagstaff, AZ: American Holistic Nurses' Association, 1996.
5. Dossey B, ed. American Holistic Nurses Association core curriculum for holistic nursing. Gaithersburg, MD: Aspen Publishers, Inc., 1997.
6. Dossey B, ed. American Holistic Nurses Association core curriculum for holistic nursing. Gaithersburg, MD: Aspen Publishers, Inc., 1997.
7. McKivergin M. The nurse as an instrument of healing. In: Dossey B, ed. American holistic nurses association core curriculum for holistic nursing. Gaithersburg, MD: Aspen Publishers, Inc., 1997.

8. von Bertalanffy L. General systems theory. New York: George Braziller, Inc., 1972.

9. Lazlo E. The systems view of the world. New York: George Braziller, Inc., 1968.

10. Dossey B, Guzzetta C. Holistic nursing practice. In: Dossey B, Keegan L, Guzzetta C, Kolkmeier L, eds. Holistic nursing: a handbook for practice. 2nd ed. Gaithersburg, MD: Aspen Publishers, Inc., 1995:18–19.

11. Kuhn C. A spiritual inventory of the medically ill patient. Psych Med 1988;6:87.

12. Tresolini CP, the Pew-Fetzer Task Force. Health professions education and relationship- centered care. San Francisco: Pew-Fetzer Health Professions Commission, 1994.

13. Guzzetta C. Holistic nursing process. In: Dossey B, Keegan L, Guzzetta C, Kolkmeier L, eds. Holistic nursing: a handbook for practice. 2nd ed. Gaithersburg, MD: Aspen Publishers, Inc. 1995:155–187.

14. Guzzetta C. Holistic nursing process. In: Dossey B, Keegan L, Guzzetta C, Kolkmeier L, eds. Holistic nursing: a handbook for practice. 2nd ed. Gaithersburg, MD: Aspen Publishers, Inc. 1995.

15. North American Nursing Diagnosis Association, NANDA nursing diagnoses: definitions and classification. St Louis, MO: North American Nursing Diagnosis Association, 1994.

16. Dossey B, Guzzetta C. Holistic nursing practice. In: Dossey B, Keegan L, Guzzetta C, Kolkmeier L, eds. Holistic nursing: a handbook for practice. 2nd ed. Gaithersburg, MD: Aspen Publishers, Inc., 1995.

17. Burkhardt M. Spirituality: an analysis of the concept. Holistic Nursing Practice 1989;3(3):69–77.

18. Patient rights. Accreditation manual for hospitals. Chicago: Joint Commission on Accreation of Health care Organizations, 1992 (suppl.spring).

19. McCloskey J, Bulechek G. Nursing interventions classifications. St. Louis: Mosby YearBook, 1995.

20. IPAKHN SURVEY (The role of a holistic nurse: an inventory of professional activities and knowledge statements). Flagstaff, AZ: American Holistic Nurses' Association, 1996.

21. Munhall P. Revisioning phenomenology: nursing and health science research. New York: National League for Nursing Press, 1994.

22. Lipowski ZJ. Physical illness, the individual and the coping process. Psych Med 1970;1:90.

23. Dossey L. Meaning and medicine. New York: Bantam, 1993.

24. Bevis EO. Accessing learning: determining worth or developing excellence—from a behaviorist toward an interpretative-criticism model. In: Bevis EO, Watson J, eds. Toward a caring curriculum: a new pedagogy for nursing. New York: National League for Nursing Press, 1990.

25. Dossey L. Healing words: the power of prayer and the practice of medicine. San Francisco: HarperSan Francisco, 1993.

26. Dossey L. Prayer is good medicine. San Francisco, CA: HarperSan Francisco, 1996.

27. Achterberg J, Dossey B, Kolkmeier L. Rituals of healing. New York: Bantam, 1994.

28. Dossey B, ed. The Amercian Holistic Nurses Association core curriculum for holistic nursing. Gaithersburg, MD: Aspen Publishers, Inc., 1997.

29. Dossey B, Fusch U, Forker J, et al. Evolving a blueprint for certification: inventory of professional activities and knowledge of a holistic nurse. J Holistic Nurs 1997;15(4):37–56.

30. Keegan L, Dossey B. Profiles on nurse healers. Albany, NY: Delmar Publishers, 1997.

CHAPTER 19

MEDICAL ACUPUNCTURE

Joseph M. Helms

BACKGROUND

Definition

Medical acupuncture is acupuncture that has been adapted for medical or allied health practices in Western countries. Acupuncture is derived from Asian and European sources and is practiced in both pure and hybrid forms. The foundation of medical acupuncture is the therapeutic insertion of solid needles in various combinations and patterns. The choice of needle patterns can be based on:

- Traditional principles, such as encouraging the flow of *Qi* (a subtle vivifying energy) through classically described acupuncture channels
- Modern concepts, such as recruiting neuroanatomical activities in segmental distributions
- A combination of traditional and modern concepts

The adaptability of classical and hybrid acupuncture approaches in Western medical environments is the key to their clinical success and popular appeal.

History and Development

In the United States, acupuncture has been increasingly embraced by practitioners and patients since the landmark 1971 *New York Times* article by James Reston describing his successful postappendectomy pain management with acu-puncture (1). Before that time, acupuncture had been practiced only in urban Asian communities, discreetly and primarily by and for Asians. In the early 1970s, widespread enthusiasm for acupuncture was fueled by reports from physician visitors to China who witnessed surgical analgesia using only acupuncture needles. Respect for the technique grew in the medical and scientific communities in the late 1970s, when acupuncture analgesia demonstrated a link to the central nervous system activities of endogenous opioid peptides and biogenic amines. Since the 1970s, guidelines for education, practice, and regulation in acupuncture have been established and implemented. Also, state, regional, national, and international societies have evolved to represent the interests of groups of practitioners.

CLASSICAL ACUPUNCTURE LITERATURE

Acupuncture is one discipline extracted from a complex heritage of Chinese medicine, a tradition that also includes massage and manipulation, stretching and breathing exercises, herbal formulae, and exorcism of demons and magical correspondences. (See Chapter 12, "Traditional Chinese Medicine," for a description of this entire system.) The earliest major source of acupuncture theory is the *Huang Di Nei Jing (Yellow Emperor's Inner Classic)*, the oldest portions of which date from the Han dynasty in the second century BC. The *Nei Jing* authors regarded the human body as a microcosmic reflection of the universe, and they believed the physician's role is to maintain the body's harmonious balance, both internally and in relation to the external environment. The *Nan Jing (Classic of Difficult Issues)* was written in the first and second centuries AD, also during the Han dynasty. This text presented a unified and comprehensive system that advanced the theories of points and channels and addressed the etiology of illness, diagnosis, and therapeutic needling. The *Zhen Jia Yi Jing (Comprehensive Manual of Acupuncture and Moxibustion)*, attributed to Huang-Fu Mi in 282 AD and based on the previous texts, is the oldest existing classical text devoted entirely to acupuncture and moxibustion (i.e., heating the acupuncture points and needles with smoldering mugwort, a dried herb).

Between the Han dynasty (206 BC–200 AD) and the Ming Dynasty (1368–1644 AD), acupuncture practice was refined and its literature underwent continual exegesis. Research, education, clinical refinement, and collation and commentary on previous classics flourished in the Ming dynasty. The *Zhen Jiu Da Cheng (Great Compendium of Acupuncture and Moxibustion)* of Yang Ji-Zhou, published in 1601, synthesized many classical texts as well as unwritten traditions of practice. This text became the most influential medical text for later generations in Asia and Europe. The *Da Cheng* was the source of acupuncture information transmitted to Europe in the seventeenth through nineteenth centuries via Latin translations by Portuguese, French, Dutch, and Danish missionaries, traders, and physicians traveling and working in China and Japan. It was also the primary source translated into French in the twentieth century.

GEORGE SOULIÉ DE MORANT

There was a flurry of primitive acupuncture experimentation by physicians in France, England, Germany, Italy, Sweden, and the United States in the first three decades of the nineteenth century. This experimentation did not renew itself in Europe until a century later and in the United States until the 1970s. The most influential impact on the development of twentieth-century European acupuncture was the work of George Soulié de Morant, a scholar–diplomat engaged in the French diplomatic service in China between 1901 and 1917. Soulié de Morant published articles and French translations of Chinese and Japanese medical texts, and, on his return to France, taught clinical applications of acupuncture to French physicians. He systematically introduced acupuncture theory from the classical texts to the French and European medical community. The commonly used terms *meridian* and *energy* both originated in his texts as translations for the two fundamental tenets of acupuncture anatomy and physiology. In twentieth-century France and in much of Europe since the 1950s, clinical acupuncture has codeveloped with biomedical science. Europe has thus served as another influence for acupuncture approaches that integrate into the practice of conventional Western medicine (2).

PRINCIPAL CONCEPTS

Classical Acupuncture

Acupuncture has evolved over two millennia, both through refinements based on treatment responses and through adaptations to changing social situations. The language in classical acupuncture texts reflects nature and agrarian village metaphors and describes a philosophy of humans functioning harmoniously within an orderly universe. The models of health, disease, and treatment are presented in terms of a patient's harmony or disharmony within this larger order; and these models involve the patient's responses to external extremes of wind, heat, damp, dryness, and cold and to internal extremes of anger, excitement, worry, sadness, and fear. Likewise, illnesses are described and defined poetically: by divisions of the *Yin* and *Yang* polar opposites (e.g., interior or exterior, cold or hot, deficient or excessive), by descriptors attached to elemental qualities (e.g., wood, fire, earth, metal, and water), and by the functional influences traditionally attached to each of the internal organs.

ANATOMY OF ACUPUNCTURE

The classical anatomy of acupuncture consists of energy channels traversing the body. The principal energy pathways are named for organs whose realms of influence are expanded from their conventional biomedical physiology to include functional, energetic, and metaphoric qualities. For example, the Kidney supervises bones, marrow, joints, hearing, head hair, and will and motivation; and the Spleen oversees digestion, blood production, blood-related functions (e.g., menstruation), and nurturing and introspection. Acupuncture anatomy is a multilayered interconnecting network of channels that establishes an interface between an individual's internal and external environments and permits energy to move through the muscles and the various organs.

The most superficial of these pathways are the *tendinomuscular meridians,* which are an interface between the organism and its external environment. These meridians provide the first defense for the body's response to climatic conditions and external traumas. The *principal meridians* travel through the muscles and provide nourishment to all tissues and vitality for animation and physical activity. The *distinct meridians* go directly from the surface of the body deep to the organs, and they allow the nourishment and the energy produced by the organs to circu-

late throughout the body. Finally, a system of pathways called the *curious meridians* creates connections among the principal acupuncture channels and serves as energy reservoirs for extreme conditions of emptiness or fullness.

These meridians and their connections form a network of energy circulation that is organized into three bilaterally symmetric plates that divide the body into six sagittal territories of influence. Each plate manifests the energy derived from four organs as it circulates in their anatomic territory of influence. Figure 19.1 represents the schematic organization of one plate in the acupuncture energy circulation. The core rectangle is the principal meridian subcircuit from which the subdivisions of energy circulation are derived: tendinomuscular meridians on the surface, distinct meridians going to the organs, and curious meridians creating connections among several principal meridian subcircuits. Figure 19.2A shows the bilateral surface tracing of one principal meridian subcircuit, and Figure 19.2B gives the organ associations, and thus the names, for these energy channels: Kidney–Heart (Shao Yin) and Small Intestine–Bladder (Tai Yang). Figure 19.3A shows the surface location of the Kidney and Bladder ten-

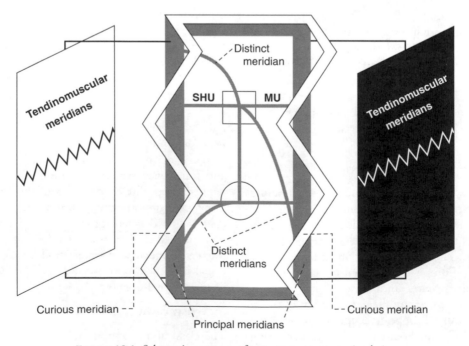

FIGURE 19.1. Schematic anatomy of acupuncture energy circulation.

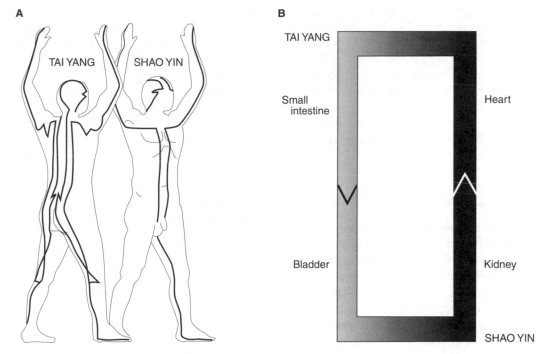

FIGURE 19.2. (A) The Shao Yin–Tai Yang meridian subcircuit. (B) Organ associations (energy channels) for the Shao Yin–Tai Yang meridian subcircuit.

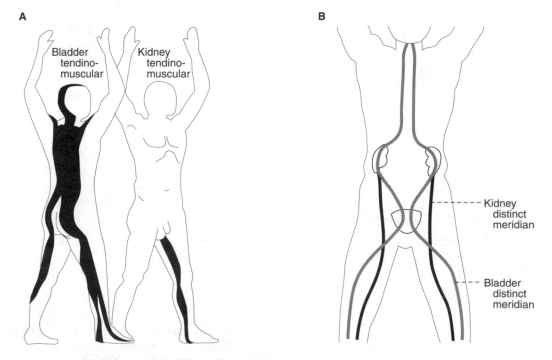

FIGURE 19.3. (A) Kidney and Bladder tendinomuscular meridians. (B) Kidney and Bladder distinct meridians.

dinomuscular meridians, associated with two of the four organs involved in the Shao Yin–Tai Yang principal meridian subcircuit, and Figure 19.3B shows the deep pathways of the distinct meridians for the same two organs. Each of the three bilaterally symmetrical subcircuits has a similar schematic organization. The anatomic territory of influence shifts with the location of its sagittal plate and the organs involved in its energy circulation.

PHYSIOLOGY AND PATHOLOGY OF ACUPUNCTURE

The classical physiology of acupuncture involves a dozen internal organs that interact to produce basic energy in blood from ingested solid and liquid nourishment. These organs then mix in the energy from inspired air and propel the transformed energy and blood through all the body's organs and tissues. The organs are divided into six parenchymal, energy-producing organs (solid, *Yin*), and six visceral, substance-transporting organs (hollow, *Yang*). These organs are coupled into groups (one *Yin* and one *Yang*) to comprise the three symmetric energy circulation plates.

Pathology in acupuncture involves an early manifestation of disharmony associated with the subtle influences of an organ, a disruption of the *Qi* flow in one of the subdivisions of the circulation network associated with an organ, or a frank disturbance in an organ's metabolic or transport function.

DIAGNOSIS AND TREATMENT IN ACUPUNCTURE

Diagnosis in acupuncture involves recognizing the level of manifestation of a disturbance. Premorbid symptomatology is organized according to the organs' subtle spheres of influence, in which early energetic and functional symptoms are linked to the organ that supervises the disturbed anatomic region or physiological function; for example, Kidney energy supervises head hair, and thus premature graying or balding reflects a deficient Kidney vitality. Obstruction of the flow of energy or blood through the principal meridians manifests as musculoskeletal pain in the territory of the channel; for exam-

ple, the Bladder principal meridian passes through the lower back, and thus lumbar pain reflects an obstruction of *Qi* and blood flow through that channel. Organ pathology is identified either in conventional biomedical terms or as a disturbance in the organ's physiological activities according to acupuncture terms; for example, nephrolithiasis is a disturbance in both Kidney and Bladder organs and spheres of influence.

Treatment in acupuncture involves the insertion of needles along the channels of the involved organs to stimulate energy circulation, which can influence the problem at its level of manifestation and thus restore energetic balance and organ function.

Modern Acupuncture

Since the late 1970s, acupuncture analgesia has been demonstrated to activate the endogenous opioid peptide system and thereby influence the body's pain regulatory mechanism by changing the processing and perception of noxious information at various levels of the central nervous system. Two model systems of acupuncture analgesia have been advanced:

Endorphin-dependent system. This involves low-frequency, high-intensity electrical stimulation of acupuncture needles (2 to 4 Hz) that is slow in onset, generalized throughout the body, and cumulative on subsequent stimulation (3).

Monoamine-dependent system. This involves high-frequency, low-intensity electrical stimulation of acupuncture needles (70 Hz or greater) that is rapid in onset, segmental, and not cumulative (3).

By combining the neurohumoral models with other observations and speculations about the mechanism of acupuncture's effect, a physiological model is created of an acupuncture needle simultaneously activating multiple systems in the body's physiology:

1. **The nervous system,** which includes peripheral afferent transmission, perivascular sympathetic fiber conduction, and the central

neurohumoral and neuropeptide mechanisms;

2. **The blood circulation system,** which transmits locally and centrally biomolecular elements and the biochemical and cellular changes stimulated by acupuncture in the periphery;

3. **The lymphatic system,** which serves as a medium for ionic flow along fascial planes and perivascular interstitial fluid circulation; and

4. **The electromagnetic bioinformation system,** which consists of static electricity on the surface, ionic migration in the interstitial fluid between the needles and as currents of injury at the needled site, and fascial and perineural semiconduction throughout the body (4).

This hybrid assemblage of descriptions creates a contemporary working model of a multisystem information network that obliges the medical acupuncture practitioner to consider not only classical paradigms to arrive at diagnostic and therapeutic decisions, but also to account for neuroanatomic and neurophysiological parameters. These considerations are of special importance in acupuncture's application in pain management, in which knowledge of dermatomal, myotomal, sclerotomal, and autonomic innervation patterns is indispensable.

PROVIDER–PATIENT INTERACTION

History and Physical Examination

In a medical acupuncture evaluation, the initial encounter with the patient is similar to that of a conventional allopathic medical interview and examination. The patient is encouraged to speak candidly and thoroughly about the presenting problems and his or her background. In addition to a conventional assessment and differential diagnosis, the practitioner explores the characteristics and behaviors of the problems in an effort to link them with the gross or subtle spheres of influence of one or several internal organs. In the case of musculoskeletal pain problems, the location of the pain is identified neuro-anatomically and according to the acupuncture channel in whose territory it lies. The goal of the interview is to identify the organs and energy circulation divisions involved in the patient's disorder, and to discern whether the association is with subtle symptoms linked to the traditional sphere of influence of the organs, with the trajectory of a meridian through a painful region, with a dense organ lesion, or with a combination of these factors.

The patient's past medical history, childhood illnesses, family history, and review of systems are elicited during the interview, and all information is tagged with the organ or meridian under whose supervision it falls. During this period, the acupuncturist poses questions of particular importance: Is there a possible cyclicity in the appearance of the symptoms? Are there seasonal exacerbations or general seasonal preferences or dislikes? Does the patient have positive or negative flavor and color affinities? How do the symptoms respond to external climatic environments? How does the lesion respond to pressure, movement, heat, or cold?

A standard physical examination appropriate for the patient and the problem is undertaken, with several additional acupuncture inspections included. The musculoskeletal evaluation includes identification of painful muscle knots and trigger points, as well as subcutaneous nodules and bands overlying contracted muscles. Specific reflex points on the front and back of the trunk—*Mu points* and *Shu points*—correspond to the organs associated with them. If any Mu or Shu points are sensitive to palpation during the physical examination, those findings are also recorded.

In acupuncture, several diagnostic somatotopic systems that microcosmically reflect the internal organs are routinely used to evaluate the balance of relative strengths and weaknesses within the organs. The systems most commonly employed are the reflex systems of the tongue, the radial pulse, and the external ear. These inspections are undertaken as part of the routine physical evaluation.

Through its color, body, coating, and surface irregularities, the tongue reflects the basic condition and underlying problem of the patient at the time of examination. Changes in tongue qualities are easily noted from week to week and often day to day. The tongue serves as an indicator of change in the patients as they evolve through illness and respond to medical interventions.

The diagnostic microsystem of the radial pulse provides another means of evaluating the patient's overall condition and of comparing the relative strengths of energetic activity in the organs and their meridians. The pulse changes from minute to minute and can therefore be used to verify whether an input had its intended effect before continuing or concluding the treatment. The pulses also serve as a subjective measurement from visit to visit, revealing the stability of the changes made through the acupuncture treatments.

Evaluation of the external ear confirms findings from the physical examination or other reflex systems, and it may indicate new directions to explore in the interview and examination. The diagnostic examination of the external ear includes visual inspection, palpation with a probe, or scanning with a battery-powered electrical resistance detector. The external ear can also be used as a treatment system, in isolation or as an adjunct to body acupuncture points.

Differential Diagnosis and Treatment Planning

Before concluding the diagnostic process, a review of past medical records, radiographs, and laboratory studies is undertaken, and appropriate new studies are requested to confirm and specify mechanical and organic disorders. From all available information, subtle and gross symptoms and characteristics are organized into affinity clusters, and patterns of disharmony are identified. The organ or organ's influence that is most disturbed is then defined, as is the *level of manifestation* of this greatest disturbance. The *energy-functional level* of disturbance involves the balance of energetic and metabolic activities of the organs and their spheres of influence, including especially their psychoemotional expressions; the *channel-structural level* involves skin, fascia, muscles, and bones; and the *organ*

level involves the metabolic or transport functions of the organs themselves. The acupuncturist then decides what division of the energy circulation network gives best access to the level of greatest disturbance.

The initial interview affords the acupuncturist an understanding of the nature of the problems and of the patient's constitutional strengths and weaknesses. The ideal diagnostic conclusion is a clear perception of the patient's health course: the presenting problems and their origins and the likely future health events. An algorithm of treatment approaches is constructed. The acupuncturist must keep in mind the goal of the overall treatment strategy while working with various tactics at each session. For example, the immediate treatment plan may address only relief of the most urgent symptoms, and longstanding problems can be addressed after change occurs in the presenting symptoms.

TREATMENT DESIGN

The first steps in treatment design are to identify the levels of manifestation of the patient's complaints and to establish an order of treating the problems. Treatment strategy involves activating the appropriate layers of the energy circulation network to address each problem in its own level of manifestation. A simple strain or sprain may need nothing more than dispersion with needles surrounding the local lesion and an activation of the appropriate tendinomuscular meridian. Musculoskeletal pain of longstanding duration will need placement of needles around one of the principal meridian subcircuits to encourage energy flow, plus local needles to focus on the site of the problem. Such a treatment may involve electrical stimulation of the points needed to move the energy through the subcircuit as well as the local points. Psychosomatic or premorbid problems may respond to the needling of several front or back *Mu* or *Shu* points, to a rarefied equilibration treatment based on more arcane models of organ and energy interactions, or perhaps to an activation of energy flow through the disturbed principal meridian subcircuit.

It is important to aim treatment at the level of manifestation of the problem being addressed. The circulation levels being activated may be changed during a series of treatments to better address the presenting problem or to introduce treatment for secondary problems. It is better to proceed slowly than with vigor, so that the patient's response to the treatment can be evaluated properly. As with any other medical intervention, factors influencing the outcome of a treatment include the patient's age, the duration and complexity of the presenting problem, presence of concurrent acute or chronic illness, medications, history of surgical interventions, lifestyle and personal health factors, and the patient's emotional state and basic vitality. The patient's attitude towards acupuncture usually does not affect the result; it is not necessary to believe in acupuncture for it to be effective.

THERAPY AND OUTCOMES

Treatment Options

The author and the majority of physician acupuncturists in the United States use the hybrid model of combining energy movement through the channels with local or focusing treatment. This model, known as *acupuncture energetics*, is derived from European interpretations of the Chinese classics and blended with neuromuscular anatomy of trigger points and segmental innervation for pain treatments. *Japanese meridian acupuncture* is most akin to the linear energy movement programs represented in this chapter, although Japanese practitioners commonly place needles more superficially than do Europeans or Americans.

Of the acupuncture systems currently practiced in the United States, *traditional Chinese medicine,* which is taught at the training colleges in China, is the most widespread. This approach to acupuncture is linked with prescribing traditional herbs as the core of the discipline and can be effective for many conditions. The acupuncture points are selected for their traditional functions to reinforce the goals of herbal therapy, rather than simply to move energy through the circulation network.

Five elements acupuncture is another widely practiced discipline, imported from England, reflecting French and other European interpretations of classical information. This approach has its greatest value assisting in the repair of problems originating in the psychoemotional sphere.

Three *somatotopic systems* have established themselves as valuable disciplines, used either as exclusive approaches to acupuncture or as adjuncts to body acupuncture. *Auricular acupuncture*, developed in France, offers a homuncular reflex organization of all body parts on the external ear. *Korean hand acupuncture* identifies a microsystem on the hand of the complete meridian circulation. *Scalp acupuncture* is yet another recent development. There are several systems of scalp acupuncture that divide cranial territories into neurological regions corresponding to cerebrocortical influences on the body structures. These somatotopic systems appear to be effective for modifying neurological problems that can be elusive to body acupuncture.

Description of Treatment

The acupuncture treatment consists of inserting fine needles into the body in patterns designed to influence the flow of *Qi* in one of the subdivisions of the energy circulation network. Usually only one energy subdivision is selected to stimulate energy movement, along with a collection of local points to focus the attention of the energy movement. Each subdivision of the circulation has a unique therapeutic point combination necessary for activation. The combinations involve the insertion of at least three needles—the energy-moving needles—that are usually in the extremities and usually run bilaterally. The focusing needles are inserted at trunk points that influence the organs being stimulated, or at muscular points tender to palpation in the region of the pain.

Needles are inserted to the depth necessary to elicit the patient's sensation of *De Qi*, or needle grab, a dull ache that radiates from the point. This can be 0.5 to 8 centimeters, depending on the location. Needles vary from 0.1

to 0.35 millimeters in diameter, and from 1 to 15 centimeters in length.

The patient is positioned comfortably, usually lying supine or prone. The acupuncture needles are inserted and are left in place for 5 to 20 minutes. It is crucial to protect the patient from energy depletion during an acupuncture treatment. The older or more fatigued the patient, the shorter the duration of the treatment must be. The energy-moving needles may be stimulated when an additional activation of the acupuncture system is desired, such as when the problem is one of deficiency according to acupuncture principles or when the patient has low vitality. This stimulation is accomplished by manual manipulation, by heating the needle with burning mugwort (moxibustion), or by connecting the needles to an electrical stimulating device.

Focusing needles can likewise be stimulated with manual, thermal, or electrical means. It is common to treat the patient using front, back, and extremity points during the course of a single treatment session. This means that the treatment is typically divided into several sections: the energy movement section using extremity points to activate flow through the meridians, and the points to focus the energy on one or several organs, or local points to influence a pain problem.

The following is an example of preventive intervention that uses the traditional influences of the organs: A 33-year-old man presents with reports of a general diminution of energy, including decreased sexual interest, increased sensitivity to cold weather, mild generalized joint aches, and a new affinity for salt. He is wearing a black T-shirt and black underpants and has significant graying at the hair on his temples (symptoms and presentation being features of Kidney influence). His medical evaluation and laboratory tests are negative. This case is a premorbid manifestation of weakness in the Kidney sphere of influence. An appropriate treatment would be to activate Kidney energy with needles and moxibustion at the *Shu* points for Kidney on the back, bilaterally, as the first section of the treatment. The second section of treatment could consist of creating an energy flow through

the *Shao Yin* (Kidney–Heart) and *Tai Yang* (Small Intestine–Bladder) principal meridian subcircuit by placing one needle in the Kidney meridian, one in the Heart meridian, and one in the Bladder meridian, bilaterally in the extremities, and manually stimulating and additionally with moxibustion. Each section would last 5 to 10 minutes and would take place in one session.

The local treatments for pain problems can be quite complex because, in addition to honoring the classical directive of encouraging the flow of *Qi* and blood through the channels that traverse the painful area, the neuromuscular anatomy must be considered. Deliberately searching for and deactivating intramuscular trigger points in the region of pain and along the myotomal distribution of the spinal segments involved in the pain is a necessary component of the local treatment. Likewise, recruiting the neurological activity of the spinal origins of the dermatomal, myotomal, sclerotomal, and sympathetic innervation of the pain problem is a common local treatment for chronic pain. In these cases, electrical stimulation is commonly used, with the frequencies ranging between 2 and 150 Hz.

For example, if the 33-year-old man described in the preceding case also has chronic lumbar pain with an occasional L5 radicular component, the acupuncture treatment will consist of an initial energy-moving section involving two needles bilaterally in the extremities on the Kidney meridian, one in the Heart meridian, one in Small Intestine, and one in Bladder. The two needles in the Kidney meridian are used to enhance the energetic activity in the subcircuit, and moxa can be applied to the other points; this section of the treatment lasts approximately 10 minutes. The second section is the local treatment for the lumbar pain and involves needles placed on the Bladder meridian (e.g., at the L2 level [somatic sympathetics for lower extremities], L4 and L5 levels [myotomal and dermatomal levels of pain], and at the S2 level [parasympathetics for lower extremities]) to recruit the spinal segments involved in his pain. Electrical stimulation at 14 or 15 Hz can be connected among these needles. This second section lasts for 20 minutes.

Schedules and Results

Patient visits are usually scheduled once weekly, although two or three weekly are not uncommon, especially during the initial stages of an acute problem. When a favorable response lasts for the entire week between visits, the interval is opened to two weeks. As the response stabilizes for a two-week period, the interval is opened again to three weeks, then four. When the symptoms are stable for four weeks, a decision is made as to whether the patient should return for a maintenance treatment in another month or six weeks, or call for an appointment only if the condition returns. Patients with chronic pain problems typically require maintenance treatments at one-month, six-week, or two-month intervals and—even when responding well to acupuncture—typically need quarterly maintenance treatments. Medical problems of lesser severity and chronicity can often be resolved adequately and do not require maintenance treatments.

Treatment Evaluation

Any change during initial treatments—even a transient exacerbation of symptoms—is considered a favorable response. No response to the initial treatment may indicate that the therapeutic input was not strong enough, that the problem is deep-seated and requires several treatments to influence, that the treatment design is inappropriate, or that the problem is inaccessible to acupuncture. An exacerbation of symptoms after the initial treatment usually indicates that the treatment decision is accurate, but that the manipulation or the duration of the needles was too extensive. An examination of diagnostic microsystems, such as the radial pulse and the tongue, is another means for the practitioner to subjectively evaluate change in the patient's condition from visit to visit, and thereby better decide if a change in treatment is indicated.

With the cumulative effect of treatments, an *enduring improvement* is the desired goal. Enduring improvement may mean a thorough resolution of the presenting problem or it may mean enabling the patient to function on a plateau of less-incapacitating discomfort. Enduring improvement may also mean that the patient requires less medication than at the time of initial presentation. Ideally, a dozen visits are scheduled to follow the course of the disorder and its response to acupuncture. Usually the extent of response can be approximated by six or eight visits, but an enduring response often requires the full schedule of visits. After the first dozen treatments, the problem and its response to acupuncture are reevaluated and the acupuncturist and patient decide about continuing intensive treatment or maintenance treatments, or abandoning the acupuncture intervention altogether.

Acupuncture treatments are as individual as the patients and their responses to acupuncture. It is common to stay with an initial treatment approach for at least three or four visits before modifying the approach. It is also common for the patient to report changes in general well-being and vitality, or a reduction in medication, before a clear change in the presenting symptoms occurs. If there is no progress by the sixth visit, the acupuncturist may consider including additional modalities to complement the acupuncture. It is best not to abandon a case that shows reasonable hope for response to acupuncture before completion of a full trial of twelve visits.

USE OF MEDICAL ACUPUNCTURE

Primary Therapy: Musculoskeletal Pain

In the United States, acupuncture has been most accepted and successful in the management of musculoskeletal pain. Acute musculoskeletal lesions, such as soft-tissue contusions, acute muscle spasms, musculotendinous sprains and strains, and the pain of acute nerve entrapments, are among the problems most frequently and successfully addressed with acupuncture. In these cases, acupuncture can legitimately serve as the initiating therapy.

Chronic musculoskeletal pain problems are also commonly and appropriately treated with acupuncture, although not usually as the only approach. Conditions likely to be responsive to acupuncture intervention include repetitive strain disorders (e.g., carpal tunnel syndrome, tennis elbow, plantar fasciitis), myofascial pain patterns (e.g., temporomandibular joint pain, muscle tension headaches, cervical and thoracic soft-tissue pain, regional shoulder pain), arthralgias (particularly osteoarthritic in nature), degenerative disk disease with or without radicular pain, and pain following surgical intervention (both musculoskeletal and visceral). In the management of chronic musculoskeletal pain, acupuncture is valuable as an adjunct to conventional therapy's pharmaceutical and invasive procedures. Other chronic pain problems commonly responsive to acupuncture include postherpetic neuralgia, peripheral neuropathic pain, and headaches from other causes.

Least Useful Indications

Although acupuncture has been established as an effective tool to treat many forms of musculoskeletal pain, its limitations must be recognized in dealing with the consequences of spinal cord injuries and cerebrovascular accidents. In these conditions, acupuncture's effectiveness is diminished, and the frequency of treatments is increased and protracted over a longer time. Furthermore, acupuncture is usually not useful for thalamically mediated pain and, apart from symptom management and general vivifying effects, is not of great value in the treatment of chronic neurodegenerative diseases.

Acupuncture as a sole therapy has not shown itself to be of substantial value in severe and chronic inflammatory and immune-mediated disorders, such as ulcerative colitis, asthma, rheumatoid arthritis, and collagen-vascular diseases, especially if those conditions have advanced to require systemic corticosteroid medication. Likewise, it is not appropriate to rely on acupuncture as the primary intervention in

chronic fatigue states or HIV disease. There can be general value, however, for the symptom control and vitality-promoting effects of acupuncture in all of these conditions. In malignancies, acupuncture can be considered as an additional therapy to combat the secondary effects of conventional therapy, and as an adjunct in pain management.

Adverse Effects

In the hands of a medically trained practitioner, acupuncture is a fairly safe and forgiving discipline. It is difficult to introduce new and lasting problems with an acupuncture treatment, even if the treatment is not designed as skillfully as an experienced provider would desire. Many patients report a sensation of well-being or relaxation following an acupuncture treatment, especially if electrical stimulation has been used. That sense of relaxation, however, sometimes evolves into a feeling of fatigue or depression that lasts for several days. Other transient psychophysiological responses can be lightheadedness, anxiety, agitation, and tearfulness.

The possible risks and complications of an acupuncture treatment are undesirable consequences of penetrating the body with a sharp instrument: syncope, puncture of an organ, infection, a retained needle. These risks can be reduced by scrupulous sterilizing or using disposable needles, acquiring good clinical skills, understanding surface and internal anatomy, and executing responsible clinical judgment. Pneumothorax is the most frequently reported and the most easily produced serious visceral complication of acupuncture needling. Pneumoperitoneum, hemothorax, cardiac tamponade, and penetration of the kidney, bladder, and spinal medulla have been reported, although infrequently.

Contact dermatitis to stainless steel needles, local inflammation, and bacterial abscesses can occur, as well as chondritis from needling points on the ear. Outbreaks of hepatitis B documented in Europe and America have been traced to single practitioners reusing unsterilized needles (5). There have been a few reports of HIV transmission through acupuncture, but these can be avoided with proper use of sterile and disposable needles.

Preventive Value

Perhaps the most fertile ground for acupuncture intervention is for disorders in their premorbid state, for problems commonly encountered by primary care providers but rarely associated with positive laboratory findings, definitive medical diagnoses, or successful therapies. These states often can be described within acupuncture diagnostic paradigms, and then modified by activating the appropriate level of energy circulation. These disorders can be loosely categorized into three groups: aesthenic states, autonomic dysregulation disorders, and immune dysregulation disorders.

Aesthenic states include ill-defined fatigue (e.g., "tired all the time," "low energy"), mild depression, stress-related myofascial symptoms (e.g., upper thoracic and cervical myofascial pain, muscle tension headache), and early functional disturbances (e.g., diminished libido). *Autonomic dysregulation disorders* may manifest as anxiety, sleep disturbances, and bowel dysfunction. *Immune dysregulation disorders* include recurrent infectious and inflammatory states without underlying frank immunodeficiency: sinusitis, pharyngitis, bronchitis, gastroenteritis, and viral illnesses.

Some conscientious patients consult the acupuncture practitioner with what may be considered from an allopathic perspective as minor symptoms, and request assistance to attain better health and vitality. In these cases, the general characteristics of the patient, the presenting symptoms, the patient's past and family medical histories, and the acupuncture examination allow the acupuncturist to identify minor imbalances in the energetic activity of the organs and energy axes. This level of subtle pathology, for which allopathic medicine has little more than lifestyle counseling to offer, is commonly overlooked in a conventional setting. The acupuncture diagnostic and therapeutic system, however, usually allows for an understanding of the

patient and the early disturbances, and an appropriate intervention can be formulated. This form of preventive maintenance is a valuable dimension of the subtle aspects of acupuncture.

Scope of Practice

Medical acupuncture is a highly adaptable discipline and is of potential therapeutic value in many pain and general medical conditions. Its use as either a primary or complementary therapy depends on the nature and severity of the presenting problem and on the training, orientation, and practice environment of the provider. The physician trained in medical acupuncture who sees patients early in the course of their disturbances can initiate treatment of a pain or medical problem with acupuncture, and introduce additional therapies if acupuncture proves insufficient as the sole treatment. The physician who receives cases later in their evolution and after conventional treatments have been initiated can add acupuncture to assist, and sometimes replace, conventional treatments.

Many patients seeking attention from acupuncture providers demand acupuncture or other unconventional interventions as the starting treatment and agree to conventional methods only later in their management. Other patients and many physicians wait until conventional therapies have been exhausted and then resort to acupuncture intervention. Acupuncture therapy is not miraculous. It has its appropriate range of applications and, like other medical interventions, yields good results in well-selected early problems and less successful results when chronicity and complexity of the presenting problems increase. Usually, the best moment to initiate acupuncture therapy is early in the evolution of a problem; however, the flexibility and adaptability of acupuncture allow it to be integrated at almost any stage of treatment.

In addition to the treatment of acute and chronic musculoskeletal pain and premorbid or functional problems, medical acupuncture can be used successfully to address many diagnosable medical conditions, although it may need to be used in collaboration with other therapies, conventional and unconventional. In the United States, the four divisions of medicine that appear most responsive to acupuncture intervention are respiratory, gastrointestinal, gynecologic, and genitourinary.

Respiratory ailments potentially accessible to acupuncture intervention include allergic rhinitis, sinusitis, and bronchitis. Gastrointestinal ailments include gastritis, irritable bowel, hepatitis, and hemorrhoids. Gynecologic problems include dysmenorrhea and infertility. Genitourinary problems include irritable bladder, prostatitis, male infertility, and some forms of impotence.

Acupuncture, particularly when applied to the external ear, has shown to be valuable in managing substance abuse problems and reducing prescription narcotic analgesics. This application for acupuncture—one of the most socially visible—has gained the respect of rehabilitation programs internationally (6).

For mental and emotional disturbances, acupuncture can be useful as a transient aid in early and acute emotional states, such as anxiety, excitability, worry, early stages of depression, and fearful states. Acupuncture should not be considered as a primary or ongoing therapy for deep-seated or chronic psychoemotional illness because its effect on these conditions is not enduring.

Adaptability: Acupuncture as Complement and Complements to Acupuncture

Acupuncture's adaptability to the changing requirements of the patient's condition extends to its adaptability when combined with other modalities of health care. This integration is an expression of the training, orientation, and creativity of the practitioner. Acupuncture can be used as the initiating therapy for many common medical problems, and it can be combined with other modalities and disciplines according to the needs of the patient and the availability of other services. In addition to allopathic pharmaceutical and surgical interventions, there are

medical modalities that particularly complement the effects of acupuncture or that acupuncture can complement. These modalities include physical medicine techniques in pain management, osteopathic manipulation, movement training, herbal therapy, homeopathic remedies, and psychiatric or psychological intervention.

Management of chronic musculoskeletal pain offers many occasions in which therapeutic modalities can be combined. A physical therapist experienced in myotherapy can extend the impact of an acupuncture treatment directed at relaxation of contracted muscles and fascial tension patterns. The conventional spray and stretch, trigger point infiltration, and transcutaneous electrical nerve stimulation techniques of physical medicine combine well with acupuncture therapy. Osteopathic manipulative therapy and its subspecialty of cranial therapy can also be productively combined with the musculoskeletal applications of acupuncture. Hatha Yoga postures assist patients with biomechanical rehabilitation and maintenance of results, and the breathing exercises assist with relaxation and stress reduction. Movement therapy, such as the Feldenkrais, Alexander, and Aston approaches, can also be useful adjunctive activities during rehabilitation.

With chronic medical problems, the traditions of herbal therapies and homeopathic remedies can be usefully combined with acupuncture treatments. Chinese herbal formulae, when prescribed according to the classical patterns of disharmony of internal organs, can serve as protopharmaceutical substrates to enhance and prolong the effects of acupuncture treatments. Herbal formulae can accomplish lasting change or maintenance that cannot be achieved with needles alone (see Chapter 12).

Homeopathic remedies are generally used in low-potency form to treat acute problems, middle-potency form to treat chronic medical problems, and high-potency form to treat problems that have a core psychoemotional disturbance. These remedies can be used to specify and enhance the acupuncture treatments and can have capability in high potency to effect enduring changes in the patient's emotional configuration. It is sometimes necessary to work in collaboration with a psychiatrist or psychotherapist who is sensitive to the acupuncture process and who can serve in a guiding role for the patient.

ORGANIZATION

Training and Quality Assurance

In the United States, acupuncture is performed by physician and nonphysician practitioners. In 35 states, the acupuncture practice is included within the scope of a physician's medical or osteopathic license, and no regulations or restrictions are imposed on medical practitioners. The other 15 states require physicians practicing acupuncture either to demonstrate evidence of participation in training programs of 200 to 300 hours or simply to register with the board of medicine with evidence of formal training. From these loose regulations of physician practitioners, it is clear that the degree of acupuncture training and experience among physicians varies from state to state and individual to individual.

The American Academy of Medical Acupuncture (AAMA) represents the education, legislation, and professional interests of physicians who are well trained in acupuncture. Full membership in the AAMA requires 220 hours of formal training and two years of clinical experience. This standard follows the physician-training guidelines established in the constitution of the World Federation of Acupuncture-Moxibustion Societies, an international society guided by the World Health Organization. The AAMA has established a proficiency examination as the first of a two-part board certification examination. Membership eligibility in the AAMA has become the standard of physician credentialing for state registration, hospital privileges, liability insurance, and third-party reimbursement. It is likely that the proficiency examination will also become a requirement for participation in managed care programs (7).

The practice of acupuncture by nonphysicians is regulated in at least 33 states, and another dozen states have statutes pending. The educational prerequisites and training requirements vary widely from state to state and have been in a flux of improvement during the past decade. There are approximately 30 colleges accredited by the National Accreditation Commission for Schools and Colleges of Acupuncture and Oriental Medicine (NACSCAOM). Most of the programs span three years of didactic and clinical training. All states except California and Nevada that license nonphysician acupuncturists recognize the national examination developed by the National Commission for the Certification of Acupuncture and Oriental Medicine. There are two main national societies together with dozens of regional, state, and local organizations that represent the interests of the licensed acupuncturist communities (8).

The World Health Organization has adopted guidelines on basic training for physician and nonphysician providers, standards for safe practice, and clinical indications for acupuncture. The training guidelines reflect the minimum hours expected in most member nations and are consistent with regulations enacted in the United States: 2500 hours for nonphysician acupuncturists and 200 hours for physicians. The basic curriculum is founded on the classical tradition of acupuncture, requiring a firm knowledge of the acupuncture points and channels and the traditional models of diagnosis and treatment. A basic knowledge of Western biomedical science is also encouraged in the curriculum (9).

Reimbursement Status

Although there is no national standard for the third-party insurance industry regarding acupuncture, many policies recognize acupuncture as a legitimate and reimbursable procedure. Because of the popular and professional demand for acupuncture services, it is likely that insurance reimbursement will become more uniform with time. Medical acupuncture, particularly as practiced by an experienced medical provider, integrates creatively into many medical disciplines. Traditional Chinese medicine integrates less smoothly into conventional settings because the herbal diagnostic model that is fundamental to traditional Chinese medicine is alien to most Western physicians' thinking.

PROSPECTS FOR THE FUTURE

The potential for medical acupuncture is just beginning to be understood. Future clinical research and utilization evaluations should clarify how best to integrate it into the conventional health care system. Medical acupuncture offers the opportunity to expand contemporary medicine in treating conditions for which current interventions are either ineffective or have undesirable secondary effects. Because of its usefulness and adaptability to so many aspects of allopathic medicine, it is probable that medical acupuncture will be integrated with increasing creativity into private and institutional practices.

REFERENCES

1. Reston J. Now about my operation in Peking. The New York Times 1971; July 26:1, 6.

2. Helms JM. Acupuncture energetics: a clinical approach for physicians. Berkeley: Medical Acupuncture Publishers, 1995:3–17.

3. Stux G, Pomeranz B. Acupuncture: textbook and atlas. Berlin: Springer–Verlag, 1987:1–26.

4. Helms JM. Acupuncture energetics: a clinical approach for physicians. Berkeley: Medical Acupuncture Publishers, 1995:71–78.

5. Norheim AJ. Adverse effects of acupuncture: a study of the literature for the years 1981–1994. J Altern Complement Med 1996;2(2):291–297.

6. Culliton PD, Kiresuk, TJ. Overview of substance abuse acupuncture treatment research. J Altern Complement Med 1996;2(1):149–159.

7. American Academy of Medical Acupuncture (AAMA), 5820 Wilshire Boulevard, Suite 500, Los Angeles, CA 90036, 213 937 5514 /fax 213 937 0959.

8. American Association of Acupuncture and Oriental Medicine (AAAOM), 433 Front Street, Catasauqua, PA 18032, 610 266 1433 /fax 610 264 2768. National Acupuncture and Oriental Medicine Alliance (NAOMA), 14637 Starr Road SE, Olalla, WA 90359, 206 851 6896 /fax 206 851 6883.

9. Helms JM. Report on W.H.O. consultation on acupuncture. Medical Acupuncture 1997;7(1).

CHAPTER 20

PHYTOMEDICINE

Tieraona Low Dog

BACKGROUND

Definition

Phytomedicine, or herbal medicine, is the science, art, and exploration of using botanical remedies to treat illness. The term *phytotherapy* describes the therapeutic application of plants. This term was coined by the French physician Henri Leclerc (1870–1955), who published numerous essays on the use of medicinal plants (1). Many consider herbal healing the oldest form of medicine. It has been used by all races, religions, and cultures throughout the world. Prehistoric records show that people of that period collected and used herbs and plants for food and medicine, and the documented use of herbal medicine dates back at least 5000 years.

General Considerations

Medical herbalism is thriving in Europe and the United States. The sale of herbal medicines in the United States is one of the ten fastest growing industries, with more than 1 billion in sales annually. Phytomedicines are sold in health food stores, pharmacies, and even grocery stores. The media coverage is extensive, and there are magazines devoted to this form of medicine. Numerous factors explain this increased use of medicinal plants for self-treatment. Although the tremendous benefits of technology that produce dramatic and specific effects (e.g., innovative drug therapies) in medicine are well recognized, the dangers of medical technology and the indiscriminate use of chemicals (e.g., preservatives, coloring agents, drugs, and chemical pollution to the environment) is straining the adaptability of our complex bodies and the environment. There appears to be a growing distrust of technology-based medicine, which has given rise to the "back to nature" movement prevalent in the United States today. Science is a double-edged sword, and its enormous influence means that we must begin to realize and address the long-term consequences of technology and its impact upon the environment and inhabitants of this world. Rising interest in herbal medicine reflects the public's attempt to create a more gentle and ecologically sensitive medicine than has been created with technology-based medicine. Yet both technology and nature must be combined wisely. Hopefully, as we learn from the past, we can take the wisdom gained to help guide our future.

When tracing the history of herbal medicine, it is difficult to distinguish it from that of medicine in general. Ancient physicians treated the sick with herbs. Their pharmacopoeias were filled with elixirs, ointments, teas, and poultices. Phytomedicine is an ancient profession that laid the foundations for what we now call modern medicine, botany, chemistry, and pharmacology. The following section covers some of the most influential historical figures of Western phytomedicine. However, the names of the unsung, unpublished, rural, and lay herbalists who kept much of the knowledge and tradition alive throughout the darkest periods of Europe are lost forever in the sands of time.

HISTORY AND DEVELOPMENT

The Egyptian Papyri Antiquarium is a 22-yard document dating from 3000 BC that contains an extensive materia medica. It is one of the oldest Western documents that lists specific conditions and specific treatments with herbal medicines. The Rig Veda, a text from India, dates from the same time period and contains approximately 750 medicinal plants. In China, the Pen T'so provided detailed information on 366 plants. The history of Chinese and Ayurvedic medicine is explored in other chapters of this book.

Around 1500 BC, the Aztecs documented in the Badianus Manuscript the use of datura, tobacco, cotton, passionflower, cochineal, and other herbs, all of which have been adopted in both European and American pharmacopeias (2). Mayan medicine included guaiacum, capsicum, and chenopodium, and South American Indians were well versed in the use of coca, curare, ipecac, and cinchona (3). Native North American people's knowledge of their flora was so complete that they used all but about a half a dozen of the indigenous vegetable drugs. Over 200 drugs that were used by one or more Indian nations have been in the United States Pharmacopeia or National Formulary (4).

When considering the history of medicine in ancient Europe, most historians usually begin with the Greek culture, which can be traced back to Helen of Troy, who is believed to have lived around 2000 BC. There was an extensive herbal pharmacopoeia during this time, much of it geared towards pain relief.

It was between 460 and 370 BC in ancient Greece when Hippocrates learned, wrote, and taught extensively about herbal medicine and healing. Blood, urine, feces, and phlegm were observed and described in terms of their substance, quality, and color. These four body fluids would come to be known as the *four humors* of Greek medicine. Hippocrates believed that there were two approaches to disease: to eliminate the symptoms that are present and to restore the patient to health. Hippocrates viewed symptomatic healing as separate from the restoration of health, or what many would now call holistic medicine. Although Hippocrates knew

more than 400 herbal and drug therapies, his primary approach to medicine was preventive in nature.

Pedacius Dioscorides was the author of *De Materia Medica*. Dioscorides was a Greek army surgeon in the service of Nero (54–68 AD) who used the opportunity of travel to study plants. His extensive *materia medica* describes more than 600 plants and plant principles. He was the first to write on medical botany as an applied science.

Another prominent figure in herbal history was Pliny the Elder (23–79 AD) who wrote 12 texts solely on medicine. These texts were part of his *Natural History*, an extensive compilation of all that was known in his time of anthropology, botany, zoology, mineralogy, geography, plants, and drugs.

Galen (131–201 AD) is considered the greatest of ancient Greek physicians after Hippocrates. He instituted an elaborate system of herbal polypharmacy and was a prolific writer, authoring more than 30 books on pharmacy. Galen was one of the first to provide a truly intelligent description on the uses of opium, hyoscyamus, hellebore, colocynth and many other herbs. It is because of his vast contribution to herbal medicine that the term *galenicals* is still used today to describe herbal simples.

When the Roman Empire fell, much of the knowledge and wisdom gained from the Greeks was lost as Europe entered the Dark Ages. The period of monastic medicine (500–1000 AD), during which the studies of Greek medical writings were taught only at European monasteries, became the only preservation of the herbal knowledge of Hippocrates, Pliny the Elder, and Dioscorides available in Europe. During the time of the great plagues of Europe, monastic medicine became more focused on the spiritual protection of the saints than in exploring the richness of the botanical medicines available. The women in the villages kept herbal medicine alive as they tended the sick and delivered the babies. Many of these village women were burned at the stake as witches because of their healing talents; *herbista*, meaning female herbalist, is an old term for a witch. Scientific exploration of medicine was in a dark slumber throughout Europe.

Meanwhile, in the Islamic world, medicine and research were flourishing. The Golden Age of Arabia (750–850 AD) was rich in the study of medicine and art. Botanical gardens were planted and herbal remedies extensively studied and harvested to supply both pharmacies and physicians. The Mohammedan era, as this period is referred to, would last until 1100 AD. In Europe, Hildegard of Bingen (1098–1179), an abbess, was carrying the torch in the darkness. Her medical writings are considered by many to be the most important scientific contribution of the Middle Ages. Hildegard of Bingen described the function of 485 plants and blended the spirit world, prayer, and medicine into a tapestry unique for her time.

The seventeenth century brought the migration of many Europeans to the New World. Although many early immigrants transported medicinal plants and seeds from their homeland to treat their ailments, they incorporated much of the indigenous *materia medica* into their own pharmacopoeia.

Samuel Thompson (1769–1843), an early American, is reputed to have learned herbal medicine from Mrs. Benton, a wise woman versed in Native American herbal lore. Thompson, who was raised on a farm in New Hampshire, became so impressed and inspired by the effectiveness of the remedies that he spent his life teaching, doctoring, and writing about herbal medicine. The Thompsonian approach to healing became widespread with its followers being primarily the common, rural folk, who gained much benefit from his simple philosophy of treatment. Samuel Thompson strongly advocated a return to the vitalist approach to medicine.

During the 1800s, drug preparations were primarily made of flowers, leaves, and roots. Medicine and botany were still closely allied. In 1850, in both Europe and America, 80% of the medicines used were derived from plants. (Today, less than 30% of our drugs are of plant origin.) The eclectic physicians of the United States were highly skilled in the use of botanical remedies and wrote detailed pharmacopoeias. Harvey Felter, John Uri Lloyd, and John King were among those well known for their teachings and writings in this area.

By the late 1800s, United States pharmaceutical companies began to gain a strong foothold in the field of medicine. As knowledge of chemistry increased, synthetic chemical drugs were developed. Aspirin was introduced by Bayer, and pharmaceutical science expanded at a rapid pace. Chemists were interested in studying chemical compounds that could be analyzed precisely and dosed in exact milligrams, with effects that could be accurately measured physiologically. The study of herbal medicine began to fall into neglect. Proprietary products became popular, and fewer physicians relied on making their own medicines. The pharmaceutical companies persuaded doctors to buy and prescribe their products conventional medicine organized around these concepts, and suppression of other practitioners, including herbalists, was intensified.

After 1910, medical schools were restructured to focus primarily on physics, chemistry, and pathology. Medicine was to become a branch of "higher" learning, available only to those who could survive the lengthy and expensive university training. Many of the medical schools that catered to minorities and women with an emphasis on herbal medicine, homeopathy, and holistic healing were closed. Fortunately, medical schools today are reconsidering the importance of psychology, sociology, and the humanities when selecting their student body, and a number of medical schools are revisiting holistic approaches and patient-centered medicine.

PRINCIPAL CONCEPTS

In phytomedicine, pathological understanding of illness is very similar to Western allopathic pathology. However, herbalists view illness within the context of the healing capacity of the whole person and then choose herbs that support the specific organ systems under stress. Most Western-trained herbalists believe that the body is a self-healing organism and that herbs should be chosen to support wellness, not simply to relieve symptoms or treat diseases. According to Simon Mills, "If we see the body, mind and spirit as a complex whole, applying a constant self-corrective force to maintain a homeostatic balance in spite of wildly varying environmental pressures, then we should use different medicines, and even redefine the term. The search is on for those agents that support homeostatic efforts, which help the body help itself" (5). Thus, therapy is directed at helping to strengthen the weakened areas of the body, often with emphasis on supporting the adrenal and nervous systems.

DIAGNOSIS

The ability to "diagnose" an illness depends on each individual herbalist's training. In the United States, most consumers who are seeking the services of an herbalist have already received a diagnosis from their health care provider and are in search of an alternative way to treat the problem. Because most lay (unlicensed) herbalists do not have access to laboratory tests or radiological or pathological studies, they rely fairly heavily on an exhaustive review of systems and history of the presenting complaint; the initial appointment with a patient often lasts between 1 and 2 hours. Physical examination may include a systematic approach to the body, including auscultation of the heart and lungs, palpation of the abdomen, and examination of the ears, nose, and throat. Some herbalists employ unorthodox techniques, such as applied kinesiology and iridology. Again, this depends on the type of training the herbalist has received, and training varies considerably by country. For example, in Europe, conventionally trained physicians frequently use herbs; whereas in the United States, this rarely is the case. In many Asian and Indian countries, herbal training is part of conventional medical education.

DISEASE CLASSIFICATION

Disease classification in phytomedicine is essentially the same as that in Western medicine. Dysmenorrhea is called just that, and herbs that support the uterus, enhance blood flow to the area, and reduce discomfort are chosen to address the problem. If the woman had significant stressors in her life, herbs for the nervous system would be included, supporting her body's overall attempts to rebalance. Therapeutic recommendations often include basic lifestyle and dietary recommendations. Some herbalists include the use of vitamins and minerals. However, the primary focus is on using herbal remedies to restore health.

As herbalist Michael Moore states, "Herbal remedies represent far more than a holistic fad or a total rejection of traditional medicine. They help to fill the overwhelming void between health and acute disease" (6). Herbal therapy is best suited for addressing a number of chronic complaints that are incompletely addressed by conventional medicine, and the many everyday minor complaints in which people seek relief from a bottle of pills. Herbalists design their protocols around assisting the body in its search for wellness rather than only blocking processes that produce disease.

David Hoffman, a British-trained herbalist, gives an example of a therapeutic approach for hypertension. He begins with the assumption that organic causes for hypertension have been explored and that the individual is living with essential hypertension. He outlines a number of herbs with hypotensive action that may be chosen based not only around their ability to reduce blood pressure, but also with an understanding of the secondary actions of the plant that may be relevant to the particular individual. For example, black cohosh (*Cimicifuga racemosa*) is hypotensive but also has antiinflammatory and antispasmodic properties and is useful for women who are suffering from hot flashes and menopausal complaints. This herb may be more suited for a 50-year-old woman with arthritis entering her menopausal years than an herb such as linden. Hoffman also discusses the use of cardiac tonics for strengthening and toning the entire system that is under "pressure." Peripheral vasodilators and diuretics are mentioned to reduce the resistance within the peripheral vessels and maintain renal perfusion. Nervines are included for addressing any stress or anxiety that may contribute to the hypertension. He then creates a formula of herbs that address these particular aspects and chooses herbs that best match a particular individuals' needs (7).

Many herbs have hypotensive properties and, through the combination of herbs addressing different aspects of the problem for a particular individual, a holistic and unique approach is created. For this reason, many herbalists do not use premade proprietary products. They create protocols based around each individual's particular need. For example, the following is a formula that might be used for a 50-year-old perimenopausal woman with hypertension and arthritis:

Black Cohosh (*Cimicifuga racemosa*): 2 parts

Hawthorn (*Crataegus* spp): 1 part

Cramp bark (*Viburnum opulus*): 1 part

Motherwort (*Leonurus cardiaca*): 1 part

The dose would be 5 mL of tincture taken three times daily. This formula provides the following:

Hypotensives: Black Cohosh, Hawthorn, Cramp bark

Cardiac tonics: Hawthorn, Motherwort

Diuretic: Hawthorn

Nervines: Motherwort, Black Cohosh

Peripheral vasodilator: Cramp bark

Antiinflammatories: Black Cohosh, Cramp bark

Estrogenic: Black Cohosh

The formula would help this woman's hypertension, perimenopausal complaints, arthritic joints, and it would help her to rest better and feel calmer throughout the day. Simultaneously, it would strengthen and protect her heart and vessels from the long-term stress of hypertension. Herbalists use the fact that one plant can have three, four, or more actions on the body. Although this often seems to frustrate pharmacists and physicians, many physicians often choose pharmaceutical medications in a similar fashion. When deciding what antidepressant to prescribe, a physician may choose the drug amitriptyline instead of fluoxetine for a depressed individual who is suffering with neurogenic pain. Fluoxetine is probably better suited for an obese individual with depression and an eating disorder. Herbalists and physicians both should

attempt to know their *materia medica* so well that they know the intricacies of each substance they prescribe.

THERAPY AND OUTCOMES

Treatment Evaluation

Most people evaluate treatment effectiveness by the way they feel when taking an herb. Most herbalists believe that the longer the condition has existed, the longer it will take to restore balance or cause change within the body. Clients who are placed on "tonifying" herbs are commonly told that they should notice some change within 8 to 12 weeks. In other conditions, such as constipation and insomnia, relief may be seen in a few days. Again, because herbalists mainly treat common complaints and chronic disorders, treatment assessment is based on the reports of symptom reduction and improved quality of life from the client. If the client presents complaining of migraine headaches, treatment efficacy is determined by the individual's report of change in frequency, intensity, and duration of headaches. If suitable results are not obtained, the herbalist usually will modify the formula.

SCIENTIFIC VALIDATION

For the past 40 years, researchers have been interested in trying to isolate the "active" constituent of a plant, which can then be studied using the same methods applied to the study of other chemical compounds. As a result, the exact mechanism of action for a number of plants has been elucidated and the understanding of phytomedicines expanded. This field of research, appropriately termed *phytochemistry*, is growing in many European countries. As science validates the use of herbal medicine, a revival of interest has occurred in both Europe and the United States. With the ability to standardize herbs—that is, to accurately measure the exact percent of active constituents within a herbal product—a new range of herbal medicines is now available to the public. Many practitioners feel more confident recommending a product if they know the exact amount of the active principle and the number of milligrams that should be prescribed daily.

As can be seen from the forgoing example, however, it may be impossible to elucidate the mechanism of action of a particular plant by analyzing all its active constituents in an isolated form on multiple conditions. Most plants contain hundreds of constituents that may be acting in concert, not individually, to create the physiological effects in those consuming them. Clinical trials that study the whole plant's activity, accounting for nature's complexity and effects on several outcomes, must be designed. This requires a shift of thinking in Western research—a movement away from the reductionist approach, looking at herbs as complete products in which the "whole is more than the sum of its parts." The study of herbal compounds, many of which contain 7, 10, or even 20 different herbs, has been even more difficult. Herbal practitioners believe that phytomedicines work synergistically and that through proper combination, the effect of a group of plants is more significant than the use of a single herb. Again, clinical trials must be conducted to evaluate the herbal "mixtures," without becoming overly fixated on identifying and evaluating each single active principle.

Little research on herbal medicine is conducted in the United States. Drug therapeutics in the United States is powerfully influenced by a large pharmaceutical industry, with the primary goal being the ability to create and market synthesized, patentable, highly active chemicals that affect the body in a specific way. Medicine that cannot be patented cannot obtain the multimillion dollar investment required for research, regardless if the substance works (8). Unfortunately, many herbs that have been used effectively for centuries by herbalists and the public remain "unproven," which many professionals incorrectly equate as "ineffective."

Most of our current research on herbal medicine is coming from Europe and Asia, where there are far fewer political, economic, or regulatory reasons for rejecting traditional (i.e., phytomedicinal) remedies. These countries deem it important to scientifically explore natural therapies, embracing or rejecting them as the data indicate (8). The *German Commission E Mono-* *graphs* are a good example of the current research conducted on phytomedicinal remedies. These monographs provide proper identification, therapeutic use, expected side effects, and safety issues of more than 100 plants. Although traditional use and medical experience is important, it is clear that we cannot rely solely on the fact that a plant was used in a certain way by Dioscorides 1000 years ago. According to Heinz Schilcher, "Uncritical acceptance of traditional reports and ancient herbals used as a revived materia medica will do more harm than good to the cause of phytotherapy" (9). He also states, "Phytotherapy in particular is a field where medical and pharmaceutical historians found much to surprise them. Tracing traditions back to their source revealed not only errors in passing on information. More often than not a plant name used today referred to a completely different species in antiquity or the Middle Ages. Exact botanical identification and description of the medicinal plant in question was the exception rather than the rule" (9).

Description of Treatment: Herbal Therapeutics

Herbal medicine can be used to treat, augment treatment, or alleviate side effects of allopathic medicines for most conditions other than serious acute illness. The following five herbs are but a few examples of some of the more popular plants and the research behind them. These herbs can help treat the following conditions: depression, anxiety, muscular tension, restlessness, insomnia, hypertension, cardiac insufficiency, upper respiratory infections, poor wound healing, sluggish immune system, intermittent claudication, impaired mental function, peripheral vascular insufficiency, vascular and Alzheimer's dementia, vertigo, macular degeneration, and Raynaud's syndrome.

St. John's Wort

St. John's wort (*Hypericum perforatum*) has received a great deal of attention lately from the media. A meta-analysis of 23 clinical trials conducted on more 1757 outpatients with mild-to-moderate depression was published in the

British Medical Journal in 1996, showing that St. John's wort extract was more effective than placebo and equally as effective as standard synthetic antidepressants (10). Following this publication, many health care practitioners in the United States have been more willing to use St. John's wort in the management of mild-to-moderate depression. Although the herb has been classified by the *German Commission E Monographs* as a monoamine oxidase inhibitor, newer studies suggest that the plant's main antidepressant effect may also be through serotonin reuptake inhibition (11). In addition to the plant's antidepressant effects, it also possesses antiretroviral activity in both in vitro and in vivo studies. It appears that hypericin and pseudohypericin interfere with the development of viral components and also directly inactivate mature retroviruses (12). This is being investigated for its possible benefit for patients with HIV. In most of the studies for depression, the dose of St. John's wort was 300 mg taken three times daily, with products standardized to contain 0.3% hypericin (13). Pediatric dosage for children 6 to 12 years of age is 250 mg daily of standardized product (14). Occasionally patients experienced gastrointestinal side effects. In light-skinned people who are sensitive to the sun, photosensitivity is a theoretical side effect. In general, St. John's wort is well tolerated and quite effective for the treatment of depression. Caution is needed when used with other psychoactive drugs, such as antidepressants and sedatives.

KAVA ROOT

Kava root (*Piper methysticum*) is found throughout the South Pacific islands, where it has been used as a slightly intoxicating, nonalcoholic beverage for thousands of years. The plant is used socially, medicinally, and ceremonially. Several clinical trials have demonstrated kava's effectiveness in easing stress, anxiety, and restlessness (15). The plant has also been used as a mild muscle relaxant and analgesic (16). The muscle-relaxing effects of kava are believed to be of supraspinal origin (17), and analgesia does not operate through opiate pathways because its effects are not reversed by naloxone (18). The

exact mechanism of action is still not well understood and the active constituents not completely identified. The limbic system appears to be inhibited by the kavapyrones present in the root, with an associated dampening of emotional excitability and a definite enhancement of mood and clarity of thought (19). Kava has also been demonstrated to increase deep sleep without affecting REM sleep (19). Kava is a viable option in the treatment of anxiety and muscle tension before turning to benzodiazepines and the tricyclic antidepressants for easing anxiety and reducing muscle tension. Sedation is not seen in the therapeutic doses recommended (20). There are minimal side effects associated with the use of the root. Weight loss and a reversible skin condition known as kava dermopathy have been reported in long-term users who consume very high doses (21). The usual dose is 200 mg three times daily. Caution is needed when used with other sedatives and psychotropic medications.

ECHINACEA

Echinacea (*Echinacea spp.*) is another popular herb in the United States and Europe. The plant is indigenous to North America and is widely exported to Europe for its medicinal uses. Echinacea is used as a stimulant to the immune system and is used for its antiviral effects. The plant's action upon the immune system is nonspecific and works primarily via the cell-mediated branch. There is an increased level of activity amongst macrophages and lymphocytes, and numbers of granulocytes are increased in the blood (22). The polysaccharides found within echinacea stimulate the secretion of tumor necrosis factor, interferon, and interleukin 1 (23). The arabinogalactans found within the roots of *Echinacea purpurea* have distinct antiviral properties. Echinacoside has bacteriostatic properties, whereas echinacin B promotes tissue granulation (24). Echinacea is a suitable herb for cold and flu-like symptoms. Physicians are reluctant to hand out antibiotics for obvious viral infections, yet there is tremendous pressure placed on the doctor to give something to the person who suffers such symptoms. Echinacea is an excellent recommendation. It stimulates the body's natural defense system and helps fight off viral infections both by direct means and through the stimulation of interferon. A meta-analysis of six double-blind, placebo-controlled and randomized studies showed an improvement in symptoms and decreased length of upper respiratory illness when echinacea was given. Echinacea for the prophylaxis of upper respiratory infections also showed positive results (25). Echinacea is well tolerated and there are few adverse reactions when applied topically to promote the healing of wounds or taken orally. The *German Commission E Monographs* state that echinacea is contraindicated in those with "progressive systemic disease states, eg. tuberculosis, leukosis, collagenosis, multiple sclerosis, AIDS, HIV infection, and other auto-immune diseases" (26) because of its immune-stimulating properties. A few adverse effects have been reported. The usual dose for echinacea is 900 mg of the root extract, 2 to 4 times a day. Echinacea can be used for treating both children and adults.

HAWTHORN

Hawthorn (*Craetagus spp.*) is a herb commonly used for the treatment of mild cardiac insufficiency (Stages I and II per the New York Heart Association classification), angina, and the aging heart that does not yet require a cardiac glycoside (27). The flavonoids and oligomeric procyanadins are believed to be the "active" constituents, but there are conflicting opinions about this (27). Hawthorn has positive inotropic, dromotropic, and chronotropic effects and negative bathmotropic effects upon the heart (27). Thus, it increases contractility, slightly increases heart rate, increases conduction velocity, and lessens the nervous-muscular irritability of the heart. The ability of hawthorn to dilate blood vessels, especially the coronary vessels, increases blood flow to the heart tissue and reduces peripheral vascular resistance. This mechanism is, in part, mediated through the inhibition of cAMP phosphodiesterase (28). The plant also reduces blood pressure and exerts angiotensin-converting enzyme activity (29). The antioxidative properties probably afford the heart a cardioprotective effect with prolonged use (30). Herbalists routinely recommend Hawthorn for those who

have cardiac risk factors but are not yet on medication, and for those with mild hypertension. Hawthorn is considered a cardiac tonic, strengthening the heart and vascular system over time. The dose when standardized to hyperoside is 12 to 15 mg daily, or 300 to 900 mg of dried extract. When the product is standardized to the oligomeric procyanidin content, the dose is 45 to 90 mg daily, or 240 to 560 mg of dried extract. Hawthorn should be taken for at least 6 weeks and is best when given in two to three doses daily (31). If using the tincture of hawthorn fruit, flower, or both, the usual dose of a 1:3 tincture (1 kg of herb to 3 liters of water/alcohol) is 5 mL, taken 2 to 3 times daily. Caution is needed if used with other cardioactive drugs, such as digitalis.

GINKGO

Ginkgo biloba comes from the leaves of the gingko tree, and it has been used and written about in the Orient for over 2000 years. The leaves have been studied for a wide number of indications, including dementia, poor memory, difficulties with concentration, cerebral insufficiency syndromes (including dizziness, headache, and tinnitus), intermittent claudication, Raynaud's syndrome, and asthma. The pharmacology of ginkgo is only partially understood. Ginkgo is an inhibitor of platelet-activating factor (PAF), which helps reduce platelet aggregation and plays a role in reducing the bronchoconstriction that accompanies asthma (32). Ginkgo also appears to have antioxidant properties, preventing lipid peroxidation, which may serve to protect vascular walls (32). Ginkgo inhibits catecholamine O-methyl transferase (COMT) and appears to stimulate the synthesis of serotonin receptors (32). This probably explains the subjective improvement in mood among elders who may have decreased serotonin receptors (33). Ginkgo prolongs the half-life of endothelium-derived relaxing factor (EDRF) (34), resulting in dilation of the arterial bed and improved peripheral circulation. A randomized placebo-controlled study found Ginkgo to be effective in increasing the pain-free walking distance in those suffering from intermittent claudication and peripheral arterial occlusive disease

(35). A study published in *Lancet* in 1991 reviewed some of the clinical studies that evaluated the use of Ginkgo in cases of cerebral insufficiency. Several of the better designed studies showed an improvement in 8 of 12 symptoms: tiredness, anxiety, dizziness, tinnitus, headache, difficulties with concentration and memory, confusion, and lack of energy (36). In addition, several small trials have shown Ginkgo to be useful in the treatment of vertigo (37) and macular degeneration (38). There is no doubt that Ginkgo has a role to play in the health of an aging population. The plant is relatively free of side effects; however, it should be used with caution in combination with other antiplatelet agents (e.g., aspirin, garlic) because bleeding time can be prolonged. Almost all of the clinical studies have used products standardized to 24% ginkgoflavonoids and 6% terpenes; the dose ranges from 40 to 80 mg three times daily. Side effects are usually dose-related, and most people can safely use doses of 120 mg daily.

Other Herbal Preparations

In addition to the herbs just described, there are several other herbal preparations that are valuable in treating several common conditions and of which practicing physicians should be aware. The best summaries of the following information are in Murray's *The Healing Power of Herbs* (1995, Prima Publishing) and Newall, Anderson, and Phillipson's *Herbal Medicines: A Guide for Health Professionals* (1996, The Pharmaceutical Press).

GARLIC

A number of studies have documented the effects of garlic, including antimicrobial and antineoplastic effects, cholesterol- and blood pressure-lowering effects, and inhibition of platelet aggregation. Stability, quality control, and standardization of the content of several active ingredients is variable from product to product, however, making treatment effects unpredictable. In general, 900 mg/day of a 1.3% alliin content product may have cardiovascular prevention effects. Caution is needed with other antiplatelet

and anticoagulants so as not to precipitate bleeding.

GINSENG

As with garlic, a considerable amount of research has been conducted on the multiple effects of ginseng. Because of these multiple effects and the variability of products derived from multiple sources (for both panax and eleutherococcus ginseng) and prepared in various ways, the reliability of these effects in actual practice is quite unpredictable. Panax ginseng is most often used as an "adaptogen" or tonic for increasing the body's resistance to stress and fatigue, to increase endurance under heavy physical activity, or to improve well-being in age-related debilitation. One of its actions is stimulation of adrenocorticotropic hormone (ACTH) from the pituitary, which in turn influences a variety of hormone levels. The usual dosage for younger individuals is between 500 and 1000 mg of the panax root, taken on an empty stomach in divided doses. This is usually continued for two to 3 weeks, with a 2-week break between courses. For sick and debilitated elderly, the recommended dosage is 400 to 800 mg/day continuously. Ginseng may interact with MAO inhibitors, stimulants (e.g., coffee, antipsychotics), and sex hormones. Those with hormone-sensitive tumors (e.g., prostate, breast) should probably avoid its prolonged use. In addition, prolonged use of high doses of ginseng has been reported to produce a "ginseng abuse syndrome," characterized by hypertension, euphoria, insomnia, nervousness, skin eruptions, and diarrhea (39).

SAW PALMETTO

In contrast to garlic and ginseng, which have multiple effects and indications, saw palmetto is claimed to be useful for one primary indication—benign prostatic hypertrophy (BPH). The fat-soluble extract of the berries inhibits the conversion of testosterone to dihydrotestosterone (DHT) and has been reported to have antiandrogen and estrogenic effects. Placebo-controlled trials and direct comparisons with finasteride (Proscar) report significant reduction in BPH symptoms without reduction in prostate size. The dosage is 160 mg, twice daily, of the extract standardized to 85–95% fatty acids. Although few side effects are reported, given its antiandrogen and estrogenic effects, prolonged use may interact with hormone replacement therapy and affect hormone-sensitive diseases.

MILK THISTLE

Milk thistle, or *Silybum marianum*, has been studied extensively in animals and humans for its hepatotoxic protective effects against various toxins, including alcohol. It appears to prolong life in advanced alcoholic cirrhosis and limit hepatic damage from viral hepatitis. The dosage is 140 mg of the standardized extract three times a day.

Concluding Remarks on Herbal Preparations

A number of other herbs have shown promising data on the importance of phytomedicine for common public health problems. Among these are:

- **Feverfew** for prophylaxis of migraine headache
- **Ginger** for motion sickness, nausea, and vomiting
- **Green tea** for prevention of carcinogenesis
- **Valerian** for improving sleep problems and anxiety, and to assist patients in withdrawal from dependency on benzodiazepines
- **Gugulipid** for the reduction of cholesterol
- **Peppermint** for the treatment of tension headache
- **Mistletoe** for improving quality of life in cancer patients
- **Horsechestnut** for the treatment of venous insufficiency
- **Evening primrose oil** for the treatment of eczema, hyperactivity, and premenstrual syndrome

Learning about these herbs and their use, indications, contraindications, safety profile, drug-herb interactions, production character,

dosing, side effects, and safety profile can help the practitioner to properly communicate with their patients about them. (See Part II of this book for reported adverse effects from the use of herbs.)

ORGANIZATION

Training and the Legal Status

There are currently no standards of education for the study of herbalism in the United States. Many of the herbal teachers and practitioners are primarily self-taught through years of study and practice. The American Herbalists Guild is currently the only professional group of herbalists in the United States. They maintain a list of herb schools and training programs available at home and abroad and have devised a "skeleton" of what most Guild members feel should constitute an acceptable curriculum of training to allow one to practice phytotherapy safely (40). Many herbal programs offer some type of certificate, using titles such as Medical Herbalist, Clinical Herbalist, Herbalist, and Master Herbalist for those who complete their course. However, there is no consistency in curricula, requirements, and length of program from school to school. Therefore, one individual may spend 400 hours of study and receive a Herbalist certificate, whereas another may receive a Master Herbalist certification after two weekends of training. This disparity creates a dilemma for the public, who cannot reliably count on the education and level of training of a particular practitioner. In addition, herbal practitioners who do not have a medical, naturopathic, or acupuncture license are technically practicing their trade illegally.

The federal government regulates the practice of medicine; this is governed by each individual state. Many states have strict consumer protection statutes, which cover "illegal" medical practices. In most states, the enforcing agency is the Board of Medical Quality Assurance and the punishment for the unauthorized practice of medicine is a misdemeanor. There have been virtually no successful prosecutions of herbalists in the United States to date; however, the risk is real for those unlicensed herbalists who see clients, diagnose, and prescribe herbal medicines. The reason there has been so little prosecution of herbalists is probably because most herbalists use gentle herbal remedies with very little risk of adverse reactions and usually not in place of conventional treatment.

With the dramatic increase in the purchase and consumption of phytomedicine in the United States, the need for well-trained, qualified herbalists is essential. Naturopathic physicians and acupuncturists have formalized study in herbal medicine, but the extent of their training in Western phytotherapy is usually limited. Schools with a standardized, formal curriculum based around the sciences and herbal medicine are needed, and individual states need to become willing to license herbalists to practice legally. Herbalists need an established scope of practice and clear guidelines for conditions that must be referred to a physician for consultation. These factors would provide the consumer with an expert in the field of phytotherapy and also would offer the medical community a referral source for patients who want responsible herbal options to pharmaceutical medications.

Reimbursement Status

Currently, there is little reimbursement available for the patient who seeks the services of an unlicensed herbalist. Even when licensed physicians prescribe herbs for a particular condition, insurance companies often refuse to reimburse the expense. Unfortunately, with the cost of herbal products rising in the United States, phytotherapy is becoming a therapeutic approach primarily for the middle class. This is unfortunate, because there is a disproportionate amount of illness among the poor compared to those with more financial resources. By not including phytotherapy as a treatment option available in conventional Western medicine, many of those who could benefit will be unable to afford it. Even more ironic is the fact that herbal medicines are generally cheaper than

most pharmaceutical drugs. However, if one is covered on a health plan in which prescriptions cost $3.00 and one must pay $10.00 for a herbal tincture, the choice becomes obvious for many.

Quality Assurance

Currently, there is no organization or government agency in the United States that certifies that a herbal product is what it claims to be. Quality control has been a problem within the herbal industry for many years, and errors abound. For example, it has been estimated that more than half of the Echinacea sold in the United States from the period of 1908–1991 was actually *Parthenium integrifolium*. An article in *JAMA* reported an incident of infant androgenization occurring secondary to the consumption of Siberian ginseng *(Eleutherococcus senticosus)* by the mother during pregnancy. The article incorrectly identified the product as panax ginseng. When investigated, it was discovered that the product the woman had taken was not Siberian ginseng at all, but was *Periploca sepium* (41). Animal studies conducted on both *Eleutherococcus* and *Periploca* have not produced any androgenic effects. The androgenization of the infant was probably totally unrelated to the herb being consumed (41).

These examples demonstrate the need for accurate identification of the plant being traded. A certificate of analysis should include the Latin name and organoleptic results (i.e., macroscopic appearance, odor, and taste), microscopic analysis, and thin layer chromatography. Reference chromatographs have been established for most herbs in common use.

The British and German pharmacopoeias have set parameters for the acceptable total ash and acid-insoluble ash contents of many commercially traded plants. The essence of these tests is that when a plant part is burned, it produces a certain amount of ash, usually in the region of 5 to 15% of the total dry weight of the sample tested. Acid-insoluble ash is that portion of the total ash content that is not soluble in acid; basically, it is any "dirt" within the sample. These tests play an important role in determining the overall cleanliness, purity, and therefore quality, of the raw material.

Microbiological assays are becoming more important as worldwide legislation tightens with regard to herbal remedies. Europe has already set limits for the total number of live microorganisms, total yeast and molds, coliform count, *Escherichia coli*, and *Salmonella* that may be present in an herbal product. Microbial counts will become an even greater issue as the number of immunocompromised individuals rises and the risk of opportunistic infection from contaminated herbs increases.

If a plant contains known active constituents, they should be properly identified and measured. In general, most herbs should be analyzed to ensure that they contain acceptable levels of active principles. It is important to know how much of the active constituent is present so that the practitioner can prescribe a safe, therapeutic dose while avoiding toxicity. Standardized extracts, in which the whole plant is used and a guaranteed level of active constituents is clearly labeled, are primarily made in Europe under strict guidelines set by the European Economic Council. Clearly, not all herbs have known actives and do not need standardization, but they should still be subjected to rigorous quality control to ensure the highest quality raw material and consistency from batch to batch using the most reasonable markers (see Chapter 6).

PROSPECTS FOR THE FUTURE

Scientific research that validates the traditional uses of many of our ancient herbal medicines is currently available. A tremendous amount of money is being spent in Germany, France, Italy, and other countries to gain new knowledge about the medicinal uses of plants. In France and Germany, phytomedicine is often prescribed by physicians in place of a pharmaceutical drug; these physicians learn about phytotherapy as part of their medical training. In these countries, ginkgo leaf is prescribed for the treatment of both peripheral vascular and cerebral vascular disease, with more than 100 million prescriptions in Europe in 1990 alone. Clearly, science is opening the door to a new, broader pharmacopoeia that encompasses both the pharmaceutical and botanical worlds.

The use of phytomedicine in today's world is as important to our well-being as it ever has been. Plants enhance our lives in many ways. Who has not paused to take in the aroma of a rose and wonder at its beauty, or experienced the healing which occurs during a walk through the woods or a field of wildflowers? Humankind has coexisted with the plant kingdom since our earliest days on the planet, evolving side by side. It is our responsibility to ensure the continued existence of all life, especially the plants that support our very life. Phytotherapy is a system of medicine that does not harm the environment (if harvesting and collection is done ethically), is available to all peoples throughout the world, is generally safer and, for the most part, far less expensive than most industrialized drugs. If we are going to achieve health care for all in the twenty-first century, Western medicine must attempt to fulfill the recommendations set by the World Health Organization, which clearly state that traditional medicines and practices need to be incorporated into the health care systems of every country. There is much to be gained and little to be lost with the incorporation of herbalism into mainstream medicine.

The rise in herb use and the increasing desire by patients to avoid many pharmaceutical drugs has put both the physician and pharmacist in a bit of a bind. Neither is adequately trained in the United States to deal with the many issues surrounding the use of plant remedies: active constituents, therapeutic dosages, interactions with other drugs, possible side effects, and the therapeutic value inherent within the plant. The sheer volume of herbal products consumed in the pursuit of health obligates the allopathic health care practitioner to expand his or her knowledge base of these practices. The practitioner musk ask: Does this therapy work? What is the risk-benefit ratio, and how does it compare to Western allopathic treatment? What are the relative costs? What therapy does the patient prefer? How does this therapy fit with the patient's view of health and illness? It seems prudent to move toward a model of integration of complementary medicines.

REFERENCES

1. Weiss R. Herbal medicine. Beaconsfield, England: Beaconsfield Publishers, Ltd, 1988.
2. Emmart EW. The Badianus manuscript, an Aztec herbal of 1552 by Martin de la Cruz and Juannes Badianus. Baltimore: Johns Hopkins Press, 1940.
3. Roys RL. The ethno-botany of the Maya. Department of Middle American Research. New Orleans: Tulane University, 1931.
4. Vogel V. American Indian medicine. Normal, OK: University of Oklahoma Press, 1970.
5. Mills S. Out of the earth—the essential book of herbal medicine. London: Penguin Books, Ltd, 1991.
6. Moore M. Medicinal plants of the desert and canyon west. Santa Fe, NM: Museum of New Mexico Press, 1989.
7. Hoffman D. The contribution of herbalism to western holistic practice. In: Tierra M, ed. American herbalism: essays on herbs and herbalism by members of the American Herbalist Guild. Freedom, CA: Crossing Press, 1992.
8. Mowrey D. The scientific validation of herbal medicine. Cormorant Books, 1986.
9. Schilcher H. Phytotherapy in paediatrics—handbook for physicians and pharmacists. Stuttgart, Germany: Medpharm Scientific Publishers, 1997.
10. Linde K, Ramirez G, Mulrow CD, et al. St. John's Wort for depression—an overview and meta-analysis of randomised clinical trials. Br Med J 1996;313:253–258.
11. Mueller WE, Schaefer C. Johanniskraut. In-vitro Studie uber Hypericum-Extract, Hypericin und Kaempferol als Antidepressive. Dtsch Apoth Z 1996;136:1015–1022.
12. Lavie G, Valentine F, Levin B, et al. Studies of the mechanisms of action of the antiretroviral agents hypericin and pseudohypericin. Proc Natl Acad Sci U S A 1989;86:5963–5967.
13. Haensgen KD, Vesper J, Ploch M. Multizentrische Doppelblindstudie zur antidepressiven Wirksamkeit des Hypericum-Extractes LI 160. Nervenheilkunder 1993;12:285–289.
14. Fach information: Helarium (R) Hypericum, hypericum extract. Neumarkt: Bionorica GmbH, 1996.
15. Lehmann E, Kinzler E, Friedemann J. Efficacy of a

16. Cawte J. Psychoactive substance of the South Seas: betel, kava and pituri. Aust N Z J Psychiatry 1985;19:83–87.
17. Fach information: Antares (R) 120, kava-kava extract. Goeppingen: Krewel Meuselbach GmbH & Co KG, 1996.
18. Jamieson DD, Duffield PH. The antinociceptive actions of kava components in mice. Clin Exp Pharmacol Physiol 1990;17:495–508.
19. Fach information: Antares (R) 120, kava-kava extract. Goeppingen: Krewel Meuselbach GmbH & Co KG, 1996.
20. Fach information: Kavasporal (R) forte, kava-kava extract. Eitorg: Mueller Goeppingen GmbH, 1996.
21. Norton SA, Ruze P. Kava dermopathy. J Am Acad Dermatol 1994;31:89–97.
22. Luettig B, Steinmuller C, Gifford GE, et al. Macrophage activation by the polysaccharide arabinogalactan isolated from plant cell cultures of Echinacea purpurea. J Natl Cancer Inst 1989:81:669–675.
23. Schulz V, Haensel R. Rational phytotherapie. Ratgaber fuer die aertzliche Praxis. 3 Aufl. Berlin: Springer Verlag, 1996:306–310.
24. Bauer R. Echinacea-Drogen-Wirkungen und Wirksubstanzen. ZaeF 1996;90:111–115.
25. Dorsch W. Klinische Anwendung von Extrakten aus Echinacea purpurea oder Echinacea pallida. ZaeF 1996;90:117–122.
26. German Commision E Monograph. Echinacea purpurea herb. Bundesanzeiger 1989;43.
27. Wichtl M. In: Bisset N, ed. Herbal drugs and phytopharmaceuticals. Stuttgart, Germany: Medpharm Scientific Publishers, 1994.
28. Schuessler M, Hoelzl J, Fricke U. Myocardial effects of flavonoids from Crataegus species. Arzneimittelforschung 1995;45:842–845.
29. Uchida S, Ikari N, Ohtaa H, et al. Inhibitory effects of condensed tannins on angiotensin converting enzyme. Jpn J Pharmacol 1987;43:242–245.
30. Schuessler M, Hoelzl J, Fricke U. Myocardial effects of flavonoids from Crataegus species. Arzneimittelforschung 1995;45:842–845.
31. Fach information: Faros (R) 300, Weissdornblaetter, -blueten-Trockenextrakt. Berlin: Lichtwer Pharma, 1996.
32. Rai GS, Shovlin C, Wesnes KA. A double blind, placebo controlled study of ginkgo biloba extract ('Tanakan') in elderly outpatients with mild to

moderate memory impairment. Curr Med Res Opin 1991;12:350–355.

33. Huguet F, Drieu K, Piriou A. Decreased cerebral 5-HT1a receptors during aging: reversal by ginkgo biloba extract (Egb 761). J Pharm Pharmacol 1994;46:316–318.

34. Klejnen J, Knipschild P. Ginkgo biloba for cerebral insufficiency. Br J Clin Pharmacol 1992; 340: 1136–1139.

35. Blume J, Kieser M, Hoelscher U. Placebokontrollierte Doppelblindstudie zur Wirksamkeit von Ginkgo-biloba Spezialextrakt Egb 761 bei austrainierten Patienten mit Claudicato intermittens. VASA 1996;25:265–274.

36. Klejnen J, Knipschild P. Ginkgo biloba. Lancet 1992;340:1136–1139.

37. Haguenauer JP, Cantenot F, Koskas H, et al. Treatment of equilibrium disorders with Ginkgo biloba extract: a multi-center double blind drug vs. placebo study. Presse Med 1986;15:1569–1572.

38. Lebuisson DA, Leroy L, Rigal G. Treatment of senile macular degeneration with Ginkgo biloba extract: a preliminary double-blind drug vs placebo study. Presse Med 1986;15:1556–1558.

39. Siegel RK. Ginseng abuse syndrome. JAMA 1979;241:1641–1715.

40. Tierra M, ed. American herbalism: essays on herbs & herbalism by members of the American Herbalist Guild. Freedom, CA: Crossing Press, 1992.

41. Awang D. Maternal use of ginseng and neonatal androgenization. J Am Med Assoc 1991;266:363.

CHAPTER 21

SPIRITUAL HEALING

Daniel J. Benor

BACKGROUND

Spiritual healing is defined as "the systematic, purposeful intervention by one or more persons aiming to help (an)other living being (person, animal, plant, or other living system) or beings by means of focused intention, by touch, or by holding the hands near the other being, without application of physical, chemical, or conventional energetic means of intervention"(1).

Spiritual healing is probably the oldest recognized therapy, used in some form in every known culture. Some of these forms include shamanism, faith healing, laying on of hands, absent (or distant) healing, and mental healing. As *shamanism* (2), it is practiced in traditional cultures, each of which dresses it in rituals and explanatory systems appropriate to its own time, place, and cosmologies. It may include meditation, prayer, chanting, and other practices, and it is often combined with herbalism. As *faith healing*, it is practiced in churches in which there is a belief that faith is required for healing. The popular press often uses faith healing as a generic term for spiritual healing. As *prani* (3) or *bioenergy healing, Qigong* (4), *Reiki* (5), *therapeutic touch* (6), *healing touch* (7), *polarity therapy* (8), *SHEN therapy* (9), and similar approaches, it is given as a laying on of hands. In Europe it is often termed *paranormal healing*, and in Eastern Europe it is termed *bioenergotherapy*. As *absent*, or *distant*, *healing*, it may be given through meditation, prayer, Reiki, LeShan, or other types of practices. *Mental healing* is the heading for reports found in the *Index Medicus*.

Spiritual healing is a generic term used in Britain and is increasingly accepted around the world, despite some lingering proprietary claims of Christian fundamentalists. For the sake of brevity in this chapter, the term *healing* is used to indicate spiritual healing. The term *spiritual healing*, first used by Lawrence LeShan, acknowledges that participation in healing opens healers and healee (10) to awarenesses of spirituality, a connectedness with aspects of self that extend beyond the physical body and reaching towards the Divine, or the *All*.

HISTORY AND DEVELOPMENT

Sixth and Seventh Century BC

Around the sixth century BC, Pythagoras, a physician as well as a mathematician, astronomer, and philosopher, considered healing the noblest of his pursuits and integrated healing into his considerations of ethics, mind, and soul. He called the energy associated with healing *pneuma*. His followers conceived of the pneuma as being visible in a luminous body, and they believed that light could cure illness. A century later,

> ... [Hippocrates] says, "It is believed by experienced doctors that the heat which oozes out of the hand, on being applied to the sick, is highly salutary ... It has often appeared, while I have been soothing my patients, as if there was a singular property in my hands

to pull and draw away from the affected parts aches and diverse impurities, by laying my hand upon the place, and by extending my fingers towards it. Thus it is known to some of the learned that health may be implanted in the sick by certain gestures, and by contact, as some diseases may be communicated from one to another" (11).

Hippocrates hypothesized a healing energy—the *vis medicatrix naturae,* or healing power of nature—as the vital force of life. He advised that physicians must identify blocking influences within individuals (and between them and the cosmos) to restore the proper flow of *pneuma.* Nature, not the doctor, heals the patient.

The theory of the greater unity of mind and body, which the Pythagoreans had advanced, was soon superseded by the Hippocratic beliefs that mind and body are dichotomous. Plato criticized this view: "If the head and the body are to be well, you must begin by curing the soul; that is the first thing . . . The great error of our day in the treatment of the human body [is] that physicians separate the soul from the body." The Hippocratic system, which was codified by Galen in the second century AD, became the standard for medical practice for many centuries thereafter.

Early Christian Era

Jesus was a great healer. The Bible and Gospels tell of numerous individual and group healings by Christ and the Apostles (1). They used touch, saliva, mud, and cloth *vehicles,* as well as words, prayers, exorcism, faith, and compassion for healing. Unfortunately, the Christian church gradually turned away from healing for a variety of reasons (12–14). It deemphasized healing in its ministries, sometimes even denying its existence other than in metaphor or mythology.

In the early Christian era, many priests apparently were selected for their healing gifts. Treatments would involve exhortations to the diseases to leave and the laying on of hands. Saint Paul, who believed that healing was a personal gift, was believed to be able to transmit

healing through objects he touched. Throughout the third century AD, the church was well known for providing healing for its members. By the fourth century, Saint Chrysostom observed that miracles were becoming rare, although healing was still being given (15). The rites for ordination of priests continued to include a prayer for healing powers, and the relics of saints and their shrines were increasingly credited with healing powers.

Seventh to Seventeenth Century AD

By the seventh century, after the conversion of Constantine to Christianity, the church exerted a domination over healing. Theological cosmologies, religious dogmas, and the hierarchy of divine power through the clergy (often used also to enhance political power) were given credence and preference over healing gifts. As in the general world views of the next 800 years, historical precedents were cited as explanations for natural events. Healing gifts were ignored, or, when outside the aegis of the church, they were often discouraged and healing practitioners persecuted. The church "looked to the practices of its past rather than to the gifts of its living members, and its rites directed greater attention to Christ's instructions to remember His last supper than to His injunction to work (or attempt to work) other miracles in His name . . . " (15). Disease was viewed as an expression of God's will that should be addressed by prayer. Healing as a deliberate and potent intervention for everyday ills was neglected.

A few shreds of healing were sanctioned within the church. The first was the ritual of *exorcism,* institutionalized in the Council of Antioch of 341. The second was the *sacrament of unction* in which the dying were anointed with holy oil.

There were few physicians, and they were too expensive for most of the populace. Apothecaries, barbers, leeches, wise women, and witches provided the primary care at the village level. Physical interventions included prescribing herbs, sweating, cupping, blood letting, and simple surgery. In parallel, magical healing powers could be sought through talismen, relics from violent deaths, elves and fairies, healing wells, as well as the laying on of hands by white witches and warlocks. These folk traditions held a strong influence through the seventeenth century and currently persist in diminished numbers (although still significant forms). Currently, untested remedies touted to cure many symptoms and illness (e.g., wearing copper bracelets, visits to shrines, and various plant and animal products) are not uncommon.

Christianity, focused on the authority of its clergy, acknowledged unusual healing gifts in particular individuals who were sanctioned as saints if not during their lives, then posthumously (15, 16).

In the seventeenth century, Paracelsus shed the first modern, holistic light on the fossilized system of medicine of the Middle Ages. He refocused the study of medicine on naturalistic observations and saw human beings as an integral part of nature, reflecting within themselves the larger cosmos outside themselves. He apparently saw auras because he reported "a healing energy that radiates within and around man like a luminous sphere" (17). He called this force *archaeus,* believing it could be effective from a distance and could cause as well as cure disease. He also believed that magnets, stars, and other heavenly bodies could influence humans via the *archaeus* force; these views persist in Western notions of *magnetic* or *sympathetic medicine* (later reinforced by Mesmer and other hypnotists).

Paracelsus further noted that a human being has a second body, which he labelled the *star,* or *sidereal, body.* He thought that the lower instincts are housed in the animal body, whereas higher instincts, such as wisdom and artistic capacity, are housed in the astral body. He believed that the etheric body motivates the physical body under the influence of the mind. He felt that both are integrally related and that both can be subject to disease (17). He also believed in a third body, a soul or eternal spark which is immortal.

Paracelsus was eccentric, hot-tempered, and impetuous. Despite his brilliant observations and conceptualizations, he alienated his contemporaries to the degree that many of his no-

tions produced far less impact than they may have otherwise. Moreover, his ideas had little chance of competing with those of two other scientists of the seventeenth century, Francis Bacon and René Descartes.

Francis Bacon led the Western world along the path of understanding the laws of science in order to *master* rather than become harmonious with nature. René Descartes revolutionized Western thinking by applying mathematical, logical concepts to analyses of the world and of humans. Descartes' thought is so much a part of current Western views that it is difficult for many to conceive of a world in which systematic, quantifiable, linear relationships do not exist among objects and among parts of objects.

Descartes' insight led to a firm dichotomizing between body (measurable) and mind (intangible) and to the assumption that body could influence mind but not the reverse. These concepts helped lead us out of the Dark Ages in the physical sciences and to search out physical causes for illness, but led to denial of the mind as a causal influence on the body. This influence has led modern science to devalue everything that is neither measurable nor verified objectively.

The West entered an industrial revolution at the time Descartes' ideas were spreading. With growing success in comprehension, manipulation, and control of the environment, the West focused more and more on a material view of the world. In medicine, this has extended to a nearly exclusive concentration on the physical aspects of disease. This focus has lead to the identification of causative agents of diseases, including bacteria, parasites, viruses, vitamins, hormones, and genetic anomalies as well as the discoveries of chemicals and mechanical interventions to treat diseases. However, the contributions of emotions, mind, relationships, and spirit are often neglected. Only a few scientists, such as Leibnitz, dared to question the view that the mind cannot influence the body; other cultures did not share this view. For example, *kahuna* healers in Hawaii were aware of the unconscious mind and of principles of suggestion many centuries before they were discovered in the West (18).

Eighteenth Century AD

At the end of the eighteenth century, Franz Anton Mesmer popularized another aspect of healing. He demonstrated that he could improve numerous symptoms with magnetic passes of his hands around patients' bodies. At first he held magnets in his hands but soon found he was just as effective without them. He hypothesized that he channeled a magnetic fluid into the patient. Although he had staunch followers, the vast majority of the medical community was critical and did not accept his findings. A commission was set up in France to study the subject, but they produced a negative report that effectively sidelined Mesmer's methods outside of mainstream medicine.

The Marquis de Puysegur introduced a form of healing similar to that of Mesmer. He demonstrated that he could influence patients by an act of will, without the use of magnetic passes and with no recourse to theories of fluids. His work with hypnosis reintroduced an appreciation of the impact of thought on the body.

Nineteenth and Twentieth Century AD

ENERGY MEDICINE

Karl von Riechenbach, a German industrialist in the middle of the nineteenth century, explored a variety of physical properties of living beings, relating them to a universal energy that he believed permeated the body. He called this force *od,* or *odyle.* Scientists such as Riechenbach, who sought to study forces within the body that seemed associated with health and disease, often went against the mainstream public opinion. Because Cartesian influence had reasoning and research to support its views, scientists with theories that contradicted conventional beliefs were ignored, ridiculed, or worse.

Wilhelm Reich, an American psychiatrist in the first half of the twentieth century, developed elaborate theories about *orgone* energy. He reported that it is a distinct form of universal energy that becomes blocked in the body because of emotional problems (19). He was persecuted and jailed in America by the government because of his views, and his books were publicly burned. Nevertheless, his adherents (Lowen, Pierrakos, and other practitioners of bioenergetics) continued to develop his ideas (20, 21).

Research in neurology supported the trend against energy medicine. Electrodes inserted in the brain can elicit specific sensations and memories. To neurologists, this is apparent proof that the mind is a product of the physical brain.

THE UNCONSCIOUS MIND

At the turn of the century, Sigmund Freud and Carl Gustav Jung clarified that the unconscious mind may be an agent for certain illnesses. This was the birth of modern psychosomatic medicine, which advocates integration of mind and body. Sir William Osler recommended that physicians seek to understand the patient who has the disease and not merely the disease that the patient has.

Modern behavioral psychology demonstrates that learning by reward and punishment, or conditioning of the unconscious mind, may produce illness. This has supported a mechanistic view of human beings, even when mental influences on physical illness is accepted. Further fragmentation of the whole self has come with the explosion of medical knowledge and specialization. No single physician today can understand all there is to know about the body. A patient, therefore, has to parcel out his or her body among various specialists. Specializations in our hospitals have added to compartmentalization of mind and body.

Modern Health Care

Many factors mitigate against the acceptance of spiritual healing as a legitimate therapy. Drug therapy is a major industry throughout the world. Private health care is another major industry that resists competition. Governments are forced by budgetary considerations to limit health care to the bare essentials of physical treatments, leaving health care professionals without time to attend to other aspects of the patient's needs.

Medical education, with its long hours and emphasis on learning volumes of information, may be teaching young physicians to neglect the more personal and spiritual side of healing. Fortunately, more medical schools are developing programs to help students develop these aspects of themselves and relate them to patient care (22).

PROVIDER–CLIENT INTERACTIONS

The Role of Diagnosis in Spiritual Healing

Many spiritual healers will ask about the healee's symptoms and medical diagnosis, if this is known. Some healers feel that they must adjust the biological energies of the healee according to their intuitively perceived assessments of the initial state of these energies. Healers of many other traditions do not require detailed information for diagnosis. They simply make themselves available as channels for energy, turning over the management of the problem to a higher power (e.g., the intuitive awareness of the healee and/or healer, God, Christ, spirit guides, guardian angels).

Healers may perceive part of the diagnostic picture but not all of it. For example, in tests of intuitive diagnosis, healers simultaneously observed a series of individuals with known diagnoses. Each drew a picture and wrote down his or her diagnostic impressions of what was observed in the auras. Then each, in turn, reported to the person observed what his or her impressions were. No one was more surprised than the healers when each of the reports was significantly different from the others' reports. The next surprise was when the people who had been given the intuitive diagnostic impressions indicated that they agreed with all but one of the "readings." All but one of the healers resonated accurately with a different facet of the problems of the people they were observing. (One healer clearly was projecting her impressions, reporting she sensed depression in most of the people she observed.) Before these studies, most of the healers had believed that they were perceiving

the whole problem when they were giving intuitive diagnostic readings (23).

Among those healers who focus on diagnosis, a pendulum or other such device may be used to help them bring intuitive information into awareness. It is generally assumed that these devices are activated by the unconscious mind of the healer, through subtle muscular movements (24–26). Clinical progress in treatment is assessed by healee subjective reports, by objective evidence of change, and by serial intuitive diagnostic impressions.

Types of Healing

LAYING ON OF HANDS

A laying-on-of-hands healing may last 5 to 30 minutes or longer. In my experience and that of others, healees usually relax and may even doze or enter deep altered states of consciousness during healings. Beneficial responses to healing may be felt immediately, especially with relief of anxiety, tension, and pain. Pain may increase briefly over the first few treatments and is often interpreted as a positive sign, apparently indicating that shifts are occurring in the processes underlying the pain; with additional treatments, a decrease in the original pain is expected. Chronic conditions may require repeated treatments, usually given at weekly intervals over several months.

DISTANT HEALING

Distant healing may be done by one or more healers who focus on the name of the person in need of healing. The distance between healer and healee is thought to be immaterial to the success of treatment; successes have been reported when healers are many miles away from their healees. There is a general belief that a group sending absent healing may be more effective than a single healer. Many healers find that the rapport established through telephone contact, a photograph, or even just a name and a summary of the problem facilitate absent healing, whereas other healers find that unconditionally accepting detachment rather than personal rapport works better and suffice with only a name for contact.

THERAPY AND OUTCOMES

Responses to Healing

Healing efficacy is unpredictable. Acute conditions, such as headaches, trauma, and infections, may respond within minutes or hours. Chronic conditions may require weekly treatments over a period of months to obtain maximum benefits. If positive effects are going to occur, one often has some indication of improvement in the first three to six sessions. A lack of effects with one healer is no indication that benefits will not be obtained with another healer. Subjective improvements are more frequent than objective ones (27). The physical disease may be unchanged, but a person's attitude may shift so that he or she lives more comfortably with his or her disabilities or seeks the meaning of the illness.

Emotional conditions, such as anxiety and depression, often respond well to healing. Poor mental attitudes, impaired self-image, long-harbored resentments and the like may improve dramatically with healing. Relationships also may improve with healing. This might be the result of healing directed to the involved parties or of healing directed to only one of them. Many healers believe that our world is more intimately linked through nonlocal awareness than is generally appreciated (28).

Spiritual awareness may be awakened during healings, bringing people in contact with a vast source of inspiration that can help them deal with their dis-eases and diseases (29–31). Many healers feel that awakening of spiritual awareness is the most important aspect of healing and that the body is a vehicle for the expression of the needs of spirit and soul. They feel that the soul chooses to be born into a particular family to learn lessons in relating with love and forgiveness to others with whom it may have had difficult relationships in previous lifetimes (32–35).

Healing into death is a major contribution of healers to conventional medical practice (36).

Conventional medicine tends to fight death and prolong life at all costs, sometime without regard for the quality of life. Spiritual healing views a peaceful death as a good healing and finds that healing often eases the transition between worlds. Survival of the spirit after physical death is assumed by many healers who claim that they channel spirits who contribute to their healing (37, 38). This type of guidance may come from the spirit guides of the healer or from spirits related to the healee.

MAJOR MODALITIES AND INDICATIONS

There are few studies on spiritual healing published in major medical journals, although over 175 controlled studies of healing have been conducted (1). The majority of these studies are published in peer-reviewed parapsychology journals. Approximately twelve of them are doctoral and master's degree dissertations. They include studies of humans, animals, plants, bacteria, yeasts, cells in laboratory culture, enzymes, and models. The following are some examples of healing studies.

Distant Healing

Distant healing is an excellent therapy for controlled, double-blind studies because it can be given with absolutely no physical or social contact between healers and healees. This factor makes it easy to maintain a blind study because no one but the experimenter assigning the patients for distant healing and the healers sending the healing will know which patients are being given the treatment.

Randolph C. Byrd, MD, studied the effects of intercessory prayer healing on patients hospitalized in a coronary care unit (CCU) (39). In a prospective, double-blind, randomized study, 192 patients were sent distant healing and 201 patients served as controls. There were no significant differences between groups on admission in degree of severity of myocardial infarction or in numerous other pertinent variables. "Intercessors" were born-again Christians who prayed daily and were active with their local church. Each CCU patient had 3 to 7 intercessors praying for him or her. Intercessors were given patients' first names, their diagnoses, and updates on their condition. "[E]ach intercessor was asked to pray daily for a rapid recovery and for prevention of complications and death, in addition to other areas of prayer they believed to be beneficial to the patient." Significantly fewer patients in the prayer group required intubation/ventilation (p < .002) or antibiotics (p < .005), had cardiopulmonary arrests (p < .02), developed pneumonia (p < .03), or required diuretics (p < .05). A multivariate analysis showed a very highly significant difference between the groups (p < .0001). Despite these differences between groups, the mean times in CCU and durations of hospitalization between groups were nearly identical. Healing appeared to reduce the severity of cardiac pathology but not shorten duration of hospitalization. This exceptionally good study is an exception in yet another way: it was published in the *Southern Medical Journal.*

Therapeutic Touch

Healing by the laying on of hands has been standardized into a treatment system called therapeutic touch by Dolores Krieger, PhD, RN, professor of nursing at New York University, and Dora Kunz, a gifted clairvoyant and healer. It is conservatively estimated that 40,000 nurses in America practice therapeutic touch. More than 90 nursing schools offer courses in therapeutic touch.

Therapeutic touch is given either with the hands lightly touching the body or as noncontact therapeutic touch, with the hands a few inches away from the body. Healers *center* their minds, focusing on the intent to help and heal while excluding other thoughts from their minds. The term *centering* comes from the potter's wheel: if the clay is in the center of the wheel, it stays there. If it is off center, centrifugal force sends it flying in all directions.

Healing and the Immune System

Healers have proposed that enhancing immune system functions (and thus strengthening the body) is one way in which healing works. Anxiety and stress bring about changes in the immune system. Changes in circulating immune proteins, such as immunoglobulins (Ig) and lymphocytes, may thus provide measures of physiological stress responses, as in the following study.

Melodie Olson and colleagues anticipated that students who were to take their professional board examinations would be highly stressed and would show changes in their immune systems which could be influenced by therapeutic touch (40, 41).

Immune system values measured after therapeutic touch treatment on the day before the exams showed significant differences for IgA and IgM (p < .05) and for a T-lymphocyte function (apoptosis, p < .05).[1] Experimental and control groups showed comparable levels of stress at the start of the study.

The authors note that confounding factors may have included nutritional changes, especially because dietary intake may have been altered before the exams, and the presence of a caring person for the experimental group that was not counterbalanced for the control group.

Pain Relief

Healers and healees report that pain is the symptom most responsive to spiritual healing. Several studies of therapeutic touch reported immediate reductions in pain from tension headaches and surgery (42–46). The following study showed effects that were of longer duration: Robin Redner et al. studied effects of a method of healing which was developed by Johnston (47). This healing method

". . . begins with the treater's assessment of the bioenergy field around the patient's phys-

---

[1] t-Tests on the mean differences between E and C groups. IgG differences nearly reached statistical significance as well (p < .06).

ical body. Using their hands, the treater senses only imbalances, (which may evidence as heat, a dense quality, or a sense of blockage), and treats the imbalance by visualizing the energy becoming balanced and free flowing. This visualization continues until the treater senses a change towards balance or the free flow of energy in that area. . . . Johnston's technique occurs entirely off the body in the patient's energy field. . . ."

Johnston's healer training includes a series of three courses. Treaters in the study had completed two or more courses and participated in weekly practice sessions for 2 years. The study introduced an *attention placebo control group*, which is intended to control for expectancy effects and for relaxation effects that occur when one receives attention from a caring person. The study also provided 30-minute interventions by two healers for four treatments during the study; compared bioenergy diagnoses with medical diagnoses; studied positive and negative moods as well as levels of anxiety; and checked outcome measures 1 week following healing.

Participants suffered from arthritis, headaches, and low back pain, and they could not have been taking narcotic medications or been receiving massage, physical therapy, acupuncture, or acupressure during the study. The 47 participants were randomly assigned to experimental or control groups, being told only that there were two intervention possibilities, but remaining blind regarding assignment. This study demonstrated significantly reduced severity of affective and sensory aspects of pain 1 week after the healing intervention on the McGill-Melzack Pain Questionnaire (each at $p < .05$) [$F(1,45) = 5.88$]. The persistence of pain reduction 1 week after healing is a significant finding over previous research on healing for pain.

On the weekly Profile of Mood Scale (POMS), the high-intensity treatment group showed increased anxiety over time, whereas the low-intensity placebo group showed less anxiety ($p < .05$) [$F(1,45) = 4.77$]. The lack of findings on the physical measurements and bioenergy evaluation may have been due to small numbers in each of the target problem categories.

Other Studies

Electrodermal response (EDR) is used as a measure of anxiety and tension and is the basis of the lie detector test. In a series of 15 experiments, William Braud and colleagues demonstrated that spiritual healing can significantly alter EDR (48). Summarizing a series including 323 sessions with 4 experimenters, 62 influencers, and 271 subjects, they found that of the 15 studies, 6 (i.e., 40%) produced significant results. Of the 323 sessions, 57% showed significant results ($p = .000023$).[2]

Studies on rodents have shown significant effects of healing for accelerating wound healing (49); reducing the rate of development of iodine deficient goiters (50); reducing the rate of development of experimentally induced amyloidosis (51); slowing the growth of tumors (52); and slowing the progression of malaria (53, 54). The last study is particularly intriguing because it dealt with healing expectations.

In an intriguing experiment using malaria-infected mice, Jerry Solfvin apparently demonstrated that the expectation of healing of illness could produce healing effects under double-blind conditions, even when no individual was specifically identified as a healer (55). Healing expectancy may be an important variable in healing effects.

Studies on plants show that rates of growth may be increased or decreased, according with the intent of the healers (56–61). The same is true of cultures of bacteria (1, 62, 63) and yeast (1, 64–67). The action of enzymes can be changed with healing interventions (46, 68–70).

An overall summary of healing research shows that of 155 controlled studies, 64 demonstrate effects at statistically significant levels that

---

[2] The . . . combined z score (for the experimental series as a whole, calculated according to the Stouffer method) and the mean effect size (Cohen's d, for the entire series). The overall z is 4.08 and has an associated $p = .000023$; the average effect size for all 13 experiments is 0.29.

could occur by chance only 1 time in a 100 or less (p $<$ .01); and another 21 at levels that could occur between 2 to 5 times out of 100 (p $<$ .02-.05) (1).

THEORETICAL BASIS FOR SPIRITUAL HEALING

Many conventional medical practitioners may find it difficult to understand (within Western scientific thought) how spiritual healing could be more than suggestion, placebo, or charlatanism. Healers explain that healing works through multiple, interdigitating levels, including body, emotions, mind, relationships (with other people and with the environment), and spirit.

Subtle Energies

Healers address the body through purported energies that surround and interpenetrate the physical body (24, 71–73). Most people can sense the energy field with their hands by holding them about an inch apart and slowly moving them further apart and then back together. These energies are thought to create certain sensations in the palms and fingers. The most common sensations people experience with this experiment are described in the following footnote, and the reader is invited to try this and write down his or her sensations before reading it.[3]

By holding one's hand opposite the hands of different people, distinct differences in sensations are felt with each person. These sensations are assumed to be stimulated by the interactions of the biological fields that surround people's hands with the biological fields of those with whom they are interacting. Healers will often practice *scanning* the entire body of healees to develop a diagnostic vocabulary of sensations through which they can identify parts of the body that are out of harmony, dis-eased (as in storing tensions or in early states of dysfunc-

tion), or diseased on a physical level (6, 37, 71). A recent article in *JAMA* claims to have refuted this ability, however (86).

Many healers consciously focus on the intent to increase energies available to healees in whom they detect energy deficits, or to draw off excess energies from healees where they sense energy congestion. Healers will also focus on enhancing the flows of energy at points at which subtle energy flows appear to be blocked.

Very sensitive people report being able to perceive these energy fields as auras of color surrounding the body (74). The colors shift constantly, reflecting the various physical, emotional, mental, relational, energy, and spiritual states of the organism. Particularly strong energy centers called *chakras* are visible along the midline of the body. (Chakra means *wheel* in Sanskrit, indicating that these energy centers were probably also perceived by sensitive people many centuries ago.) Healers find that the changes in the colors of the *chakras* reflect states of health and illness in parts of the body near the relevant *chakra*, and that projecting healing to a *chakra* that appears abnormal can restore the energy body and improve health (74). The perceptions of auras is reported by healers even with their eyes closed. Most healers assume that clairvoyance (intuitive perception rather than visual perception) is involved.

Intuitive Perceptions

Some healers report hearing words, sometimes medical diagnoses, when they are tuning in energetically to a healee. Occasionally healers report they can smell particular odors or taste odd tastes when they scan a person's body and that these, like the tactile or visual sensations, are associated with disease states. It would appear that the mind uses various ordinary sensation modalities in bringing these sensations into conscious awareness and in interpreting them as meaningful information (75).

The healee's emotional and physical states are reported by many healers as mirrored feelings

---

[3] Most people report they feel warmth, light pressure (like a gentle bubble, or like two identical poles of weak magnets being pushed together), tingling (like a mild electrical current), vibration, or cold.

within themselves, sometimes labeled as *telesomatic reactions*. These reactions are used by psychics in *clairsentient* "readings" (76). One must not put too great credence in such readings, as Macbeth learned to his detriment. Healers may have intuitive impressions of the origins of emotional difficulties in traumas that occurred many years before scanning the healee. Alternatively, spiritual healing may awaken awareness of early traumas in healees. Intuitive emotional awareness can be particularly helpful when there are emotional tensions underlying physical problems. For example, a healer gave healing to a 40-year-old woman with low back pain. She spontaneously started to recall sexual abuse in her early teenage years. Working through this long-buried emotional trauma brought about healing in her back pain, which had been present for many years and unresponsive to conventional therapies.

Intuitive diagnostic awareness suggests that healing may be affected by a transfer of information rather than by transfers of energy. This theory is supported by reports of healing from great distances, with no apparent diminution of effect as occurs with conventional energies over increasing distances (28, 77–79).

An overall theory to explain healing may arise out of Einstein's observation that energy and matter are interconvertible. Quantum physics has confirmed that, on a microscopic level, what appears to our senses as a solid, material world can be equally well described and defined in terms of energies. Biology and medicine have been slow to consider that the body, which they address as matter, may also be addressed as energy (24–26).

INDICATIONS FOR TREATMENT

Spiritual healing has been used most often as a last-resort treatment, when all conventional therapies have had little or no affect. This is unfortunate, because healers report that when spiritual healing is given early in the course of an illness, it is effective more quickly and profoundly. If there is neither urgency nor a known effective conventional medical treat-

ment, healing should be considered as an initial treatment because it has no known harmful effects. Healing can always be used as a complement to other therapies. Although no formal studies have been conducted, anecdotal reports indicate that healing can lessen the need for various medications and therapies (e.g., antihypertensives, antidiabetics) and that it can reduce side effects of conventional treatments, such as cancer chemotherapy and radiotherapy. Although healing may not always improve the physical condition being treated, it often improves a person's ability to deal with his or her conditions. Through its relaxation effects, it can contribute to the management of many conditions.

Healing is not recommended as an alternative to medications. Injudicious discontinuation of medications with healing for diabetes, epilepsy, and hypertension, for example, has been reported to worsen these conditions (sometimes drastically). Conversely, when given as a complement to medicinal therapies, the attending doctor should be alerted that lower doses of medication may be needed. There are reports of diabetics who went into insulin shock after receiving healing when their doctors were not advised about it; there are also reports of reduced need for tranquilizers, pain medications, and sleeping pills.

The preventive use of healing has not been explored in a serious way. Casual studies of healing to prevent influenza (38); to prevent bovine foot and mouth disease; and to ease the course of anticipated difficult pregnancy, labor, and delivery (80) suggest it may be a promising preventive treatment for some conditions. More research is needed.

Healing may be highly cost-effective. Michael Dixon, a general practitioner (internist) in England, invited a healer to treat 25 patients with a broad range of problems for whom he had nothing more to offer but palliative, maintenance medications. In 6 months the healer saved the equivalent of $1,500 in medication costs alone. She also reduced the numbers of return visits. His impression was that if healing had been given earlier on in the course of illness, there would have been further savings in referrals to specialists (81).

Prohibitions against healing practitioners and against cooperation of physicians with healers are common, varying widely from state to state in America and other countries. Apart from the need to discipline exploitative charlatans, suppression of healing practices is unreasonable if one considers the research available and the apparent lack of harmful effects.

ORGANIZATION

Training

Healing is an art that can be enhanced with training and practice. Most caring people can develop a measure of healing ability through the intent to help and heal, through meditation, study under experienced healers, and practice. How good a healer will become with study is similar to the development of any other gift, such as playing the piano. There are people who are born with a highly developed gift for spiritual healing and others in whom a great gift develops spontaneously or with study. Some achieve excellent or credible results with application and practice, and others remain mediocre despite their best efforts.

Healing is an excellent complement to most other therapies. Many conventional and complementary therapists develop their own healing gifts (82). My own preference is to combine counseling/psychotherapy with healing, because each complements the other so well. Healing may bring about spontaneous releases of old emotional hurts, and then psychotherapy can help people to deal with these. Psychotherapy may raise anxieties and emotional traumas from the past, and healing helps to assuage the stresses and hurts of these. Healing also opens spiritual dimensions of awareness, which are helpful to people in dealing with their problems (24–26, 28, 83).

The exact nature and format for training in healing varies with the healing model being used. For some, healing is primarily an energetic intervention. Healers provide laying on of hands or absent healing alone. Some feel that healing should be left to a higher power, both within

and beyond the healee. Despite these differences, one may learn the basics of healing in a few hours or days. These basics include:

1. Holding a caring intent to heal in one's awareness (both mind and heart).
2. Centering one's mind and maintaining a focus on Step 1.
3. Developing awareness of and trust in one's intuitions.
4. Opening oneself to connect with a power greater than oneself, and inviting the healee (overtly or quietly) to do the same (84, 85).

Regardless of theoretical preferences, there are great advantages to programs that organize ongoing mentor and/or peer supervision (37). There are endless lessons to learn and pitfalls to stumble into, as with psychotherapy. It is prudent to have other professionals to turn to for discussing one's work.

Duration of programs vary from a single weekend to 2 to 4 years. Clearly the longer one studies, the broader and deeper will be one's knowledge.

Certification and Licensure

Certification is given by some, but not all, schools. Among the more responsible schools are the Barbara Brennan School of Healing (P.O. Box 2005, East Hampton, NY, 11937), the LeShan Method Consciousness Research and Training Project (315 E. 68 Street, Box 9G, New York, NY, 10021), and the International SHEN Therapy Association (3213 West Wheeler Street, No. 202, Seattle, WA, 98199). In several countries (e.g., England, Holland, Norway, South Africa), healers have written and subscribed to codes of conduct. There is no licensure for spiritual healing in the Western world. In America, many healers obtain licenses to touch as masseurs, chiropractors, or the like. Another alternative has been to offer healing within a religious setting. I have heard of licensure for healers in several East European countries but have seen no official documentation on this. Their requirements include courses in basic anatomy and physiology; demonstration of intuitive diagnostic abilities to correlate with medical diagnoses; and demonstration of healing abilities with physical problems for which no treatment is being received and in which spontaneous improvement is highly unlikely. Licensure is said to be *nonexclusive*—that is, those healers who qualify have the distinction and recognition of having met the required standards. Those who have not qualified are not prohibited from practice. Because a mother kissing away a child's hurt and children who have healing abilities are not uncommon, a nonexclusive licensure appears advisable.

Fees vary but are usually modest. Some healers treat without charge. Others request donations. Beware of healers who charge large fees, especially if they require payment in advance for a series of treatments. In England, a growing number of healers work in doctors' offices and hospitals, where they may be paid by the National Health Service.

PROSPECTS FOR THE FUTURE

Prospects for the future of spiritual healing are promising. Much of the reluctance to consider healing derives from lack of knowledge about the research database or fear of charlatans and frauds (a fear that, in this author's opinion, is overblown). Healers must form professional organizations if they are to attain greater professional acceptance. This has been possible in England and Holland, and is clearly a manageable challenge in other countries. The lack of side effects with healing, combined with its potency as a complement to other therapies and probable cost-effectiveness, make it one of the most promising of complementary therapies.

REFERENCES

1. Benor DJ. Healing research, volume I. Spiritual healing: does it work? Science says, yes! Southfield, MI: Vision Publications, 1999.
2. Krippner S, Welch P. Spiritual dimensions of healing: from native shamanism to contemporary health care. New York: Irvington, 1992:22.
3. Ramacharaka Y. The science of psychic healing. Chicago: Yogi Publishing Society, 1934.
4. Cohen KS. The way of Qigong: the art and science of Chinese energy healing. New York: Ballantine, 1997.
5. Rand WL. Reiki: the healing touch, first and second degree manual. Southfield, MI: Vision, 1991.
6. Krieger D. Accepting your power to heal: the personal practice of therapeutic touch. Santa Fe, NM: Bear & Co., 1993.
7. Hover-Kramer D, ed. Healing touch: a resource for health care professionals. Albany, NY: Delmar, 1996.
8. Sills F. The polarity process: energy as a healing art. Longmead, England: Element, 1989.
9. Pavek RR. Handbook of SHEN. Sausalito, CA: SHEN Therapy Institute, 1987.
10. LeShan L. The medium, the mystic and the physicist: toward a general theory of the paranormal. New York: Ballantine, 1974(a); British edition— Clairvoyant reality. Wellingborough, England: Thorsons, 1974.
11. Harvey D. The power to heal: an investigation of healing and the healing experience. Wellingborough, Northamptonshire, England: Aquarian, 1983:35.
12. Bek L, Pullar P. The seven levels of healing. London: Century, 1986.
13. MacManaway B, Turcan J. Healing: the energy that can restore health. Wellingsborough, England: Thorsons, 1983.
14. Rose L. Faith healing. London: Penguin, 1971:27–29.
15. Rose L. Faith healing. London: Penguin, 1971:30.
16. Leuret F, Bon H. Modern miraculous cures: a documented account of miracles and medicine in the 20th century. New York: Farrar, Straus and Cudahy, 1957.
17. Coddington M. In search of the healing energy. New York: Warner/Destiny, 1978.
18. Long MF. The secret science behind miracles. Marina del Rey, CA: DeVorss, 1976.
19. Mann WE. Orgone, Reich and Eros: Wilhelm Reich's theory of life energy. New York: Touchstone/Simon and Schuster, 1973.
20. Lowen A. Bioenergetics. New York: Penguin, 1975.
21. Pierrakos JC. Core energetics: developing the capacity to love and heal. Mandocino, CA: Life Rhythm, 1987.
22. Benor DJ. Medical student health awareness: the Louisville program for medical student health awareness. Complementary Therapies in Medicine 1995;3(2):93–99.
23. Benor DJ. Intuitive diagnosis. Subtle Energies 1992;3(2):41–64.
24. Benor DJ. Healing research, volume II. Southfield, MI: Vision Publications. In press.

25. Bird C. The divining hand: the five hundred year old mystery of dowsing. New York: E.P. Dutton, 1979.

26. Leuret F, Bon H. Modern miraculous cures: a documented account of miracles and medicine in the 20th century. New York: Farrar, Straus and Cudahy, 1957.

27. Strauch I. Medical aspects of "mental" healing. International Journal of Parapsychology 1963;5(2):135–165.

28. Benor DJ. Healing research, volume IV. Southfield, MI: Vision Publications. In press.

29. Benor DJ. Healing research, volume III. Southfield, MI: Vision Publications. In press.

30. Dossey L. Healing words: the power of prayer and the practice of medicine. New York: HarperSanFrancisco, 1993.

31. Walton J. Spiritual relationships: a concept analysis. Journal of Holistic Nursing 1996;14(3):237–250.

32. Dethlefsen T. Voices from other lives: reincarnation as a source of healing. New York: M. Evans/Lippincott, 1977.

33. Markides KC. Fire in the heart: healers, sages and mystics. London: Arkana/Penguin, 1991.

34. Motoyama H. Karma & reincarnation. London: Piatkus, 1992.

35. Norwood R. Why me? Why this? Why now? London: Century, 1994.

36. The Doctor-Healer Network Newsletter, 1993–4, Issue no. 4.

37. Brennan B. Light emerging. New York: Bantam, 1993.

38. Edwards H. Thirty years a spiritual healer. London: Herbert Jenkins, 1968.

39. Byrd RC. Positive therapeutic effects of intercessory prayer in a coronary care population. South Med J 1988;81(7):826–829.

40. Olson M, Sneed N, LaqVia M, et al. Stress-induced immunosuppression and therapeutic touch. Alternative Therapies 1997;3(2):68–74.

41. Olson M, Sneed N. Anxiety and therapeutic touch. Issues in Mental Health Nursing 1995;16:97–108.

42. Keller E, Bzdek VM. Effects of therapeutic touch on tension headache, pain. Nursing Research 1986; 2(1)101–104. (Keller: Unpublished M.A. Thesis, University of Missouri 1983).

43. Meehan TC. An abstract of the effect of therapeutic touch on the experience of acute pain in postoperative patients. Unpublished Ph.D. Thesis, New York University, 1985.

44. Meehan TC. Therapeutic touch and postoperative pain: a Rogerian research study. Nursing Science Quarterly 1993;6(2):69–78. (Doctoral dissertation, New York University, 1985.)

45. Meehan TC, Mersmann CA, Wiseman ME, et al. The effect of therapeutic touch on postoperative pain. Pain 1990;Suppl:149.

46. Wirth DP, Brenlan DR, Levine RJ, Rodriquez CM. et al. The effect of complementary healing therapy on postoperative pain after surgical removal of impacted third molar teeth. Complementary Therapies in Medicine 1993b;1:133–138.

47. Redner R, Briner B, Snellman L. Effects of a bioenergy healing technique on chronic pain. Subtle Energies 1991;2(3):43–68.

48. Braud W, Schlitz MA. Methodology for the objective study of transpersonal imagery. Journal of Scientific Exploration 1989;3(1):43–63.

49. Grad B, Cadoret RJ, Paul GK. The influence of an unorthodox, method of treatment on wound healing in mice. International Journal of Parapsychology 1961;3:5–24.

50. Grad BR. Some biological effects of laying-on of hands: a review of experiments with animals and plants. Journal of the American Society for Psychical Research 1965(a);59:95–127 (Also reproduced in Schmeidler G, ed. Parapsychology: its relation to physics, biology, psychology and psychiatry. Metuchen, NJ: Scarecrow, 1976).

51. Snel F, Hol PR. Psychokinesis experiments in casein induced amyloidosis of the hamster. European Journal of Parapsychology 1983;5(1):51–76.

52. Snel F, van der Sijde PC. Effects of paranormal healing on tumour growth. Journal of Scientific Exploration 1995;9(2):209–221.

53. Solfvin GF. Psi expectancy effects in psychic healing studies with malarial mice. European Journal of Parapsychology 1982(b);4(2):160–197.

54. Snel FWJJ, van der Sijde PC. The effect of retroactive distance healing on babesia rodhani (rodent malaria) in rats. European Journal of Parapsychology 1990–1991;8:123–130.

55. Solfvin GF. Psi expectancy effects in psychic healing studies with malarial mice. European Journal of Parapsychology 1982(b);4(2):160–197.

56. Barrington MR. Bean growth promotion pilot experiment. Proceedings of the Society for Psychical Research 1982;56:302–304.

57. Nicholas C. The effects of loving attention on plant growth. New England Journal of Parapsychology 1977;1:19–24.

58. Macdonald RG, Hickman JL, Dakin HS. Preliminary physical measurements of psychophysical effects associated with three alleged psychic healers. Research Brief, July 1, 1976. (Summary in Metuchen NJ. Research in Parapsychology. London: Scarecrow, 1977.)

59. Saklani A. Psi-ability in shamans of Garhwal Himalaya: preliminary tests. Journal of the Society for Psychical Research 1988;55(81):60–70.
60. Saklani A. Psychokinetic effects on plant growth: further studies. In: Henkel LA, Palmer J. Research in Parapsychology 1989;1990:37–41.
61. Scofield AM, Hodges DR. Demonstration of a healing effect in the laboratory using a simple plant model. Journal of the Society for Psychical Research 1991;57:321–343.
62. Nash CB. Psychokinetic control of bacterial growth. Journal of the Society for Psychical Research 1982;51:217–221.
63. Nash CB. Test of psychokinetic control of bacterial mutation. Journal of the American Society for Psychical Research 1984;78(2):145–152.
64. Barry J. General and comparative study of the psychokinetic effect on a fungus culture. Journal of Parapsychology 1968;32:237–243.
65. Cahn HA, Muscle N. Towards standardization of 'laying-on' of hands investigation. Psychoenergetic Systems 1976;1:115–118.
66. Haraldsson E, Thorsteinsson T. Psychoknetic effects on yeast: an exploratory experiment. In: Weiner DH, Radin DI, eds. Research in parapsychology. Metuchen, NJ and London: Scarecrow, 1973:20–21.
67. Tedder WH, Monty ML. Exploration of long-distance Pk: a conceptual replication of the influence on a biological system. In: Weiner DH, Radin DI, eds. Research in parapsychology. Metuchen, NJ and London: Scarecrow, 1981:90–92.
68. Edge H. The effect of laying on of hands on an enzyme: an attempted replication. In: Weiner DH, Radin DI, eds. Research in parapsychology. Metuchen, NJ and London: Scarecrow, 1980:137–139.
69. Rein G. An Exosomatic effect on neurotransmitter metabolism in mice: a pilot study. Second International Society for Parapsychological Research Conference. Cambridge, England, 1978.
70. Rein G. A psychokinetic effect of neurotransmitter metabolism: alterations in the degradative enzyme Monoamine Oxidase. In: Weiner DH, Radin DI, eds. Research in parapsychology. Metuchen, NJ and London: Scarecrow, 1986:77–80.
71. Brennan B. Hands of light. New York: Bantam, 1987.
72. Chopra D. Quantum healing: exploring the frontiers of mind/body medicine. London/New York: Bantam, 1989.
73. Gerber R. Vibrational medicine. Santa Fe, NM: Bear, 1988.
74. Brennan, Kunz D, van Gelder D. The personal aura. Wheaton, IL: Quest/Theosophical, 1991.
75. Benor DJ. Further comments on 'loading' and 'telesomatic reactions'. Advances 1996;12(2):71–75.
76. Benor DJ, Mohr M. The overlap of psychic 'readings' with psychotherapy. Psi Research 1986;5(1,2):56–78.
77. Dossey L. But is it energy? Reflections on consciousness, healing and the new paradigm. Subtle Energies 1992;3(3):69–82.
78. Dossey L. Healing words. HarperSanFrancisco, 1993:169–195.
79. Dossey L. Prayer is good medicine. HarperSanFrancisco, 1996.
80. Turner G. I treated plants, not patients (Part 2 of 4-Part Series). Two Worlds 1969;(Aug):232–234.
81. Dixon M. A healer in GP practice. The Doctor-Healer Network Newsletter 1994;7:6–7.
82. Benor DJ. Spiritual healing: a unifying influence in complementary therapies. Complementary Therapies in Medicine 1995;3(4):234–238.
83. Benor DJ, Benor R. Spiritual healing, assuming the spiritual is real. Advances 1993;9(4):22–30.
84. Goodrich J. The psychic healing training and research project. In: Fosshage J L, Olsen P. Healing: implications for psychotherapy. New York: Human Sciences, 1978:84–110.
85. LeShan L. The medium, the mystic and the physicist: toward a general theory of the paranormal. New York: Ballantine 1974(a);British edition: Clairvoyant reality. Wellingborough, England: Thorsons, 1974.

CHAPTER 22

MASSAGE THERAPY

Tiffany Field

BACKGROUND

Definition

The word *massage* has its origins in many languages, including the French word *masser* (literally meaning *to shampoo*), a Greek word that means *to knead,* a Hindu word that means *to press,* and an Arabic word that means *to press softly.* Massage is defined as the hand manipulation of body tissues to promote wellness and to reduce stress and pain. The therapeutic effects of massage are from its impact on the muscular, nervous, and circulation systems.

Massage therapy sessions usually combine several techniques, including Swedish massage (stroking and kneading), Shiatsu (pressure points), and neuromuscular massage (which generally involves pressure by the therapist in all areas of the body, not just tender pressure points) (1). Oils are typically used, and aromatic essences are often added for an additional effect. Massage sessions may also feature soft background music to enhance relaxation.

History and Review of Literature

The practice of massage has been used for thousands of years, before recorded time. The word *massage* can be found in many classic texts, including the Bible and the Vedas. As early as 400 BC, Hippocrates talked about the necessity for physicians to be experienced in rubbing. Ancient records from China and Japan refer to massage therapy. Massage was also widely used by other early cultures, including by Arabs, Egyptians, Indians, Greeks, and Romans. During the Renaissance, massage spread throughout Europe. Swedish massage was developed in the early nineteenth century by Henry Lind.

Key published works include volumes by M. Beck, *A Theory and Practice of Therapeutic Massage* (2); L.J. Chaitow, *Soft Tissue Manipulation* (3); T. Field, *Touch* (4); N. Hollis, *Massage for Therapists* (1); L. Lidell, *The Book of Massage: The Complete Step by Step Guide to Eastern, Western Techniques* (5); and C. Maxwell-Hudson, *A Complete Book of Massage* (6). Most of the books provide directions for performing various massage techniques, with accompanying photographs or drawings.

PRINCIPAL CONCEPTS

Many people in the field of massage therapy assume that the world is a stressful place, and that the stress experienced manifests in the body from tense muscles to unhealthy postures to disorganized physiology, all of which lead to sleep problems, mental illness, immune dysfunction, and other chronic diseases. Massage therapy is believed to alleviate these problems by reducing stress, improving depressed mood states, improving sleep, and reducing pain. Recently, discussions about massage therapy have centered on wellness and how massage therapy can be used to prevent many stress-related problems and illnesses. Aside from taking a physical and medical history, massage therapists are not involved in diagnosing clients. Generally, the client presents to the massage therapist's office with a diagnosis already made by a physician.

Therapeutically, massage is believed to affect all body systems, from circulation to metabolism. Massage therapists claim that massage improves the elasticity and tone of the skin, relaxes muscles, alleviates aches and pains in muscles and joints, facilitates respiration, enhances digestive processes, decreases blood pressure, and increases circulation of blood and lymph (1). Recently, based on research data, massage therapy was noted to enhance wellness by reducing stress hormones and, in turn, improving immune function (7).

PROVIDER–CLIENT INTERACTION

The optimal massage therapist–client interaction is brief and nonverbal. Aside from history-taking and inquiring about the patient's diagnosis or complaint, the therapist typically only needs to rule out contraindications and to request feedback from the clients as to how much pressure they prefer. Most therapists then discourage verbal interaction; it is not their specialty, and quiet massage sessions are often more relaxing.

Most types of massage feature standard techniques that can be presented as a package to most clients. Occasionally, therapists will need to shift from techniques that involve pressure (e.g., Swedish, Shiatsu) to nonpressure techniques (e.g., the Trager method, which involves moving the limbs). For example, if the patient has fibromyalgia (pain all over the body with an unknown etiology), massage techniques involving pressure may exacerbate the pain of the condition.

THERAPY AND OUTCOMES

Treatment Options

There are many options for massage therapy. There are different types of therapists, different types of massage, and different places to get massage therapy. The client makes all of these

decisions and, if unsatisfied, can make other choices. Most massage therapy practices are run by trained massage therapists, physical therapists, and nurses who offer massage therapy (now called nurse massage therapists). Typically, people go to a therapist who has been recommended and who practices the client's technique of choice. Determining the technique of choice is probably best done by simply trying a massage in various techniques. Research will also help document the specific techniques that are effective for the client's specific condition.

Many practitioners work out of private clinics; some have treatment rooms in their own homes. Massage therapists may also work in spas, athletic clubs, hair salons, hotels, airports, and even at car washes in some cities. Finally, massage therapists are often hired to come to a client's home with a portable table or chair. Massage therapy used to be practiced routinely in hospitals (as recently as the 1950s); unfortunately, it is rarely seen in hospitals today.

Types of Massage Techniques

Treatment options include choosing the type of massage (e.g., Swedish or Shiatsu); typically, several techniques are combined. Many techniques are similar and involve stroking, kneading, stretching, and relaxation. Generally, the client has some choice about the type of music used during the session and the type of aroma to be added to the massage oil. In some wellness centers and commercial programs—The Great American Backrub in New York and Unwind in Miami—clients can choose between table massage, which typically involves removing clothing and applying oils, or chair massage, which can be done without removing clothing.

Swedish Massage

There are five basic techniques in Swedish massage:

1. **Effleurage** is stroking, which can be superficial or deep and of varying pressure. Deep stroking is usually done in a direction toward the heart, reputedly to help circulation; a more superficial stroking is done on the return motion away from the heart.

2. **Petrissage** is a kneading motion in a circular pattern using the fingers and thumbs. It is intended to stimulate the muscle tissue and the deeper circulation of the limbs as well as venous flow, which is made possible by its vigorous movement.

3. **Friction** involves deeper muscle stimulation by using rolling, ringing, and compression movements. The therapist uses the palm or the heel of the hand and sometimes even the elbow and forearm to accomplish these movements. A variation of this technique is practiced in China. The therapist is suspended from a bar above the client, enabling him or her to use his or her feet for these friction movements.

4. **Tapotement** is percussion that involves rhythmic movements, such as slapping, beating, and tapping in a quick vigorous fashion. It is designed to stimulate deeper muscles.

5. **Vibration** is accomplished by the therapist's hands or an electric vibrator to facilitate relaxation.

Swedish massage techniques are typically found in spas, hotels, and athletic clubs. Swedish massage is usually performed with the client on a massage table, on the floor, or on a chair. Typically, baby oil, vegetable oil, or an aromatic natural oil is used. These oils are stroked and kneaded on all parts of the body. The various movements (e.g., effleurage, petrissage) are done up and down the back, and across the shoulder and neck muscles, the backs of the legs, feet, arms, and hands. Stroking on the front of the client is done across the stomach, the front of the legs and arms, and the face and forehead. Therapists will generally inquire if there is a body part the client prefers is not touched; that part as well as the private parts are covered, typically with a towel or sheet, at all times.

ACUPRESSURE (SHIATSU)

Acupressure, or Shiatsu (*shi* for finger, *atsu* for pressure), is a prolonged and heavy pressure that is often combined with Swedish massage. Usually the therapist uses only the balls of his or her thumbs and occasionally the palms or the elbows. The therapist's movements follow a diagram of key pressure points called *tsubos*. These points are reputedly located along meridians in which the energy flows. *Yang* meridians flow down the body from head to foot; *ying* meridians flow up the body from the feet to the head. The therapist reputedly makes an assessment to determine if the client has more ying or yang, and then applies pressure along the opposite meridian as indicated (e.g., the yang meridian if the client has more ying).

Various mechanisms have been described for the Shiatsu effect, including an increase in vagal activity (the slowing of the heart caused by the vagus nerve), which also slows circulation and relaxes the patient. Others say that stress and muscle spasms are reduced by the increase in glucose released in the body (1).

NEUROMUSCULAR MASSAGE

In neuromuscular massage, the therapist applies even more pressure than in the other types of massage. Neuromuscular massage is intended to reach the deeper connective tissues, tendons, ligaments, and nerves. The therapist typically performs this technique using the pads of his or her thumbs, fingers, or both. This technique requires greater strength on the part of the therapist.

Treatment Evaluation

Based on existing research, clients normally show immediate effects, including improved mood state and affect and decreased anxiety and stress hormone levels (e.g., salivary cortisol). These effects have been highly significant and based on observations of the client, self-reports by the client, and saliva assays of cortisol. In addition, changes in EEG recorded before and after the session suggest increased alertness (8). Longer-term changes have also been evaluated after 4 to 6 weeks of treatment. These changes include a decrease in depression; improved sleep patterns; lower stress, as measured by urinary cortisol, norepinephrine, and epinephrine levels (9); and enhanced immune function (e.g., an increase in natural killer cells) (7).

The effects of massage have also been noted

on clinical measures that are specific to different conditions or considered by clinicians to be good measures of improved clinical condition. For example, increases in pulmonary function, including peak airflow, have been noted in children with asthma (10), and decreased blood glucose levels have been reported in children with diabetes after a month of massage (11). Another example is significant weight gain in premature infants who are given 10 days of massage (12). These changes are unique to the given conditions and are not expected to occur generally across medical conditions.

Many of these noted changes are reported in research that compares treatment and control groups or that compares massage with other forms of treatment. Massage therapists are more likely to assess treatment effects based on the presence or absence of various obvious symptoms or from the client's reporting a decrease in symptoms. Currently, massage therapists are not collecting physiological or biochemical measures, although they are being encouraged to do so. Usually therapists alter their treatment if there is no therapeutic effect. However, usually the client elects to discontinue the treatment or seek treatment elsewhere if desired changes do not occur, unless the client feels the treatment was indicated just for making him- or herself feel better.

USE OF THE SYSTEM FOR TREATMENT

Major Indications

The primary indications of massage therapy are for wellness and stress and pain reduction. However, there are many other ways in which massage therapy is clinically useful.

PAIN REDUCTION

Pregnancy and Labor

In many countries, such as India, pregnant women are massaged several times daily for relaxation and to reduce their anxiety levels (13). This therapy is considered beneficial for both the woman and her fetus. We have been teaching the partners of pregnant women to massage the women during pregnancy and labor (14). Ultrasound images taken after the massages show positive responses from the fetus. Most of them "like the massage," as is seen by their smiles on ultrasound. When we coded fetal movements, we found a normalization of activity level. This may be associated with reduced anxiety and depression in the mothers.

Burn Patients

Debridement (i.e., skin brushing) is an extremely painful medical procedure used for severe burn patients. Patients usually have significant anxiety in anticipation of the pain. Massage therapy is being used to reduce anticipatory anxiety before debridement and to indirectly alleviate pain during the procedure. Following a 5-day, 30-minute treatment before debridement, burn patients experienced lower anxiety and an associated decrease in cortisol levels (15). Pain had also decreased by the fifth day of massage treatment, as had depression (probably because of the decrease in pain). Postburn patients, who experience not only pain but itching, reported a decrease in both (15).

Chronic Pain: Fibromyalgia

In a study on fibromyalgia syndrome, subjects were randomly assigned to one of three therapies—massage therapy, transcutaneous electrical stimulation (TENS), or transcutaneous electrical stimulation with no current (SHAM TENS)—for 30-minute treatment sessions, twice weekly for 5 weeks (16). The subjects receiving massage therapy reported lower anxiety and depression, and their cortisol levels were lower immediately after the therapy sessions on the first and last days of the study. The TENS subjects showed similar changes, but only after therapy on the last day of the study. The massage therapy group improved on a dolorimeter measure of pain, and they reported less pain, less stiffness and fatigue, and fewer nights of difficult sleeping. Thus, massage therapy was the most effective therapy with these fibromyalgia patients.

MODELS FOR UNDERLYING MECHANISMS OF TOUCH AND PAIN RELIEF

Pain alleviation has most frequently been attributed to the "gate theory" (17). This theory suggests that pain can be alleviated by pressure or cold temperature because pain fibers are shorter and less myelinated than are pressure and cold temperature receptors. The pressure or cold temperature stimuli are received before the pain stimulus, the "gate" to the brain is closed, and thus the pain stimulus is not received.

Another potential theory for pain alleviation through massage therapy relates to quiet (restorative) sleep deprivation. There seems to be a connection between quiet sleep deprivation and pain. During quiet sleep, somatostatin is normally released. In the absence of quiet sleep, somatostatin is not released and pain is experienced. Also, substance P, which is notable for causing pain, is released in the absence of restorative sleep. One of the leading theories for the pain associated with fibromyalgia syndrome is the production of substance P because of restorative sleep deprivation (16). With this in mind, it is interesting that the subjects in a fibromyalgia syndrome study experienced more quiet sleep and less pain following the massage therapy treatment period (16).

ALLEVIATING DEPRESSION AND ANXIETY

Bulimia in Adolescents

Adolescents with the eating disorder bulimia (overeating and self-induced vomiting) also experience severe depression. After 1 month of massage, bulimic adolescents had fewer depressive symptoms, lower anxiety levels, and lower urinary cortisol levels (18). Their eating habits also improved, and they had a less distorted body image in the short term; long-term effects need to be assessed in a follow-up study.

Chronic Fatigue Syndrome

In one study, chronic fatigue syndrome subjects who had high scores on the Beck Depression Inventory were randomly assigned either to a massage therapy or to a SHAM TENS control group (19). On the first and last days of the study, the massage therapy group had lower depression and anxiety scores and lower salivary cortisol levels than did the SHAM TENS group. Longer-term effects (last day versus first day) indicated that the massage therapy group had lower depression, fewer somatic symptoms, more hours of sleep, lower urinary cortisol levels, and elevated urinary dopamine levels than did the SHAM TENS group.

STRESS REDUCTION

Job Stress

In a job-stress study, medical school staff and faculty were give a 15-minute massage during their lunch periods in massage chairs in their offices (8). These sessions involved the massage therapist applying deep pressure in the back, shoulders, neck, and head regions. Rather than being more sleepy than usual after their midday massage, the subjects reported that they experienced heightened alertness, similar to a "runner's high." EEG recordings before, during, and after the massage sessions showed that alpha waves significantly decreased during massage, which is in contrast to the significant increase in alpha levels that occurs during relaxation and sleep. This decrease in alpha waves, combined with increased theta and decreased beta waves, suggested a pattern of heightened alertness. A math computation task showed that computation time was significantly reduced and the computation accuracy increased following the massages, suggesting that 15-minute massages during the lunch period enhance alertness and cognitive performance.

"Grandparent" Volunteers Massaging Infants

Elderly people are noted to suffer from touch deprivation. In an attempt to decrease this situation, volunteer "grandparents" were recruited to massage abused infants (20). The grandparents also benefited from giving the massages. Their depressed mood decreased following a 1-month period of massaging the infants; they also experienced increased self-esteem and decreased cortisol levels. The effects these volunteers experienced from *giving* massage were compared with the effects they experienced when *receiving* massage themselves. In a counterbalanced design, these volunteers gave infants massages for 1 month and then received massages for 1 month. The volunteers benefited more from giving the massage than from receiving the massage. Their affect and self-esteem improved, as did their lifestyle habits: they reported drinking fewer cups of coffee daily, they made more social phone calls, and they made fewer trips to the doctor's office.

MODELS UNDERLYING TOUCH ALLEVIATING STRESS AND DEPRESSION

In all of the above studies, the participants' depressed mood was decreased and anxiety levels and stress hormones (e.g., norepinephrine, epinephrine, cortisol) were reduced. One potential mechanism is suggested by a recent study measuring frontal EEG activation following massage in depressed adolescents (21). The individual's shift to a more positive mood is notably accompanied by shifts from right frontal EEG activation (normally associated with sad affect) to left frontal EEG activation (normally associated with happy affect) or at least to symmetry (midway between sad and happy affect). In this study on depressed adolescent mothers and their infants, right frontal EEG activation (noted in chronically depressed adults and also observed in the depressed mothers and infants in our study) was shifted towards symmetry following a 20-minute massage (21). The many chemical and electrophysiological changes previously discussed may underlie the decrease in depression noted following massage therapy.

An associated potential mechanism may be the increase noted in vagal activity following massage therapy. The nucleus ambiguous branch of the vagus (i.e., the "smart" vagus) stimulates facial expressions and vocalizations, which could contribute to less depressed affect and in turn could feedback to effect less depressed feelings.

IMMUNE DISORDER: HIV-POSITIVE ADULTS

In a study on HIV-positive adults, natural killer cells and natural killer cell cytotoxicity increased following 20 days of massage (7). Twenty-nine gay men, 20 of whom were HIV-positive and 9 of whom were HIV-negative, were massaged for 1 month; 11 of the HIV-positive men served as their own controls by being compared when they were receiving versus not receiving massage. Major immune findings for the effect of the month of massage included a significant increase in the number of natural killer cells, natural killer cell cytotoxicity, and subsets of CD8 cells. There was no change in HIV disease progression markers (i.e., CD4; CD4 to CD8 ratios), possibly because the HIV-positive men were already severely immunocompromised. Major neuroendocrine findings, measured via 24-hour urines, included a significant decrease in cortisol and nonsignificant trends showing decreased catecholamines. Significant decreases in anxiety and increases in relaxation were significantly correlated with increases in the number of natural killer cells. Elevated stress hormones (e.g., catecholamines, cortisol) are noted to negatively affect immune function. The increase in cytotoxic capacity associated with massage therapy probably derives from the decrease in these stress hormones following massage therapy.

OTHER INDICATIONS

Massage has demonstrated effects on a number of other conditions that physicians and other health care practitioners may want to consider. These include use in the intensive care unit for stress and pain management (22); prevention of perineal trauma during childbirth (23); pressure ulcers (24); low back pain (25); muscle soreness from exercise (26, 27, 28, 29); cancer pain (30); and to improve maternal–infant bonding (31).

These are some areas of improved function noted following massage therapy. In addition to each clinical condition being marked by unique changes, there was also a set of common findings. Across most of the studies, decreases were noted in anxiety, depression, and stress hormones (cortisol and catecholamines). Increased parasympathetic activity may be the underlying mechanism for these changes. The pressure stimulation associated with touch increases vagal activity, which in turn lowers physiological arousal and stress hormones (cortisol levels).

The amount of pressure is critical because light stroking is generally aversive, much like a tickle stimulus. Decreased cortisol levels lead to enhanced immune function. Parasympathetic activity is also associated with increased alertness and better performance on cognitive tasks. Given that most diseases are exacerbated by stress and given that massage therapy alleviates stress, receiving massages should probably be ranked with diet and exercise on any list of health priorities, as it was in India around 1800 BC.

Major Contraindications

Some massage therapists have warned of contraindications for massage (1). There is little research examining particular contraindications. These contraindications include the following:

1. **Infectious or contagious skin conditions.** There is concern that massage may spread the infection from the infected area to other parts of the body as well as to the therapist.
2. **High fever.** Massage therapy may further increase body temperature.
3. **Scar tissue, open wounds, and burn areas.** Massaging is contraindicated with new wounds because the healing tissue is fragile. This might be qualified by the recency of the scar tissue because burn areas can benefit from massaging with cocoa butter to reduce itching.
4. **Varicose veins or phlebitis.** There is the possibility that a dislodged blood clot might result in pulmonary embolus, but no systematic research or case reports have examined this.
5. **Tumors and infected lymph nodes.** Massage therapy may cause metastases by loosening cells from tumors. It is advisable not to directly massage a tumor, although it is unlikely that massage would cause cells to break off any more than they would from daily exercise. However, most cancer treatments contribute to skin sensitivity, and patients receiving chemotherapy often feel too sick to be touched.
6. **Low platelet count.** Rigorous massage may cause bruising.

ORGANIZATION AND TRAINING

Currently, there is considerable variability from school to school regarding training standards and from state to state regarding licensing standards. Training requirements vary—from providing specialized training as a certification program for already-licensed professionals (e.g., nurses) to extensive programs designed to be professional degrees. Some states have extensive licensing requirements, whereas other state legislatures have been lobbied by professional groups to prevent the licensure of massage therapists. National organizations do not agree on standards: some suggest licensing is a minimal standard and others suggest not requiring licensure. Although massage therapy has been practiced since before recorded time, the standards and professional activities of the field are in their infancy and need further development. See Chapter 2 for states that license massage therapists.

PROSPECTS FOR THE FUTURE

Massage therapy appears to have common positive effects on many clinical conditions. These effects seem to involve facilitating parasympathetic activity, leading to more organized physiology, lower stress hormones, and enhanced immune function. In addition, increased parasympathetic activity enables greater alertness and improved cognitive performance. Finally, measures of several clinical conditions appear to be affected; for example, reduced glucose levels in diabetes and improved pulmonary function in asthma. These changes may also result from increased parasympathetic activity and reduced stress hormones.

Further research is needed not only for replication purposes, but also for investigation of associated disease processes. In addition, research is needed on those conditions massage therapists have cautiously labeled contraindications. Finally, cost-benefit analyses are needed to help justify further support for research and efforts to convince insurance companies and health maintenance organizations that massage therapy should be covered. An example of the cost-effectiveness of massage therapy taken from our research is that $4.7 billion in medical costs could be saved yearly if all prematurely born infants were massaged. That figure was derived from 470,000 infants born prematurely each year being massaged and discharged 6 days early (as they were in a study [32] at a hospital cost savings of $10,000 per infant). Further, the massage program could be offered by senior citizen volunteers, who would also benefit both health- and cost-wise. In the study in which we used senior citizen volunteers as the massage therapists for the infants, the senior citizen therapists had lower stress hormones and fewer trips to the doctor's office following 1 month of massaging infants (20). Similar cost-effectiveness figures are likely to emerge for other conditions because they too benefit significantly from the stress reduction effects of massage therapy.

The token level of research funding currently provided by the massage therapy professional societies and the federal government will not support adequately designed research protocols. Until respectable funding levels are achieved for the field of massage therapy, it will remain alternative. Tremendous potential exists for massage therapy, however, and realization of this potential will contribute to improved health and reduced costs for many.

REFERENCES

1. Hollis N. Massage for therapists. Oxford: Blackwell, 1987.
2. Beck M. The theory and practice of therapeutic massage. New York: Milady, 1988.
3. Chaitow LJ. Soft tissue manipulation. Wellingborough: Thorsons, 1988.
4. Field T. Touch in early development. Hillsdale, NJ: Lawrence Erlbaum Associates, 1995.
5. Lidell L. The book of massage: the complete step by step guide to eastern, western techniques. London: Ebury, 1984.
6. Maxwell-Hudson C. A complete book of massage. London: Doiling-Kindersley, 1988.
7. Ironson G, Field T, Scafidi F, et al. Massage therapy is associated with enhancement of the immune systems cytotoxic capacity. Int J Neurosci 1996;84: 205–218.
8. Field T, Ironson G, Pickens J, et al. Massage therapy reduces anxiety and enhances EEG pattern of alertness and math computations. Int J Neurosci 1996;86:197–205.
9. Field T, Morrow C, Valdeon C, et al. Massage reduces anxiety in child and adolescent psychiatric patients. J Am Acad Child Adolesc Psychiatry 1992;31:124–131.
10. Field T, Henteleff T, Hernandez-Reif M, et al. Children with asthma have improved pulmonary function after massage therapy. J Pediatr 1998;132:854–858.
11. Field T, Hernandez-Reif M, LaGreca A, et al. Glucose levels decreased after giving massage therapy to children with diabetes mellitus. Spectrum 1997;10:23–25.
12. Field T, Schanberg SM, Scafidi F, et al. Tactile/kinesthetic stimulation effects on preterm neonates. Pediatrics 1986;77:654–658.
13. Older J. Touching is healing. New York: Stein and Day, 1982:86.
14. Field T, Hernandez-Reif M, Taylor S, et al. Labor pain is reduced by massage therapy. J Psychosom Obstet Gynecol 1997;18:286–291.
15. Field T, Peck M, Krugman S, et al. Massage therapy effects on burn patients. J Burn Care Rehabilitation 1998;19:241–244.
16. Sunshine W, Field T, Schanberg S, et al. Massage therapy and transcutaneous electrical stimulation effects on fibromyalgia. J Clin Rheumatol 1996; 2:18–22.
17. Melzack R, Wall PD. Pain mechanisms: a new theory. Science 1965;150:971–978.
18. Field T, Schanberg S, Kuhn C, et al. Bulimic adolescents benefit from massage therapy. Adolescence 1998. In press.
19. Field T, Sunshine W, Hernandez-Reif M, et al. Chronic fatigue syndrome: massage therapy effects on depression and somatic symptoms in chronic fatigue syndrome. J Chronic Fat Syn 1997; 3:43–51.
20. Field T, Hernandez-Reif M, Quintino O, et al. Elder retired volunteers benefit from giving massage therapy to infants. J Appl Gerontol 1998; 17:229–239.
21. Jones N, Field T, Davalos M. Massage attenuates right frontal EEG assymetry in one-month-old infants of depressed mothers. Infant Beh Devel 1998 (in press).
22. Dunn C, Sleep J, Collett D. Sensing an improvement: an experimental study to evaluate the use of aromatherapy, massage, and periods of rest in an intensive care unit. J Adv Nurs 1995;21:34–40.

23. Labrecque M, Marcoux S, Pinault JJ, et al. Prevention of perineal trauma by perineal massage during pregnancy: a pilot study. Birth 1994;21:20–25.

24. Olson B. Effects of massage for prevention of pressure ulcers. Decubitus 1989;2:32–37.

25. Pope MH, Phillips RB, Haugh LD, et al. A prospective randomized three-week trial of spinal manipulation, transcutaneous muscle stimulation, massage and corset in the treatment of subacute low back pain. Spine 1994;19:2571–2577.

26. Rodenburg JB, Steenbeek D, Schiereck P, et al. Warm-up, stretching and massage diminish harmful effects of eccentric exercise. Int J Sports Med 1994;15:414–419.

27. Smith LL, Keating MN, Holbert D, et al. The effects of athletic massage on delayed onset muscle soreness, creatine kinase, and neutrophil count: a preliminary report. J Orthop Sports Phys Ther 1994;19:93–99.

28. Viitasalo JT, Niemela K, Kaappola R, et al. Warm underwater water-jet massage improves recovery from intense physical exercise. Eur J Appl Physiol 1995;71:431–438.

29. Weber MD, Servedio FJ, Woodall WR. The effects of three modalities on delayed onset muscle soreness. J Orthop Sports Phys Ther 1994;20:236–242.

30. Weinrich SP, Weinrich MC. The effect of massage on pain in cancer patients. Appl Nurs Res 1990; 3:140–145.

31. White-Traut RC, Nelson MN. Maternally administered tactile, auditory, visual, and vestibular stimulation: relationship to later interactions between mothers and premature infants. Res Nurs Health 1988;11:31–39.

32. Field T, Schanberg S, Cafidi F, et al. Tactile/kinesthetic stimulation effects on preterm neonates. Pediatrics 1986;77:654–658.

CHAPTER 23

QIGONG

Ching-Tse Lee and Ting Lei

"With Regard to Chi Circulation: If it is deep, it is stored; if it is stored, it is extended; if it is extended, it can move downward; if it moves downward, it can be fixed; if it is fixed, it can be consolidated; if it is consolidated, it can sprout."

—From an ancient script carved on a jade ornament more than 2000 years ago

BACKGROUND

Definition

Qigong is a major branch of Traditional Chinese medicine (TCM). It is a generic term used to denote methods used to cultivate, regulate, and harness *chi* (vital energy) for general self-preservation and health, healing, self-defense, longevity, and, particularly, spiritual development. *Chi* means vital energy and *gong* means function, or work; thus, *qigong* literally means the function of *chi*. The theoretical background of qigong is deeply rooted in classical Chinese cosmology, which views the human being as a microcosmic energy system synergistically embedded in the macrocosm (e.g., the ecological environment). These micro- and macrocosms constitute a unified energy field, and energy is constantly interchanged between them based on the operational principle of homeostasis. From TCM's point of view, how to maintain *chi* homeostasis is the *modus vivendi* for health, and how to attain it at a higher level is the *modus operandi* of healing.

As far as healing is concerned, beneficial effects can be achieved by the following:

1. Applying the *extrinsic chi* (the vital energy transmitted from other people) and/or infusing healers' *intrinsic chi* (the vital energy generated by the practitioner) to restore the patient's energy to a healthy state.
2. Performing movement-oriented qigong to direct and speed up intrinsic *chi* flow through the ailed areas.
3. Mobilizing the power of the mind (intention/imagination/visualization) to move internal *chi* through the blocked areas.
4. Practicing meditation to allow the energy to perform its natural health and healing function.

Dynamic and meditative qigong exercises that generate and preserve energy also strengthen the body, mind, and spirit and prevent diseases (1). For health or healing, qigong is holistic by engaging mind, body, and spirit in *chi* cultivation. As such, qigong exercises are neither merely body movements nor relaxation responses per se. Rather, an altered state of consciousness and an action consciousness may be aroused while performing meditative-oriented and movement-oriented qigong exercises, respectively. Given the human organism as a homeostatic system, these two forms of consciousness provide feedback for self-regulation (2). Furthermore, qigong operating on the spiritual dimension entails transcendental consciousness that engages the practitioner to interact with the environment at a higher level, which may facilitate the healing process (3).

History and Development

An archaeological finding of a porcelain vase with a drawing of a human figure holding a seemingly meditative qigong posture shows that qigong was performed approximately 5000 years ago. The word *chi* first appeared in inscriptions carved on bones and tortoise shells that have been dated back three millennia. Although we now realize the effects of ecological factors on health and illness, the basic understanding of the etiology of human illness during this period was shamanic in nature.

The theoretic foundations of currently practiced TCM are primarily based on *The Yellow Emperor's Classic of Internal Medicine,* which made sketchy references to qigong healing (4). The excavation of the tomb (*Mawangtui,* Chinese for a feudal king's graveyard) of an officer from the first century BC provided the missing link of this important branch of Chinese healing arts. Among the excavated materials most pertinent to health and healing are scrolls of 44 drawings of qigong postures, with short commentaries and a collection of medical texts that preceded similar material found in *The Yellow Emperor's Classic of Internal Medicine* (5). The *chi* and meridian theories recorded in these texts are basically the same as those of contemporary TCM. Detailed analyses of these materials indicate that qigong was an integral part of the healing arts at that time. The drawings found in this tomb are the most comprehensive documents of the ancient qigong exercises ever recovered.

These ancient exercises can be divided into three categories. The first group, designed for health promotion, included some animal forms, such as the bear, bird, and monkey. The second group depicted breathing exercises to use extrinsic energy for health and healing purposes. The third group included movement forms specifically designed for healing. Patients performed these exercises to guide and facilitate *chi* circulation in various parts of the body, thereby eliminating pains and ameliorating disease.

The development of the qigong healing arts in TCM history followed two major paths. The first path refers to the tradition of self-healing style of qigong (SHQ, or internal gigong), including movement-oriented qigong, meditation-oriented qigong, and breathing exercise-oriented qigong. The second path, which refers to healing provided by qigong practitioners (external qigong), arrived during the modern era. The development of these two branches of qigong is described briefly in the following subsections.

SELF-HEALING STYLE OF QIGONG

Movement-Oriented Qigong

This form of qigong first appeared as simple body movements performed by individuals to facilitate energy circulation and healing. It gradually evolved into dancelike sequences of qigong movements, such as Tai *chi* chuan (6), wild goose (7), and soaring crane qigong (8). These gentle, supple, and slow movements channel energy through the blocked and stagnated areas, thus eliminating discomfort in the affected areas and restoring the normal physiological functions.

Meditation-Oriented Qigong

In contrast to movement-oriented qigong, meditation-oriented qigong stresses inner serenity, control of one's own microcosmic energy, and a connection with the macrocosmic energy system. This modality is performed in a sitting, standing, or sleeping position. Body movement is kept to a minimum so that it does not disrupt the working of the mind. The major emphasis of this modality is to restore the homeostasis of the energy system through harmonizing *yin* and *yang* energy, clearing the obstruction in energy circulation, and obtaining an optimal amount of energy through meditation. The theoretical foundation of this practice can be traced back to I-Ching and Lao-tzu (9), both of which referred to *chi*. Meditative qigong is implied in some of the passages of these works. Following the path of Lao-tzu, Chuan-tzu expanded the delineation of *chi* to include the *chi* generated by breathing. In so doing, references were made to breathing qigong exercises as well as to meditation, relaxation techniques, and massage.

The curative effects of meditation qigong became known in modern China after Chiang (10) published a book describing his own experiences with meditation. Chiang claimed to have completely cured himself of tuberculosis and of the related internal hemorrhage with meditation. He experienced energy circulation in both the governing meridian and conception meridian, which are located in the midline of the front and the back of the body—the so-called microcosmic orbit circulation.

Breathing-Oriented Qigong

Because fresh air has long been considered a source of vital energy, breathing exercises were designed to increase energy levels, strengthen various vital organs, and expel the sick *chi*. Breathing exercises were practiced by ancient sages. For the purpose of strengthening and invigorating energy, one should practice daily breathing exercises, preferably in the morning hours. For healing purposes, the overnight stagnated *chi* should be intentionally exhaled in a prolonged manner to expel the sick *chi*, and then the morning fresh air should be wholeheartedly inhaled and stored in the body. This should be done several times a day and for as long as it takes to store sufficient energy in the body. Then, and only then, can the individual attempt to use his or her *intention* to move the stored energy to attack the illness.

The practice of breathing-oriented qigong clearly marks the birth of mind–body medicine. Master Huang-zhen of the Tang dynasty (11) was credited as the inventor of this method. During the same time period, Sung integrated breathing exercises with vocalization and created what is now known as the six-word method, which entails the production of the

following six sounds—*shu, kir, su, tzua, fou,* and *shie*—a combination that is thought to ameliorate disease of the liver, heart, lung, kidney, spleen, and triple burner, respectively. *Triple burner* is a TCM term describing the three sections of the body: the upper burner (chest), the middle burner (stomach area), and the lower burner (lower abdomen). This method, and a modified version of it, are still being practiced today (12).

PRINCIPAL CONCEPTS

Assumption about Nature and Mankind

The theoretic foundation of qigong is representative of TCM. It postulates that human beings, aside from having a concrete and observable physical body, also possess a subtle microcosmic energy system that synergistically connects with the macrocosmic system. *Chi* constantly flows through the meridian system in a balanced mode. Within a human being's subtle energy system, a myriad of *chi* unceasingly flows through the body via a complex matrix of networks called meridians, which are set in a predetermined circadian sequence and homeostatic pattern (13–15). *Chi* functions to protect the individual from pathogens; nourish the body through the conversion of nutrient substances; activate physiological activities, including all internal and external movements; retain all body substances; and eliminate biological waste products. Disturbances of this energetic system may lead to deviation from homeostasis, which results in physiological and mental dysfunction, deterioration of health, and eventually disease.

If the disturbed condition persists, illness may ensue. According to the model just described, *chi* disturbance is the beginning of the unfolding of an illness (Fig. 23.1). The appearance of physical signs of discomfort marks the second stage of disease development. Qigong diagnosis of energy disturbances allows the condition to be corrected at the beginning of disease development, thus preventing the unfolding of the disorder. Because the detection of energy imbalance requires training and awareness of *chi*, diagnostic methods have been developed to

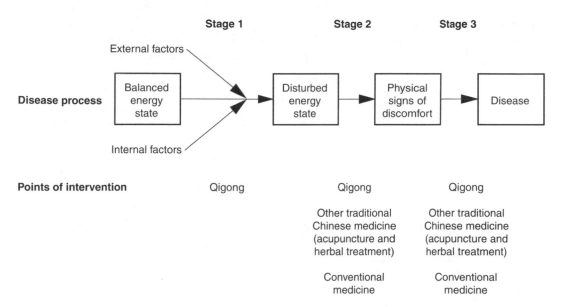

FIGURE 23.1. Development of disease and points of intervention.

allow the healer to make inferences from the energy system's conditions. TCM physicians have developed methods, such as acupuncture, moxibustion, and complex herbal prescriptions, to restore the subtle energy system for healing and health purposes. These approaches are described in Chapter 12, "Traditional Chinese Medicine." They are designed to treat the illness at the second stage of its development, that is, at the appearance of signs and symptoms. In general, this is the stage at which conventional medicine is most effective in treating disease. The advances of medical science in understanding pathophysiological and biochemical mechanisms, inventing fine-grained technology for diagnosis, and developing pharmaceutical agents account for the efficacy of the Western approach at this stage.

Pathogenesis and Etiology

According to TCM theory, the causes of illness are generally attributed to both external and internal factors. External climatic factors, such as wind, cold, heat, moisture (dampness), dryness, and heat (fire), are able to cause imbalances in the energy and meridian systems and thereby interrupt normal physiological functions, which results in ailments. Furthermore, it is hypothesized that wind, heat (fire), moisture (damp-

ness), dryness, and coldness can affect the energy and function of the liver, heart, spleen, lung, and kidney, respectively. When these organs are affected, the color of the skin, face, and tongue may turn yellow, red, green, white, and gray, which indicates the corresponding malfunction of liver, heart, spleen, lung, and kidney. Injuries, poison, parasites, and plagues are also recognized as external etiological factors.

Two groups of internal factors can affect the energy balance. The first group relates to emotional imbalance, which is also recognized by psychosomatic medicine as an important factor in affecting health. Acute emotional outbursts and chronic states of anger, joy, worry, sadness, and fear may affect the meridian system and disturb the function of the liver, heart, spleen, lung, and kidney, respectively. The second group relates to an abnormal lifestyle, such as excessive eating and drinking, overwork or exhaustion, and a sedentary style of living (boredom, inactivity, and sometimes depression).

Chi imbalances caused by external and internal factors may affect the body on three levels:

1. Superficial level (skin, hair, and muscle).
2. Meridian level.
3. The internal organs deep inside the body.

For example, with chronic exposure to wind, a person may first develop superficially sensitive skin and muscle, then subsequent diseases of the internal organs, such as liver and kidney dysfunction. Chronic elevated anger state (e.g., Type A personality) may result in changing of facial color from normal to red; disturbances of the heart meridian; and illness associated with the heart meridian, such as hypertension and heart disease.

Diagnosis

One of the unique features of qigong healing is that the qigong health provider can use his or her trained and expanded awareness directly to detect energy imbalance. Energy disturbances can be diagnosed with the hand, qigong meridian examination method, visual or mental inspection, or a combination of these methods. Most qigong healers tend to use the first two methods for diagnostic purposes. To perform hand diagnosis, the diagnostician brings his or her hand close to the patient's body and scans the patient's energy field. A normal variation of energy distribution, activity level, and other energy characteristics in healthy individuals may be noticed.

With this information, the diagnostician proceeds to pinpoint the manifestation of en-

ergy disturbances on the meridian and organ systems with the qigong meridian acupressure method and other physical examination techniques. Complementary to this direct detection of energy disturbances are the well-developed TCM diagnostic methods, which rely on ordinary human behavior sensation, perception, and cognition to diagnose and infer energy disturbances. Visual inspection, questioning, listening (smelling), and palpation are used to collect physical and behavioral signs of discomforts and abnormalities. The diagnostic results are categorized into four dialectic patterns, which are comprised of eight bipolar factors (Table 23.1). These four patterns are *yin/yang*, fullness/emptiness, hot/cold, and interior/exterior. Metaphorically speaking, at the physiological level, *yin/yang* is analogous to the parasympathetic/sympathetic dyad. At the neural level, this pattern is analogous to the inhibition/excitation relationship. Fullness/emptiness represents excess or deficient energy. Cold/hot represents the thermal properties of the various human physiques. Interior/exterior demonstrates the peripheral, or core, components of the human body. Under normal circumstances, the energy system maintains a harmonious *yin/yang*, fullness/emptiness, and hot/cold relationship

Table 23.1. Patterns of Illness	
Yang	Agitated, restless, active, hot body, red face, yellow tongue, rough voice, talkative, coarse breathing, dry mouth, thirsty, likes cold drinks, constipated, strong and slippery pulse, putrid odor
Yin	Quiet, withdrawn, slow, weak, tired, pale face and tongue, low and weak voice, shallow breathing, acid odor, loss of appetite, likes warmth and touch, dislikes cold, cold limbs, empty and weak pulse
Fullness	Hot body, red face, loud voice, heavy breathing, dislikes cold, irritable, excessive phlegm, stomach distention, constipation, red face and eyes, thick tongue, strong pulse
Emptiness	Physically weak, lean, chronically ill, tired, depressed, shallow and slow breathing, loss of appetite, frequent perspiration, urinary incontinence, weak movement of bowels, weak and thin pulse
Hot	Agitated, red face and eyes, yellow tongue, feverish and sweating, thirsty, likes cold drinks, red urine, dry stool, strong and rapid pulse
Cold	Dislikes cold, likes warmth and hot drinks, pale face, purple or green tongue, cold hands and feet, not thirsty, clear phlegm, clear urinary output, scanty and watery stool, slow and/ or tight pulse
Exterior	Fever, dislikes cold wind, headaches, neck and body aches, weak limb and joint pain, sweating, running nose, coughing and sneezing
Interior	Thirsty, chest pain, vomiting, nausea, diarrhea, stomach pain, organ malfunctions

inside and outside the body. However, external and internal factors may derail this intricate harmony, thus affecting first the exterior part of the body and later the interior organ systems.

Therapy

Based on the results of *chi*, energy, and TCM diagnoses, the healer is ready to suggest appropriate treatment methods. The patterns of disturbed energy and the principles and methods of treatment are shown in Table 23.2.

Specifically, qigong meridian massage (QMM) can be used to replenish the deficient energy in a particular meridian; the healer can apply pressure on the affected area *along* the direction of energy flow. To deplete excessive energy, pressure can be applied on the affected area *against* the direction of the energy flow. To facilitate energy flow in a blocked area, the

healer can press, massage, or knead the area. To disperse energy concentrated in certain areas, a rotating movement can be used, starting from the center of the affected area and working toward the peripheral region. The healer can also use this rotating motion to move energy into a deficient area by starting from a peripheral area and working toward the center of the targeted area.

The same treatment principles used for QMM also apply to the extrinsic-*chi* treatment method, with the exception that the healer performs the healing at a distance. After self-preparation, the healer then uses his or her finger, fingers, or palm to project energy toward the patient's energy field. Once the healer feels the connection between his or her energy and the patient's, the patient's energy can be guided to flow in the natural direction to replenish energy deficiency, or against the natural direction to release blocked or stagnated energy. The healer

Table 23.2. Energy Disturbances and Methods of Qigong Treatment

ENERGY DISTURBANCES	PRINCIPAL OF TREATMENT	METHOD OF TREATMENT
Uneven energy field	Balance	By healer, qigong meridian massage, or movement and meditation qigong
Leakage of energy	Seal	By healer, meditation qigong
Scattered energy	Solidify	By healer, meditation qigong
Solidified energy	Disperse	By healer, movement qigong
Sick energy	Expel	By healer, breathing, and movement qigong
Collapsed energy	Replenish	By healer, breathing, and meditation qigong
Stagnated energy flow	Facilitate	By healer, movement qigong
Wrong direction of energy flow	Reverse	By healer, movement and meditation qigong
Excessive energy	Release	By healer, breathing, and movement qigong
Deficient energy	Replenish	By healer, breathing, movement, and meditation
Yin	Balance	By healer, *yang* type qigong
Yang	Balance	By healer, *yin* type qigong
Hot	Balance	By healer *yin* type qigong
Cold	Balance	By healer, *yang* type qigong
Wet	Balance	By healer, *yang* type qigong
Dry	Balance	By healer, *yin type qigong*

Table 23.3. Types of Self-Healing Qigong (SHQ)	
TYPE	EFFECT
Movement-oriented qigong	Restores and regulates the energy system through specific dance-like movement exercises
Meditation-oriented qigong	Relaxes the mind and allows *chi* to return to its naturally balanced state; employs the mind to perform self-healing
Breathing qigong	Emphasizes the role of breathing in replenishing, releasing, or storing *chi* for healing and health

can also infuse his or her own energy into the patient's energy system or drain excessive energy out of the patient's system by intention (i.e., volition with a sense of direction, and with clear formulation and deliberateness).

The application of intrinsic *chi* to heal also adheres to the aforementioned principles. With the healer's finger placed on an acupoint or with his or her palm on a particular location, intrinsic *chi* is infused into the patient's body. This intrinsic *chi* method is frequently combined with QMM to correct the condition of *chi* deficiency. The patient may also be prescribed SHQ as a primary healing modality (Table 23.3).

PROVIDER–PATIENT INTERACTION

The qigong health provider can assume the role of healer, teacher, or both. As a healer, he or she serves the client in a role similar to that of the health provider in conventional medicine. This novel way of understanding the etiology of diseases should be explained to the client, and the patient should be taught to lead a new way of life—to live in harmony with oneself, others, the immediate environment, and the universe. In this sense, the qigong health provider should also serve as a model of sound living.

Patient-Assessment Procedures

HISTORY-TAKING

A detailed record of the patient's history is established. Dates of visits, general patient information, and source of referral are recorded in the patient's chart. The provider then continues to establish the patient's history by interviewing

the patient in an empathic and friendly atmosphere concerning his or her major complaints and relevant minor complaints. The record of the presenting health problem includes descriptions of the onset of the problem, the circumstances in which it developed, its manifestation(s), and treatment history. The symptoms are described in terms of location, nature, quantity and severity, timing of occurrence, factors that have aggravated or relieved them, and associated complaints.

A comprehensive health history of the patient is taken as well. Childhood illnesses, accidents, injuries, or falls are most relevant. Patients are asked to describe in detail how accidents and injuries have occurred; these early experiences may damage their meridians and result in latent manifestation of health problems. History-taking is also the right time to gather the patient's family health history for future reference. The patient's current health status and psychosocial history are recorded as well.

CHI AND THE PHYSICAL EXAMINATION

The body weight, body height, and other pertinent information, such as blood pressure and laboratory test results, are recorded in the patient's chart before *chi* and physical examination. For a complete checkup of the energy system, the patient should lay on his or her back with palms facing up. The healer starts the examination from the top of the patient's head. By bringing his or her hand close to the patient's head, the healer may sense the patient's energy field. Thereafter, the healer's hand moves down to check the energy condition of the eyes, nose, ears, neck, chest, stomach, bladder, and extremities. This process is repeated as needed. Once this phase of the examination is complete, the healer examines the patient's general energy condition while the patient is lying down on his or her stomach. Aside from the general condition of the energy system, the healer notes the energy condition of the meridian systems.

During this phase of examination, the healer notes the nature of the energy conditions. Is the energy active, piercing, even, hot, wet, or dry? Can the energy be detected at a distance or at close range? When the energy checkup is complete, the healer should have a good idea of the patient's energy conditions. After completing the energy examination, the healer then proceeds to perform a physical examination to investigate the impact and severity of the energy disturbances on exterior and/or interior parts of the body as well as on the meridian system. The healer should first pay attention to any injuries, open sores, tender and stiff areas, and any discomforts, and then conduct a general physical examination. This should be done by applying TCM diagnostic methods as described in Chapter 12, "Traditional Chinese Medicine." If the healer feels that laboratory and other tests are required, he or she should ask the patient to consult with the primary care physician.

At the end of the general examination, the healer should proceed to narrow the examination down to the location of energy disturbances or to the location with which the patient has complaints. For example, if the patient complains of headaches and the healer finds energy imbalances in this area, the healer should determine the nature of the energy disturbances. To pinpoint meridian problems, finger or fingernail pressure can be applied to various locations in the head region. If the patient shows aversive reactions or avoidance behavior to pressure on acupoints of the gallbladder, bladder, or governing meridians, the healer needs to examine the whole meridian system to determine other problem areas within that system.

Differential Diagnosis

DISEASE CLASSIFICATION

Most patients in the West who visit alternative medicine clinics come with a well-diagnosed illness made by conventional medicine physi-

cians. This provides an excellent opportunity for a dialectic synthesis of mainstream and alternative medicine. The qigong healer can take advantages of both systems to prescribe a better course of treatment. However, the physician should be aware of the cultural differences in devising a disease classification system (16–18).

TCM attributes pathogenesis and etiology of illness to the derailment of the energy system's homeostatic state; thus, practitioners of this modality have developed a system of disease classification different from that of the symptom-driven (disease-oriented) system of conventional medicine. According to TCM, pathology is the end product of this derailed energy system. Therefore, the first order of business in TCM is to correct the energy condition rather than to remedy pathology. With this theoretic orientation, TCM has developed a scheme to classify symptoms into patterns of illness according to the eight principles of four dialectic opposites (*yin/yang*, cold/hot, fullness/emptiness, and interior/exterior). Table 23.1 presents a representative sample of symptoms that correspond to the patterns of illness.

Each one of the patterns represents a deviation from the individual's harmonious energy state. For example, the pattern of emptiness shows a lack of energy, weak body and voice, loss of appetite, and weak pulse. To heal this patient, the practitioner must strengthen the energy system. The illness seen in a fullness pattern indicates that the patient has excessive energy buildup and is also possibly invaded by sick *chi*. This patient is physically strong, speaks with a loud voice, and has breathing that is heavy and loud. Other symptoms of this pattern are dislike of the cold, constipation, difficult urination, very strong pulse, and a tongue that is red and tight. The healer should release the patient of the sick *chi* and allow the normal energy to carry out the physiologic functions.

By the same token, the cold pattern should be treated with warming methods, such as infusing *yang* energy to the patient, performing qigong exercises to enhance energy, or prescribing warm herbal soup. The hot (fire or fever) pattern should be treated with modalities that cool and neutralize this pattern.

These principles have also been used to more specifically classify disturbances at the level of energy fields, meridians, and internal organs. Chi disturbances are described in terms of these principles as well as other characteristics (Table 23.2). The afflicted meridian systems are categorized as suffering from *yin* or *yang*, excess or deficiency, and cold or hot, and their associated symptoms are manifested in the interior or exterior body parts. If the energy disturbance continues, it can cause organ dysfunction; such disorders can then be categorized accordingly. Thus, liver disorders may be attributed to deficient or stagnated liver energy (or liver fire), and respiratory problems may be caused by deficient lung energy; invasion of cold, wind, or fire to the lung system; or ingestion of excessive *yin* vegetables and cold drinks. (The term *fire* is used here symbolically. Its metaphoric meaning includes extraordinary energy of heat and/or fever, without any connotation of inflammation.)

THERAPY AND OUTCOMES

Treatment Patterns

Drawing from the unique features of ailments that are intimately related to the general conditions of the energy system, as indicated in Table 23.1, qigong healers generally adhere to the eight previously described principles to prescribe treatment plans: *yin/yang*, hot/cold, fullness/emptiness, and exterior/interior patterns.

Treatment Options

Patients who are looking for qigong treatments have two options. The first option is to visit a qigong clinic that uses the traditional healer–client approach. The practitioner serves primarily as a healer, and he or she may also assume the role of teacher to instruct self-healing techniques. The second patient option is to look for classes or groups that offer instruction on SHQ.

Description of Treatments/ Interventions with Case Examples

The healer should treat the general conditions of the patient before attending to specific prob-

lems. For example, if the patient's energy is scattered and unstable (e.g., in the case of severe anxiety), the healer needs to consolidate the patient's energy before other health problems are treated. The healer should ask the patient to sit straight on a chair with neck, shoulders, and lower back relaxed, chin slightly pulled in, and a smile on his or her face. This posture allows for the natural flow of energy.

The healer then asks the patient to place his or her hands on the navel area with closed eyes, which allows the energy to return to the *chi* (Dantian) reservoir that is located near the navel area. Then, the healer places his or her hand near the navel area of the patient for approximately 1 minute and uses the power of the mind to consolidate the patient's energy. The healer may have to repeat this consolidation technique several times to achieve the desired effects. In a case of severe anxiety, the healer should also encourage the patient to practice sitting meditation at home in the same posture at least once a day until the next visit. The guiding principle for meditation is that it should be practiced in a relaxed manner. When the mind is not calm, the patient should stop meditating, but the patient should return to meditation when the mind is more relaxed. Otherwise, the patient may be so frustrated that he or she will stop the exercise altogether.

One of the frequently encountered energy problems is the uneven distribution of energy around the body. This may lead to the manifestation of physical illness on one side of the body and a general feeling of off-centeredness in mental and behavioral responses. For example, some patients tend to have health problems on the right side of the body, such as headaches, back pains, and skin problems. When this type of patient is asked to sit in a quiet and relaxed manner, his or her body tends to tilt to one side. In this case, the healer should correct this energy imbalance before treatment of any related health problems begins. To balance the patient's energy, the healer places his or her hand near the base of the patient's spine and moves up slowly towards the head and over it, and then moves the hand to the front of the body. At any given time, when the healer detects uneven distribution of an energy field, he or she moves the hand several times around that region to make sure that the distribution of that energy field is rectified. Once this is accom- plished, the healer can proceed to treat specific problems in the local areas. The following two cases describe treatment methods.

CASE EXAMPLES

CASE 1: HYPERTENSION

A 40-year-old man who is studying for a college degree presents with a 2-year history of essential hypertension. He notes that medications for his hypertension are near the maximum dosage level and that he dislikes their cognitive side effects. After taking the medication, he cannot concentrate on his studies. He wants to find an alternative treatment so that he can finish his degree. Laboratory tests, including a computerized axial tomography scan and renal studies, do not reveal any pathological conditions.

Chi examination indicates that this patient has excessive energy in the head and chest regions. The physical examination does not reveal any significant clinical problems. However, the practitioner notices that his face and eyes are very red, and his tongue is cherry-red. His pulse is very strong and fast. He likes cold beverages and hates hot drinks. His muscles around the neck and shoulders are extremely tight. He also suffers from occasional numbness in his thumbs as well as the fourth and fifth fingers. QMM examination further reveals that the patient is very sensitive to pressures around the wrist and fifth finger. He is also quite sensitive to pressures exerted on the lung meridian near the pectoral area, elbow, and thumb, which indicates that chi disturbances have already invaded his meridian systems and affected cardiovascular function.

The healer observes that the patient is suffering from a yang pattern of illness, with disturbances in the heart and lung meridians. In this case, the healer should first release the excessive energy in the head and chest area, then harmonize the yang and correct the heart and lung meridians. The healer can use his or her hand to move the excessive energy in the head to the front and down to the lower part of the body, thus balancing the energy distribution. QMM should also be applied to balance the heart and lung meridian energy. In addition, the healer should instruct the patient on SHQ breathing exercises to release excessive energy. Treatment results in improved concentration even with continued use of the medications.

CASE 2: DEPRESSION

A 45-year-old woman presents complaining of depression and suicidal ideation. She is cared for by a psychiatrist but hates the side effects of her antidepressant medication. She rarely has a good conversation with her husband because of his busy schedule. She complains of losing her appetite, waking up at approximately 4 AM without being able to fall sleep again, suffering shortness of breath, and lacking motivation to do anything. She is grossly underweight. Her face is pale, her tongue is pale with a yellowish tint, and her pulse is very weak. Chi examination reveals that she has a very weak energy field, although the energy is quite evenly distributed around her body. This is a severe case of emptiness pattern. The color of the tongue and shortness of breath may suggest minor problems in the liver and lung meridians. QMM examination of the acupoints along these two meridians indicates that the upper chest area is very sensitive to pressures, which suggests an accumulation of stagnant energy in the lung meridian area.

To treat the patient, the healer uses external chi for approximately 1 minute to replenish the patient's energy. Afterward, the patient is given QMM to clear the blockage in the lung meridian to facilitate energy flow. The patient is then taught movement qigong to practice at home for approximately 20 to 30 minutes a day. These qigong exercises should ideally be done in the morning to harness the morning yang energy. Breathing exercises to rectify energy conditions should also be taught and practiced. Continued treatment and regular practice result in improved mood and sleep, as well as less bothersome side effects from medication.

Treatment Evaluation

EXPECTED CHANGES IN THE PATIENT

Effective qigong treatment results in restoration of the energy field back to a healthy state, correction of meridian functions, improvement and elimination of complaints and signs of discomfort, and amelioration of illness.

How the Magnitude of Change Is Assessed

The healer relies primarily on *chi* and TCM examination methods to monitor changes in the patient. Simple measures may also be used to monitor physiological changes, such as blood pressure, heart rate, muscle tension, and peripheral and core temperature. Whenever it is necessary, the patient should be followed by conventional physicians for laboratory and diagnostic tests to validate and monitor significant changes in the pathological conditions. The frequency and severity of complaints represent major variables in determining continuation of treatment. Unfortunately, subjective reports may not be sufficient grounds for treatment termination because ordinary human sensation and perception may not be sensitive to the subtlety of the disease-causing energy disturbances. However, failure of objective signs to improve may mean that aspect of the disease is refractory to qigong treatment and requires other interventions.

Time Period in Which Changes Occur

Changes in the overall energy field may occur in a relatively short period of time. The exterior expression of the illness, such as the color of the skin, face, and tongue, is also very responsive to changes. Red and pale facial color may change to normal pink color during the first treatment session, largely caused by changes in microcirculatory functions (19–21). Yellow and gray will take longer because of the severity of *chi* disturbances. Physical signs and discomfort related to exterior components of the body may take on average four weekly treatments to show significant changes. The affected meridian systems may require approximately eight treatments to regain normal function. When *chi* disturbances invade the interior components of the human body and result in diseases of internal organs, the observable improvements may not take place until after 3 months of treatment. For chronic illness, such as arthritis, liver disorders, and cancer, significant changes may not occur until one half a year to a year after beginning the treatment. External healing techniques used by qigong healers generally tend to produce changes faster than SHQ techniques alone.

USE OF THE SYSTEM FOR TREATMENT

Qigong is one approach within Traditional Chinese Medicine and is therefore usually delivered in the context of TCM, which includes dietary changes, acupuncture, herbal medicine, and manipulation. However, the use of both external and internal qigong produces effects on its own and may be the treatment of choice for certain conditions. From the Western perspective, qigong looks like a combination of relaxation, breathing, and exercise, and so it would be expected to help conditions that these behaviors are known to benefit: respiratory disorders, neuromuscular problems, psychological problems like depression, and certain physiological conditions such as hypertension and fatigue. From the perspective of TCM, however, qigong provides a major way to alter and balance *chi*, thus making it ideal for several conditions in both early and late stages. Fortunately, a considerable amount of research has been conducted on qigong in China and elsewhere that can serve as a guide to its major indications (6, 20).

Major Indications Based on Approach

MOST USEFUL AS A PRIMARY APPROACH

Regular qigong practice increases respiratory volume and improves oxygen uptake and carbon dioxide exchange (19). It is therefore not surprising that qigong is an effective treatment of asthma and emphysema (21). Increased microcirculation (22, 23) and reduced reactive catecholamine production and sensitivity (24) seem to occur with prolonged qigong practice, with effects on cardiovascular disease including increased cardiac output (24), reduced heart rate (25), and ischemia (22, 23). Enhanced lipolysis

(26, 27), improved lipoprotein levels (28), reduced hypertension (29), and increased aerobic conditioning (25, 30) may also contribute to the prevention of or improvement in cardiovascular disease.

Qigong has been shown to produce significant improvements in neurological and psychological function. These include improvements in memory (31) and learning capacity (32), reductions in anxiety, fatigue (30), and hyperactivity (33), improvements in nerve function (34), and changes in EEG patterns (5), typical of some types of meditation.

Slowed or reversed effects of aging have also been reported in several studies, including increases in bone density (33, 35) and estradiol levels in aging women (36), and improved respiratory, cardiovascular function, balance, and other age-related effects in normal elderly (5). Some studies have also suggested increased resistance to infection (37, 38). Finally, reduced side effects from chemotherapy and radiation during cancer treatment have also been reported with qigong use (39). While many of these effects are well documented, others are based on preliminary research or are done in China where the quality of clinical research is inconsistent. These findings are consistent, however, with demonstrated effects from studies done in the West from exercise, breathing, and relaxation techniques when applied intensively.

CONTRAINDICATIONS AND ADVERSE EFFECTS

Chinese qigong practitioners warn that inappropriately applied qigong therapy can be harmful. A so-called adjustment or adaptation phenomenon is commonly reported in which a number of unpleasant symptoms, such as muscle aches, pain, fatigue, and other symptoms, can occur from qigong (1, 22, 40). These symptoms are usually minor and temporary but do need to be managed properly. Qigong exercises, if applied vigorously and consistently, need to be adapted and individualized to the patient's needs and conditions. For example, some types of qigong exercises (such as those similar to tai *chi* or practices that focus on forehead concentration) may increase sympathetic tone and be contraindicated for those with anxiety, hypertension, and angina (38).

The *Chinese Classification of Mental Disorders-2* describes a qigong deviation syndrome (QDS) characterized by specific abnormal *chi* movement and manifesting in symptoms such as malaise, headache, insomnia, abdominal distension, and other symptoms. Xu (41) has pointed out that some schools of qigong emphasize producing rapid changes by using suggestion and autosuggestion techniques. These approaches can increase the risk of anxiety, depression, hallucinations, and psychological disturbances similar to inappropriate application of hypnosis. The appropriate application of qigong in any serious manner requires detailed understanding of the patient's condition, predispositions, and skill and training on the part of the practitioner. Unfortunately, few qigong practitioners in the West have this training or work in an environment that can assure the safe and skilled application of qigong as a therapy for serious diseases. The physician is in a unique position to provide such an environment by assuring that minimum requirements for application of qigong therapy are arranged. Some of the requirements for such application are discussed below.

ORGANIZATION

The qigong perspective presented in this chapter is a dialectic synthesis of both TCM and conventional medicine. As such, the basic training involved in both TCM and conventional medicine is necessary, but not sufficient, training for a postconventional qigong healer. To that end, some specific prerequisites, requirements, and curriculum components should also be taken into account.

Training

PREREQUISITES AND REQUIREMENTS

Qigong is not simply a therapeutic technique, but a healing art. It requires talent and temperament as well as training. Talent includes sensitivity or receptivity to *chi* and the ability to comprehend the rationale underlying qigong practice. Like hypnotizability and many other abilities, sensitivity and receptivity to *chi* may be inherently different for each individual. To be sure, this skill is not an all-or-none nonverbal intelligence, but a characteristic that differs in degrees among individuals. Students with higher sensitivity to *chi* have greater potential to become more competent healers. Along the same line, the ability to understand the subtlety involved in qigong is also necessary for becoming a true healing artist. Performing qigong without a deep grasp of its theoretical foundation would mean that the qigong movements would be ungrounded gestures lacking significance.

Temperament refers to empathy and humanistic and humanitarian devotion. As a transcendental philosophy of life, Taoism, the philosophical foundation underlying qigong, helps people reflect upon the purpose of our existence, for which human connection and compassion play a very important role. Enlightened by this teaching, qigong healers view their profession as a calling to help human beings become integrated with nature (namely, heaven and earth, metaphorically speaking) by means of *chi*—to return to integrity and balance and to make whole the *sine qua non* of healing (42). Qigong as a healing art aims for the integration of body, mind, and spirit. To serve this purpose, qigong healers themselves must have integrity of sound body, mind, and spirit. The sound spirit presupposes the temperamental factor already mentioned.

Curriculum Components

Given qigong as a culture-embedded medicine, a general understanding of the traditional Chinese cultural context, especially the world view, seems necessary. This learning is better achieved in a course like medical anthropology because the anthropological point of view is nonjudgmental and intersubjective (43, 44) and thus helpful for students to assimilate the new knowledge and to accommodate this knowledge with their original world view. A well-designed course of medical anthropology in this regard should put the "old wine in a new bottle"; that is, examine and reconstruct the classical contents of Chinese cultural context from a posttraditional perspective.

For further development of the qigong curriculum, what has been presented so far in this chapter may provide a rough guideline. In addition, some components of the qigong training program include the following:

1. Introduction of the traditional point of view, which distinguishes tradition from traditionalism (this is essential).
2. Integration from a dialectic synthesis of TCM and modern science.
3. Relaxation theory and practice.
4. Significance of regulating the body.
5. Basic posture of regulating the body (rooting, centering, and balancing).
6. Choice of positions in qigong exercise.
7. Introduction to the action of consciousness, implicit consciousness, and mindful/mindless qigong.
8. Tactics of generating conscious awareness, holding attention within, and stopping of thoughts.
9. Strategies for developing inner serenity and control over involuntary functions.
10. How to solicit transcendent intuition and understand it.
11. How to best use this symbolism by relating to Jungian theory.
12. Different approaches to qigong respiration.
13. General keys to regulating normal respiration.
14. Duration and other training requirements.

At present, Zou Du University in the Hai Ding District in Beijing offers a two-year training course for potential practitioners, and Tianjin University in Hebei province also offers four quarterly medical qigong classes yearly. Short-term workshops and seminars have also been provided by TCM colleges, such as the Qigong Institute of the TCM Academy of Shanghai, and universities, such as the Beijing Institute of Technology and Beijing University of Agriculture and Engineering in China. Both the duration of training and the training requirements vary according to the goals and backgrounds of the students. Given that qigong is a form of TCM, Western students may need a longer duration of training and more training requirements to reach the same goals. The curriculum components listed previously are geared for trainees of qigong healers.

Quality Assurance

Until recently, few well-designed studies of medical qigong's efficacy have been recognized by mainstream researchers. To demonstrate medical qigong's efficacy by ruling out the placebo effect and other alternative explanations, a double-blind and well-controlled design is necessary according to the standards of conventional medicine. Admittedly, this evaluative process is not sufficient because the conventional approach is generally reductionistic, mechanistic, and outcome-oriented. As such, it is less likely to evaluate a whole picture of the vital organism as well as the therapeutic process involved. To that end, *Geisteswissenschaften*—the German term for holistic human studies—should be applied to explore the therapeutic phenomena observed in the medical qigong process. *Geisteswissenschaften* includes phenomenology, hermeneutics, and so forth and is especially useful for carrying out studies that are embedded in the Chinese cultural context (2, 45, 46). Unfortunately, few researchers use this approach to conduct the study of qigong.

Moreover, longitudinal follow-up of qigong healing is also required to confirm the long-term effect. Otherwise, qigong therapy may just work like a drain opener, which can only open the clogged drain for a while but cannot keep the water flowing forever. As far as we know, most longitudinal follow-up studies of qigong and other TCM modalities have continued for only 6 months. Because the efficacy of qigong healing remains to be confirmed and the operational mechanism of qigong needs to be demonstrated, quality assurance is difficult and often filled with controversy. Still, for the sake of the patients' physical, psychological, and financial concerns, such measures should be attempted.

LICENSURE AND CERTIFICATION

In the past two decades, there has been a rapid rise in the popularity of medical qigong as a form of therapy in China, where the official position has been "not to publicize and not to deny." This position means they accept but do not advocate it. On November 19, 1989, the Chinese Ministry of Public Health introduced on a trial basis 14 regulations regarding medical qigong, and the Central Traditional Chinese Medicine Bureau tightened its control over qigong masters (47). Some of these regulations may be adapted to other countries, as shown in the following list:

1. If a person provides treatment by emitting *chi*, he or she has to apply to the medicine section or the medical administration for approval to practice. If the treatment of 30 cases of the same kind is statistically confirmed as effective by the authorities, a certificate will then be issued to the applicant to provide such specific type of treatment.
2. The treatment effect must be demonstrated longitudinally as well. Moreover, not only should the treatment outcome be examined, but the processes of learning and providing service need to be monitored as well. The best way to do this is to require students to be interns or apprentices in a qigong hospital and clinic for a certain period of time before taking the license examination. During their internship they can build up the 30 clinical cases under supervision for their examination, and their case reports can be used by their affiliated hospital or clinic as partial fulfillment for the evaluation of that institution.

Unfortunately, not even such minimum requirements are present in the West.

LEGAL STATUS AND REGULATION

Medical and public health authorities can employ qigong masters who have been qualified under the aforementioned regulations to perform qigong therapy. Should qigong be used to treat disease, a full medical record must be kept to evaluate its long-term effectiveness.

Medical qigong activities must be documented reliably without selection bias. Misleading readers of advertisements by relating superstition with therapy is deemed a violation of professional ethics. All advertisements and promotion materials about medical qigong should be approved by medical and public health authorities.

Anyone found to have contravened these regulations is warned, fined, and suspended or banned from practice. These actions are enforced by the medical and public health authorities in conjunction with appropriate medical associations. All healers who have been in medical qigong practice before the introduction of these regulations must apply for approval of such practices.

Unfortunately, no such regulation of qigong practice occurs in the West except to prevent qigong practitioners from practicing medicine without a license. Thus, anyone can hold themselves out as a qigong "master" without proof of training or competence. Patients and physicians should ask for documentation of training and certification.

PROFESSIONAL SOCIETIES AND CONTINUING EDUCATION

The China Research Society of Qigong Science is the major professional qigong association in China. Professional societies at local levels are numerous, and a quarterly journal, *China Qigong,* is published at Bei Dai He Qigong Hospital. As of 1990, the circulation of each issue was approximately 80,000. In general, the associations or societies have sanction power, provide peer-review and referral services, and organize conferences for scholarly exchange and workshops or seminars for continuing education. Any workshop or seminar has to be preapproved by the academic committee of the professional association, and official credits are issued to the participants.

Reimbursement Status

In China, fees charged for qigong treatment are supposed to be reasonable and worked out jointly by the authorities and the local consumer council. Exorbitant charges are prohibited. As discussed earlier, qigong healers claim to call on cosmic and divine power, which resides at a higher level than the secular level, to help human beings. The aim of qigong healers is to help people relate to the *intention*, or *mind*,

part of the body-mind-spirit tripartite system because the mind plays the most important role in qigong practice (48). The mind provides the direction for the flow of the *chi*, and purer intentionality induces better direction. Empirical research (49) has also revealed that theta waves were lower and beta waves were higher during qigong practice that incorporated concentrative mind focus versus qigong practice that employed nonconcentrative mind focus. During concentrative mind focus, any ideas other than helping the patient would distract the healer's mind and misguide the *chi* flow. However, the survival of qigong therapy as a profession is certainly dependent on financial support. Fees for service should be based realistically to maintain the positive interaction between qigong therapists and their clients. Concerning reimbursement status of qigong therapy, it could be commensurate with that of physical therapy.

No reimbursement for qigong generally occurs in the West except as part of other treatments. In those cases, it is usually treated as part of physical therapy.

Relation with Conventional Medicine

As purported earlier, TCM–based qigong therapy and conventional medicine can be integrated in a dialectic synthesis. Conventional medicine is viewed as a thesis built on reductionism originating from Auguste Comte, mind/body dualism initiated by René Descartes, the concept of mechanic physics constructed by Issac Newton, and analytic philosophy and logical positivism. In contrast, being rooted in TCM, qigong therapy is holistic in nature. In that sense, after it differentiates complex phenomena into separate and simpler parts for analysis, it weaves them together as a whole web. The thread that connects every part is *chi*, which manifests itself in different forms within each segment of the mind-body-spirit tripartite system. In so doing, it is able to see not only each single tree in the forest, but also a bird's-eye view of the whole forest.

In addition, qigong is better understood by quantum physics than the Newtonian mechanical concepts that explain conventional medicine. This is because quantum physics recognizes aspects of reality beyond Newtonian mechanics and consequently helps to illuminate some of the mechanisms underlying qigong. In a similar vein, the methodology commonly employed in mainstream medical research is insufficient for the exploration of qigong therapy. The fact that conventional research methodology has difficulty assessing the observations seen in qigong therapy and practice is often used as a justification for refuting qigong.

PROSPECTS FOR THE FUTURE

Qigong has a long, time-tested track record as a therapeutic tool that has prevailed among a billion people in China. Its long-lasting prevalence cannot be attributed completely to its medical value because economic, cultural, and other contextual factors also play an important role. As such, distinguishing the medical *sine qua non* of qigong from other contributing factors seems to be indispensable for its application to other sociocultural contexts. For that purpose, a scientific approach to the study of qigong is needed in modern global world culture.

The scientific approach suggested previously integrates both natural and social scientific methodology. The inclusion of natural sciences into the research design here obviously requires no justification, whereas the main reason for taking social sciences into account is to comprehend the cultural, social, psychological, and spiritual factors involved in qigong treatment. Given qigong as a synergistic system of body, mind, and soul, these factors have been much less attended to compared with the scientific aspects of this modality, so they need to be affirmed in the future. The few available empiric studies addressing the issues related to the mind-body connection can be seen in the work of Omura and Beckman (37), Sancier and Hu (50), and Tsai et al. (22). Among these studies, the work of Tsai et al., in which the psychological variable—ability to function—was observed and measured, can serve as a model for further research along this line. Specifically, Tsai et al. evaluated the qigong program's efficacy according to patients' subjective improvements, which were graded according to the Karnofsky scale. Patients' subjective feelings were recorded faithfully, thereby indicating the patients' sense of well-being.

As pointed out previously, the identification of the operational mechanisms underlying qigong treatment is important for assuring the consistency of this modality's quality as well as for demystification purposes. To that end, both process-oriented and outcome-oriented research design should be taken into account. So far, most studies have been outcome-oriented, so researchers have not been able to monitor how the potential mechanisms work. Instead, the researchers can merely infer the mechanisms indirectly from the final results. To design process-oriented research, idiographic methodology is more appropriate than is nomothetic methodology. The former requires each subject to be observed intensively across different occasions of the temporal dimension and extensively across various situations on the spatial dimension. In contrast, the latter methodology collects data only at one point of time, but uses large sample and quantitative analyses so that general rules can be drawn. A complete research design needs both methodologies, as demonstrated by Lee and Lei (40). Without the idiographic methodology, the subject remains in the black box; and without the nomothetic methodology, the research result cannot be generalized to other populations. To fully understand qigong, multiple research methods across the full domains of knowledge, as described in Chapter 4, are needed.

Process-oriented study and idiographic design also help to verify the principal concepts of the qigong system that have been presented earlier, especially the stage model of disease development shown in Figure 23.1. Many of those concepts are either metaphysical or metaphoric (e.g., *yin/yang*) and thus short of empiric substantiation. To substantiate these theoretic concepts, careful observations of the disease development at every step along the way are indispensable. After TCM theory is empirically verified, it can be synthesized dialectically with conventional medicine, and both should be included hierarchically into postconventional medicine.

Integrated postconventional medicine is based both on quantum physics that goes over and beyond the metaphysics of TCM and on Western medicine's materialistic world view. To carry on both postconventional medicine's theoretic reconstruction work and empiric studies to verify dialectically synthesized postconventional medicine is a mission for contemporary medical students and scientists.

Author's Note: The authors wish to acknowledge the collegial support of Profs. Ellen D. Ciporen, Ronald Doviak, Sadie Chavis Bragg, and Antonio Perez, without which the present chapter could not have been completed on time.

REFERENCES

1. Lee CT, Lei T. All rivers flow to the sea: encountering with energy through Qigong without acupuncture. The Fourth World Conference on Acupuncture, Sept. 20–23, 1996, New York.
2. Lei T. Geisteswissenschaften of Sittlichkeit and political Umwelt: Sinnverstehen in the East. Pacific Focus 1990;5(1):19–59.
3. Benson H. Timeless healing: the power and biology of belief. Edgartown, MA: S&S Scribner, 1996.
4. Veith I. Huang Ti Nei Ching Su Wen: the yellow emperor's classic of internal medicine. Berkeley, CA: University of California, 1972.
5. Lin CP, ed. Chinese qigongology. Beijing, China: Beijing College of Athletic Education, 1988 (in Chinese).
6. Cheng MC, Smith RW. Tai chi: the supreme ultimate exercise for health, sport, and self-defense. Rutland, VT: Charles E. Tutle, 1967.
7. Yang MJ, Tian CW. Dayan Gong. Beijing, China: Renmin Weisheng, 1983 (in Chinese).
8. Chao ZS. The crane qigong. Beijing, China: Renning Weishing, 1984.
9. Blofeld J. The quest for immortality. London: Unwin, 1979.
10. Chiang WC. Yin si tzu's meditation method for health. Taipei, China: Jian Shan Mei, 1964.
11. Fang CY. The complete work of Chinese qigong. Chielin, China: Chielin Science and Technology Publishing, 1989 (in Chinese).
12. Guo L. New qigong method for cancer treatment. Beijing, China: Ton Shin Publishing, 1994.
13. Kaptchuk, Ted J. The web that has no weaver: understanding Chinese medicine. Congdon & Weed, 1983.

14. Kendall DE. Understanding traditional energetic concepts. In: Green E, ed. Energy fields in medicine. Kalamazoo, MI: The John E. Fetzer Foundation, 1989.
15. Wong ST. Complete work of Chinese acupuncture and moxibustion. Vols. 1 and 2. Honan, China: Honan Science and Technology Publishing, 1988.
16. Kleinman A. Patients and healers in the context of culture. Berkeley, CA: University of California Press, 1980.
17. Kleinman A. Rethinking psychiatry. New York: The Free Press, 1988b.
18. Kleinman A, Lin T, eds. Normal and abnormal behavior in Chinese culture. Holland: Reide, 1981.
19. Xie HC. The scientific basis of qigong. Beijing, China: Beijing Institute of Technology, 1988 (in Chinese).
20. Lim YA, Boone TF, Flarrity JR, Thompson WR. Effects of qigong on on cardiorespiratory changes: a preliminary study. Am J Chinese Med 1993;21(1):1–6.
21. Lin CP, Lu H. Modern research of clinical qigong. In: Lin CP, ed. Chinese qigongology. Beijing, China: Beijing College of Athletic Education, 1988 (in Chinese).
22. Tsai TJ, Lai JS, Lee SH, et al. Breathing-coordinated exercise improves the quality of life in hemodialysis patients. J Am Soc Nephrol 1995;6(5): 1392–1400.
23. Mou FF, Shi Z, Hsu G, Chao GL. Study of qigong on bulbar conjunctiva microcirculation disorder of persons entering highlands. J Microcir 1994; 4(4):18–20.
24. Wang CX, Xu DH, Qi YH, Kuang AK. The beneficial effect of qigong on the hypertension incorporated with coronary heart disease. J Gerontol 1988;8(2):83.
25. Ganlante L. Tai chi: the supreme ultimate. York Beach, ME: Samuel Weiser, 1981.
26. Galbo H. Hormonal and metabolic adaptation to exercise. New York: Thieme-Stratton, 1983.
27. Hetzler RK, Knowlton RG, Kaminsky LA, Kamimori GH. Effect of warm-up on plasma free fatty acid responses and substrate utilization during submaximal exercise. Res Quart Exer Sports 1986; 57:223–228.
28. Liu GL, Cui RQ, Li GZ, Huang CM. Changes in brainstem and cortical auditory potentials during qigong meditation. Am J Chin Med 1990; 18(3–4):95–103.
29. Mou FF, Yen ZF, Li CY, Chao GL. Study of qigong's bi-directional regulation and its mechanism. Chin J Modern Dev Trad Med 1991; 10(6):353–356.

30. Jin P. Efficacy of tai chi, brisk walking, meditation, and reading in reducing mental and emotional stress. J Psychosom Res 1992;36(4):361–370.

31. Abrams AI. Cited in Lin CP, Lu H. Modern research of clinical qigong. In: Lin CP, ed. Chinese qigongology. Beijing, China: Beijing College of Athletic Education, 1988.

32. Collier RW. Cited in Lin CP, Lu H. Modern research of clinical qigong. In: Lin CP, ed. Chinese qigongology. Beijing, China: Beijing College of Athletic Education, 1988.

33. Xu D, Wang C. Clinical study of delaying effect on senility of hypertensive patients by practicing yang jing yi shen gong. Presented at the Proceedings from the Fifth International Symposium on Qigong. Shanghai, China; 1994:109.

34. Hwang MG. Qigong therapy on neurological system. In: Lin CP, ed. Chinese qigongology. Beijing, China: Beijing College of Athletic Education, 1988 (in Chinese).

35. Hu SH, Shen YM. An observation of senior qigong practitioners' bone density. Qigong 1992;13(3):99–100.

36. Ye M, Zhang RH, Wu XH, Wang Y, Shen JQ. Relationship among erythrocyte superoxide dismutase (RBC-SOD) activity, plasma sexual hormones (T, E2), aging and qigong exercise. Presented at The Third International Symposium on Qigong. Shanghai, China; 1990.

37. Omura Y, Beckman SL. Application of intensified (+) qigong energy, (å) electric field, magnetic field, electric pulse, strong shiatsu massage or acupuncture on the accurate organ representation areas of the hands to improve circulation and enhance drug uptake in pathological organs. Acupunct Electrother Res 1995;20:21–72.

38. Omura Y, Lin TL, Debreceni L, et al. Unique changes found on the qigong master's and patient's body during qigong treatment. Acupunct Electrother Res 1989;14:61–89.

39. Zhang QC, Hsu, HY. AIDS and Chinese medicine. Long Beach, CA: OHAI Press, 1990.

40. Lee CT, Lei T. The impact of vital energy exercise on physiological and psychological variables. Presented at the Eastern Psychiatric Association's 66th Annual Meeting. Boston; March 31–April 2, 1996.

41. Xu SH. Psychophysiological reactions associated with qigong therapy. Chin Med J 1994;107(3):230–233.

42. Weil A. Spontaneous healing. New York: Alfred A. Knopf, 1996.

43. Geertz C. Interpretation of culture. New York: Basic Books, Inc., 1973.

44. LeVine RA. Properties of culture: an ethnographic view. In: Shweder RA, LeVine RA, eds. Cultural theory. Cambridge, England: Cambridge University Press, 1984.

45. Kleinman A. Illness narratives. New York: Basic Books, 1988a.

46. Lei T. Being and becoming moral in a Chinese culture: unique or universal? Cross-cultural Res (formerly Beh Sci Res) 1994;28(1):59–91.

47. Tang KC. Qigong therapy—its effectiveness and regulation. Am J Chin Med 1994;12(3–4):235–242.

48. Yang JM. The root of Chinese chi kung. Jamaica Plain, MA: Yang's Martial Arts Association (YMAA), 1996:85–168.

49. Pan WX, Zhang LF, Xia Y. The difference in EEG theta waves between concentrative and non-concentrative qigong states. J Trad Chin Med 1994;14(3):212–218.

50. Sancier KM, Hu BK. Medical application of qigong and emitted qi on humans, animals, cell cultures, and plants: review of selected scientific research. Am J Acupuncture 1991;19(4):367–377.

CHAPTER 24

BIOFEEDBACK THERAPY

Judith A. Green and Robert Shellenberger

BACKGROUND

Definitions

A patient presents with tachycardia. A heart rate monitor is attached to her finger, so that she can see moment-to-moment changes in heart rate for the purpose of learning to lower her heart rate. This is biofeedback. To facilitate treatment, the patient is taught breathing and relaxation exercises as well as other techniques for reducing sympathetic arousal. The patient uses these techniques to alleviate and prevent the symptom. This is biofeedback therapy.

BIOFEEDBACK

Biofeedback is the use of instrumentation to monitor, amplify, and feed back physiological information, so that a patient can learn to change or regulate the process being monitored. Biofeedback instrumentation may provide elaborate computer feedback or may be as simple as a thermometer taped to the finger; the feedback may be visual or auditory and may be analog, digital, or graphic. Feedback instrumentation provides accurate measurement and immediate meaningful information. The most commonly used biofeedback instruments and feedback modalities are as follows:

- **Electromyograph (EMG):** feedback of striate muscle tension
- **Thermal:** feedback of peripheral blood flow, which is monitored as skin temperature

- **Electroencephalograph (EEG):** feedback of brain waves
- **Electrodermal response (EDR):** feedback of sweat gland activity, measured from the patient's fingers
- **Perineometer:** feedback of contraction of anal sphincter and pelvic floor muscles

The patient may receive feedback from two or three of these instruments, depending on the disorder being treated. For example, treatment of a stress-related disorder with somatic and autonomic nervous system components includes EMG and thermal (blood flow) feedback.

BIOFEEDBACK THERAPY

Biofeedback therapy is the use of biofeedback instrumentation in conjunction with other therapeutic procedures for the clinical goals of symptom and medication reduction, enhanced quality of life, and prevention. An expert in neuromuscular rehabilitation describes biofeedback therapy as "an interaction between the therapist and the patient, with the biofeedback instrument functioning as an observer and partner" (1).

In biofeedback therapy, these clinical goals are achieved through *psychophysiological self-regulation*, a term that accurately describes the process in which mental, emotional, and physiological strategies and skills are learned and *used* by the patient. The feedback of information assists the patient in gaining self-regulation and physiological control. Biofeedback instrumentation is a useful tool during the learning process.

When biofeedback instrumentation is used in treatment, the feedback of physiological information may be the primary therapeutic procedure or it may be complementary to other therapeutic procedures. The relative importance of the biofeedback component depends on the disorder being treated, the particular needs and therapeutic goals of the patient, and the training of the therapist. For example, in the treatment of epilepsy for seizure reduction, EEG feedback is the primary therapeutic tool. In contrast, in the treatment of chronic myofascial pain exacerbated by depression, a variety of therapeutic procedures are used, including cognitive therapy, stress management, and EMG feedback. In this case the biofeedback component, EMG feedback, has an important complementary role in treatment.

Furthermore, a simple definition of biofeedback therapy as a single treatment entity is inaccurate. Biofeedback therapy is used in a variety of applications, from physical injury and disease to stress-related disorders in adults and children. It is used in a variety of settings, from hospital to classroom. These applications and settings necessitate different therapeutic procedures, and clinicians develop therapeutic techniques that are unique to their specialty and practice. For this reason, an official document of the Association for Applied Psychophysiology and Biofeedback on clinical efficacy refers to "biofeedback therapies" (2). In this chapter, we describe the principles and procedures of biofeedback therapy in broadest terms, noting briefly the many variations related to treatment goals for specific disorders.

Health care professionals who use biofeedback in treating patients within their specialty continue to refer to themselves by licensure or specialty—nurse, physical therapist, physician, psychologist. We use the term *biofeedback therapist* to refer to professionals who use biofeedback within their specialty and to clinicians who have specialized in biofeedback therapy and are certified through the Biofeedback Certification Institute of America (BCIA).

Biofeedback therapy is unique among medical treatments because the treatment is self-regulation that is achieved through skills that are learned and used by the patient. Successful treatment involves instrumentation feedback, counseling, and coaching by the therapist, and training and practice by the patient.

In summary, biofeedback therapy is behavioral medicine. It is a skills-oriented, multimodal approach in which the treatment protocol is tailored to the individual needs of the patient, self-responsibility is encouraged, and a successful outcome depends on the patient's use of self-regulation skills and strategies.

History and Development

In the mid-1960s, the concept that information feedback enhances learning was not new (nor was the concept of physiological feedback). In that decade, however, several researchers in the United States independently developed instrumentation for monitoring and feeding back physiological information, and they unexpectedly established the foundation for a new therapy. These researchers were of different backgrounds—some worked solely with operant conditioning in animal labs and viewed biofeedback from an operant conditioning model, others worked with human subjects and viewed biofeedback from a self-regulation model. Their common interest was to demonstrate and explore the extent to which subjects can change or regulate physiological processes governed by the autonomic and somatic nervous systems.

In 1969, Barbara Brown, a pioneer in EEG feedback, organized the first conference at which the term *biofeedback* was coined and the national organization, the Biofeedback Research Society, was formed. In 1976, the name of the organization was changed to the Biofeedback Society of America, and in 1988 the membership voted for a more comprehensive name, the Association for Applied Psychophysiology and Biofeedback (AAPB). These changes reflect the evolution of the field from research to clinical applications.

The possibility that humans can gain some control over normally unconscious and autonomic processes seemed unlikely to practitioners trained in traditional medicine and Western science, and skepticism was common. The development of biofeedback instrumentation enabled the scientific demonstration and investigation of psychophysiological self-regulation not previously possible. It soon became apparent that biofeedback is a powerful tool for helping patients alleviate a variety of symptoms, and the new procedure moved rapidly from the research laboratory to the clinic. Biofeedback therapy evolved as clinicians learned to effectively combine biofeedback and therapeutic procedures.

Early clinical research that launched biofeedback into clinical use includes treatment of migraine headache (3), tension headache (4), torticollis (5), hypertension (6), Raynaud's Disease (7), muscular dysfunction of cerebral palsy (8), neuromuscular disorders (9), and epilepsy (10). The simplicity and logic of feedback prompted a rapid development.

By the early 1980s, clinicians in many fields (e.g., primary care, family practice, neurology, psychotherapy, neuromuscular rehabilitation, alcohol and drug rehabilitation, dentistry, pain management) had incorporated biofeedback procedures into their practice, either acting as the therapist or working in conjunction with a biofeedback therapist. Biofeedback therapy evolved from an interaction of these disciplines, which continues to enliven and broaden the field today. Key references for biofeedback therapy are as follows:

- Biofeedback and Self-Regulation, Volumes 1–21 (11)
- Biofeedback and Self-Control, Volumes I–IV (12)
- Basmajian: *Biofeedback—Principles and Practice for Clinicians* (13)
- Birk: *Biofeedback: Behavioral Medicine* (14)
- Blanchard and Andrasik: *Management of Chronic Headache: A Psychological Approach* (15)
- Brown: *Stress and the Art of Biofeedback* (16)
- Green and Green: *Beyond Biofeedback* (17)
- Green and Shellenberger: *The Dynamics of Health and Wellness* (18)
- Hatch: *Biofeedback: Studies in Clinical Efficacy* (19)
- Peper: *Mind/Body Integration* (20)
- Schwartz: *Biofeedback: A Practitioner's Guide* (21)

- Shellenberger and Green: *From the Ghost in the Box to Successful Biofeedback Training* (22)
- Amar and Streifel: *Standards and Guidelines for Biofeedback Applications in Psychophysiological Self-regulation* (23)

MODELS AND TREATMENT EVALUATION

The model of biofeedback used in research is an important issue in the history of the field. In early biofeedback research, two inappropriate models were often used—we refer to these as the *operant conditioning model* and the *drug model*. Both are based on the model of scientific research in which the independent variable is isolated and its specific effects are determined (22).

Although there is still debate as to the most appropriate model for studying biofeedback, we feel that the operant conditioning and drug modes are erroneous, often leading to false-negative results. The fundamental error in these models is the assumption that the biofeedback instrument itself, or a characteristic of the instrument such as feedback, is the independent variable, and that this independent variable should have specific physiological effects. This is analogous to attempting to isolate the specific effects of a mirror or scalpel blade. Biofeedback instrumentation is like a mirror; the instrument and information are useful, but in themselves have no specific symptom-reducing effects. Because operant conditioning and pharmaceutical research are not concerned with self-regulation, these models do not use self-regulation as the independent variable and the main focus of study.

In an effort to isolate the nonexistent specific effects of biofeedback, researchers using the drug model attempted to eliminate the so-called placebo effects and thereby isolate and measure effect of "biofeedback." This was done by eliminating all variables except instrumentation feedback that might enhance self-regulation and symptom alleviation, such as home training and cognitive skills. Researchers using the operant conditioning model referred to the information feedback as a "reward." Because this model assumes that behavior is controlled by rewards, as seems true in laboratory animals, researchers often failed to facilitate self-control in subjects. Both models assumed that the specific effects come from the instrument and not from the individual; this led to erroneous control groups and research designs and limited learning to a trial-and-error strategy. Neither model viewed the treatment as self-regulation based on learned skills. These models led to minimal training, used symptom reduction as the outcome measure rather than skills acquisition *and* symptom reduction, and led to misleading conclusions. When the independent variable is a skill that must be learned for effective treatment, these research protocols generate misleading results because they hinder rather than enhance self-regulation skills and symptom reduction. In summary, these research models are not appropriate for clinical biofeedback and the demonstration of clinical efficacy.

Today clinical research protocols are comprehensive and, in general, a skills model of biofeedback therapy is used. Although research is no longer needed to determine the value of information feedback per se, it continues to refine and enhance training procedures. We include this brief discussion of models, however, because a reviewer of the research on biofeedback, or on any treatment, must critically assess the model being used.

PRINCIPAL CONCEPTS

Principles of Psychophysiological Self-Regulation

The principles that underlie biofeedback therapy are related to the interaction of mental/emotional and physiological processes. We describe four basic principles that are the foundation of psychophysiological self-regulation. By virtue of these principles, health is not merely a matter of good fortune—humans can learn and use self-regulation skills for overcoming illness and maintaining health.

MIND–BODY INTERACTION

The fact that mental images, cognitions, and emotions effect physiological processes has long been recognized in Western medicine as the basis of psychosomatic illness. But anyone who has experienced the instantaneous stress response upon stepping on a harmless garden hose perceived as a snake knows well the effect of the mind on the body. Biofeedback therapy uses this mind-body interaction for promoting health. In teaching mind-body interaction to children, we simply say that everyone has a mind-body team and explain that in biofeedback therapy we train the whole team—that is, mind and body. Biofeedback is an excellent tool for learning psychophysiological self-regulation because the instrumentation provides accurate and immediate information that both verifies mind-body interaction and guides the patient during training.

MECHANISMS

The neurophysiological mechanisms that enable mind-body interaction are fairly well understood and are referred to as the cortical-limbic-hypothalamic-pituitary-adrenal axis. These neuronal pathways in the brain and nervous system mediate mental processes and concomitant physiological responses. A perceived threat—whether to the body or to the ego, real or imagined, severe or mild—triggers physiological reactions. This mind-body interaction affects the stress response and the development of stress-related symptoms. However, these same pathways allow the body to respond to stress-reducing and health-enhancing emotions and mental processes, and ultimately enable psychophysiological self-regulation. Through these mechanisms, mental regulation of the autonomic nervous system occurs, as do all activities that are directed by the mind, whether of the striate voluntary system or the autonomic nervous system. Mind-body interaction is the *sine qua non* of biofeedback therapy, and feedback facilitates regulation of this interaction.

HOMEOSTASIS

When biofeedback was evolving into a clinical tool in the 1970s, health professionals learning about the new procedure occasionally asked, "What kind of snake oil is this?" This question arose because many types of symptoms were responding to treatment. One explanation for this success is *homeostasis*—the body's ability to maintain a "steady state." Hundreds of homeostatic mechanisms allow the body to adapt to changes in the internal and external environments and to return to normal. We explain this principle to our patients by stating that "the body knows how to be healthy." Bernard Cannon, who originated the term, wrote, "When we are afflicted and our bodily resources seem low, we should think of these powers of protection and healing which are ready to work for bodily welfare" (24). Cannon referred to "the wisdom of the body." Unfortunately, there are many ways in which humans disrupt healthy homeostasis, including chronic stress, poor lifestyle habits, drug abuse, and injury. When the body is unable to maintain healthy homeostasis, symptoms appear.

We explain to our patients that although stress "pushes the body off-balance," relaxation brings balance back. The ability to relax deeply and to achieve low arousal is a fundamental skill in the treatment of many disorders because relaxation facilitates return to healthy homeostasis and thus promotes healing. This appears to be true, regardless of the direction in which the body is off-balance. For example, hypoglycemia and hyperglycemia are both improved through relaxation training (25). The body's ability to return to healthy homeostasis explains why so many symptoms are alleviated through seemingly simple relaxation procedures and why people with certain conditions tend to recover without conventional medical treatment.

CONSCIOUSNESS

Consciousness facilitates control, and feedback facilitates consciousness. It is not possible to control behavior and physiological processes of which one has no awareness; therefore, being conscious is fundamental to change.

For example, Mrs. Jones comes to the clinic with raised and tense shoulders; she does not relax and drop her shoulders because she is not conscious of the tension. Although she is conscious of the headache, the muscle tension habit is unconscious. Through biofeedback and other procedures, Mrs. Jones becomes conscious of muscle tension, learns to relax, and develops a new habit. Consciousness facilitates control.

The value of information feedback in this process is analogous to removing the blindfold from a person attempting to play darts while blindfolded—that is, making an impossible task possible. Biofeedback removes mind-body "blindfolds." The trainee (patient) uses information from the instrumentation and the therapist's coaching to become aware of subtle mind-body processes, to learn how to change them and, finally, to gain control of them.

SELF-RESPONSIBILITY AND VOLITION

As we say to our patients, the first three principles (i.e., mind-body interaction, homeostasis, and consciousness) are true, but without the fourth principle—self-responsibility and volition—self-regulation will not occur. Psychophysiological self-regulation occurs only when the patient assumes self-responsibility and uses willpower to learn, practice, and apply self-regulation skills and strategies. From the viewpoint of the autonomic nervous system, so named because of its apparent autonomy from the mind, volition is essential. To create change in this system (e.g., warming cold hands, lowering blood pressure) the patient must intervene, using volition and skills. In neuromuscular rehabilitation, when patients work to retrain muscles and regain function, the importance of willpower is obvious. Because lack of self-responsibility and willpower is the nemesis of successful outcome, biofeedback therapists continually motivate, encourage, and inspire their patients to "go the distance." A patient who is self-motivated and is an enthusiastic *partner* with the therapist may succeed; a patient who is not, or who hoped for a "quick fix," may not succeed.

Principles Applied: Thermal Feedback

These principles and the process of biofeedback are illustrated in Figure 24.1, which demonstrates a patient learning to relax and increase peripheral blood flow through thermal feedback. Blood flow is monitored and fed back to the trainee as skin temperature. Stress induces vasoconstriction, resulting in reduced blood flow in the periphery and decrease in skin temperature; relaxation induces vasodilation, re-

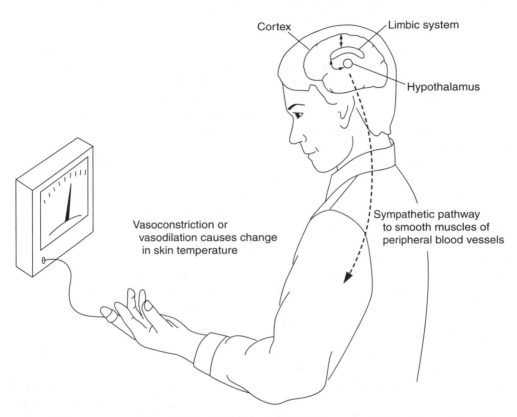

FIGURE 24.1. The trainee uses skin temperature (blood flow) feedback as a guide while learning to relax and increase peripheral blood flow. Neurophysiological pathways mediate mind–body interaction.

sulting in increased blood flow in the periphery and an increase in skin temperature. Peripheral skin temperature therefore reflects both vasomotor activity and emotional/mental states of arousal and relaxation. Anyone who is a "vascular responder" is aware of having unusually cold hands when about to perform in some way.

To learn to relax and increase blood flow in the periphery, the patient uses thermal feedback and a variety of strategies taught by the therapist, including relaxed deep breathing, autogenic training phrases, imagery, and a kinesthetic experience of heaviness in the limbs. Feedback of finger temperature guides the patient and indicates progress in relaxing and increasing pe-

ripheral blood flow. Patients are impressed by the responsiveness of peripheral blood flow to the mind (mental activity). For example, when the mind wanders from the relaxation procedure to a confrontation with a colleague, temperature drops—an excellent psychophysiological demonstration.

Thermal feedback is a tool for relaxation training because increased blood flow in the periphery is a correlate of generalized relaxation. In addition, increase in peripheral blood flow is a treatment for Raynaud's disease and for the vascular pathology of diabetes and arthritic conditions, and it is useful in the treatment of other illnesses with a vascular component, such as migraine headache and hypertension. With increased awareness of stress and relaxation, and with practice, the patient learns to relax and to reduce or prevent symptoms.

The simplicity of this feedback modality belies the complexity of the process and significance of results. Cortical, limbic, hypothalamic, and autonomic processes are regulated through relaxation and counter the extensive physiological effects of the stress response. Without these four principles, psychophysiological self-regulation would not be possible. In addition, therapists rely on important principles of learning, such as generalization (i.e., transfer of training) and mastery, to ensure successful outcome. Patients are trained to master skills, so that they can transfer learning from the clinic to any symptom-triggering situation. Patients are also taught to anticipate triggers and to prevent stress. These principles underlie the ability of humans to achieve a significant degree of psychophysiological self-regulation, implying that we do not have to be passive victims of chronic stress and illness. We can learn to be active in recovery and proactive in maintaining health and wellness.

Etiology of Health and Illness

Biofeedback therapists accept a biopsychosocial, or multicausal, etiology of health and illness. The biopsychosocial approach describes the complex interaction of biological, psychological, and social variables in health and illness, recognizing that in a given disorder one variable may have the greatest effect (although all are important). For example, a car accident victim with chronic pain from physical injury brings to biofeedback therapy a host of psychological and social factors that influence the injury, the experience of pain, and therapeutic outcome. Another example is a gastric ulcer patient experiencing a flare-up during times of stress— biological factors (*Helicobacter pylori*) and psychological factors with physiological components (stress-induced vasoconstriction and thinning of the mucosa) interact. Stress-related illnesses and organic disorders that are sensitive to stress, such as epilepsy and asthma, illustrate

the importance of psychosocial factors in the etiology of illness; likewise, physical disorders, such as cardiovascular disease resulting from obesity or smoking, illustrate that strong social and psychological forces play a causal role.

Based on the biopsychosocial etiology, a distinction can be made between *simple* and *complex* disorders (18). Simple disorders are stress-related and are not the result of complex biopsychosocial factors; they are easily treated with relaxation and stress management techniques. Complex disorders necessitate more extensive therapy.

Diagnosis

Biofeedback therapists who are credentialed to diagnose do so based on standard diagnostic procedures used in the therapist's specialty. When the therapist is not credentialed to make a diagnosis, the patient is requested to obtain a medical diagnosis before therapy if a diagnosis has not been made. In neuromuscular rehabilitation, biofeedback instrumentation is used to assess and diagnose reflex patterns and functional capacity. Experts in this specialty are becoming sophisticated in the use of surface EMG for these purposes and subsequent treatment (26, 27). Although biofeedback therapy does not include medical procedures for diagnosis, therapists continually assess psychological, social, and physical factors that contribute to the symptom or illness.

Therapy

The principles of psychophysiological self-regulation naturally focus biofeedback therapy on mind-body skills and therapeutic procedures that enhance these skills. Furthermore, the goals of biofeedback therapy reach beyond symptom reduction and include improved self-image and self-efficacy, improved quality of life, and skills and resources for health and wellness. The biopsychosocial approach to health and illness automatically leads to a repertoire of therapeutic procedures for addressing the multicausal nature of complex disorders. In summary, the multicausal etiology of psychosomatic and organic disorders necessitates a multimodal biopsychosocial treatment, such as biofeedback therapy, in which remediation of causes and symptoms is the focus.

PROVIDER–PATIENT INTERACTION

Patient Assessment Procedures

HISTORY-TAKING AND PHYSICAL DIAGNOSIS

For most applications of biofeedback therapy, history-taking provides an opportunity for the therapist and patient to examine psychosocial and physical factors involved in the symptom. It also sets the stage for mind–body work. In addition to the verbal history, we use a lengthy inventory that the patient completes at home. The inventory includes symptom history and causes, medications, previous treatments, and impact of the symptom on various activities. The inventory also assesses symptom triggers, stress signs, Type A behaviors, dietary patterns, physical exercise and relaxation activities, assertiveness, goals, and self-image. In our practice, the patient also completes the Cornell Medical Index (28) and the State-Trait Anxiety Scale (29). These inventories are used for treatment design and provide a doorway for addressing psychosocial issues. Intake procedures vary according to the application and preferences of the clinician and are appropriate to the specialty in which biofeedback is used. For example, in neuromuscular rehabilitation, other procedures (e.g., tests of range of motion) are used to assess type and degree of dysfunction.

Finally, some clinicians use a procedure known as the stress profile, or psychophysiological profile, to assess the patient's mode of responding to stress. In a typical profile, EMG, finger temperature, EDR, and heart rate are monitored without feedback while the patient alternately relaxes and experiences a variety of stressors, such as an unexpected loud noise, thinking of a stressful situation, or solving a math problem mentally (23). The profile is a useful teaching tool, and the patient may begin therapy by training on the modality that is most responsive to these stressors. Many biofeedback therapists are knowledgeable about criteria for differential diagnosis but do not diagnose unless qualified to do so.

Determining Treatment

In biofeedback therapy, initial treatment procedures are determined by the presenting symptom and the immediate needs of the patient. The treatment of simple stress-related disorders incorporates standard procedures (e.g., diaphragmatic breathing, autogenic training, progressive relaxation) that are the foundation for relaxation skills and stress management. Treatment protocols for complex psychophysiological disorders include standard procedures and psychotherapy, whereas protocols for treatment of epilepsy or fecal incontinence are unique to these disorders.

THERAPY AND OUTCOMES

Treatment Options

Patients who choose biofeedback therapy receive one or more types of biofeedback training and, in most applications, some type of home practice is required. The options are the range of therapeutic procedures available to the patient based on clinical goals, therapist skill, and specialty. The therapist and patient may decide together on the most effective procedures for meeting the patient's goals. The patient may also be referred to another type of treatment, and it is not uncommon to work with a patient who is referred by another therapist and continues therapy with that therapist.

Description of Treatments and Interventions

Patient education is an important ingredient in biofeedback therapy. Patient education covers the following:

- **The symptom** (in our clinic we use handouts, anatomy charts, *The Merck Manual*, and other resources)
- **The effects of stress, relaxation, and lifestyle on the symptom**

- **The principles of psychophysiological self-regulation and biofeedback procedures**

We also recommend books related to the patient's goals and use a variety of handouts to facilitate training. In addition to biofeedback, the treatment protocol may include other procedures, such as breathing exercises, autogenic training, progressive relaxation, short relaxation techniques, the quieting response, the relaxation response, visualization, stress inoculation training, desensitization, cognitive restructuring, dialogue techniques, and stress management techniques (e.g., time management and assertiveness training). We conscientiously foster hope and positive expectations—essential ingredients for compliance and successful outcome—as we teach and train our patients.

Biofeedback therapists create therapeutic procedures as needed, and they continually seek psychological, social, and physical strategies that aid in recovery and prevention. The therapy is skills-oriented and involves training; the patient learns the therapeutic procedures. To ensure generalization and mastery, home training is required, and patients may be given audio tapes of the relaxation procedures to use at home. An individualized relaxation and visualization tape may also be made for the patient. Temperature feedback is used primarily for home training programs and is possible because the feedback devices are inexpensive and effectively monitor autonomic nervous system activity. Fortunately, one of the best indicators of sympathetic nervous system activity, blood flow in the periphery, is easily measured and amenable to home training. Children are trained in the same manner as adults but often earn prizes for completing homework and achieving behavioral goals (30).

Table 24.1 provides specific examples of biofeedback therapy. These examples, however, can

Table 24.1. Biofeedback Clinical Procedures Used in Certain Disorders

	MIGRAINE	LOW BACK PAIN	EPILEPSY	ASTHMA IN CHILDREN
Teaching concepts	Principles of biofeedback Stress and relaxation response Physiology of symptom	Principles of biofeedback Body mechanics and posture	Principles of EEG feedback Neurophysiology of seizure; triggers	Principles of biofeedback Relaxation response Anatomy of lungs
Relaxation strategies	Diaphragmatic breathing Autogenics with thermal feedback Body scan Short relaxation procedures	Diaphragmatic breathing Progressive relaxation Body scan Short relaxation stretching		Diapharagmatic breathing Bellows breathing Autogenic with thermal feedback
Biofeedback training	Thermal feedback; finger placement	EMG feedback—low back, bilateral, static and dynamic	EEG feedback	Thermal feedback for relaxation EMG feedback on forehead Respirometer
Stress management	*	*	*	As needed
Cognitive strategies	Countering perfectionism and Type A behavior as needed			Changing self-image
Other	Dietary change Assertiveness training as needed	Postural alignment Ergonomics Referral to physical therapy	Lifestyle counseling Behavioral management	Visualization: desensitization to the allergen "clean up and inspection" tour of lungs

*Time management, stress inoculation, and desensitization as needed.

only capsulate treatment protocols and cannot capture the richness of a therapy in which human interaction, teaching, learning, and individual needs are paramount.

Treatment Evaluation

EXPECTED CHANGES

In biofeedback therapy, many changes are expected and nurtured: symptom and/or medication reduction, symptom prevention, increased knowledge of symptom dynamics including biopsychosocial factors, increased knowledge of the dynamics of stress and relaxation, development of a variety of skills involving knowledge, practice, and application. In addition, some patients achieved enhanced sense of self-responsibility and self-efficacy, enhanced self-image, more healthful lifestyle habits, and enhanced quality of life.

UNEXPECTED CHANGES

The unexpected changes that occur during therapy are often as significant and informative as the expected changes. For example, a woman undergoing biofeedback for chronic reflux had a long-standing case of eczema on her hands clear up after mastering temperature (bloodflow) training. Unusual and unexpected results of self-regulation training are not rare (although rarely published), demonstrating the potentials of mind-body interaction and the ability of the body to heal.

ASSESSING THE MAGNITUDE OF CHANGE

Symptom Reduction and Prevention: The Treatment Effect

Symptom reduction and prevention are the primary goals of therapy. In most applications, the patient has a well-documented history of a recurrent or ongoing symptom, such as headache or hypertension. Symptom change is usually assessed by the patient through "symptom charting." Symptom charts are comprehensive enough to track key dimensions of the symptom, such as duration and intensity of headache

and medication use, and are simple enough to encourage compliance in charting. In addition, days absent from work, physician visits, and related indices can be recorded. In assessing behavioral change in children, parents and teachers may keep behavioral records.

Developing Skills: The Training Effect

When treatment is a skill, one cannot assess the treatment effect without assessing the training effect: did the patient learn the necessary skills? Biofeedback instrumentation simultaneously feeds back information to the trainee and continually measures the physiological processes being monitored. Measurement enables comparison of baseline and ending readings within and across clinic sessions. Simple temperature feedback devices enable the patient to keep records of home training.

In many applications, training goals or learning criteria are used as indicators of successful training. For example, the ability to increase finger temperature 1°F per minute indicates successful training in relaxation and blood flow control. Although biofeedback therapists use guidelines and goals for training, individual differences necessitate variation in the criteria for successful training.

After it became evident that a training effect is important for successful outcome, we developed a *mastery model* of training that emphasizes the importance of both learning a skill and mastering it, meaning that the skill can be used during challenging circumstances (13). For example, a patient with Raynaud's disease may be able to increase finger temperature easily in the clinic and at home, indicating that the skill is learned; maintaining finger temperature while shopping in the freezer section of the grocery store indicates mastery. Mastery is assessed through *mastery tasks* in the clinic or in the daily environment. For some patients, life presents many mastery tasks, and these patients demonstrate mastery by overcoming life stressors and coping in healthful ways. Patients' reports of success or failure during life challenges provide ongoing assessment of the training effect.

Changes in cognitions, emotions, and personality traits can be assessed with standard pre-

and post-measurements, although verbal report and clinical observation are usually the primary sources of information regarding these variables as well as changes in quality of life, lifestyle, self-image, and self-efficacy.

TIME PERIOD

There are three time periods of interest in bio-feedback therapy: one relating to the training effect, one to mastery, and one to the treatment effect. Each time period varies according to the patient's disorder, the patient's compliance, and the type of feedback used. In the treatment of uncomplicated stress-related disorders using EMG and thermal feedback, the time period for learning self-regulation strategies and relaxation skills may be only 2 to 4 sessions when the patient practices at home; learning to relax quickly during stressful situations may take another 2 to 4 weeks of training and practice; significant reduction or elimination of the symptom may take longer. In our experience, children learn faster than adults and require fewer therapy sessions for stress-related disorders.

Patients may learn needed skills and achieve a degree of mastery while in therapy; however, the greatest change in symptoms may occur after termination of therapy. If the patient continues to use self-regulation strategies and skills, improvement will continue. For this reason, patients need not continue therapy until the treatment effect is achieved; once the skills are learned, the patient continues on his or her own with follow-up sessions as needed. Self-responsibility is an important underlying principle of psychophysiological self-regulation.

Treatment of long-term disorders with an organic component, such as epilepsy, may be lengthy. In this case, a minimum of 3 months (36 sessions) of EEG feedback training is common (31). Neuromuscular reeducation using EMG feedback for treatment of congenital disorders, such as cerebral palsy, may also be lengthy (8). In all cases, however, biofeedback therapists seek ways of helping the patient develop and use self-regulation skills outside the clinic. For example, a variety of behavioral strategies can reduce seizure rate and, in treating epilepsy, the patient is instructed to use these strategies in daily life (32).

EVALUATING CHANGE

As biofeedback evolved into biofeedback therapy, research with patients raised an important question: is statistically significant change clinically significant? This is a continuing question in medical research. Clearly, the answer is "not necessarily." In biofeedback therapy, the significance of changes in the physiological processes being monitored are evaluated by accompanying clinical results, not on changes in their absolute values. For example, some therapists use 94°F to 96°F as the training goal for finger temperature in treating migraine headache and hypertension (33, 34), but symptom reduction may occur in patients who do not reach this goal and patients who reach this goal may not experience symptom reduction (19). As in most medical treatments, change is evaluated by clinical effects—what works.

Behavioral changes are also evaluated by the ability of the patient to maintain the new behavior and cope with mastery tasks. Biofeedback therapists help patients transform procedures for symptom relief into lifelong skills.

ALTERING TREATMENT

Treatment is altered according to the needs of the patient. It is common to begin therapy for the presenting symptom and discover an important secondary symptom or psychosocial issue that must be addressed. When the biofeedback therapist has a repertoire of skills, changing therapeutic strategies is possible. In some cases, the therapist refers the patient to another specialist and/or recommends other treatment.

Treatment is also altered when a component appears to be ineffective despite the patient's attempted use; in this case, other strategies are introduced. Treatment is altered, or may be terminated, when the patient fails to comply with home-training instructions. Failure to comply is addressed frankly, and the patient and therapist decide on a strategy to improve compliance. Therapists may introduce simpler techniques, create short-term goals, or reexplain the rationale and expected changes. We emphasize that self-regulation is similar to taking a medication—if not used, it will not work. Biofeedback therapists continually explore ways to improve therapy.

USE OF THE SYSTEM FOR TREATMENT

Biofeedback therapy has matured in the past two decades and is currently a primary or complementary treatment for many disorders. Once efficacy has been established, the approach (whether it is primary or complementary) depends on patient desires, effectiveness of conventional therapy, likelihood of success, and other factors. For example, biofeedback therapy may be selected as the primary therapy by patients seeking a nonpharmacologic approach to their condition.

Major Indications

PRIMARY APPROACH

In l989, a select committee of biofeedback clinicians and researchers from several institutions accepted the task of assessing the clinical efficacy of biofeedback therapy for a variety of disorders. This group concluded that biofeedback therapy is primarily indicated for the following disorders in adults and children: Raynaud's disease/syndrome; certain types of fecal incontinence; urinary incontinence; muscle contraction headache; migraine headache; irritable bowel or spastic colon syndrome; essential hypertension; asthma; several neuromuscular disorders; epilepsy in certain patients; and attention deficit disorder (2).

The committee found that biofeedback therapy is also effective for anxiety disorders, disorders of intestine motility, enuresis, insomnia, motion sickness, myofascial pain, temporomandibular joint pain and mandibular dysfunction, some types of chronic pain, such as rheumatoid arthritic pain, and stroke rehabilitation.

COMPLEMENTARY APPROACH

Biofeedback therapy may be considered complementary when the patient is being treated by a primary health care professional, particularly when the illness necessitates traditional medical intervention, as in epilepsy, asthma, and diabetes. The synergistic interaction of two or more therapies can be highly efficacious and enables the patient to receive specialized yet complementary treatment. When biofeedback therapy benefits the patient but is not a specific treatment of the patient's disorder, it may be considered complementary. For example, cancer patients may benefit greatly by the relaxation and stress management components of biofeedback therapy. These skills improve quality of life and enhance the patient's sense of control; when used with desensitization training, these skills may help the patient overcome the side effects of chemotherapy, such as conditioned vomiting (35). Relaxation skills are also combined with visualization. Visualization may effect immune system functioning (36, 37) and relaxation may promote healing through homeostatic mechanisms. Anyone coping with a life-threatening illness or stressful life circumstance could benefit from biofeedback therapy.

Least Useful Indications

Relaxation and stress management skills, coupled with increased sense of self-responsibility and self-control, are useful and may bring relief to many patients. However, biofeedback therapy is least useful for treating chronic conditions in which structural damage has occurred. As a behavioral medicine, biofeedback therapy is also least useful for treating infectious disease, although evidence suggests that relaxation and stress reduction enhance the immune system (37, 38); therefore, biofeedback therapy may, under some circumstances, help patients with an impaired immune system. Biofeedback therapy is also less useful for patients who cannot or will not invest the necessary time and effort in training; it may be of limited use for patients who have difficulty developing internal awareness.

Contraindications

There are no recognized contraindications for biofeedback therapy because the therapy is non-pharmacological, noninvasive, and promotes homeostasis. An incompetent therapist or faulty instrumentation may hinder successful outcome, but the components of biofeedback therapy are not contraindicated or dangerous for any condition. However, because relaxation can induce homeostatic change, patients who use medications to maintain homeostatic balance (e.g., insulin for diabetes, antihypertensives) must be treated with caution. In this case, the patient must conscientiously monitor his or her condition and adjust medications accordingly. Schwartz (1) lists several psychiatric disorders that are assumed to be contraindicated for biofeedback therapy, but no data are available.

Occasionally, a patient experiences emotional or physical discomfort (e.g., dizziness, floating sensations, body disorientation, anxiety) when attempting to relax. We have worked with seven patients who became anxious in the first relaxation exercise. Six patients reported a traumatic experience while undergoing ether anesthesia in childhood, and one patient had encephalitis as a child and recalled the panic of losing consciousness. With coaching, these patients were able to disassociate relaxation and panic and continued therapy. These reactions are rare and do not constitute a contraindication, yet therapists should be cautious and immediately interrupt a relaxation procedure when necessary. By monitoring finger temperature during initial training, the therapist can detect autonomic arousal even when the patient appears to be relaxed.

Prevention

Preventing both the onset of illness and symptom recurrence is facilitated through psychophysiological self-regulation. Biofeedback procedures and self-regulation skills for prevention can be taught in many settings—hospitals, outpatient clinics, schools, and corporations. Soaring health costs necessitate these types of preventive measures. Biofeedback procedures may also be useful in preventing symptoms secondary to a known disease. For example, patients diagnosed with diabetes mellitus type I could learn to increase blood flow in hands and feet and use the

skill regularly. This training might prevent or retard the development of vascular pathology in the extremities. As a treatment, biofeedback therapy is uniquely preventive in two aspects: patients learn how to prevent symptoms (e.g., preventing a migraine headache during the aura) and biofeedback therapy facilitates healthy homeostasis and thus reduces the likelihood of symptom onset and recurrence.

Scope of Therapy

Throughout this chapter, the broad scope of biofeedback therapy and the mechanisms for this have been discussed: the mind-body interaction and neuronal pathways underlying this interaction, the universality of stress and its impact on the body, homeostasis and the power of relaxation, the value of information feedback, and people's ability to gain a degree of psychophysiological self-regulation through training and practice. The broad application of biofeedback therapy for stress-related disorders and for disorders exacerbated by stress is explained by the fact that physiological processes that respond to stress also respond to stress reduction, returning the body to healthy homeostasis. Furthermore, the principles of psychophysiological self-regulation underlie the unusual cases of recovery from organic disease. Finally, the usefulness of feedback in enhancing inner awareness and proprioception underlies the applications of biofeedback therapy for neuromuscular disorders.

ORGANIZATION

Training

PREREQUISITES AND REQUIREMENTS

Biofeedback therapists should be licensed in their profession and/or certified in clinical biofeedback by an accrediting agency. In the United States, the Biofeedback Certification Institute of America (BCIA) is the only certification agency, established in 1981. For certification, BCIA requires 200 hours of formal training from an approved institution in the following areas: didactic education in biofeedback, personal experience with biofeedback, and supervised clinical biofeedback experience (39).

Clinicians applying for certification must have at least a bachelor's degree in an approved health care field, and applicants must complete 30 clinical hours supervised by a certified therapist.

CURRICULUM

The BCIA requires the following for biofeedback therapists: introduction to biofeedback; preparing for clinical intervention; neuromuscular intervention (general); neuromuscular intervention (specific); central nervous system interventions (general); autonomic nervous system interventions (general); autonomic nervous system interventions (specific); biofeedback and distress; instrumentation; adjunctive techniques and cognitive interventions; and professional conduct. There are several avenues for training in these areas, ranging from academic classes to training given by private corporations to seminars given by the Association of Applied Psychophysiology and Biofeedback (AAPB) and other organizations. Training programs are assessed and approved by the BCIA.

Quality Assurance and Certification

The current credential for biofeedback clinicians is certification. To be certified, the applicant must meet educational and training requirements and must pass a written and a practical (instrumentation) exam, all of which are established and administered by the BCIA. Certification is granted for 4 years. Recertification is based on continuing education credits and/or retaking the written examination when sufficient credits have not been earned or when certification has expired. The primary objective of the BCIA is to provide a standard in biofeedback that can be accepted as reliable and valid evidence that the individual provider has attained minimum specific professional competency. A Register of certified individuals is published annually. Certification as a specialist in EEG feedback and in nontherapeutic stress

management education are also provided by the BCIA.

Legal Status and Regulation

Legal recognition of biofeedback therapy as a treatment entity varies by state. Generally, it is considered under mental health provisions, and biofeedback therapists follow the guidelines and procedures established in their state for health professionals. Biofeedback therapists who are licensed in another specialty follow the guidelines and procedures established for their specialty and for biofeedback therapy.

Professional Societies and Continuing Education

The AAPB is an international society that serves its members and the public through publications, oversight committees, working committees for the advancement and acceptance of the field, annual meetings, seminars and workshops, and peer review. Thirty-seven state societies and six international chapters serve some of these functions and hold regional meetings that provide continuing education credit. AAPB comprises six interest sections: EEG, surface EMG, instrumentation, allied professionals, pediatric biofeedback, and education.

Reimbursement Status

Biofeedback therapy is covered by many third-party payers and by worker's compensation in several states. The range of coverage varies with the provider and policy and may exclude certain disorders. With the advent of managed care, restrictions on fees, number of sessions, and the provider have increased. Like other therapeutic modalities, biofeedback therapy is scrutinized by third-party payers and intermediary organizations with an aim at reducing short-term costs. It is our experience, however, that some insurance companies are willing to evaluate coverage on a case-by-case basis and often preauthorize treatment. We anticipate increased coverage as long-term cost-effectiveness studies are completed, and as the value of covering preventive medicine is recognized.

Current CPT treatment codes for biofeedback applications are as follows:

90901—Biofeedback training by any modality

90911—Biofeedback training, anorectal, including EMG and/or manometry

90875—Individual psychophysiological therapy incorporating biofeedback training by any modality (face to face with the patient)

ICD classification for biofeedback—other individual psychotherapy (biofeedback)

Relations with Conventional Medicine

Most practitioners of conventional medicine understand the effects of stress and psychological factors on physical health. It is estimated that 70 to 80% of physician visits are for stress-related disorders. Physicians and other practitioners who inform themselves of the applications and principles of biofeedback therapy readily appreciate the potential of the therapy. Patients who request biofeedback therapy are usually encouraged by their physician to pursue treatment, and some physicians routinely refer patients to biofeedback therapy.

The introduction of behavioral medicine into medical school curricula is increasing and has been well received by medical students and interns (40). This sets the foundation for the incorporation of biofeedback therapy into mainstream medicine.

PROSPECTS FOR THE FUTURE

In 1976, pioneers in the field predicted that in the twenty-first century it will be taken for granted by every school child that mind and body interact (17). The implication is that both lay persons and health care professionals will understand and use mind-body interaction for health. This is becoming true, and biofeedback therapy is becoming an integral part of mainstream medicine. In addition, the use of psychophysiological self-regulation procedures for prevention is becoming more common.

Currently, there are powerful social, economic, and political forces working against health and self-responsibility, including a "quick-fix" mentality that permeates the culture, industries that promote "worseness" habits (e.g., smoking, alcohol), a medical model that focuses on biological rather than psychosocial causes of illness and treatments, and increasing violence and stress. Today, the soaring cost of conventional medicine affects complementary treatments as third-party payers employ cost-containment and managed-care procedures. Nonetheless, the prospects for biofeedback therapy are good. The potential of this therapy for cost-containment and prevention are clear.

We anticipate a bright future in which patients and health care practitioners are partners, medical clinics house a variety of treatment facilities, clinicians work together as a treatment team, and biomedical engineers develop user-friendly instrumentation to feed back parameters that are not accessible today, such as blood sugar levels and white blood cell counts.

In the past two decades, the role of the mind in illness and health has been reinstated in both psychology and medicine. Currently, mind and body are seen as integrated systems. In parallel, medical treatments are becoming integrated, bringing together psychological and physiological forces for health. As the biopsychosocial approach to illness and wellness is adopted, a "whole person" and "whole society" approach to treatment and prevention will evolve, ultimately bringing together the most powerful ingredients of conventional and nontraditional treatments into a comprehensive and integrated prevention and treatment system.

REFERENCES

1. Fogel ER. Biofeedback-assisted musculoskeletal therapy and neuromuscular re-education. In: Schwartz M, ed. Biofeedback: a practitioner's guide, 2nd ed. New York: Guilford Press, 1995: 560.
2. Shellenberger R, Amar P, Schneider C, Turner J. Clinical efficacy and cost-effectiveness of biofeed-

back therapy. Wheat Ridge, CO: Association for Applied Psychophysiology and Biofeedback, 1994: 2–4.

3. Sargent J, Walters D, Green E. Psychosomatic self-regulation of migraine headaches. Sem Psychiatry 1973;5:415–428.

4. Budzynski TH, Stoyva JM, Adler CS, Jullaney DJ. EMG biofeedback and tension headache: a controlled outcome study. Psychosom Med 1973;35: 484–496.

5. Brudny J, Grynbaum B, Korein J. Spasmodic torticollis: treatment by feedback display of the EMG. Arch Phys Med Rehabil 1974;55:49–53.

6. Patel C. Yoga and biofeedback in the management of hypertension. Lancet 1973;2:1053–1055.

7. Surwit RS. Biofeedback: a possible treatment for Raynaud's disease. In Birk, ed. Biofeedback: behavioral medicine. New York: Grune & Stratton, 1973:123–130.

8. Finley W, Niman C, Standley J, Ender P. Frontal EMG-biofeedback training of athetoid cerebral palsy patients: a report of six cases. Biofeedback Self Regul 1976;1:196–198.

9. Basmajian J. Muscles alive. Baltimore: Williams & Wilkins, 1974.

10. Sterman MB, Friar L. Suppression of seizures in an epileptic following EEG feedback training. Electroenceph Clin Neurophysiol 1972;33:89–95.

11. Biofeedback Self Regulation. New York: Plenum Press, 1976–1996.

12. Biofeedback Self Control. Chicago: Aldine Press, 1970–1974.

13. Basmajian JV. Biofeedback—principles and practice for clinicians. Baltimore: Williams & Wilkins, 1979.

14. Birk L, ed. Biofeedback: behavioral medicine. New York: Grune & Stratton, 1973.

15. Blanchard EG, Andrasik F. Management of chronic headache: a psychological approach. New York: Pergamon Press, 1992.

16. Brown B. Stress and the art of biofeedback. New York: Harper & Row, 1977.

17. Green E, Green A. Beyond biofeedback. New York: W.W. Norton, 1977.

18. Green JA, Shellenberger, RD. The dynamics of health and wellness. Chicago: Holt, Rinehart & Winston, 1991.

19. Hatch JP, ed. Biofeedback studies in clinical efficacy. New York: Plenum Press, 1987.

20. Peper E, Ancoli S, Quinn M, eds. Mind/body integration. New York: Plenum Press, 1979.

21. Schwartz M, ed. Biofeedback: a practitioner's guide, 2nd ed. New York: Guilford Press, 1995.

22. Shellenberger R, Green J. From the ghost in the box to successful biofeedback training. Greeley, CO: Health Psychology Pubs, 1996.

23. Streifel S, ed. Standards and guidelines for biofeedback applications in psychophysiological self-regulation. Wheat Ridge, CO: AAPB, 1995.

24. Cannon WB. The wisdom of the body. New York: WW. Norton, 1932:228–229.

25. Schultz J, Luthe W. Autogenic training. New York & London: Grune & Stratton, l965.

26. Cram JR, ed. Clinical EMG for surface recordings. Nevada City, CA: Clinical Resources, 1990.

27. Donaldson CS, Skubick DL, Clasby RG, Cram JR. The evaluation of trigger point activity using dynamic EMG techniques. Am J Pain Management 1994;4(3).

28. Cornell Medical Index. New York: Cornell University Medical College, 1974.

29. Spielberger CE, Gorsuch RL, Lushene R. State-trait anxiety inventory. Palo Alto, CA: Consulting Psychologists Press, Inc., 1968.

30. Green JA. Biofeedback therapy with children. In: Rickles W, Sandweiss J, Grove D, Criswell E, eds. Biofeedback and family practice medicine. New York: Plenum Press, 1983:121–144.

31. Sterman MB. Epilepsy and its treatment with EEG feedback therapy. Ann Behav Med 1986;8:21–25.

32. Reiter J, Andrews D, Janis C. Taking control of your epilepsy. Santa Rosa, CA: Basics Publishing, 1987.

33. Fahrion SL. Autogenic biofeedback treatment for migraine. Mayo Clin Proc 1977;52:776–784.

34. Green E, Green A, Norris P. Self-regulation training for control of hypertension. Prim Cardiol 1980;6:126–137.

35. Burish TG, Jenkins RA. Effectiveness of biofeedback and relaxation training in reducing the side effects of cancer chemotherapy. Health Psychol 1992;11:17–23.

36. Rider MS, Achterberg J, Lawlis GF, et al. Effect of immune system imagery on secretory IgA. Biofeedback Self Regul 1990;15:317–333.

37. Gruber B, Hersh, S, Hall N, et al. Immunological responses of breast cancer patients to behavioral interventions. Biofeedback Self Regul 1993;18: 1–22.

38. Peavey B, Lawlis F, Goven, A. Biofeedback-assisted relaxation: effects on phagocytic capacity. Biofeedback Self Regul 1985;l0:33–47.

39. Biofeedback Certification Institute of America. l996: Wheat Ridge, CO.

40. Anderson GL, Lovejoy D. Behvioral medicine training for primary care physicians. Biofeedback 1996;24:10–11.

CHAPTER 25

HYPNOTHERAPY

Ian Wickramasekera

BACKGROUND

General Definitions and Descriptions

Hypnosis is a form of cognitive information processing in which a suspension of peripheral awareness and critical analytic cognition can lead to apparently involuntary changes in perception, memory, mood, and physiology (1). One hundred years ago, hypnotherapy was an alternative form of therapy in which a patient was induced into a trancelike state, followed by suggestions for the relief of clinical symptoms. Today, hypnotherapy almost always involves adding hypnotic procedures to standard psychological, medical, or dental treatment. It is usually used by those who are already licensed by their state to diagnose and treat disorders within the scope of their medical, psychological, or dental license. This chapter focuses on the use of hypnosis with established forms of psychological therapy, such as psychodynamic psychotherapy or cognitive behavior therapy (CBT), to treat psychological, somatic, or organic symptoms. As our understanding of the neuroendocrine and immune links between mind and body grows (2), it appears that all diseases are psychophysiological in nature. Today, hypnotherapy is essentially a form of psychophysiological therapy (1, 3). There is growing empirical evidence that the addition of hypnosis to an established form of psychotherapy, such as CBT or behavior modification, may increase its long-term clinical efficacy even for some chronic intractable diseases like obesity (4, 5). For example, Kirsch (6) reported from a meta-analysis of eight studies (Fig. 25.1) that hypnosis can double the efficacy of CBT for obesity and that efficacy increases during long-term follow-up (two years). Earlier, a famous meta-analysis by Smith et al. (7) found that the addition of hypnosis to psychodynamic psychotherapy significantly increased its efficacy over all other types of nonhypnotic psychotherapies.

History and Development

Hypnotic phenomena have been reported in all cultures across the world, across all periods of recorded human history, and in various culturally conditioned forms. Manifestations of hypnotic behavior have typically occurred in either a religious or a healing (medical) context. Although hypnosis did not originate over 200 years ago in France with the physician Anton Mesmer (1734–1815), Mesmer deserves recognition as the first person known to propose a naturalistic rather than a demonic explanation of hypnotic phenomena. Borrowing from contemporary physics, Mesmer formulated a theory of hypnotic phenomena based on (animal) magnetism radiating from himself.

The last 75 years of experimental research has clearly established that the bulk of hypnotic phenomena resides in the hypnotized person's natural hypnotic ability, not in any projection from the hypnotist (8). In controlled experiments conducted more than 200 years ago by the French Academy of Sciences, no evidence

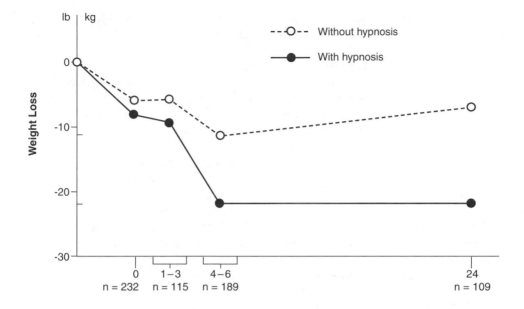

FIGURE 25.1. Weight loss as a function of assessment interval and inclusion of hypnosis in treatment. (Adapted with permission from Kirsch I, Montgomery G, Sapirstein G. Hypnosis as an adjunct to cognitive-behavioral psychotherapy: a meta-analysis. J Consult Clin Psychol 1995;63(2):214–220.)

of projected animal or other magnetism was found. However, the Academy did not deny the empiric efficacy of Mesmer's cures. They concluded that Mesmer was wrong with respect to the mechanism of hypnotic behavior but correct about its clinical efficacy. The French Academy of Sciences alternatively proposed that the mechanism of Mesmer's cures was mere imagination. The Academy was partly right with respect to the hypothesized mechanism of imagination in that it proposed to account for the clinical efficacy of hypnosis. However, it was erroneous with respect to the implication that the potency of imaginative and cognitive effects is trivial. Recent work in cognitive neuroscience has made it clear that the effects of cognitions on biology are very significant (9).

The French Academy's report temporarily hurt the scientific study of hypnosis. In coining the term *hypnotism* (or *nervous sleep*), English physician Braid proposed another naturalistic mechanism of explanation for hypnosis. Braid went on to demonstrate its clinical efficacy in

medical practice. This second hypothesized mechanism of hypnotic behavior has also been proved false by controlled electroencephalographic (EEG) studies of hypnosis in the last 50 years. Hypnosis is definitely not sleep stages 4, 3, or 2 (10).

The third naturalistic, but pathologic, explanation of the mechanism of hypnotic clinical efficacy was proposed by the eminent French neurologist Charcot (1835–1893) in Paris. Charcot's towering scientific reputation and clinical genius resuscitated the scientific and clinical status of hypnosis. According to Charcot, hypnosis was associated with a psychopathologic phenomenon (hysteria) and abnormal central nervous system function. Bernheim, Professor of Medicine at Nancy, France, challenged Charcot's theory and proposed a fourth theory—that hypnosis was caused by the normal behavioral phenomenon of increased suggestibility.

The modern systematic study of hypnosis in the experimental psychology laboratory can be dated to the psychologist Clark Hull, whose research at Yale University led to the 1933 publication of *Hypnosis and Suggestibility*, a classic text. More recently, the eminent experimental psychologist E.R. Hilgard (8) of Stanford University has made major contributions to establishing the scientific credibility of hypnosis with quantitative empirical studies of individual differences in hypnotic ability as well as a theory of hypnosis as "divided consciousness" (11).

Many physicians and psychologists are unaware that in 1955 the British Medical Association cautiously recommended the teaching of hypnosis in medical schools and its use in clinical practice. In 1958, the American Medical Association made a similar recommendation. In 1960, the American Psychological Association officially recognized the American Board of Psychological Hypnosis (ABPH) and its authority to examine and certify diplomates with advanced competence in either experimental or clinical hypnosis. There are now similar national boards identifying advanced competence in medical and dental hypnosis.

Model: Mind-Body Interaction

In 1979, a model of mind-body interaction, in which hypnotic ability was a central component and beliefs were hypothesized to have biologic consequences, was proposed (1, 3, 12–14). There is now evidence from cognitive neuroscience that causality operates in both a top-down and a bottom-up sense (9). Recent empiric neuroscience work has been specifying the neuroendocrine and immune links between cognitions, emotions, and biology (2). There is growing evidence that beliefs may have biologic consequences through neuroendocrine and immune mechanisms (1, 3, 12–14). In fact, in highly hypnotizable persons and under certain conditions (e.g., during stress, highly supportive environments), beliefs can have potent, specific, and reliable biologic consequences that range from allergic reactions, warts, or congenital skin diseases to changes in mammary glands, proneness of the skin to burn or be burnt, and the inhibition of bleeding (1, 12, 15). Converging evidence shows that if threatening beliefs are

blocked from consciousness, under some circumstances they may drive somatic symptoms (1, 3, 12, 14, 16–18) like chronic pain, insomnia, and irritable bowel syndrome; these circumstances may include major life changes, times of low social support, or the individual having a high Marlowe-Crowne score (an operational definition of repression [19]).

These physiologic effects in highly hypnotizable subjects can be more specific and rapid than the effects of drugs. For example, one study (20) demonstrated that it is possible under hypnotic control for an individual to demonstrate significant increases in peripheral skin temperature in one hand and significant decreases concurrently in the other hand. There is no drug that can have such concurrent and specific selective effects on the human body.

Hypnosis and the High-Risk Model of Threat Perception

In highly hypnotizable and motivated persons, hypnosis results in apparently involuntary changes in perception, memory, and mood; these changes can have profound behavioral and biologic consequences (1, 3, 14). This perception of changes occurring without effort or involuntarily is the litmus test of true hypnosis (21, 22). At a baseline level, there are large individual differences in people's response to hypnotic suggestions. There appears to be an association between a patient's measured hypnotic ability and the clinical efficacy of hypnotherapy for several somatic and psychologic symptoms (5, 23, 24). There is evidence from the high-risk model of threat perception (HRMTP) (1, 3, 12–14, 16, 25) that high and also low hypnotic abilities, in interaction with conscious or unconscious negative affect, may be risk factors for several psychophysiologic disorders and some psychological disorders (1, 12, 14, 25). "Highs" will develop a mix of psychological (e.g., anxiety, depression) and somatic (e.g., pain, sleep) symptoms, but "lows" will develop mainly somatic symptoms during trauma or stress (1, 12, 14).

The HRMTP predicts that persons who are high in hypnotic ability will be at risk for stress-related disorders because of their hypersensitivity to the perception of threat; a superior capacity for operant conditioning; an ability to keep secrets from self (e.g., the ability to block memory and perception, as in posthypnotic amnesia and surgical hypnoanalgesia); a propensity to surplus pattern recognition (their tendency to see meaning in apparently randomly distributed events); and a tendency to surplus empathy (their tendency to absorb the emotions of others, with indistinct interpersonal boundaries). The following symptoms have been found to be related to a patient's measured baseline hypnotic ability: migraine pain intensity (26); experimental pain intensity (27); facial pain intensity (28); intensity of chronic urticaria (29); atopic eczema (30); severity of clinical and dental phobias (31, 32); negative moods (33, 34); major depression (35); posttraumatic stress disorder (36, 37); dissociative disorders (38, 39); predisposition to nightmares (40); EEG–defined insomnia (3); substance abuse and bulimia (35); moderate and morbid obesity (3, 41); and nausea and vomiting during pregnancy (42).

This vulnerability of highly hypnotizable persons is probably related to peculiarities in their perception, memory, and mood that amplify negative affect (14, 16). A subset of patients who have chronic somatic complaints that are unresponsive to standard medical or surgical therapy are high or low in hypnotic ability (14). Hypnotic ability is related, in a dose-response manner, to sympathetic electrodermal reactivity (EDR) during experimentally-induced cognitive stress, and hypnotizability interacts with experimentally-induced cognitive stress (16) to drive up EDR in chronic pain patients. High hypnotizability also appears related to alterations in immune function (43). There is evidence that low hypnotic ability during stress may be a risk factor for somatic symptoms associated with pathophysiology (14, 44–46). These symptoms include chronic pain, morbid obesity, response to cardiac surgery, chest pain, and insomnia. It appears that these low hypnotizable patients, because of their rigidly skeptical cognitive style and denial of psychological causation, have limited psychological coping skills, are hyposensitive to psychosocial threat, and delay seeking diagnostic investigation of their symptoms (1, 14, 41). High hypnotic ability is related to sympathetic hyperactivity, and low hypnotic ability is related to dysregulation of the parasympathetic nervous system during stress or trauma (19, 41).

PRINCIPAL CONCEPTS

Despite prior controversy, sophisticated signal processing techniques have shown that, under baseline conditions and during and after hypnotic induction, there are systematic EEG differences between carefully selected high and low hypnotizable subjects (47). It is worth noting that these electrophysiologic differences exist in the frontal and temporal cortex, and that they distinguish between high and low hypnotizable subjects at baseline before any hypnotic induction. These converging data are consistent with the hypothesis that high and low hypnotizables have different cognitive styles and process information very differently both outside of and within hypnosis (1, 3, 12, 14), and that using biofeedback to increase theta EEG waves may at least temporarily increase hypnotic ability (48, 49). Recent work suggests that measuring baseline frontal and temporal theta waves may provide an electrophysiologic test of hypnotic ability.

Hypnotizability and hypnosis have also been shown to be related to the ability to verbally alter a variety of basic physiologic, electrophysiologic, and conditioning phenomena (operant and respondent) during hypnosis. For example, Klein and Spiegel (50) and Whorwell et al. (51) showed that hypnotizability or hypnosis could stimulate and inhibit both gastric acid secretion and a colonic motility index. In a controlled study, Ruzyla-Smith et al. (43) showed that hypnotizability was related to alterations in B cells and helper T cells of the immune system. Black (52) and Zachariae et al. (53) showed that high hypnotic ability was related to the inhibition of the Mantoux reaction to tuberculin, and that during hypnosis the Mantoux reaction could be selectively increased in one arm and decreased in the other. For persons who are highly hypnotizable, hypnotic analgesia is as effective as morphine and more effective than acupuncture (54, 55). Also, naloxone does not block the mechanism of hypnotic analgesia (56, 57). It has been found that hypnotically suggested visual hallucinations alter cortical EEG event-related potentials and not simply verbal reports (58–60). High hypnotic ability can increase the rate of acquisition of learning in both operant (61–65) and Pavlovian conditioning (2) situations. Hence, it is not surprising to find that high hypnotic subjects respond more rapidly to various types of short-term psychotherapy (66, 67) and appear to learn both adaptive and maladaptive responses rapidly and unconsciously (1, 3, 12, 13, 19).

PROVIDER-PATIENT INTERACTIONS

Hypnotizability

Hypnotherapy is the use of hypnosis for treatment and is usually added to some established form of psychosocial diagnosis and therapy (65), such as psychodynamic psychotherapy (7), behavior therapy (65, 85), or biofeedback therapy (65). It appears that a hypnotic induction can potentiate verbal instructions in any social influence situation (65, 86–88). After a hypnotic induction, a variety of psychological techniques, such as age regression (psychodynamic therapy), guided imagery, systematic desensitization (behavior therapy), or the delayed or immediate feedback of biologic information (biofeedback), may reduce specific clinical symptoms (89). The clinical efficacy of blocking or recovering painful, fantasized, or real memories or altering experimental pain perception is related to hypnotic ability (11). The hypnotic induction ritual increases, at least moderately, the following factors:

1. Suggestibility
2. Imagery and fantasy ability
3. Access to primitive modes of information processing
4. Access to early childhood memories and fantasies
5. Tolerance for logical incongruities (e.g., "trance logic," which is the acceptance of

the suggestion that a person is in two different places at the same time)
6. Alteration or inhibition of cognition; selective amnesia
7. Creativity
8. Alterations in the perception of sensory events and muscular response

Empirical evidence exists showing that most of these eight factors can be increased to some degree by a hypnotic induction ritual particularly for persons who have high hypnotic ability (90, 91). Hypnotic ability, like absorption, appears to be a normally distributed stable trait (8, 92), with a .71 test-retest correlation after 25 years. It also appears to be partly genetically based (93, 94).

Hypnotizability associated with a "nonvolitional" response to hypnotic suggestions (22) is not compliance, conformity, gullibility, or social desirability (8, 14). Nor is hypnotizability correlated significantly with any other known personality variable measured on any standard personality tests, such as the Minnesota Multiphasic Personality Inventory (MMPI), California Personality Inventory (CPI), Neuroticism Extroversion Openness (NEO) Personality Inventory, Eysenck Personality Inventory, or the Meyers Briggs Inventory (8, 14). Hypnotic ability is an essential, but not a sufficient, condition to demonstrate the aforementioned eight alterations in perception, memory, and mood. The highly hypnotizable person must also be motivated to participate in the hypnotic induction and to respond to the verbal instructions in hypnosis (22, 65).

Tests of Hypnotizability

There are a number of tests of hypnotizability, each of which has strengths and weaknesses. Hypnotic depth measurements made by clinicians 150 years ago are generally in agreement with psychometrically more reliable and valid procedures developed in the last 50 years. For example, the estimates of the percent of people in the general population with high hypnotic ability and those with low hypnotic ability are similar (68, 69).

STANFORD HYPNOTIC SUSCEPTIBILITY SCALE, FORM C

Currently, the gold standard in the measurement of hypnotic ability is the Stanford Hypnotic Susceptibility Scale, Form C (69, 70). However, the Stanford Form C has many difficult cognitive items, and its distribution of scores is not normal, but it taps a broader range of hypnotic abilities than do other tests. Its use in routine clinical practice is not practical for several reasons. First, this test can be given to only one patient at a time, and it takes nearly one hour to administer. Second, its use in a clinical practice requires a skilled clinician, and it can generate a high rate (29–31%) of negative side effects (e.g., temporary headache or disorientation, nausea), even with otherwise healthy college students (71, 72).

HARVARD GROUP SCALE OF HYPNOTIC SUSCEPTIBILITY, FORM A

For clinical research, there are several reasons to use the Harvard Group Scale of Hypnotic Susceptibility, Form A (73) (HGSHS:A) with congruent subjective validation (21). The Harvard scale was found to correlate .68 (p < .0001) with the gold standard in a recent study (70), and other studies have also found correlations as high as .84 (74). It was found that the HGSHS:A correctly classified more than 80% of highly hypnotizable persons (74). Group testing with the addition of subjective validation criteria (21) permits a skilled technician working under the supervision of a clinician to test 5 to 10 patients in 1 hour with a minimal rate (less than 3%) of negative side effects (e.g., temporary headaches and disorientation, nausea). Using the Harvard scale, Crawford et al. reported a 5% rate of similar negative side effects in normal college students (71).

After being tested on the Harvard scale, the bulk of patients (85%) in a behavioral medicine clinic reported temporarily increased comfort and relaxation. Approximately 5% of these patients even reported immediate temporary relief of their presenting clinical symptom or symptoms. This nonspecific therapy response is brief, but it grabs the patient's attention and improves

general compliance. The Harvard scale correlates (r = .74) with the Stanford, Form C (75), which has been used extensively in large-scale longitudinal and cross-sectional studies of the stability and genetics of hypnotic ability. The Harvard scale has norms on large cross-cultural non-patient samples (69) and even on patients (14, 35, 76, 77). Also, this scale has high reliability, and its validity can be increased by using congruent, subjective scoring procedures (21, 78). Using a technician to administer the Harvard scale avoids contaminating the clinician–patient relationship with "failed" test suggestions. Failed test suggestions are hypnotic suggestions the patient could not experience. In clinical research today, the Harvard scale, along with subjective scoring, has many merits as a first test of hypnotizability. The patient's score can tell what disorders and types of symptoms (somatic or psychological) this patient is at risk for and what the mean rate of therapeutic response will be to learning-based treatments (e.g., biofeedback, cognitive behavior therapy).

HYPNOTIC INDUCTION PROFILE

For purposes of rapid routine clinical screening, the Hypnotic Induction Profile (HIP) (79) has many merits. It is a brief test (10 minutes) that is minimally challenging to the patient and presents hypnosis as a subtle perceptual alteration involving a capacity for attention, responsiveness, and concentration that is inherent in the person and can be tapped by the examiner (79). The HIP has two components: the eye roll sign and the induction (IND). The eye roll sign appears to correlate .34 (p < .001) with the Stanford, Scale C (69). The eye roll is a biologic marker of hypnotic potential but not necessarily of typical hypnotic performance. The IND score on the HIP correlated at .63 with the Stanford, Form C, and when depth ratings from the two scales were compared, the correlation was .78 (80). The aforementioned considerations suggest that the HIP may be a useful, brief measure of hypnotic ability in clinical demonstrations and in routine clinical practice. Its limited acceptance by the research community is a constraint on its use in clinical research.

ABSORPTION TEST

All the previously mentioned tests of hypnotizability involve a standardized hypnotic induction and one or more behavioral or verbal report measures of response to standardized hypnotic suggestions. The absorption test involves neither a hypnotic induction nor an actual measure of response to standardized suggestions (81). The absorption test is a short (10 minute) paper-and-pencil test that correlates moderately with the Harvard and Stanford tests. It inquires about the frequency of naturally occurring hypnotic-like experiences (e.g., the ability to use fantasy and to ignore distractions in everyday life). On some theoretical and empirical grounds, it can be considered a good measure of true hypnotic ability and one of the most difficult cognitive tests of hypnotic capacity (22).

Absorption is a personality trait that is normally distributed, is stable (30-day retest, r = .91), and appears—like hypnotic ability—to be partly genetically based in monozygotic twins reared apart (82) and independent of context effects (83). Like hypnotic ability (1, 12, 14, 16, 25), absorption has also been shown to be a risk factor for several stress-related disorders, such as nonorganic chest pain (45) and somatic complaints in family medicine, as well as morbid obesity (41), nightmares (40), and anticipatory nausea and vomiting secondary to chemotherapy (84).

Absorption appears to provide a nonintrusive measure of hypnotic ability, particularly at the high (above 75%) and low (below 25%) ends of the scale. This test can be given to a patient before a clinical session to obtain a primitive estimate of the patient's hypnotic ability. I suspect that absorption will predict, for example, response to several clinical interventions like acupuncture, guided imagery, noncontact therapeutic touch, herbal therapy, massage, and so forth (1).

WICKRAM EXPERIENCE INVENTORY

Another brief (24 item) paper-and-pencil test called the Wickram Experience Inventory (1) also correlates moderately with measured hypnotic ability and very highly with the absorption scale. Persons who answer "True" to more than 18 of these questions generally have moderate-to-high hypnotic ability. The paper-and-pencil test avoids the large problem of noncompliance with standardized behavioral tests (e.g., Harvard, Stanford) of hypnosis that is encountered with medical-surgical patients (19).

CLINICAL APPLICATIONS OF HYPNOTIZABILITY MEASURES

Estimating the Patient's Hypnotic Ability

The ability to accurately estimate a patient's hypnotic ability noninvasively can have great value in clinical practice. It enables the clinician who is familiar with the empirical literature regarding the base rates of hypnotic ability in specific syndromes (e.g., bulimia) to make more accurate predictions about a specific patient during the initial sessions. The therapist's knowledge of both the patient's cognitive style and the empirical base rates of certain verbally reported experiences and potential behaviors are predictive: individuals who have high hypnotic ability can be told, "you can wake up without an alarm at a preselected time without training; you can find meaning in randomly distributed events or stimuli; you are likely to cry at movies; you are hypersensitive; you can fall asleep easily in a variety of places; you are too empathic; you are prone to mood swings, you spend time in fantasy; you have had several extrasensory perception (ESP) experiences." Persons who have low hypnotic ability can be told, "you are skeptical and pragmatic; you are practical; you rarely day dream; you need to be shown, not just told; and you seldom recall even night dreams." With persons of high or low hypnotic ability, these therapist verbalizations may grasp the patient's attention and interest, enhancing the therapeutic rapport in the critical first few sessions of therapy. Some patients may feel the therapist is "reading their mind." Rapport with the patient may potentiate the therapist's ability to influence the patient's perceptions, memories, and moods about the past, present, or future (19, 86–88). The skilled therapist can often make accurate predictions and postdictions about the patient's present, future, and past life experiences, based on the patient's (high or low) hypnotic ability, that help the patient to very quickly feel deeply understood. The patient is likely to see the therapist as having specialized knowledge, wisdom, and understanding. A patient is more likely to follow the instructions of such a highly credible therapist. The induction of a sense of hope, trust, and mysterious power is sometimes a prerequisite to mobilize a demoralized patient who has chronic disease. This perception of strength and wisdom can be used to help the patient take the initial steps to become an active participant in his or her own rehabilitation. It is done through a hypnotic induction and later through training in self-hypnosis, and it can be confirmed by objective quantitative biological feedback (1, 65).

Estimating How Often the Patient Uses the Hypnotic Mode of Information Processing

It is also useful to know how often your patient typically uses the hypnotic mode of information processing, particularly during stress in everyday life. High hypnotic ability is a cognitive style that has predictable consequences for health and disease (1, 3, 12, 65). I recommend the use of a technician to administer either a formal test, such as the Harvard scale, or even a paper-and-pencil test, such as the absorption test or the Wickram Experience Inventory (1), to secure a quick measure of hypnotizability. The information from the tests is useful even if the clinician never labels the interventions used as hypnotic. For the patient who easily and often uses the hypnotic mode of information processing, the ritual of writing a prescription for an active medication (e.g., benzodiazepine, beta-blocker) can be a type of waking hypnotic induction. The ritual of prescription writing and delivery can be used to secure eye contact with the patient and to give direct, clear, and simple verbal suggestions to potentiate the effects of even small quantities of sleep, pain, or anti-anxiety medication (1). In the case of the patient who has high hypnotic ability, special care should be taken during the interview and patient education to avoid inadvertently delivering negative suggestions that may contribute to iatrogenic illness. If the patient of high hypnotic ability is interpersonally engaged in a negative way, he or she can be a formidable antagonist—one who is creatively resistant and who can even negate the clinical efficacy of specific chemical and surgical procedures of scientifically proven potency (1).

Matching Patient Hypnotizability to Therapy

The ability to use hypnotizability measures to match clinical procedures with patient characteristics has great clinical potential (89). It is essentially matching the patient's cognitive style to specific, empirically validated therapy procedures to maximize the clinical outcome. For example, a patient who has high hypnotic ability but is technologically and quantitatively minded and skeptical of hypnosis should get delayed biofeedback (1, 3, 89). Delayed biofeedback involves the therapist verbally instructing the patient to relax with eyes closed while withholding immediate biologic (e.g., EMG) feedback. The feedback can be provided after 4 to 5 minutes of passive relaxation to confirm the objective changes in physiology. This reduces skepticism and objectively builds the highly hypnotizable patient's faith in his or her ability to alter one's physiology. Immediate auditory EMG feedback can initially interfere with muscle relaxation learning of highly hypnotic subjects (1, 121). Labeling the procedure as delayed biofeedback rather than hypnosis enables the therapist to access instructionally the patient's hypnotic ability while avoiding the mobilization of the patient's skepticism. The patient who has low hypnotic ability can learn to decrease his or her frontal EMG signal (muscle relaxation) most rapidly with immediate EMG biofeedback (1, 121). If a patient with low hypnotic ability has a strongly positive attitude toward hypnosis, hypnotic suggestions can be given along with the immediate biofeedback training procedure, thus capitalizing on the separate placebo or non-specific components of both biofeedback and hypnosis (1, 48, 65). This approach enables the therapist to rationally use both ability and motivational components in hypnotic performance. Although the ability component may not be altered permanently or significantly, the motivational component may be potentiated, attenuated, or neutralized through creative use of labeling procedures and the instructional manipulation of implicit or explicit expectancies. Hence, there are good clinical and scientific reasons (e.g., matching cognitive styles with therapy procedures) to unobtrusively estimate every patient's hypnotic ability in routine clinical practice, especially when dealing with chronic stress-related disease (1, 3). Many stress-related diseases may be driven by high or low hypnotic ability (1, 12).

If a patient has low hypnotic ability but has a positive attitude toward hypnosis, certain psychophysiologic procedures may temporarily increase hypnotic ability. In fact, these pretreatment procedures may be indicated for the majority of patients because only approximately 10% of the population is estimated to have high hypnotic ability. These procedures include sensory restriction, EMG, and EEG theta wave feedback training (1, 3, 48, 49, 65). Both alpha wave and frontal EMG feedback training concurrently increase theta wave production. These procedures are the pretreatment procedures of choice for all patients who have low or moderate hypnotic ability. They probably work by temporarily inducing a relative inhibition of the patient's skeptical-critical-analytic-cognitive functions, which potentiates the therapist's verbal instructions (1, 48, 49, 65).

Summary of Clinician Assessment

The clinician should start by making two assessments. First, he or she should determine with a simple visual analogue rating scale how positively, neutrally, or negatively the patient feels about hypnosis, and how much hypnotic ability (high, moderate, or low) the patient thinks he or she has. Attitudes and self-predictions of hypnotic ability modestly predict hypnotic performance. If the patient has a negative attitude toward hypnosis, the specific sources of the negativity should be investigated. For example, is the negativity based on misinformation (e.g., fear of unconsciousness—I will blurt out private information) or on a humiliating personal experience with stage hypnosis? These negative attitudes can be neutralized by counter-information from the therapist, a high credibility source with whom the patient has rapport. Second, it is necessary to get a valid and reliable measure of

hypnotic ability. This test measure can enhance rapport through therapist statements that seem uncannily accurate in a predictive and/or postdictive sense, even if hypnotic procedures are never used in therapy. If the patient has low or high hypnotic ability, clinical interventions can be planned more economically and rationally than if the information on hypnotic ability was unavailable. For example, long hypnotic inductions and elaborate suggestions are redundant with high hypnotic ability subjects. Patients with low hypnotic ability require biofeedback or sensory restriction procedures before hypnotic induction to temporarily increase their hypnotic response (1, 48, 49).

Therapy and Outcomes

Description of Treatments

Hypnotizability and Clinical Efficacy in Specific Hypnotherapy

Specific hypnotherapy is the use of hypnosis with persons who have high measured hypnotizability. Several empirical studies have shown a correlation between measured hypnotizability and the clinical efficacy of hypnosis for treating asthma, acute and chronic pain, obesity, and warts (5, 24, 28, 95–99). Hypnotizability has also been found to be related to the clinical efficacy of hypnotherapy for severe itching of chronic urticaria (29), pain of atopic eczema (30), obesity (100), smoking cessation (101), allergic skin reactions (52), migraine headaches (102), acupuncture (54), and aversive medical procedures (103).

Nonspecific Hypnotherapy

It is likely that the label hypnosis (9) and the relaxation and sensory restriction components of the hypnotic induction ritual can elicit a temporary increase in hypnotic ability (1, 49, 88, 104, 105) in some persons of low or moderate hypnotic ability. It is theorized that the label hypnosis can activate cognitive motivations, positive attitudes, and placebo expectancies that are independent of baseline hypnotic ability (106). However, it is not commonly observed that motivated but low hypnotizable persons volunteer for major surgery with hypnosis as the only mode of anesthesia.

Treatment Evaluation

Hypnotic induction has been shown to potentiate the effects of psychodynamic psychotherapy (7) and CBT for treating pain, insomnia, hypertension, and—most notably and surprisingly—for the long-term efficacy of obesity therapy (4, 6) (see Figure 25.1). This is noteworthy because there is evidence that obesity is an increasing problem in the United States (107), and long-term weight loss is rare except with surgery (108). The Kirsch (6) and Levitt (5) studies challenged a previous literature review (24), which concluded that the efficacy of hypnosis is limited to involuntary or autonomically mediated symptoms (e.g., pain, asthma, warts). In controlled studies, hypnotic induction and therapy effectively reduced insomnia (109), severe

nausea and vomiting secondary to chemotherapy (110), refractory irritable bowel syndrome (111–113), fibromyalgia (114), allergies (115), and severe burn pain (116). However, the most intriguing findings involved metastatic breast cancer patients—those who used self-hypnosis for pain control in addition to group psychotherapy and standard medical management compared with those who used standard medical management alone (117) (Fig. 25.2). The delayed mechanisms through which hypnosis and group psychotherapy presumably altered neuroendocrine and immune function in this study remain to be explicated.

Hypnosis may also be effective in identifying and uncovering unconscious threatening perceptions and memories that drive somatization and autonomic nervous system dysregulation (1, 3, 14, 16–19, 25, 46). Hypnosis may uncover unconscious real or fantasized trauma. There are clinical reports and controlled studies indicating that hypnosis can influence basic autonomic, neuroendocrine, and immune mecha-

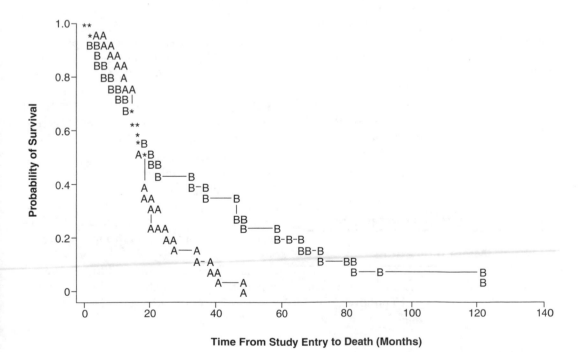

FIGURE 25.2. Kaplan-Meier survival plot of metastatic breast cancer patients in psychosocial treatment study. A = control (N = 36); **B** = treatment (N = 50); * = overlapping control and treatment probabilities of survival. Some points represent more than one patient. (Adapted with permission from Spiegel D, Bloom JR, Kraemer HC, et al. Effect of psychosocial treatment on survival of patients with metastatic breast cancer. Lancet 1989;2:888–891.)

nisms that are implicated in physical healing (23, 43, 51, 90). The efficacy of hypnosis has been measured in terms of clinical examinations, clinical rating scales, reductions in medications, reduced hospitalization, and changes in biomedical tests (e.g., event-related brain potentials, Mantoux test skin reactions, gastric motility index). Generally, the response of acute clinical symptoms (acute pain, anxiety) to hypnosis has a rapid onset. However, randomized controlled prospective studies of adjunctive hypnotherapy have suggested that for chronic diseases, such as metastatic breast cancer (117) and obesity (4, 5), positive effects could be delayed for several weeks or months (1, 3, 4, 12, 13).

In summary, hypnotic ability has been shown to be related specifically to the clinical efficacy of hypnosis. The hypnotic induction ritual is related in a nonspecific way that amplifies the therapy response to a variety of stress-related disorders, even when baseline hypnotic ability is not measured before intervention. Because high hypnotic ability appears to be a risk factor (i.e., contributes to the etiology of the disorder) for several stress-related disorders (1, 3, 12, 16, 25), it is also likely that the hypnotic induction component in these nonspecific hypnotherapies may enhance their clinical efficacy by positively recruiting and redirecting the hypnotic mechanisms of risk that contributed to the development of the stress disorder in the first place (1, 3, 13, 14). In many cases, the negative recruitment of high hypnotic abilities may have contributed to the stress-related disease (1, 3) and therefore can be used to help alter the illness.

USE OF THE SYSTEM FOR TREATMENT

Major Indications

Hypnosis is particularly indicated if the patient has high hypnotic ability and a positive attitude toward hypnosis for treating any clinical condition in which an alteration of perception, memory, or mood can reduce the intensity of a psychological or somatic symptom and/or provide information about the etiology of a disorder. For example, a chronic pain patient with high hypnotic ability and a positive attitude toward hypnosis will profit from suggestions that alter present or future pain perception, blur the memory of past pain, and provide ego strengthening to elevate mood and increase the patient's perception of self-efficacy. Hypnosis appears to be particularly effective for involuntary or autonomically mediated symptoms, such as headache pain, asthma, warts, and irritable bowel syndrome (24, 51, 112, 118). Hypnosis may be effective for patients with moderate or even low hypnotic ability on a temporary or nonspecific basis (placebo basis) if they have positive but realistic attitudes toward hypnosis. Moderate and low hypnotic ability subjects are likely to profit from hypnosis if methods that temporarily increase baseline hypnotic ability, such as theta EEG, frontal electromyographic (EMG) biofeedback, or sensory restriction, are added to hypnotherapy (1, 48, 49, 65, 105, 119).

If there is a need to increase rapport and intensify positive transference reactions, hypnosis may be indicated (64, 87, 104, 120). On a specific or temporary basis, hypnosis may also amplify imagery, memory, and mood (90). All the aforementioned indications should be constrained by professional diagnostic and therapeutic judgments regarding the psychodynamics and psychopathology of each clinical case. Attention should also be paid in each case to the patient's specific pathophysiology, issues of timing, and perceptions of hypnosis. The clinician should cautiously plan therapeutic suggestions.

The following case study illustrates the use of hypnosis in the psychophysiological psychotherapy of a somatization disorder.

Case Examples

CASE 1

Jane went to her internist complaining of shortness of breath that occurred mainly during the night, frequent chest pains, and chronic insomnia. She has also rushed herself to the emergency room more than 25 times in the last 12 months because she thought that she was having a heart attack. She has had the aforementioned symptoms for more than 1 year and denies any premorbid psychiatric or significant medical history. Multiple biomedical tests ordered by her internist and six medical specialists (e.g., cardiologists, endocrinologists, neurologists) have produced no evidence of any pathophysiology. Results from multiple psychiatric interviews and conventional psychological testing were negative for any psychopathology. Jane was then referred for both evaluation with the high-risk model of threat perception and psychophysiologic psychotherapy.

During her initial interview, Jane mentioned that she had dated the same boyfriend for 4 years. She wanted to get married and start a family, but each time she suggested this, he offered a different excuse. She loved him, but he had kept her in a holding pattern for 4 years. Jane made it clear that although this was not an arrangement she would choose, she was not notably unhappy with it. Most somatizing patients are skeptical of psychological explanations and need to be shown, not told, about what bothers them.

On the Harvard test, her hypnotizability was in the high range (11/12). But on all the other high-risk factors—catastrophizing, negative affectivity, Marlowe-Crowne scores, major life change, hassles, social support, and coping skills—the patient's scores were in the normal range. These findings explain all the prior negative findings for psychopathology from the psychiatric clinical interviews and the standard psychological tests. The patient had no conscious awareness of mental distress (e.g., anger, depression). However, hypnotic ability cannot be measured by a psychiatric interview or any conventional psychological test (hypnotic ability is statistically orthogonal to all personality test measures except absorption). Highly hypnotizable persons can keep secrets from their minds but not their bodies (19). A psychophysiologic stress profile (1, 3, 16, 25, 65) of the patient revealed an abnormal respiratory pattern and an elevated and highly variable heart rate response that occurred only during standardized cognitive stress. This abnormal autonomic reactivity was absent under resting baseline conditions.

Uncovering the hypothesized unconscious perceptions or cognitions that were driving the atypical respiration and heart rate responses during psychosocial cognitive stress was the next step. While her physiologic responses were monitored, Jane was hypnotized and asked to talk about and visualize several salient psychosocial topics (e.g., relationship with parents, boyfriend, or specific close friends; medical evaluations). Only on the topic of her relationship with her boyfriend did we observe an amplified autonomic reactivity (episodic inhibition of respiration) and elevated (120 bpm) and variable (55–120 bpm) heart rate that was associated with a verbal report of anger and even rage at her boyfriend. She reported during hypnosis feeling choked or strangled in the relationship. After the termination of the boyfriend topic, her physiology abruptly returned to normal. She had total spontaneous amnesia to both her autonomic nervous system (ANS) reactions and her specific emotional reactions to her boyfriend.

When I told Jane that her relationship with her boyfriend was perhaps distressing her more than she realized, she was incredulous and burst out laughing. The next step was to show her, on the monitoring instruments, the ANS changes produced by thoughts, memories, and images of her boyfriend when she was not hypnotized. The topic of her boyfriend reliably elicited ANS abnormalities, but to a lesser degree during waking psychotherapy than during hypnosis. She began to recognize during psychotherapy the extent to which she felt frustrated by, trapped by, and angry at her boyfriend. Within a few weeks, her clinical symptoms reduced in both intensity and frequency, and she began to explore alternative social and dating relationships. She was also able, in a few weeks, to phase off all the psychotropic and sleep medications she had used to cope with the sympathetic activation that was driven by her unconscious rage at her boyfriend.

All cases are not this simple. Many somatizing patients are addicted to narcotic, sleep, or psychotropic medications or have had multiple unsuccessful surgeries. They are angry, demoralized, skeptical, and bitter, and they continue to press for a strictly medical solution to their exclusive somatic symptoms. The difficult part is finding the unconscious factors maintaining the somatic stress response and showing, not just telling, the patient how these stressors drive somatic symptoms. The electronic instruments used in psychophysiologic psychotherapy track the biologic correlates of unconscious, threatening psychological events (3, 17, 18, 25, 46). In amplifying these biologic correlates so that they become recognizable to the patient, these instruments operate as truth detectors rather than lie detectors.

Contraindications

The major contraindications to hypnosis are poor psychodiagnostic and psychotherapeutic skills of the therapist and, particularly, countertransference problems in the therapist. Everything that occurs in psychotherapy occurs with more rapid onset when hypnotherapy is used, and so the clinician should be skilled in psychotherapy (1). Also, high hypnotic ability poses a risk for appropriate physician-patient boundaries. The therapist should examine his or her motives for adding hypnosis to psychotherapy as well as the patient's motives for requesting hypnosis. Is the patient looking for a magical cure in which the patient is not an active participant? Is the patient looking for some fantasied or real history of abuse that legitimizes a passive victimlike role in psychotherapy and life? Is the patient's ego stable and integrated enough to do abreactive, regressive, or uncovering psychodynamic work? Certain diagnoses, such as borderline personality, major dissociative disorders, and paranoid reactions, require great clinical skill when hypnosis is used.

ORGANIZATION

Training and Quality Assurance

A therapist should not treat a patient with hypnosis for any condition for which the therapist would not treat that patient without hypnosis. For example, the pain of a brain tumor or fractured bone should not be treated exclusively with hypnotic analgesia. Hypnosis is simply an adjunct to the treatment process and is seldom a permanent treatment in and of itself. Hence, persons who are candidates to be trained to use hypnotic techniques in clinical practice must be licensed professionals in psychology, medicine, or other health-related professions. They should recognize the scope of their diagnostic competence. Psychologists should not treat brain tumors, and neurologists should not treat dissociative disorders. The American Society of Clinical Hypnosis, the Society for Clinical and Experimental Hypnosis, and the International Society of Hypnosis have established codes of ethics that define and limit the persons who can be taught hypnosis. The American Boards of Hypnosis identify clinicians with advanced competence in psychological (American Board of Psychological Hypnosis), medical (American Board of Medical Hypnosis), and dental (American Board of Dental Hypnosis) hypnosis. Information about board-certified clinicians can be secured by calling or writing to The American Society of Clinical Hypnosis in Des Plaines, Illinois (telephone: 847–297–3317; 2200 E. Devon Avenue, Des Plaines, 60018).

Legislative bodies have not imposed a licensing structure on hypnosis and hypnotherapy as an adjunctive treatment modality restricted to health care providers. Individuals who are unlicensed and untrained in health care professions advertise hypnotherapy for many symptoms despite the fact that they are not licensed to diagnose and treat somatic or psychological disorders. In highly hypnotizable persons who are not correctly diagnosed, hypnosis can mask organic disease (e.g., pain of brain tumor) or a serious mental disorder (according to the *Diagnostic and Statistical Manual of Mental Disorders* [DSM-IV]). Because hypnosis and hypnotherapy are not restricted by law, there is no effective way to censure or police unlicensed individuals other than through public education. For example, using people with high hypnotic ability and a history of trauma for entertainment is always hazardous, but there is currently no legislative restriction on irresponsible people to keep them from abusing others in this way.

Reimbursement Status

The use of hypnosis as an adjunct to medical, dental, and psychotherapy procedures is covered by many (but not all) insurance companies and is included in CPT diagnostic codes used in medicine and psychotherapy. Outside of this, hypnosis is generally not reimbursed.

PROSPECTS FOR THE FUTURE

It appears that one of the most promising applications of hypnosis is in the primary prevention of somatization disorders and stress-related diseases (1, 14, 19, 25, 65). This may involve 50% of all patients seen by primary care medicine (122). Somatization has been called "one of medicine's blind spots," (123) and an editorial described it as medicine's "unsolved problem" (124). One of the most promising diagnostic and therapeutic applications of hypnosis is with psychophysiologic psychotherapy (1, 3, 16, 19, 25) for somatization disorders. As our understanding of the intricate connections between mind and body grows, hypnosis will likely play a key role in the treatment of disease and in improvement in quality of life. With its extensive theoretical, experimental, and empirical base, hypnosis is both a complement and an occasional alternative to conventional treatments. The role of hypnosis will also expand as new techniques for enhancing hypnotic ability in the general population are further developed.

REFERENCES

1. Wickramasekera I. Clinical behavioral medicine: some concepts and procedures. New York: Plenum, 1988.
2. National Academy of Science Institute of Medicine Report. Behavioral influences on the endocrine and immune systems. Washington DC: National Academy Press, 1989.
3. Wickramasekera I. Assessment and treatment of somatization disorders: the high risk model of threat perception. In: Rhue J, Lynn S, Kirsch I, eds. Handbook of clinical hypnosis. Washington, DC: American Psychological Association, 1993: 587–621.
4. Kirsch I, Montgomery G, Sapirstein G. Hypnosis

as an adjunct to cognitive-behavioral psychotherapy: a meta-analysis. J Consult Clin Psychol 1995;63(2):214–220.
5. Levitt EE. Hypnosis in the treatment of obesity. In: Rhue JW, Lynn SJ, Kirsch I, eds. Handbook of clinical hypnosis. Washington, DC: American Psychological Association, 1993:511–532.
6. Kirsch I. Hypnotic enhancement of cognitive-behavioral weight loss treatments—another meta-reanalysis. J Consult Clin Psychol 1996;64(3): 517–519.
7. Smith ML, Glass GV, Miller TI. The benefits of psychotherapy. Baltimore: John Hopkins University Press, 1980.
8. Hilgard ER. Hypnotic susceptibility. New York: Harcourt, Brace and World, 1965.
9. Sperry R. Mind-brain interaction. Neuroscience 1980;5:195–206.
10. Evans FJ. Hypnosis and sleep: techniques for exploring cognitive activity during sleep. In: Fromm E, Shor RE, eds. Hypnosis: developments in research and new perspectives, 2nd ed. New York: Aldine, 1979:139–183.
11. Hilgard ER. Divided consciousness: multiple controls in human thought and action. New York: Wiley, 1977.
12. Wickramasekera I. A model of the patient at high risk for chronic stress related disorders: do beliefs have biological consequences? Paper presented at the Annual Convention of the Biofeedback Society of America, San Diego, CA, 1979.
13. Wickramasekera I. A model of people at high risk to develop chronic stress related somatic symptoms: some predictions. Prof Psychol: Res Prac 1986;17(5):437–447.
14. Wickramasekera I. Somatization: concepts, data and predictions from the high risk model of threat perception. J Nerv Ment Dis 1995;183(1):15–23.
15. Barber TX. Changing "unchangeable" bodily processes by (hypnotic) suggestion: a new look at hypnosis, cognitions, imagining, and the mind-body problem. Advances 1984;1(2):6–40.
16. Wickramasekera I, Pope AT, Kolm P. On the interaction of hypnotizability and negative affect in chronic pain: implications for the somatization of trauma. J Nerv Ment Dis 1996;184:628–635.
17. Wickramasekera I. On the interaction of two orthogonal risk factors, 1) hypnotic ability and 2) negative affectivity (threat perception) for psychophysiological disregulation in somatization. Second Symposium on Suggestion and Suggestibility, University of Rome, Italy, 1994.
18. Wickramasekera I. Somatic psychological symptoms and information transfer from implicit to explicit memory: a controlled case study with pre-

dictions from the High Risk Model of Threat Perception. Dissociation 1994;7(3):153–166.

19. Wickramasekera I. Secrets kept from the mind but not from the body or behavior. Advances 1998;14:81–98.

20. Maslach C, Marshall G, Zimbardo PG. Hypnotic control of peripheral skin temperature: a case report. Psychophysiology 1972;9:600–605.

21. Kirsch I, Council JR, Wickless C. Subjective scoring for the Harvard Group Scale of Hypnotic Susceptibility, Form A. Int J Clin Exp Hypn 1990;38:112–124.

22. Woody EZ, Bowers KS, Oakman JM. A conceptual analysis of hypnotic responsiveness: experience, individual differences, and context. In: Fromm E, Nash MR, eds. Contemporary hypnosis research. New York: Guilford Press, 1992: 3–33.

23. Brown DP. Clinical hypnosis research since 1986. In: Fromm E, Nash MR, eds. Contemporary hypnosis research. New York: Guilford Press, 1992:427–458.

24. Wadden TA, Anderton CH. The clinical use of hypnosis. Psychol Bull 1982;91:215–243.

25. Wickramasekera I, Davies T, Davies M. Applied psychophysiology: a bridge between the biomedical model and the biopsychosocial model in family medicine. Prof Psychol: Res Prac 1996;27(3):221–233.

26. Andreychuk T, Skriver C. Hypnosis and biofeedback in the treatment of migraine headaches. Int J Clin Exp Hypn 1975;13(3):172–183.

27. DeBenedittis G, Paneral AA, Villamirqa MA. Effects of hypnotic analgesia and hypnotizability on experimental ischemic pain. Int J Clin Exp Hypn 1989;37(1):55–69.

28. Stam H, McGrath P, Brooke R, Cosire F. Hypnotizability and the treatment of chronic facial pain. Int J Clin Exp Hypn 1986;34:182–191.

29. Shertzer CI, Lookingbill CI, Lookingbill DP. Effects of relaxation therapy and hypnotizability in chronic urticaria. Arch Dermatol 1987;123:913–916.

30. H'ajek P, Jakoubek B, Radil T. Gradual increase in cutaneous threshold induced by repeated hypnosis of healthy individuals and patients with atopic eczema. Percept Mot Skills 1990;70:549–550.

31. John R, Hollander B, Perry C. Hypnotizability and phobic behavior: further supporting data. J Abnorm Psychol 1983;92(3):390–392.

32. Kelly SF. Measured hypnotic response and phobic behavior. A brief communication. Int J Clin Exp Hypn 1984;32(1):1–5.

33. Crowson JJ, Conroy AM, Chester TD. Hypnotizability as related to visually induced affective reactivity. Int J Clin Exp Hypn 1991;39(3):140–144.

34. Velten E. A laboratory task for induction of mood states. Behav Res Ther 1968;18:79–86.

35. Pettinati HM, Kogan LG, Evans FJ, et al. Hypnotizability of psychiatric inpatients according to two different scales. Am J Psychiatry 1990; 147(1):69–75.

36. Spiegel D, Hunt T, Dondershine H. Dissociation and hypnotizability in post-traumatic stress disorder. Am J Psychiatry 1988;145:301–305.

37. Stutman RK, Bliss EL. Post-traumatic stress disorder, hypnotizability, and imagery. Am J Psychiatry 1985;142(6):741–743.

38. Braun GG, Sachs RG. The development of multiple personality disorder: predisposing, precipitating, and perpetuating factors. In: Kluft RP, ed. Childhood antecedents of multiple personality. Washington, DC: American Psychiatric Press, 1985:37–64.

39. Putnam FW. Diagnosis and treatment of multiple personality disorder. New York: Guilford Press, 1989.

40. Belicki K, Belicki D. Predisposition for nightmares: a study of hypnotic ability, vividness of imagery, and absorption. J Clin Psychol 1986; 42:714–718.

41. Wickramasekera I, Price D. Morbid obesity, absorption, neuroticism and the high risk model of threat perception. Am J Clin Hypn 1997; 34(4):291–302.

42. Apfel RJ, Kelley SF, Frankel FH. The role of hypnotizability in the pathogenesis and treatment of nausea and vomiting of pregnancy. J Psychosom Obstet Gynecol 1986;5:179–186.

43. Ruzyla-Smith P, Barabasz A, Barabasz M, Warner D. Effects of hypnosis on the immune response: B-cells, T-cells, helper and suppressor cells. Am J Clin Hypn 1995;38(2):71–79.

44. Greenleaf M, Fisher, S, Miaskowski C, DuHamel K. Hypnotizability and recovery from cardiac surgery. Am J Clin Hypn 1992;35(2):119–128.

45. Saxon J, Wickramasekera I. Discriminating patients with organic disease from somatizers among patients with chest pain using factors from the high risk model of threat perception. Meeting of the Society for Experimental and Clinical Hypnosis. San Francisco, CA, October 1994.

46. Wickramasekera I, Wickramasekera II I. EMG correlates in hypnosis: recall of a repressed memory: A case report. Dissociation. In press.

47. Graffin NF, Ray WJ, Lundy R. EEG concomitants of hypnosis and hypnotic susceptibility. J Abnorm Psychol 1995;104(1):123–131.

48. Wickramasekera I. The placebo effect and medical instruments in biofeedback. J Clin Eng 1977;2(3):227–230.

49. Wickramasekera I. On attempts to modify hypnotic susceptibility: some psychophysiological procedures and promising directions. Ann N Y Acad Sci 1977;296:143–153.

50. Klein KB, Spiegel D. Modulation of gastric acid secretion by hypnosis. Gastroenterology 1989; 96:1383–1387.

51. Whorwell PJ, Houghton LA, Taylor EE, Maxton DG. Physiological effects of emotion: assessment via hypnosis. Lancet 1992;340:69–72.

52. Black S. Inhibition of immediate-type hypersensitivity response by direct suggestion under hypnosis. Br Med J 1963;6:925–929.

53. Zachariae R, Bjerring P, Arendt-Nielsen L. Modulation of type I immediate and type IV delayed immunoreactivity using direct suggestion and guided imagery during hypnosis. Allergy 1989; 44(8):537–542.

54. Knox VJ, Gekoski WL, Shum K, McLaughlin DM. Analgesia for experimentally induced pain: Multiple sessions of acupuncture compared to hypnosis in high-and low-susceptible subjects. J Abnorm Psychol 1981;90:28–34.

55. Stern JA, Brown M, Ulett A, Sletten I. A comparison of hypnosis, acupuncture, morphine, Valium, aspirin, and placebo in the management of experimentally induced pain. Ann N Y Acad Sci 1977;296:175–193.

56. Barber J, Mayer DJ. Evaluation of the efficacy and neural mechanism of a hypnotic analgesia procedure in experimental and clinical dental pain. Pain 1977;4:41–48.

57. Goldstein A, Hilgard ER. Lack of influence of the morphine antagonist naloxone on hypnotic analgesia. Proc Natl Acad Sci USA 1975;72: 2041–2043.

58. Blum GS, Nash J. Posthypnotic attenuation of a visual illusion as reflected in perceptual reports and cortical event-related potentials. Acad Psychol Bull 1981;3:251–271.

59. Spiegel D, Cutcomb S, Ren C, Pribram K. Hypnotic hallucination alters evoked potentials. J Abnorm Psychol 1985;94:249–255.

60. Spiegel D, Barabasz AF. Effects of hypnotic instructions on P300 event-related-potential amplitudes: research and clinical applications. Am J Clin Hypn 1988;31:11–17.

61. King DR, McDonald RD. Hypnotic susceptibility and verbal conditioning. Int J Clin Exp Hypn 1976;24:29–37.

62. Webb RA. Suggestibility and verbal conditioning. Int J Clin Exp Hypn 1962;10:275–279.

63. Weiss RL, Ullman LP, Krasner L. On the relationship between hypnotizability and response to verbal operant conditioning. Psychol Rep 1960;6: 59–60.

64. Wickramasekera I. The effects of hypnosis and a control procedure on verbal conditioning. Paper presented at the annual meeting of the American Psychological Association, Miami, FL, 1970.

65. Wickramasekera I. Biofeedback, behavior therapy and hypnosis. Chicago: Nelson Hall, 1976.

66. Larsen S. Strategies for reducing phobic behavior. Dissertation Abstracts International 1966;26: 6850.

67. Nace EP, Warwick AM, Kelley RL, Evans FJ. Hypnotizability and outcome in brief psychotherapy. J Clin Psychiatry 1982;43:129–133.

68. Bates BL. Individual differences in response to hypnosis. In: Rhue JW, Lynn SJ, Kirsch I, eds. Handbook of clinical hypnosis. Washington, DC: American Psychological Association, 1993:23–54.

69. Perry C, Nandon R, Button J. The measurement of hypnotic ability. In: Fromm E, Nash MR, eds. Contemporary hypnosis research. New York: Guilford Press, 1992:459–490.

70. Kurtz RM, Strube MJ. Multiple susceptibility testing: is it helpful? Am J Clin Hypn 1996; 38(3):172–184.

71. Crawford HJ, Hilgard JR, Macdonald H. Transient experiences following hypnotic testing and special termination procedures. Int J Clin Exp Hypn 1982;30:117–126.

72. Hilgard ER. Sequelae to hypnosis. Int J Clin Exp Hypn 1974;22:281–298.

73. Shor RE, Orne EC. Harvard Group Scale of Hypnotic Susceptibility, Form A. Palo Alto, CA: Consulting Psychologists Press, 1962.

74. Green J, Lynn S, Carlson B. Finding the hypnotic virtuoso—another look. Int J Clin Exp Hypn 1992;50:68–73.

75. Bowers KS. Hypnosis for the seriously curious. Monterey, CA: Brooks/Cole, 1976.

76. Jupp JJ, Collins JK, McCabe MP. Estimates of hypnotizability: standard group scale versus subjective impression in clinical populations. Int J Clin Exp Hypn 1985;33(2):140–149.

77. Pettinati H, Horne RL, Staats JM. Hypnotizability in patients with anorexia nervosa and bulimia. Arch Gen Psychiatry 1985;42:1014–1016.

78. Kumar VK, Geddes M, Pekala RJ. Behavioral and subjective scoring of the Harvard group scale of

hypnotic susceptibility: further data and an extension. Am J Clin Hypn 1996;38(3):191–199.

79. Spiegel H, Spiegel D. Trance and treatment: clinical uses of hypnosis. New York: Basic Books, 1978.

80. Frischholz EJ, Tryon WW, Vellios AT, et al. The relationship between the Hypnotic Induction Profile and the Stanford Hypnotic Susceptibility Scale, Form C: a replication. Am J Clin Hypn 1980;22:185–196.

81. Roche SM, McConkey M. Absorption: nature, assessment, and correlates. J Pers Soc Psychol 1990;59(1):91–101.

82. Tellegen A, Lykken DT, Bouchard TJ Jr, et al. Personality similarity in twins reared apart and together. J Pers Soc Psychol 1988;54(6):1031–1039.

83. Nadon R, Hoyt IP, Register PA, Kihlstrom JF. Absorption and hypnotizability: context effects reexamined. J Pers Soc Psychol 1991;60:144–153.

84. Challis GB, Stam HJ. A longitudinal study of the development of anticipatory nausea and vomiting in cancer chemotherapy patients: the role of absorption and autonomic perception. Health Psychol 1992;11(3):181–189.

85. Bolocofsky DN, Spinter D, Coulthard-Morris L. Effectiveness of hypnosis as an adjunct to behavioral weight management. J Clin Psychol 1985;41:35–41.

86. Wickramasekera I. Goals and some methods in psychotherapy: hypnosis and isolation. Am J Clin Hypn 1970;13(2):95–100.

87. Wickramasekera I. Reinforcement and/or transference in hypnosis and psychotherapy: a hypothesis. Am J Clin Hypn 1970;12(3):137–140.

88. Wickramasekera I. Effects of "hypnosis" and task motivational instructions in attempting to influence the "voluntary" self-deprivation of money. J Pers Soc Psychol 1971;19(3):311–314.

89. Zillmer EA, Wickramasekera I. Biofeedback and hypnotizability: initial treatment considerations. Clin Biofeedback Health 1987;10(1):51–57.

90. Holroyd J. Hypnosis as a methodology in psychological research. In: Fromm E, Nash MR, eds. Contemporary hypnosis research. New York: Guilford Press, 1992:201–226.

91. Shames VA, Bowers PG. Hypnosis and creativity. In: Fromm E, Nash MR, eds. Contemporary hypnosis research. New York: Guilford Press, 1992: 334–363.

92. Piccione C, Hilgard ER, Zimbardo PG. On the degree of stability of measured hypnotizability over a 25-year period. J Pers Soc Psychol 1989; 56(2):289–295.

93. Morgan AH, Hilgard ER, Davert EC. The heritability of hypnotic susceptibility in twins: a preliminary report. Behav Genet 1970;1:213–224.

94. Morgan AH. The heritability of hypnotic susceptibility in twins. J Abnorm Psychol 1973;82: 55–61.

95. Barabasz AF, Barabasz M. Effects of restricted environmental stimulation: enhancement of hypnotizability for experimental and chronic pain control. Int J Clin Exp Hypn 1989;37:217–231.

96. Collison DA. Which asthmatic patients should be treated by hypnotherapy. Med J Aust 1975;1: 776–781.

97. Ewer TC, Stewart DE. Improvement in bronchial hyperresponsiveness in patients with moderate asthma after treatment with a hypnotic technique. Br Med J 1986;1:1129–1132.

98. Hilgard ER, Hilgard JR. Hypnosis in the relief of pain. Los Altos, CA: William Kaufmann, 1975.

99. Murphy AI, Lehrer PM, Karlin R, et al. Hypnotic susceptibility and its relationship to outcome in the behavioral treatment of asthma: some preliminary data. Psychol Rep 1989;65(2):691–698.

100. Andersen MS. Hypnotizability as a factor in the hypnotic treatment of obesity. Int J Clin Exp Hypn 1985;33:150–159.

101. Barabasz AF, Baer L, Sheehan DV, Barabasz M. A three year clinical follow-up of hypnosis and restricted environmental stimulation therapy for smoking. Int J Clin Exp Hypn 1986;34:169–181.

102. Cedercreutz C. Hypnotic treatment of 100 cases of migraines. In: Frankel FH, Zamansky HS, eds. Hypnosis at its bicentennial. New York: Plenum Press, 1978.

103. Wall VJ, Womack W. Hypnotic versus active cognitive strategies for alleviation of procedural distress in pediatric oncology patients. Am J Clin Hypn 1989;31(3):181–189.

104. Wickramasekera I. Effects of sensory restriction on susceptibility to hypnosis. J Abnorm Psychol 1970;76:69–75.

105. Wickramasekera I. Effects of EMG feedback training on susceptibility to hypnosis: preliminary observations (summary). Proceedings, 79th Annual Convention of the American Psychological Association 1971;6:783–784.

106. Kirsch I. Changing expectations: a key to effective psychotherapy. Pacific Grove, CA: Brooks/ Cole, 1990.

107. Kuczmarski RJ. Prevalence of overweight and weight gain in the United States. Am J Clin Nutr 1992;55:495S–502S.

108. Brownell KD, Rodin J. The dieting maelstrom: is it possible and advisable to lose weight? Am Psychologist 1994;49(9):781–791.

109. Stanton HE. Hypnotic relaxation and the reduction of sleep onset insomnia. Int J Psychosomat 1989;35(1–4):64–68.

110. Walker LG, Dawson AA, Pollet SM, et al. Hypnotherapy for chemotherapy side effects. Br J Exp Clin Hypn 1988;5(2):79–82.

111. Harvey RF, Hinton RA, Gunary RM. Individual and group hypnotherapy in treatment of refractory irritable bowel syndrome. Lancet 1989;1:424–425.

112. Whorwell PJ, Prior A, Faragher EB. Controlled trial of hypnotherapy in the treatment of severe refractory irritable bowel syndrome. Lancet 1984;2:1232–1234.

113. Whorwell PJ, Prior A, Colgan SM. Hypnotherapy in severe irritable bowel syndrome: further experience. Gut 1987;28:423–425.

114. Haanen HCM, Hoenderdos TW, Romunde LKJ, et al. Controlled trial of hypnotherapy in the treatment of refractory fibromyalgia. J Rheumatol 1991;18(1):72–75.

115. Madrid A, Rostel G, Pennington D, Murphy D. Subjective assessment of allergy relief following group hypnosis and self-hypnosis: a preliminary study. Am J Clin Hypn 1995;38(2):80–86.

116. Patterson DR, Goldberg ML, Ehde DM. Hypnosis in the treatment of patients with severe burns. Am J Clin Hypn 1996;38(3):200–212.

117. Spiegel D, Bloom JR, Kraemer HC, Gottehil E. Effect of psychosocial treatment on survival of patients with metastatic breast cancer. Lancet 1989;2:888–891.

118. Whorwell PJ. Hypnotherapy in irritable bowel syndrome. Lancet 1989;1:622.

119. Barabasz AF, Barabasz M, eds. Clinical and experimental restricted environmental stimulation: new developments and perspectives. New York: Springer-Verlag, 1993.

120. Fromm E, Nash MR, eds. Contemporary hypnosis research. New York: Guilford, 1992.

121. Qualls PJ, Sheehan PW. Electromyograph biofeedback as a relaxation technique. A critical appraisal and reassessment. Psychol Bull 1981;90(1):21–42.

122. De Gruy F. Mental health care in the primary care setting. Washington, DC: National Academy Press, 1996.

123. Quill TE. Somatization disorder: one of medicine's blind spots. JAMA 1985;254:3075–3079.

124. Lipowski ZJ. Somatization: medicine's unsolved problem (Editorial). Psychosomatics 1987;28:294–297.

CHAPTER 26

BEHAVIORAL MEDICINE

G. Randolph Schrodt, Jr. and Allan Tasman

BACKGROUND

Definitions

Behavioral medicine is "the application of the theory and practice of modern behavioral sciences to the theory and practice of modern medicine" (1). Behavioral medicine is deeply rooted in conventional medicine, especially through its emphasis on the scientific method and empirical research. In distinction to conventional medical practice, however, health and illness are not conceptualized in either predominantly biological or physical terms. In addition, behavioral medicine is frequently not taught in medical schools, not used extensively in hospitals, and not reimbursed by health insurance.

Clinicians who practice in a behavioral medicine model distinguish between a patient's *disease* and his or her *sickness*. Conventional Western medical training and clinical practice have focused predominantly on the *objective* aspects of tissue/organ pathology and pathophysiology (disease). Behavioral medicine offers a paradigm that incorporates the *subjective* experience, which includes the personal *meaning* and cultural and interpersonal *context* of illness and healing, as well as the associated behavioral responses to physical illness (sickness). Moreover, these attitudes, emotions, and behaviors are also considered to be critical factors in the etiology of disease.

Behavioral medicine is a multidisciplinary field concerned with the development and clinical evaluation of interventions that enhance patients' "active, informed and responsible roles in understanding the precursors of their illnesses, the disease process itself, the management of recovery, and the subsequent adoption of beneficial life routines" (2).

History and Development

The origins of behavioral medicine within psychiatry stem from studies of psychosomatic illnesses. After World War II, this research was based on an understanding of psychopathology from the psychoanalytic theoretical perspective, which predominated at the time. These studies focused on discerning whether particular physical illnesses that had no known etiology at that time, such as rheumatoid arthritis, asthma, and ulcerative colitis, were caused by psychological stress (3). This interest in the possible relationship between mental functioning and physical illness stimulated a variety of changes in psychiatric practice. One change was the development of general hospital-based psychiatric units (4). The development of these units allowed for better integration of psychiatry into general medicine and a focus on patients whose illnesses appeared to lie at an intersection of psychological and physical etiologies. Coincident with the development of these units was the evolution of consultation/liaison programs in psychiatry, which focused on patients whose primary disorder was a physical one, but in whom the stress of the physical illness precipitated psychiatric problems (5).

These events of the 1940s and 1950s influenced the work of George Engel, who coined the word *biopsychosocial* to reflect the importance of understanding the multifactorial interactions of biological, psychological, and social influences in a patient's presentation (6). The natural evolution of a biopsychosocial approach has included a focus on illnesses whose origins are clearly behavioral. Early behavioral medicine programs that developed in the 1960s focused on such issues as smoking cessation and weight loss as adjuncts to the treatment of patients who had significant smoking- or obesity-related illness or risk for disease.

In more recent decades, behavioral medicine programs have begun to focus on the importance of self-monitoring, self-care, self-awareness, and compliance with treatment for patients who have a wide range of physical problems (7). Using predominantly psychosocial treatment methods, which are described later in this chapter, modern behavioral medi-

cine programs provide intervention for patients who have severe chronic illnesses such as cancer (8–10), cardiovascular disease (11–13), chronic pain (14–18), diabetes (19, 20), and rheumatologic diseases (21–23). Cognitive-behavioral psychotherapies have come to play a more predominant role in behavioral medicine programs than have psychoanalytic-derived therapeutic interventions (24).

Principal Concepts of the System

Treatment of sickness is facilitated when both the patient and clinician share a common conceptual model that can provide a guide for treatment interventions. Figure 26.1 is a graphic representation of a basic cognitive-behavioral medicine model that may be introduced to the patient early in the course of treatment. This model emphasizes the interrelationship between stressful life events, cognitive processes, emotional and physiological reactions, and behavior.

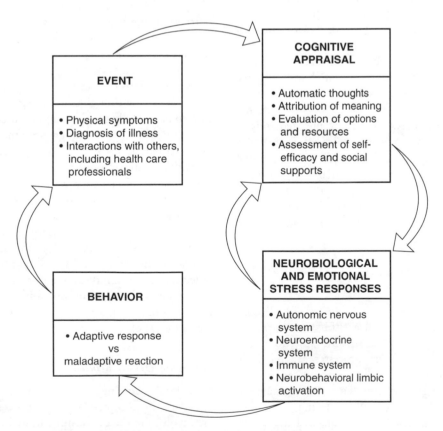

FIGURE 26.1. The cognitive-behavioral medicine model.

STRESSFUL LIFE EVENTS

The initial premise of the cognitive-behavioral model is that emotions, physical reactions, and behaviors are not triggered by events per se, but rather by the individual's cognitive appraisal of these events (25–27). Therefore, until a life event, symptom, or disease process is perceived, processed, and the meaning is established, the person generally does not experience an emotional reaction or behave differently. Any situation (health-related or otherwise) may constitute an event in this model. Events may include actual or imagined situations (e.g., visiting the doctor's office or anticipating the results of a diagnostic test), as well as past, present, or future experiences (e.g., the memory of a painful examination, shortness of breath, or expectations of future impact on one's family after being diagnosed with cancer).

Mind–body research has focused on a variety of stressful life events that appear to have particular relevance to health and illness. Studies have shown that disruptions of interpersonal relationships, such as the death or serious illness of a spouse or child, are often associated with a strong negative impact on health and well-being (28). Other stressful events, including divorce or separation, social isolation, loss of a job, financial problems, or *role strain*—that is, the competition between various life demands—may also lead to adverse health effects (29,30). However, regardless of the pathogenic potential of stressful life events, individuals vary considerably in host *susceptibility*. A growing body of research suggests that an individual's thinking style may be the critical mediating factor in the stress response.

COGNITIVE APPRAISAL: YOUR THINKING MAY BE KILLING YOU

Several factors can influence an individual's cognitive appraisal of an event. First, *awareness* of an event is required. In some situations, the early stages of disease processes are relatively asymptomatic (e.g., heart disease or cancer) and do not trigger cognitive/emotional/behavioral reactions because the illness is not perceived. Likewise, some behaviors (e.g., a diet high in saturated fats or unprotected sex) do not intuitively suggest potential adverse health effects. Unless an individual is informed of the potential negative implications of a situation or behavior, change is unlikely. This is the fundamental principle of personal and public health education efforts.

Unfortunately, information alone is often insufficient to change ingrained attitudes, beliefs, and behaviors. In some cases, psychological defense mechanisms, such as denial or repression, may diminish an individual's awareness of a potentially dangerous situation. However, these defense mechanisms may not always be maladaptive. For example, women undergoing chemotherapy for breast cancer tolerate the procedure best if they are able to employ distraction and other cognitive avoidance techniques (31). Likewise, patients who have chronic pain disorders often find relief if they can employ these same approaches (16,17). Nevertheless, even patients who have breast cancer or chronic pain need to be aware of and informed about their illness and treatment options to be effective partners in the healing process.

The conscious awareness of an event usually triggers *automatic thoughts*. Automatic thoughts and mental images occur rapidly and are often not subjected to close scrutiny or logical analysis (25–27). These thoughts and images often appear to be a totally plausible and accurate representation of reality, although they may in fact be distorted or incorrect. For example, some individuals misinterpret epigastric pain as indigestion when in fact they are having a myocardial infarction. In contrast, patients who have somatization and anxiety disorders may catastrophize the significance of relatively minor somatic sensations. In each case, the subjective *reality* of the symptom is different than the objective evidence indicates, and this subjective perception will trigger emotional and behavioral responses that are markedly different from those based on an objective evaluation.

Changing Health-Related Behaviors

Behavioral medicine researchers have begun to elucidate the complex cognitive processes that are involved in the establishment, maintenance, and change of health-related behaviors (32–34).

The process of changing a behavior (e.g., stopping smoking or drinking) or initiating a new behavior (e.g., exercise, measuring blood sugar levels each day, learning to meditate) involves a series of cognitive assessments and decisions that ultimately determine behavioral intent and motivation. Readiness to change behavior can be seen to involve movement through various stages:

1. Precontemplation (not thinking of change)
2. Contemplation (considering change but not actively trying)
3. Preparation (early steps are taken and trial efforts to change are made)
4. Action (initiation of behavioral change)
5. Maintenance (continued change for more than 6 months) (32)

Some of the cognitive processes involved in these transitions include personal risk assessment, perception of costs versus benefits of change, expectations of outcome, and compatibility with sociocultural norms. Positive or negative feedback from others after initiating new behaviors also can be a powerful influence in this process. In many cases, an individual's *conclusion* regarding a health behavior may appear illogical, even ridiculous to the health care professional or others. In fact, research suggests that most people evaluate risk predominantly from an emotional rather than logical point of view (35). This may partly explain how an individual could insist on drinking bottled spring water but not wear a car seat belt, despite the fact that he or she is more likely to die from a motor vehicle accident than from drinking contaminated tap water.

As the patient and clinician explore thinking processes through the course of treatment, basic organizing themes or *schemas* begin to emerge (25–27). Schemas are deeper cognitive structures, which may operate outside of one's usual conscious awareness. They include the fundamental rules or assumptions that act as templates for screening, filtering, processing, and evaluating the significance of experiences. Stressful situations and life events, particularly health- or illness-related events, may activate latent maladaptive schemas, such as, "I don't function well under stress," "I'm not a real man

if I can't work," or, "It's a sign of weakness to ask for help." These basic beliefs and assumptions influence the perception of events and increase the frequency of distorted automatic thoughts.

Chronic Illness

Chronic illness is commonly associated with a pervasive sense of *helplessness* (7, 34). Even patients who demonstrate effective coping during acute illnesses may be overwhelmed by unrelenting pain or other symptoms; the need for ongoing medical care; uncertainty of outcome, relief, or cure of symptoms; and the disruption of normal lifestyle patterns and relationships resulting from chronic illness.

Not all patients who have chronic illness, however, adopt this posture of helplessness. Seligman (36) has focused on the value of *optimism* in effectively dealing with illness. In his and other researchers' studies of attributional style (how people explain the causes of events), they have identified a distinct difference in how optimistic individuals think about stressful life events compared with pessimists (36–38).

Pessimists tend to interpret negative events in global ("I'm useless to my family. . . . I can't do anything anymore"), personalized ("I'm weak"), and persistent ("It'll never get better") terms. This outlook is associated with a diminished sense of *self-efficacy* (20), decreased effort when confronted with problems, and a hopeless outlook for the future. In contrast, optimistic individuals view negative life events as more specific ("This illness will require that I make some modifications in my work load"), externalized ("I am not my illness"), and variable ("I can influence the outcome of this illness"). Compared with their more optimistic peers, persons who have a pessimistic explanatory style at age 25 are predicted to have poorer health status in later life (38).

Stress Hardiness

Certain attitudes appear to convey a type of immunity to the negative impact of stressful life events and situations. Kobasa and her colleagues (39) have identified three characteristic attitudes of *stress hardiness: control, challenge,* and *commit-*

ment. An increased sense of personal control is generally associated with improved tolerance of stressful events. Some events, however, such as undergoing surgery, are not under direct personal control. However, even in these cases, an ability to discriminate between events that can be controlled and those that cannot be controlled, and to focus one's efforts on the former, appears to be the most effective (and least distressing) problem-solving strategy (40). Stress-hardy individuals also perceive problems as challenges rather than burdens or overwhelming obstacles. As demands increase, they exhibit greater effort toward the identification of possible solutions and alternatives as well as the design of problem-solving strategies. Finally, a deep sense of commitment to a personal or higher purpose provides meaning and coherence in the midst of chaos and uncertainty (41).

Although it is difficult to compartmentalize the mechanism of action of most alternative and complementary therapeutic techniques, it is apparent that many involve the modification of cognitive processes. The basic doctor-patient relationship, psychotherapy, educational efforts, and even the healing aspects of visualization, ritual, and spirituality may all be understood as powerful tools that modify an individual's perception of reality and basic belief systems.

EMOTIONAL AND NEUROBEHAVIORAL REACTIONS: THE BODY'S INNER DIALOGUE

When an individual interprets an event or situation as dangerous, the *stress response* is activated (42,43). The stress response is a complex, coordinated cascade of neurobehavioral activation that has evolved as a basic survival mechanism. The most basic threat is to one's life or health. However, *danger* thoughts may also extend to other vital interests, such as the welfare of loved ones, self-esteem, or financial security (26). In this respect, the use of the stress response for survival and well-being is straightforward. The capacity to predict and detect danger enhances the likelihood of success in negotiating the complexities of daily life. In fact, the absence of automatic thoughts of danger can be of great clinical significance. For instance, some adolescents display a distorted sense of invulnerability and omnipotence, and as a result, the actual dangers of drug use, reckless driving, and unprotected sex are not recognized.

The main neurophysiological components of the stress response involve increased release of corticotropin-releasing factor (CRF) from the hypothalamus, the activation of the sympathetic nervous system via the locus ceruleus/noradrenergic system in the brainstem, and the release of neuropeptides from various areas of the brain (42, 43). Increased CRF release activates the pituitary-adrenal axis and has other peripheral effects, including a major role in immunosuppression. The immune system and the brain communicate via hormones, neurotransmitters, and peptides such as cytokines, which results in reciprocal modulation of activity (28, 44, 45).

Specific Responses

Physiological features of the stress response include increased energy production (gluconeogenesis and lipolysis), increased muscle tension, increased respiratory rate, and increased cardiovascular tone (elevated blood pressure and heart rate). Neurobehavioral reactions include increased arousal, alertness, scanning, and vigilance. Emotional tone is altered, with increased subjective anxiety and apprehension. As suggested in Figure 26.1, even the cognitive functions of perception, retrieval, and analysis of information regarding the environment are altered (26). Essentially, the individual is prepared to *fight, flee, freeze,* or *faint.* Physiological activity that is relatively insignificant to immediate survival, such as feeding or reproduction, is suppressed so that all resources can be redirected toward coping with the threat.

In many circumstances, this stress response has positive adaptive value. Increased apprehension and an impulse to flee would probably be a rational reaction to turning a corner and walking into an unfamiliar dark alley in a major city. Likewise, when the *threat* is time-limited, such as engaging in a sporting competition or driving on a busy interstate highway, the increased alertness and neuroendocrine and autonomic arousal may be beneficial.

Unfortunately, the characteristics of this innate alarm system evolved within an environment very distinct from that of contemporary culture. The instinct to run when threatened may enhance the likelihood of survival if one is being chased by a saber-toothed tiger, but this instinct is clearly maladaptive if the threat is a physician who wants to discuss a health problem. The freeze reaction may protect a deer in the forest from hunters, but it is a poor adaptive response if its paralyzing effect prevents a diabetic person from testing blood sugar levels or self-injecting insulin. Furthermore, chronic activation of the stress response system appears to be a major etiological factor in many chronic illnesses, such as cardiovascular disease; immune system disorders; and psychiatric illnesses, including depression, panic disorder, and addictions (7,42–45). When the chronic stress is a chronic illness, neurobehavioral stress reactions may exacerbate the initial medical problem and impair adaptive coping behavior (13, 22, 46, 47).

Relaxation Response

The *relaxation response* is characterized by decreased arousal of the autonomic and central nervous system, lowered musculoskeletal and cardiovascular tone, and altered neuroendocrine function associated with restoration and repair of tissues (48). The relaxation response is elicited by a variety of mental states and techniques that are described in more detail later in this chapter and in other sections of this volume. In general, the relaxation response is associated with a general quieting of the usual flood of thoughts, daydreams, inner conversations, judgments, sensations, and emotions that characterize the waking consciousness. This state of consciousness is typically first elicited by focusing attention on a repetitive word or sound (e.g., mantra); stimulus (e.g., staring at a mandala or a flame); or behavior (e.g., one's breathing). Second, when intrusive thoughts, sensations, or feelings enter into awareness, the individual adopts a passive, *observer* attitude and gently redirects focus back to the meditative word or sound (41).

Mind–Body Interaction

Although the concepts of stress and the relaxation response are well characterized and useful for patient education and clinical practice, it is an oversimplification to suggest that states of consciousness and associated neurobehavioral responses fit neatly into these two discrete categories. Walsh (49) has emphasized the need for researchers to take a more discriminating approach to defining, mapping, and comparing altered states of consciousness. For example, different forms of meditation are associated with variations in the level of arousal, concentration, awareness of the environment, and emotional responsiveness (49). Other researchers have identified differential effects of stress management strategies (e.g., biofeedback, hypnosis, meditation) with different medical disorders (14, 50, 51). Nevertheless, the intimate relationship between mental processes and physiological responses is well established and remains a fundamental principle of behavioral medicine theory and practice.

BEHAVIORAL RESPONSES: TYPES OF COPING

Behavior is the observable response of an individual to life events, and it may be generally classified as adaptive (restoration of homeostasis, or movement toward growth) or maladaptive (perpetuation of sickness). As discussed in the preceding sections, behavior is largely determined by the individual's appraisal of the situation and level of emotional/physiological arousal. However, there are other *environmental contingencies* that are critical in determining an individual's health or illness-related behavioral responses.

There is general consensus that certain behaviors are associated with health and well-being, such as eating a healthy diet; regular exercise; moderation in alcohol use; abstinence from hard drugs and unsafe sex; participation and meaningful involvement with family, friends, and community rituals; or the practice of meditation or prayer. Moreover, when an individual is ill, other behaviors may be required, such as regularly taking medication, self-monitoring practices, physical therapy or other rehabilitation programs, and keeping appointments with health care providers. Each of these behaviors appears to be relatively straightforward, and yet many, if not most, people do not adhere to these recommendations.

It is common for some individuals to simply lack the skills or experience needed to perform the expected behavior. When they then attempt the behavior, they experience frustration rather than success. This lack of positive reinforcement decreases the likelihood of trying again. In some cases, the critical factor in failure to change behavior is an external barrier, such as prohibitive cost or lack of transportation. At times, an individual may be cognitively/affectively inclined to perform a behavior, but family, friends, and others strongly oppose it. This may be related to the fact that the behavior is incompatible with sociocultural standards (e.g., participation in an alternative therapy approach such as meditation or biofeedback) or that other barriers exist (e.g., lack of insurance coverage).

In certain situations, family and friends may inadvertently enable the continuation of a behavior, such as alcoholism or overeating, by failing to address the problem or by making excuses for the individual. With chronic illness, some individuals may unconsciously adopt the *sick role.* Typically, when someone behaves in a way that identifies them as *sick,* they are (temporarily) allowed certain privileges, such as the right to seek care and support from health care providers and family, and are relieved of certain responsibilities. In chronic illness, however, the sick role may be maladaptive in that it provides a disincentive for recovery. The medico-legal designation of impairment and compensation for disability may actually create a reward for illness behavior.

When an individual is anxious and distressed, instinctive behavioral responses may be activated, including inhibition (e.g., avoidance, phobias); compulsive behavior (e.g., addictions, binging and purging [in bulimia], compulsive handwashing); or search for safety (e.g., agoraphobia, repeated requests or demands for diagnostic tests, clinging dependency on others). In many cases, the anxious patient's decision-making may be inflexible and repetitive, and the behavioral repertoire is limited and poorly adaptive.

PROVIDER-PATIENT INTERACTION

Doctor-patient interactions in behavioral medicine are guided by certain fundamental tenets of the therapeutic relationship. The interaction is characterized by collaboration and shared responsibilities. The doctor's role includes:

1. Providing an expert knowledge base and clinical practice of medical and behavioral sciences, including taking a careful clinical history and ordering appropriate tests (e.g., physical examination, psychometric testing, laboratory studies).
2. Guiding the diagnostic and treatment process toward the identification of specific problems, goals, and therapeutic options.
3. Serving as a teacher (providing didactic instruction or assigning reading or other self-help homework) and coach (providing encouragement and suggestions) for the patient.

The patient is encouraged to:

1. Actively participate in the healing process.
2. Begin an educational process and exploration of both the disease and the sickness.
3. Engage in self-help activities to modify dysfunctional attitudes and behaviors.
4. Assume responsibility as captain of the health care team.

Nonspecific therapist characteristics of warmth, respect, and equanimity under pressure appear to influence therapy outcomes (52). The effective behavioral medicine therapist is both pragmatic and flexible and takes an active role in structuring the therapy agenda (25–27). The treatment plan is problem-oriented and has specific, measurable short- and long-term goals and objectives. In general, the focus of behavioral medicine is on current problems in functioning. However, there are circumstances in which exploration of past events, such as traumatic experiences, is indicated, particularly in the latter stages of treatment after acute symptom relief has been achieved. Throughout therapy, the therapist gives and elicits feedback about improvement, strategies, and reactions to the treatment.

Although behavioral medicine is frequently practiced in a traditional one-to-one doctor-patient format, treatment may involve a *multidisciplinary team* of different specialists who have distinct skills. The involvement of family and significant others is recognized as critical to the healing process. The concept of *healing community* is perhaps best illustrated by the frequent use of group therapies in behavioral medicine.

THERAPY AND OUTCOMES

Treatment Options

PSYCHOTHERAPEUTIC STRATEGIES

Effective cognitive-behavioral therapy (CBT) is based on a clear formulation of each individual case, and a comprehensive treatment plan that focuses on the patient's specific problems and goals. However, therapy is also guided by certain generic objectives:

1. Establish a collaborative partnership with the patient.
2. Assist in development of enhanced self-awareness and self-monitoring.
3. Teach the patient methods of relaxation to decrease physiological arousal.
4. Help the patient identify the relationship between events; automatic thoughts; and affective, physiological, and behavioral responses.
5. Promote the patient's ability to *respond* rather than *react* to stressful situations.
6. Guide the patient in cultivating a more integrative, realistic, and adaptive set of attitudes.
7. Encourage the development of effective problem-solving strategies and other behavioral skills that enhance the patient's sense of mastery and self-efficacy.
8. Support the practice of health enhancement and relapse prevention strategies.

Cognitive Techniques

A variety of techniques can be used to guide the patient in the identification and modification of automatic thoughts that influence health behaviors and coping with chronic disease (Table 26.1). *Self-monitoring exercises,* such as keeping a journal and thought recording, can enhance awareness of negative, distorted thoughts and maladaptive *self-talk. Imagery, visualization techniques,* and *role playing* may be helpful for patients who have difficulty identifying automatic thoughts, and these techniques can provide an

Table 26.1. Cognitive Techniques
Agenda setting
Guided discovery
Identification of automatic thoughts
Testing of automatic thoughts
Thought recording/keeping a journal
Modifying cognitive distortions
Educational reading
Imagery and visualization techniques
Role playing
Developing rational alternatives
Changing schemas

opportunity to consider different strategies for thinking through a difficult situation.

With an enhanced ability to monitor thought processes, the patient can work on developing rational alternatives based on a realistic assessment of problems and options. Patients are encouraged to consider their automatic thoughts as *hypotheses* that can be tested and modified as they acquire more accurate information, learn new skills, and refine coping strategies. A cognitively-oriented health care professional can also encourage an alternative, more flexible set of attitudes about dealing with stressful situations (e.g., patience, self-control, *letting go*). Peer-group therapy with others who are dealing with similar issues (e.g., chronic pain, cancer, addictions) provides an excellent opportunity to compare personal experiences, attitudes, and belief systems. Many individuals are more willing to acknowledge and adopt the attitudes and behaviors of a peer who is successfully coping with a similar problem than to accept the advice of a health care professional. Although cognitive techniques are often very effective in modifying schemas, sustained change is greatly facilitated by a concurrent change in habitual behavior patterns that reinforce those attitudes and beliefs.

Behavioral Techniques

Most patients can identify maladaptive behaviors that interfere with their activities of daily living or medical treatment. Limitations or complete avoidance of certain activities; exces-

Table 26.2. Behavioral Techniques
Behavioral analysis
Activity scheduling
Self-monitoring
Exposure techniques
Behavioral rehearsal
Skills training

sive behavior (e.g., taking too much pain medication, overeating); or interference with normal interpersonal interactions are commonly observed in clinical settings. Table 26.2 lists a variety of behavioral techniques that can be employed to facilitate adaptive coping and lifestyle modification. A *behavioral analysis* is usually done early in the course of treatment to establish a baseline frequency of behaviors that are targeted for change. For example, a patient who has an eating disorder may be instructed to keep a food diary (a record of the time of, location of, and amount eaten at meals; degree of hunger; and associated environmental triggers such as stress), whereas a patient in cardiac rehabilitation may be instructed to record the number of miles walked each day. Patients frequently observe that carefully tracking and recording information about their behavior result in greater depth of awareness and understanding, and can lead to a significant decrease in maladaptive behavior. Not only are the data collected useful in the development of practice exercises, but they can also help with identifying distorted cognitions as well as be used to monitor progress in treatment.

Many patients find that having a *written list of coping strategies* enhances their ability to deal with pain, anxiety, or other severe symptoms. Patients usually report that it is difficult to concentrate, remember, and make decisions when they are in severe distress. Likewise, it is hard to develop creative solutions to problems or consider alternatives in this state. The therapist can assist the patient in the development of a specific protocol of coping behaviors for different situations. With repeated practice and refinement, patients learn to modulate their thoughts, feelings, and behavioral responses in actual situations.

It is not uncommon to find that patients struggling with chronic illness have certain basic deficits in assertiveness, effective communication, time management, and problem-solving skills. For example, many patients are frustrated after an appointment with their doctor because "he didn't spend much time with me," or "I left with unanswered questions." *Skills training* usually involves both didactic instruction and homework practice. For instance, the therapist may suggest that the patient observe the behavior of another group member, read material on the topic of assertiveness, write down a list of concerns and questions to ask the doctor, rehearse what he or she intends to ask with a friend, and practice this new behavior in an actual situation (e.g., at the next appointment with the doctor).

One of the most useful skills that a patient can learn is the development of an *action plan*. Many patients are aware that they should modify their behavior, and they may even initiate efforts to change, only to find that it is more difficult than they imagined. An action plan is a detailed analysis of specific goals (e.g., "I plan to learn yoga and practice it three times a week"); supports (e.g., "I will sign up for the class with my sister"); resources/barriers (e.g., child care, cost of class, transportation); and specific actions to be taken (e.g., "I will call tomorrow about when the next class starts").

Relaxation Techniques

Behavioral medicine programs generally provide instruction in one or more methods of relaxation training, such as progressive muscle relaxation (53), diaphragmatic breathing, autogenic training (54), or biofeedback (55). The mastery of one or more of these techniques provides the individual with a readily available tool to use in situations when autonomic nervous system arousal makes coping difficult. In addition to eliciting the physiological benefits of the relaxation response, advanced relaxation techniques, such as self-hypnosis, guided imagery, and meditation, can be used to augment the effectiveness of traditional cognitive-behavioral approaches, such as imagery, desensitization, cognitive restructuring, and adaptive self-statements

(41,56–58). A more detailed description of the use of relaxation techniques in behavioral medicine can be found in the references and in other chapters in this volume. However, the following cases illustrate how behavioral techniques can help the patient cope with stressful life events.

CASE EXAMPLES

CASE 1

When he was initially seen, Mr. M was a 50-year-old married white man who was referred to the psychiatry and behavioral medicine service by his neurosurgeon. The referral and subsequent hospitalization was precipitated by an emergency call from Mr. M's wife after he made statements to her threatening suicide and voicing homicidal thoughts toward individuals at the workmen's compensation insurance company with whom he had been dealing over approximately the past 10 months since he injured his back at work. Frustrated by continued delays and paperwork, and developing a growing sense of paranoia about "being messed with," he had threatened over the telephone to "come down there and blow someone's head off so you'll listen to me and get me some help."

Mr. M had worked for 25 years at his company, and he was noted to be a diligent, highly regarded employee by his employers. Approximately 10 months before his psychiatric hospitalization he had injured his back lifting a box at work. Subsequent work-up revealed herniations of three lumbar discs, and he underwent L2–L5 fusion without complications. However, despite the surgery, narcotic analgesic medication, and regular physical therapy, Mr. M continued to experience severe back pain that radiated down both legs.

The first several days of hospitalization focused on the completion of a comprehensive biopsychosocial evaluation, including reevaluation by his neurosurgeon and a consultation with an anesthesiologist specialist in pain management. Psychological testing revealed severe depression (Beck Depression Inventory score of 44 of a highest possible score of 63) (59), but no evidence of psychosis or significant personality disorder. Mr. M also demonstrated extreme hopelessness (Hopelessness Scale score of 15 of a highest possible score of 20) (60), which is considered to be a significant risk factor for suicide. On the Survey of Pain Attitudes (SOPA) (61), the patient exhibited a profound sense of loss of control over his pain, a belief that only surgery or medication could provide relief, and a pervasive belief that his pain was unfair and that his family and health care providers did not understand either the extent of his pain or the degree of his disability.

In individual psychotherapy sessions, Mr. M's history and basic schemas began to emerge. His father died when Mr. M was 12 years old, and as the oldest child he needed to start working to help support his family. Years later, one brother died in an alcohol-related car accident, and another brother committed suicide after years of dealing with drug abuse that he developed while in combat in Vietnam. Mr. M acknowledged a sense of guilt that he "could have done something" to have prevented their deaths. He attributed his depression to the injury, and also believed that the injury caused his inability to now be a "good provider" for his family.

The early phases of treatment included collaboration between Mr. M and the treatment team in the development of a detailed problem list and treatment plan. Drug therapy was begun with an antidepressant (sertraline [Zoloft]) and a nonsteroidal anti-inflammatory agent (nabumetone [Relafen]), and Mr. M also began a series of epidural blocks performed by the anesthesiologist.

Mr. M was seen in individual and marital cognitive-behavioral psychotherapy and began attending a chronic pain management group that met twice a week. Initially, the focus of therapy centered on his hopelessness, agitation, anxiety, and suicidal and homicidal thoughts. For several days, Mr. M was encouraged to keep a pain log, which is an hourly record of pain intensity as well as associated thoughts, feelings, activities, and the effects of pain relief interventions. In both individual and group sessions, Mr.

M learned of the basic mechanisms and pathophysiology of chronic pain, and through the various self-monitoring assignments he began to identify factors (thoughts, emotions, social situations) that either intensified or relieved his pain. The therapy sessions were augmented with homework assignments that included readings and worksheets from the book *Managing Pain Before It Manages You* (62). His wife was actively involved in the educational and treatment process, and she provided feedback regarding his behavior at home and suggestions regarding his unrealistic expectations of both himself and others. Gradually, Mr. M's insomnia, nightmares, and mood improved, and he was discharged to the partial hospitalization program after 10 days.

For the next six months, Mr. M attended a weekly chronic pain management group, augmented by several marital sessions with his wife. In group therapy, he learned techniques of relaxation, including diaphragmatic breathing, meditation, and visualization. He further developed and refined his pain control *toolbox,* including a self-directed exercise program of water walking at a nearby heated pool, as well as communication and assertiveness skills that he was able to use when dealing with his physicians, attorneys, and workmen's compensation company representatives.

The therapy group provided support and an opportunity to rehearse skills in dealing with his ongoing disability hearings, and provided feedback and challenge to his negative and helpless attitudes. For example, soon after joining the group, Mr. M came in very depressed about the upcoming Thanksgiving holiday. With support from the group, he was able to identify his distress at not being "a good grandfather" because he would not be able to throw the football with his grandsons. Furthermore, he expected that he would be "a burden" to the entire family because of his pain, intolerance of "all the noise," and his inability to participate in all the preparations and activities. Other group members shared their similar thoughts and feelings, but challenged his assumptions and rigid beliefs about what others would think or feel. They suggested that he could go out in the yard with his grandsons even if he couldn't join the game, and that later he could play a board game with them. If he should experience an exacerbation of pain or become fatigued, he could go and rest briefly. Mr. M came to the next group meeting in an excellent mood and with an overall diminished pain level, and he reported his great sense of accomplishment in dealing with the holiday.

Over the next months he continued to develop a more flexible and realistic attitude regarding his abilities and limitations, and showed greater creativity in solving problems as they arose. He also returned to his church and began volunteer work visiting members who were homebound due to illness, an activity he found exceptionally rewarding. A year after his initial hospitalization, he still attends group therapy approximately once a month, and he is doing well. As he is apt to tell new members, "I still hurt, but I don't suffer anymore."

CASE 2

Ms. C is a 47-year-old married white woman who had previously had a baseline mammogram at age 40 on the recommendation of her gynecologist, but had not had a follow-up and had only irregularly done breast self-examinations (an example of only partially effective public education efforts). After watching a TV show on breast cancer, Ms. C again scheduled a mammogram, and she was subsequently referred to a general surgeon after a suspicious 1.5-cm mass was identified. The surgeon performed a biopsy the next day that revealed infiltrating ductal carcinoma. When the surgeon called Ms. C to discuss the biopsy results, he referred her to the hospital's cancer resource center, and she was contacted that day by a trained volunteer who was a breast cancer survivor herself. Ms. C and her husband were invited to come to the center and view a computer-assisted multimedia program on the surgical, medical, reconstructive, and psychosocial options available for the treatment of breast cancer before her appointment the next day with her surgeon. The cancer center volunteer offered to serve as a navigator, or guide, through the maze of the health care system and to coordinate the various services that Ms. C and her family might find useful.

Ms. C and her husband met with the surgeon to discuss treatment alternatives. Together, they agreed on lumpectomy with axillary node dissection, which is a breast-conserving surgery that is equally effective compared with total mastectomy for early stage cancer, but is associated with better postoperative body image and sexual functioning (31,46). After meeting with the surgeon, Ms. C consulted with a nurse clinician to discuss the details of the upcoming surgical procedure and postoperative care (see reference 40 for further discussion of the benefits of presurgical psychological preparation).

Two days later, Ms. C arrived at the hospital early in the morning and successfully underwent surgical resection of the tumor. Ms. C's state legislature had previously passed a law requiring insurance carriers to provide coverage for 48-hour postoperative hospital care in uncomplicated breast cancer surgery. This allowed Ms. C and her family to meet again with the nurse clinician regarding wound care and home instructions. It also provided an opportunity for the volunteer navigator to accompany Ms. C to one of several breast cancer support groups held weekly at the hospital. Although initially somewhat reluctant to attend a group dealing with such a personal matter, Ms. C was favorably influenced by information on the group provided by a video she watched in her hospital room, a pamphlet provided by the volunteer, and the strong recommendation of her doctor.

Following surgery, a course of radiotherapy (5 days per week for 5 weeks), followed by chemotherapy (doxorubicin [Adriamycin] and cyclophosphamide [Cytoxan]) for the next several months were prescribed. The cancer support group focused on case management, referral for consultation when indicated, patient education, emotional support, and the development of coping skills (9,10,31,46). For example, Ms. C consulted a hypnotherapist before beginning chemotherapy and was thus able to manage the nausea and vomiting with the techniques she learned (63). Later, she and her husband met with a marital therapist to discuss Mr. C's anxiety about sexual activity and irrational fear that he could cause a recurrence of cancer by touching her breasts.

Treatment Evaluation

There are three main outcome measures that are the focus of behavioral medicine practice and research: objective clinical outcomes, cost-effectiveness, and the subjective experience of the patient. First, objective clinical outcomes are necessary if behavioral medicine (or other complementary therapies) are to be considered viable alternatives or adjuncts to conventional medical care. Does this treatment reduce symptoms? Does this treatment improve the functional status of the patient's activities of daily living, ability to work, and so on? How does this treatment compare in effectiveness to other established treatments?

Although modifications of traditional double-blind, placebo-controlled studies may be necessary, behavioral medicine research is conducted using objective, reliable measures of clinical outcome, which are comparable to those measures used in studies of conventional therapies. However, because the scope of behavioral medicine extends beyond the basic organic pathology of disease, data about the patient's environment, thoughts and belief systems, associated physiological subsystems, and behavior, including relationships with others, are all elements of behavioral medicine outcome studies.

Second, the cost-effectiveness of behavioral medicine interventions is a critical variable in treatment evaluation. Research suggests that behavioral medicine treatments actually reduce overall medical costs, particularly with conditions such as chronic pain, asthma, and diabetes (15, 64, 65). There is an increasing awareness of both the high frequency of occurrence and increased cost and morbidity associated with untreated anxiety and depressive disorders that coexist with many chronic medical conditions (13, 16, 19, 66–68). Again, research now supports the cost-effectiveness of programs designed to identify and treat patients who have such conditions (69, 70).

Third, behavioral medicine outcome research has focused on the subjective experience of illness and medical treatment. Hospital administrators and insurance carriers may refer to this dimension as customer satisfaction. From the patient's viewpoint, the important questions are, "Was I treated with dignity and respect?" and "Would I recommend this treatment to my friends or family?"

ORGANIZATION

In recent years, there has been a progressive reintegration of psychiatry (including behavioral medicine) and general medicine. Professional psychiatric organizations have joined with other medical specialty groups to lobby for legislation mandating parity for *cognitive services* and mental health coverage for all patients. Departments of psychiatry within medical schools have refocused the curriculum for medical students and psychiatric residents to emphasize the developments in mind–body medicine. Psychiatric and behavioral medicine research has begun to establish both the clinical efficacy and cost-effectiveness of these approaches, and as a result there is an expanding presence of behavioral medicine services within general medical settings. However, despite these advancements, behavioral medicine services are still not covered by health insurance programs to the same extent as are more traditional medical treatments, such as surgery or the prescription of medication, even when benefits have been demonstrated.

PROSPECTS FOR THE FUTURE

Behavioral medicine is still significantly underused in the treatment of patients who have severe medical illness. However, because the origins of this treatment approach come from the practice of general psychiatry, the integration of behavioral medicine techniques into conventional medicine may be easier than that of alternative or complementary approaches, which have originated outside of standard medical practice. This is because conventional medical practitioners will probably offer less resistance to a treatment approach that is already perceived as part of the system. Further, the clinical effectiveness of behavioral medicine interventions, especially cognitive-behavioral therapies, in the treatment of patients with chronic medical illnesses should stimulate the growth of behavioral medicine programs. Health promotion and disease prevention is a natural area for expansion and integration of behavioral medicine programs within the general medical environment.

Behavioral medicine programs are useful adjuncts in the treatment of patients who have severe illnesses. Improved compliance with treatment, greater self-esteem, and better quality of life have all been demonstrated when behavioral medicine interventions are used in conjunction with standard medical treatment. Perhaps the greatest opportunity for the future, in light of these findings, is the integration of behavioral medicine techniques with standard medical practice to form a new alternative system of health care delivery (71).

Research attempting to elucidate the mechanisms of action of behavioral medicine interventions is in its infancy. Particularly exciting is the developing area of psychoneuroimmunologic research, which investigates the relationship between psychological status and immune functioning (44, 45). These and other areas of mind–body medicine offer promising new approaches to our understanding of human health and illness.

REFERENCES

1. Elkes J. Self-regulation and behavioral medicine: The early beginnings. Psych Ann 1981;11(2): 15–30.
2. Elkes J. The emerging understanding of mind-body relationships and physical health. New York: The Institute for the Advancement of Health, 1989.
3. Alexander F. Psychosomatic medicine. New York: WW Norton, 1950.
4. Schneck JM. United States of America. In: Howells JG, ed. World history of psychiatry. New York: Brunner/Mazel, 1975:432–475.
5. Schwab JJ, Brosin HW. Handbook of psychiatric consultation. New York: Appleton-Century-Crofts, 1968.
6. Engel GL. The need for a new medical model: a challenge for biomedicine. Science 1977;196: 129–136.

7. Tunks E, Bellissimo A. Behavioral medicine: concepts and procedures. New York: Pergamon Press, 1991.

8. Fawzy FI, Fawzy N, Hyun C, et al. Malignant melanoma: effects of an early structured psychiatric intervention, coping, and affective state on recurrence and survival 6 years later. Arch Gen Psych 1993;50:681–688.

9. Fawzy FI, Fawzy NW, Arndt LA, Pasnau RO. Critical review of psychosocial interventions in cancer care. Arch Gen Psychiatry 1995;52:100–113.

10. Speigel D, Bloom JR, Kraemer HC, Gottheil E. Effect of psychosocial treatment on survival of patients with metastatic breast cancer. Lancet 1989;2:888–891.

11. Gould KL, Ornish D, Scherwitz L, et al. Changes in myocardial perfusion abnormalities by positron emission tomography after long-term, intense risk factor modification. JAMA 1995;274:894–901.

12. Linden W, Chambers L. Clinical effectiveness of non-drug treatment for hypertension: a meta-analysis. Ann Behav Med 1994;16(1):35–45.

13. Shapiro PA. Psychiatric aspects of cardiovascular disease. Psych Clin North Am 1996;19(3): 613–629.

14. Integration of behavioral and relaxation approaches into the treatment of chronic pain and insomnia. NIH Technol Assess Statement; October 16–18, 1995:1–34.

15. Flor H, Fydrich T, Turk DC. Efficacy of multidisciplinary pain treatment centers: A meta-analytic review. Pain 1992;49:221–230.

16. Gatchel RJ, Turk DC, eds. Psychological approaches to pain management. New York: Guilford Press, 1996.

17. Keefe FJ, Dunsmore J, Burnett R. Behavioral and cognitive-behavioral approaches to chronic pain: recent advances and future directions. J Consult Clin Psych 1992;60:528–536.

18. Koenig TW, Clark MR. Advances in comprehensive pain management. Psychiatr Clin North Am 1996;19(3):589–611.

19. Jacobson AM. The psychological care of patients with insulin-dependent diabetes mellitus. N Engl J Med 1996;334:1249–1253.

20. Anderson BJ, Wolf FM, Burkhart MT, et al. Effects of peer-group intervention on metabolic control of adolescents with IDDM: Randomized outpatient study. Diabetes Care 1989;12:179–183.

21. Baumstark KE, Buckelew SP. Fibromyalgia: clinical signs, research findings, treatment implications, and future directions. Ann Behav Med 1992; 14:282–291.

22. Moran MG. Psychiatric aspects of rheumatology. Psychiatr Clin North Am 1996;19(3):575–587.

23. White KP, Nielson WR. Cognitive behavioral treatment of fibromyalgia syndrome: a followup assessment. J Rheumatol 1995;22:717–721.

24. Slater MA, Weickgenant AL, Dimsdale JE. Behavioral medicine. In: Tasman A, Kay J, Lieberman JA, eds. Psychiatry. Philadelphia: WB Saunders, 1997:1500–1512.

25. Beck AT, Rush AJ, Shaw BF, Emery GD. Cognitive therapy of depression. New York: Guilford Press, 1979.

26. Schrodt GR Jr, Wright JH, Breen KJ. Practical applications of cognitive-behavioral therapy in anxiety disorders. In: den Boer JA, ed. Clinical management of anxiety. New York: Marcel Dekker, 1997:151–177.

27. Wright JH, Beck AT. Cognitive therapy. In: Hales RE, Yudofsky SC, Talbott JA, eds. The American Psychiatric Association textbook of psychiatry. 2nd ed. Washington, DC: American Psychiatric Press, 1995:1083–1113.

28. Calabrese JR, Kling MA, Gold PW. Alterations in immunocompetence during stress, bereavement, and depression: focus on neuroendocrine regulation. Am J Psychiatry 1987;144:1123–1134.

29. House JS, Landis KR, Umberson D. Social relationships and health. Science 1988;241:540–545.

30. Brown GW, Harris TO. Life events and illness. New York: Guilford Press, 1989.

31. Glanz K, Lerman C. Psychosocial impact of breast cancer: a critical review. Ann Behav Med 992;14(3):204–212.

32. Prochaska JO, Velicer WF, Rossi JS, et al. Stages of change and decisional balance for twelve problem behaviors. Health Psychology 1994;13(1):39–46.

33. Leventhal H, Diefenbach M, Leventhal EA. Illness cognition: using common sense to understand treatment adherence and affect cognition interactions. Cogn Ther Res 1992;16(2):143–163.

34. Bandura A, Adams NE, Beyer J. Cognitive processes mediating behavioral change. J Personality Social Psychol 1977;35:123.

35. Redelmeier DA, Rozin P, Kahneman D. Understanding patients' decisions: cognitive and emotional perspectives. JAMA 1993;270:72–76.

36. Seligman M. Learned optimism. New York: Knopf, 1991.

37. Peterson C. Explanatory style as a risk factor for illness. Cogn Ther Res 1988;12:119–132.

38. Peterson C, Seligman MEP, Vaillant GE. Pessimistic explanatory style is a risk factor for physical illness: a thirty-five year longitudinal study. J Personality Social Psychol 1988;55:23–27.

39. Kobasa S. Stressful life events, personality and health: an inquiry into hardiness. J Personality Social Psychol 1979;37:1–11.

40. Johnston M, Vogele C. Benefits of psychological preparation for surgery: a meta-analysis. Ann Behav Med 1993;15(4):245–256.

41. Kabat-Zinn J. Full catastrophe living: using the wisdom of your body and mind to face stress, pain, and illness. New York: Delacorte Press, 1990.

42. Chrousos GP, Gold PW. The concepts of stress and stress system disorders: overview of physical and behavioral homeostasis. JAMA 1992;267: 1244–1252.

43. Folkow B. Physiological organization of neurohormonal responses to psychosocial stimuli: implications for health and disease. Ann Behav Med 1993;15(4):236–244.

44. Stein M, Miller AH, Trestman RL. Depression, the immune system, and health and illness. Arch Gen Psychiatry 1991;48:171–177.

45. Ader R, Felten D, Cohen N, eds. Psychoneuroimmunology. 2nd ed. San Diego: Academic Press, 1990.

46. Moyer A, Salovey P. Psychosocial sequelae of breast cancer and it treatment. Ann Behav Med 1996; 18(2):110–125.

47. Helz JW, Templeton B. Evidence of the role of psychosocial factors in diabetes mellitus: a review. Am J Psychiatry 1990;147:1275–1282.

48. Benson H. The relaxation response. New York: William Morrow, 1975.

49. Walsh R. Mapping and comparing states. In: Walsh R, Vaughan F, eds. Paths beyond ego. Los Angeles: Tarcher/Perigee, 1993.

50. Lehrer PM, Carr R, Sargunaraj D, Woolford RL. Differential effects of stress management therapies in behavioral medicine. In: Lehrer PM, Woolford RL, eds. Principles and practice of stress management. 2nd ed. New York: Guilford Press, 1993.

51. Flor H, Birbaumer N. Comparison of the efficacy of electromyographic biofeedback, cognitive-behavioral therapy, and conservative medical interventions in the treatment of chronic musculoskeletal pain. J Consult Clin Psychology 1993;61: 653–658.

52. Wright JH, Davis D. The therapeutic relationship in cognitive-behavioral therapy: patients' perceptions and therapists' responses. Cognitive Behav Pract 1994;1:25–45.

53. Jacobson E. Progressive relaxation. Chicago: University of Chicago Press, 1938.

54. Luthe W. Autogenic therapy. New York: Grune & Stratton, 1969.

55. Schwartz MS. Biofeedback. New York: Guilford Press, 1995.

56. Rossi EL, Cheek DB. Mind-body therapy: methods of ideodynamic healing in hypnosis. New York: WW Norton, 1988.

57. Samuels M, Samuels N. Seeing with the mind's eye: The history, techniques and uses of visualization. New York: Random House, 1975.

58. Kabat-Zinn J. An outpatient program in behavioral medicine for chronic pain patients based on the practice of mindfulness meditation: Theoretical considerations and preliminary results. Gen Hosp Psychiatry 1982;4:33–47.

59. Beck AT, Ward CH, Mendelson M, et al. An inventory for measuring depression. Arch Gen Psychiatry 1961;4:561–571.

60. Beck AT, Weissman A, Lester D, Trexler L. The measurement of pessimism: the hopelessness scale. J Consult Clin Psychol 1974;42:861–865.

61. DeGood DE, Shutty MS. Assessment of pain beliefs, coping, and self-efficacy. In: Turk DC, Melzack R, eds. Handbook of pain assessment. New York: Guilford Press, 1992.

62. Caudill MA. Managing pain before it manages you. New York: Guilford Press, 1995.

63. Genuis ML. The use of hypnosis in helping cancer patients control anxiety, pain, and emesis: a review of recent empirical studies. Am J Clin Hypnosis 1995;37:316–325.

64. Cohen S, Kessler RC, Gordon LU, eds. Measuring stress: a guide for health and social scientists. New York: Oxford University Press, 1995.

65. Caudill MA, Schnable R, Zuttermeister P, et al. Decreased clinic use by chronic pain patients: response to behavioral medicine interventions. J Clin Pain 1991;7:305–310.

66. Friedman R, Sobel D, Myers P, et al. Behavioral medicine, clinical health psychology, and cost offset. Health Psychology 1995;14(6):509–518.

67. Frasure-Smith N, Lesperance F, Talajic M. Depression following myocardial infarction: impact on 6-month survival. JAMA 1993;270:1819–1825.

68. Sherbourne C. Comorbid anxiety disorder and the functioning and well-being of chronically ill patients of general medical providers. Arch Gen Psychiatry 1996;53:889–895.

69. Pallack MS, Cummings NA, Dorken H, Henke CJ. Effect of mental health treatment on medical costs. Mind/Body Med 1995;1:7–12.

70. Smith GR, Rost K, Kashner TM. A trial of the effect of a standardized psychiatric consultation on health outcomes and costs in somatizing patients. Arch Gen Psychiatry 1995;52:238–243.

71. Gordon JS. Manifesto for a new medicine: your guide to healing partnerships and the wise use of alternative therapies. Reading, Mississippi: Addison-Wesley, 1996.

CHAPTER 27

ORTHOMOLECULAR MEDICINE AND MEGAVITAMIN THERAPY

Alan R. Gaby

BACKGROUND AND DEFINITION

Orthomolecular medicine is the use of molecules normally present in the body for the prevention and treatment of disease. In 1968, Linus Pauling, PhD, introduced the concept of *orthomolecular medicine* (1), a term he invented to denote "the right molecules." It was Pauling's contention that adjusting the concentrations of molecules (e.g., vitamins, minerals, amino acids, hormones, and metabolic intermediates) that are normally present in the body is one effective approach to the prevention and treatment of disease. Orthomolecular medicine is both a concept and a treatment modality. Practitioners who use orthomolecular medicine believe that increasing or decreasing the concentration of certain naturally occurring molecules can have a beneficial effect on various disease processes.

Some treatments that are considered orthomolecular are also well accepted in the practice of medicine. For example, the management of phenylketonuria includes dietary changes designed to reduce the concentration of phenylalanine; vitamin B_6–dependent seizures are controlled by large-dose supplementation of vitamin B_6; and insulin injections are given to diabetics who have a deficiency of (or resistance to) insulin. More recently, there has been growing acceptance of the idea that administering folic acid and vitamin B_6 may reduce the risk of cardiovascular disease by lowering homocysteine concentrations (2). Other orthomolecular treatments are more controversial, such as the use of large doses of niacinamide to treat schizophrenia or the use of vitamin C to treat the common cold and other viral illnesses (3).

The rationale for using orthomolecular therapies may differ from one treatment to another, and some of the theoretical reasons for using meganutrient therapy are covered in this chapter. However, not all orthomolecular treatments have a clear rationale; some have been developed primarily through empirical observation. In many cases, nutrient doses have also been derived empirically, and the optimal doses may still be unknown.

In some cases, an orthomolecular treatment is nothing more than replacement therapy, as with the use of vitamin C to treat scurvy. In other cases, natural substances are used in doses beyond those normally required to correct a deficiency. However, it is sometimes difficult to distinguish between replacement therapy and "purposeful loading." For example, supraphysiological doses of insulin may be needed not only to correct insulin deficiency, but also to overcome insulin resistance. And, although elevated serum concentrations of homocysteine can result from deficiencies of vitamin B_6 or folic acid, some patients need higher-than-normal amounts of these vitamins to compensate for genetic defects in homocysteine metabolism.

Although all physicians practice orthomolecular medicine to some extent, only a small minority of them consider it their primary treatment modality. However, interest in this approach has been increasing because of the growing body of scientific literature documenting the effectiveness of various natural substances. In addition, these substances may often be safer and less expensive than conventional drugs and surgery.

Meganutrient Therapy: Theoretical Aspects

Orthomolecular medicine frequently involves the use of vitamins, minerals, amino acids, and other substances in amounts greater than the Recommended Dietary Allowance (RDA). It is important to recognize that the RDAs were designed to prevent nutritional deficiency diseases in the majority of the healthy human population. In formulating the RDA, the Committee on Dietary Allowances did not address the issue that larger doses of nutrients might produce benefits that extend beyond merely preventing deficiency.

The RDA by definition applies only to healthy individuals, not to those with physical or mental illness (4). Some individuals may become ill simply because they have higher-than-normal nutritional requirements that are not met by their diet. Extreme examples of this can be seen in the various inborn errors of metabolism that result in nutrient-dependency syndromes. For example, individuals with primary hyperoxaluria develop multiple calcium oxalate renal stones (which can progress to renal failure) unless they receive massive doses of pyridoxine (vitamin B_6). Although most of the well-characterized nutrient-dependency syndromes are rare, it is likely that milder versions of these or similar conditions are prevalent in a larger proportion of the population.

In addition to correcting nutritional deficiencies and dependencies, nutrients exert pharmacological effects that may be clinically useful. For example, ascorbic acid at high concentrations in vitro is both virucidal (5) and antibacterial (against *Mycobacterium tuberculosis, Escherichia coli,* and *Pseudomonas aeruginosa*) (6, 7). The concentrations of ascorbic acid that produce these antimicrobial effects are obtainable in vivo by intravenous administration of vitamin

C. Vitamin B_6 (in lozenge form) can prevent dental caries by shifting the balance of oral flora (8).

Pharmacological doses of nutrients also have the capacity to alter human biochemistry by activating or inducing the synthesis of enzymes, by inhibiting enzyme breakdown, or by other mechanisms. For example, vitamin B_6 can inhibit the endogenous synthesis of oxalate, thereby reducing the risk of calcium oxalate urolithiasis (9). Large doses of vitamin E inhibit platelet aggregation, which may be valuable in the prevention of cardiovascular disease (10). Magnesium has been shown to exert a bronchodilating effect in asthmatics (11). Some nutrients serve as precursors for neurotransmitters, prostaglandins, and other biologically active compounds. Thus, administration of tryptophan and choline have been shown to increase the concentrations of serotonin and acetylcholine, respectively (12). Supplementation with specific essential fatty acids has produced antiinflammatory effects, probably by altering the ratio of certain prostaglandins (13).

Other biochemical or physiological abnormalities that may be indications for nutrient supplementation include malabsorption, defective transport of nutrients into cells or across the blood-brain barrier, or a genetically abnormal enzyme that has a reduced affinity for its cofactor (usually a vitamin or mineral) (14). Disease processes (or the drugs used to treat them) may also increase nutritional requirements.

Thus, high-dose nutrient therapy can exert a wide range of physiological and pharmacological effects. These diverse actions have been listed to help create a conceptual framework that can be used to explain the observed benefits of orthomolecular treatments. It should be noted, however, that orthomolecular medicine is still in its infancy, and there are still many unknowns concerning mechanisms of action, choice of appropriate patients for treatment, and optimal nutrient doses.

The Practice of Orthomolecular Medicine

A growing number of physicians in the United States are using meganutrient therapy for the prevention and treatment of a wide range of medical conditions. Some of these clinical applications are theoretical, some are supported by anecdotal reports or uncontrolled studies, and other clinical applications have been documented by double-blind, placebo-controlled trials. Although the scientific documentation of orthomolecular medicine is increasing, the amount of research in this field is still small compared with many areas of orthodox medicine, such as drug therapies. And, although some orthomolecular treatments have not been subjected to rigorous controlled trials, many physicians have been impressed with their effectiveness.

It should be noted that orthomolecular physicians often use a combination of nutrients that have each been studied individually but usually not together. For example, there is evidence that coenzyme Q_{10} (CoQ_{10}), taurine, and magnesium are each valuable in the treatment of congestive heart failure (CHF) (15–17). The physician might prescribe all three of these nutrients, hoping for an additive or synergistic effect.

PROVIDER-PATIENT INTERACTION

In orthomolecular medicine, history taking, physical examination, and laboratory tests are largely the same as those done in a conventional medical setting. However, a physician practicing orthomolecular medicine may also seek additional information. For example, a patient with asthma might be questioned about symptoms of carpal tunnel syndrome because both conditions often respond to vitamin B_6. The physical examination would include observation for signs of nutritional deficiency (e.g., white spots on the fingernails, which may indicate zinc deficiency, or follicular hyperkeratosis, which suggests vitamin A deficiency). Certain laboratory tests may be used to help guide the treatment plan or to identify adverse effects. For example, whole-blood serotonin measurements can be used to predict which hyperactive children will respond to vitamin B_6, and erythrocyte copper levels may be measured in conjunction with high-dose zinc therapy because zinc supplementation can induce copper deficiency (18).

Although the classification of diseases in orthomolecular medicine is essentially the same as in conventional medicine, the treatment plans are often different. For example, a conventional physician is likely to treat rheumatoid arthritis with nonsteroidal anti-inflammatory drugs, corticosteroids, and antirheumatic drugs. An orthomolecular physician is likely to use essential fatty acids, zinc, copper, and dietary modifications, as well as prescription medications if the response is unsatisfactory. In most cases, nutrients can be administered concomitantly with conventional therapy. However, in some cases, the dosages of prescription medications must be adjusted (e.g., with a diabetic patient whose insulin requirement is reduced by supplementation with chromium and other nutrients). Nutritional therapy sometimes produces clinical improvements that are significant enough to obviate the need for conventional drug therapy.

At present, there are no established standards as to which treatments are most appropriate for which conditions. However, there now exists a substantial body of scientific research and clinical data from which practitioners can draw. The process of determining appropriate therapy is based largely on scientific research and clinical experience, just as it is in conventional medicine. Unlike many areas in conventional medicine, there generally are not data from large multicenter clinical trials on combination nutritional therapies as used in practice.

ORTHOMOLECULAR THERAPY AND OUTCOMES

Evaluation of treatment outcomes is also similar to that in conventional medicine. For example, bone densitometry studies would be used to monitor the effectiveness of an orthomolecular treatment for osteoporosis. The time period over which changes are expected to occur varies with the nature and severity of the illness, the age of the patient, and other well-known factors in conventional medicine. As in conventional medicine, changes in the treatment plan depend mainly on response to therapy, side effects, and cost.

USE OF THE SYSTEM FOR TREATMENT

This chapter's scope does not permit a comprehensive review of the field of orthomolecular medicine. Therefore, several medical conditions have been selected to illustrate the therapeutic potential of orthomolecular medicine. Practitioners interested in incorporating nutrient therapeutics into their practices should become familiar with the biochemical actions of the various nutrients, their clinical indications and toxicity, and their interactions with drugs and other nutrients (19).

Congestive Heart Failure

Conventional treatment for congestive heart failure (CHF) focuses primarily on minimizing the consequences of a failing myocardium but does little to improve the health and functionality of the heart muscle. Supplementing the patient with nutrients that have been shown to enhance cardiac function may help improve conventional therapy.

COENZYME Q_{10}

CoQ_{10} is a component of the electron transport chain, which is involved in the production of adenosine triphosphate (ATP). A deficiency of CoQ_{10} would be expected to impair energy-dependent processes, including myocardial contractility. The concentrations of CoQ_{10} in both plasma and myocardial tissue are significantly lower in patients with ischemic heart disease or dilated cardiomyopathy than in healthy controls (20, 21). Furthermore, the level of CoQ_{10} has been found to decrease progressively with increasing severity of heart disease.

Administration of 100 mg/day of CoQ_{10} to patients with cardiomyopathy resulted in a significant increase in mean left ventricular ejection fraction (from 41 to 59%) and a more than fivefold increase in survival time, compared with published survival statistics (22). In a double-blind trial, 641 patients with CHF were randomly assigned to receive placebo or CoQ_{10} (2 mg/kg/day) for one year. Conventional therapy was continued in both groups. The number

of patients requiring hospitalization for heart failure was 38% less in the CoQ_{10} group than in the placebo group (p < 0.001). The incidence of pulmonary edema was about 60% lower in the CoQ_{10} group than in the placebo group (p < 0.001) (23). CoQ_{10} therapy has also been reported to improve edema, pulmonary rales, dyspnea, and other manifestations of CHF (15).

TAURINE

Taurine constitutes more than 50% of the free amino acid pool in the heart. Taurine has been shown to have a positive inotropic effect and antiarrhythmic activity and to regulate the transport of calcium and potassium across myocardial cell membranes. Oral administration of taurine reduced the extent of cardiac lesions in genetically cardiomyopathic hamsters (24) and reduced the severity of experimentally induced CHF in rabbits (25).

In human studies, seven patients with CHF resulting from valvular disease received 2 g of taurine twice daily. Before treatment with taurine, all patients were restricted in activity and all had experienced worsening heart failure despite treatment with digitalis and diuretics for at least four weeks. Marked improvement was noted in 5 of 7 patients within 3 to 21 days after administration of taurine. These patients improved from New York Heart Association functional class III to class II within 4 weeks, and improvement was maintained with continued taurine supplementation (up to 12 months) (26). In a double-blind study, 58 patients with CHF received taurine (2 g, 3 times daily) or a placebo for 4 weeks. Administration of taurine resulted in significant improvements in dyspnea, edema, palpitations, cardiothoracic ratio on chest x-ray, and New York Heart Association functional class, whereas no significant improvements were seen in the placebo group (16).

MAGNESIUM

Magnesium also plays an important role in cardiac health. It functions as a vasodilator, calcium-channel blocker, and cofactor for the synthesis of ATP. In animal studies, magnesium deficiency resulted in focal myocardial necrosis.

In humans with cardiomyopathy, myocardial concentrations of magnesium were 65% lower than in healthy individuals, although serum levels were normal (17).

Although there have been no controlled trials of magnesium therapy for CHF, the author has seen dramatic results using parenteral magnesium. One patient, a 55-year-old man with a 15-year history of cardiomyopathy, was in the final stages of heart failure, being kept alive only by a continuous infusion of dobutamine in an intensive care unit. At the time, his life expectancy was thought to be hours or days. However, after administration of a single intramuscular injection of magnesium sulfate (1 g), the patient almost immediately experienced a marked improvement, which became even more pronounced following additional magnesium injections. The dobutamine infusion was successfully discontinued and the patient was able to return home, where he lived for two more years. During that time, he would rapidly decompensate if he did not receive a magnesium injection every fourth day. Although there are no randomized controlled trials of these three agents in combination for CHF, physicians using orthomolecular medicine will use this information from the scientific literature to put together combination therapies for CHF using nutrients and endogenous substances.

Osteoarthritis

Another example of how orthomolecular treatments are developed can be seen in arthritis. In the 1940s, William Kaufman, MD, administered niacinamide (900 to 4000 mg/day) to several hundred patients with osteoarthritis. In most cases, joint range of motion increased (as measured by goniometry) and symptoms, such as pain and stiffness, were reduced. Results were usually apparent three to four weeks after the initiation of treatment. Thereafter, progressive improvement occurred with continued treatment, but a gradual return of symptoms was noted if treatment was discontinued (27, 28).

Kaufman's observations recently have been confirmed in a double-blind trial. Seventy-two patients with osteoarthritis were randomly as-

signed to receive niacinamide (500 mg, 6 times daily) or a placebo for 3 months. Compared with the placebo, administration of niacinamide resulted in significant improvements in joint mobility and in overall severity of arthritis. Niacinamide-treated patients showed a reduction in erythrocyte sedimentation rate and were able to decrease their anti-inflammatory medications (29).

The delayed onset of action of niacinamide and the gradual return of symptoms on discontinuation of treatment suggest that niacinamide does more than merely relieve the symptoms of osteoarthritis. Apparently, this vitamin somehow controls the disease process. Nonsteroidal anti-inflammatory drugs, however, may actually accelerate the progression of osteoarthritis (30). At the present time, the mechanism of niacinamide's action is not known.

Niacinamide should be administered in at least three divided doses because it has a rapid half-life. On rare occasions, hepatotoxicity has developed with high-dose niacinamide. Therefore, liver enzymes (aminotransferases) should be monitored periodically, and patients should be advised to watch for nausea (an apparent early warning sign of niacinamide hepatotoxicity). Note that niacinamide causes liver damage less frequently than does niacin (nicotinic acid). When used appropriately, niacinamide is well tolerated and appears to be safer than nonsteroidal anti-inflammatory drugs.

Glucosamine sulfate, a compound that occurs naturally in the body, has also been shown to be effective in the treatment of osteoarthritis. Glucosamine sulfate is a precursor for the synthesis of the proteoglycans that make up joint cartilage and has also been shown to inhibit the degradation of proteoglycans (31). In one study, 20 patients with osteoarthritis of the knee received glucosamine sulfate (500 mg, 3 times daily) or a placebo for 6 to 8 weeks. Glucosamine sulfate was significantly more effective than placebo in relieving symptoms of pain, joint tenderness, and swelling. The results were rated as excellent in all 10 patients receiving glucosamine sulfate, whereas all 10 patients given placebo rated the results as fair or poor (32).

In another study, 40 patients with osteoarthritis of the knee received, in double-blind fashion, either glucosamine sulfate (500 mg, 3 times daily) or ibuprofen (1.2 g/day) for 8 weeks. The rate of improvement was slower in the glucosamine sulfate group, but the degree of improvement increased in that group as the study progressed. By the eighth week, glucosamine sulfate was significantly more effective than ibuprofen (33). Other studies have confirmed the effectiveness of glucosamine sulfate against osteoarthritis (34, 35). This compound appears to act directly on the disease process, reversing tissue degeneration and stimulating the production of healthy joint cartilage (36). Glucosamine sulfate is generally well tolerated and has not been reported to cause serious side effects or significant changes in standard laboratory parameters. An orthomolecular treatment for osteoarthritis of the knee may involve a combination of the previously mentioned and other compounds.

Gingivitis

Three small studies of nutritional therapy in gingivitis combine to provide another useful treatment. Thirty healthy volunteers participated in a double-blind study of the effect of folic acid on gingival health. Each participant rinsed his or her mouth twice daily with 5 mL of a 0.1% solution of folic acid or placebo. After 60 days, gingival inflammation (as assessed by the gingival index and bleeding index) was significantly less in the folic acid group than in the placebo group (37). Similar results were obtained after oral administration of folic acid (4 mg/day) (38).

CoQ$_{10}$ also appears to play a role in the prevention and treatment of gingivitis. Gingival biopsies have revealed subnormal concentrations of CoQ$_{10}$ in 60 to 96% of patients with periodontal disease (39, 40). Eighteen patients with periodontal disease received either CoQ$_{10}$ (50 mg/day) or a placebo for three weeks in a double-blind trial. All 8 patients receiving CoQ$_{10}$ improved, whereas only 3 of 10 patients receiving placebo showed improvement (p < 0.01) (41). Orthomolecular physicians have

found that combining these two approaches is very helpful in treating gingivitis.

Fatigue

Fatigue, which has many causes, is a common and often difficult problem to treat. Vitamin B$_{12}$ has long been used as a general "tonic" to relieve fatigue and to enhance well-being. Although vitamin B$_{12}$ injections are widely used, most physicians believe that the benefits are purely a placebo effect. The efficacy of vitamin B$_{12}$ as a tonic was investigated in a 1973 double-blind study. Twenty-eight individuals complaining of fatigue (all of whom had normal serum levels of vitamin B$_{12}$) received intramuscular injections of vitamin B$_{12}$ (hydroxocobalamin; 5 mg twice weekly) or a placebo, each for two weeks. Compared with placebo, vitamin B$_{12}$ treatment produced significant improvements in general well-being (p = .006) and happiness (p = .032). Improvements in fatigue (p = .09) and appetite (p = .073) were of borderline statistical significance (42). Other studies have not always shown benefit.

Another compound that has been found to be useful in the treatment of fatigue is potassium magnesium aspartate. It is thought that fatigue may in some cases be a result of inefficient mitochondrial energy production and, because of key roles in this process, potassium magnesium aspartate might be expected to improve mitochondrial function. Magnesium is involved in the synthesis of ATP and potassium in the stabilization of membranes. Aspartate serves as a substrate for the tricarboxylic acid (Krebs) cycle, and there is evidence that aspartate promotes the facilitated transport of potassium and magnesium into mitochondria.

Three double-blind, placebo-controlled studies that included a total of nearly 3000 patients have evaluated the effect of potassium magnesium aspartate (usually 1 g twice daily) in the treatment of fatigue. An improvement in symptoms was reported by 75 to 91% of patients receiving active treatment, compared to only 5 to 25% of patients given placebo (43–45). The author's experience is that a combination of these treatments, along with others, can significantly help many patients who have fatigue of unknown etiology.

Kidney Stones

Approximately 75% of the kidney stones that occur among Americans consist wholly or partly of calcium oxalate. Magnesium is known to inhibit the formation of calcium oxalate crystals (46), and vitamin B_6 has been reported to reduce urinary oxalate levels, apparently by reducing its endogenous synthesis (47). In one study, 55 patients with recurrent kidney stones received 500 mg/day of magnesium (in the form of magnesium hydroxide) for up to 4 years. Urinary magnesium increased and remained elevated during the entire treatment period. The mean number of stone recurrences was reduced by 90%, and 85% of the patients remained stone-free (48). In another study, 149 patients with recurrent stone formation were given 300 mg of magnesium oxide (equivalent to 180 mg of magnesium) and 10 mg of vitamin B_6 daily for 4.5 to 6 years. During this period, the mean stone formation rate decreased by 92.3%, from 1.3 to 0.1 stones per person per year (49). More research is needed, but the treatment is inexpensive and safe, warranting use for those with recurrent stones.

Osteoporosis

The effects of calcium, vitamin D, and estrogen on osteoporosis prevention are well known. However, several other nutrients also appear to play an important role in osteoporosis prevention. Magnesium, which constitutes up to 1% of bone ash, regulates calcium transport and bone mineralization. In one study, magnesium deficiency was demonstrated in 16 of 19 women with osteoporosis (50). Thirty-one postmenopausal women with osteoporosis received magnesium (250–750 mg/day) for 1 year. During that time, bone density increased in 22 women (71%) and remained stable in another 5 (51).

Vitamin K is required for the synthesis of osteocalcin, the bone protein that promotes

mineralization of bone. In one study, the mean serum vitamin K concentration was significantly lower (by 56%) in patients with a history of vertebral crush fractures than in age-matched controls (52). In a clinical trial in Japan, supplementation with vitamin K markedly reduced bone loss in postmenopausal women (53).

Trace minerals also appear to play a role in osteoporosis prevention. Postmenopausal women treated with calcium plus trace minerals (e.g., zinc, copper, and manganese) for 2 years showed a 1.48% increase in mean bone mineral density (BMD), whereas mean BMD decreased by 1.25% in women receiving calcium alone. Calcium plus trace minerals, but not calcium alone, was significantly more effective than placebo in preventing bone loss (54). In another study, administration of copper (3 mg/day) significantly reduced bone loss relative to placebo (55). There is evidence that other nutrients (including folic acid, vitamin B_6, vitamin D, boron, silicon, and strontium) may also be important for osteoporosis prevention (56, 57). Although these studies are small and the nutrients have not yet been evaluated in combination, the ability to monitor bone loss allows the physician to determine when the nutrients are effective in individual patients.

Orthomolecular Psychiatry

Nutrient therapy has shown potential in the treatment of schizophrenia, depression, dementia, and other psychiatric disorders.

SCHIZOPHRENIA

In 1962, Hoffer and Osmond reported that administration of large doses of niacin or niacinamide (usually 3–6 g/day) to schizophrenic patients significantly reduced the incidence of readmission to the hospital (58). Follow-up studies by other groups produced equivocal or negative results, and the use of megavitamins for schizophrenia has remained controversial. Hoffer later found that ascorbic acid enhanced the effect of niacinamide. More recently, Kanofsky reported that administration of large doses of ascorbic acid (up to 6 g/day) resulted in dramatic improvements in some schizophrenics (59). After 40 years of experience with megavitamin therapy, Dr. Hoffer has stated, "I can confidently tell the family of an acute schizophrenic that there is a 95% chance he or she will be back to normal in two years, and if chronic schizophrenic there is a 65% chance of [becoming] normal in ten years" (60). Because schizophrenia is a serious condition that is often refractory to treatment, controlled clinical trials using the orthomolecular approach are urgently needed, and sedative use in carefully monitored patients seems warranted.

DEPRESSION

Depression is often treated in conventional medicine by drugs designed to increase the concentration or the effect of serotonin, norepinephrine, or other neurotransmitters. Supplementation with the precursors of these neurotransmitters may have an effect similar to those of antidepressant drugs. Tryptophan, the precursor to serotonin, has been used with some success in the treatment of depression. Administration of niacinamide in combination with tryptophan appears to enhance the effectiveness of the latter, possibly by increasing the conversion of tryptophan to serotonin (61). Tyrosine, the precursor to norepinephrine, is also reportedly effective for some patients with depression (62). However, the efficacy of tryptophan and tyrosine has been inconsistent. Buist developed an algorithm to help predict which patients are most likely to respond to each of these amino acids (63).

DEMENTIA

Several naturally occurring compounds are being used to treat dementia. In one study, 12 of 16 elderly patients with dementia and polyneuropathy had low levels of vitamin B_{12} in the cerebrospinal fluid (CSF). However, only three of these patients had low serum levels of the vitamin. Parenteral administration of vitamin B_{12} was associated with clinical improvement (64). This study suggests that vitamin B_{12} deficiency (localized to the brain and central nervous system) may play a role in the etiology of some cases of dementia. Furthermore, serum

vitamin B_{12} measurements may fail to identify this abnormality in many cases. Because obtaining CSF is an invasive procedure, and because vitamin B_{12} injections are safe and inexpensive, I recommend a therapeutic trial of intramuscular vitamin B_{12} injections (1000 mcg weekly for 6 weeks). If effective, the treatment is continued as needed. Other compounds that are reportedly of value in the treatment of dementia include phosphatidylserine (65), L-acetylcarnitine (66), and nicotinamide adenine dinucleotide (NADH) (67). Clearly, much more research is needed before a completely rational administration of nutrient therapies is achieved. Currently, there are few documented ways to help identify which patients will benefit from specific nutrient therapies. However, an increasing number of functional and serum tests are developing that may aid in a more rational and objective use of orthomolecular medicine in the future.

Intravenous Nutrient Therapy

Because nutrients almost always work in concert, many physicians practicing orthomolecular medicine feel that a therapeutic trial of nutrient loading is a useful approach to many patients with refractory conditions. Intravenous nutrient therapy is becoming increasingly popular among physicians practicing nutritional medicine. Although there are few controlled trials to support this treatment approach, the results are in many cases obvious and dramatic. A combination treatment consisting of magnesium, calcium, B vitamins, and vitamin C was described by John Myers, MD, in the 1970s and is currently being used by more than 1000 physicians in the United States. The author has administered more than 15,000 of these treatments, without observing any serious adverse reactions.

Because there is the potential for vasovagal, allergic reactions and drug interactions, treatment must be administered carefully and professionally and all patients monitored. The so-called Myers cocktail has aborted acute asthma attacks and migraines in a matter of minutes or even seconds. I have found it valuable in the treatment of some cases of chronic fatigue, depression, fibromyalgia, acute or chronic urticaria, allergic rhinitis, acute infection, congestive heart failure, occlusive peripheral vascular disease, and angina pectoris. Information on this intravenous protocol and its proper administration is available (68).

Recent studies have shown that intravenous administration of magnesium can rapidly relieve acute attacks of asthma (69) and migraine (70). Otherwise, most of the observations on intravenous nutrient therapy, though highly enthusiastic, are anecdotal. Unfortunately, blinded trials are difficult to perform because intravenously administered magnesium produces an unmistakable sensation of warmth.

Large intravenous doses of vitamin C (sometimes in combination with other nutrients) have been used to treat acute viral hepatitis, mononucleosis, and other infections. Although no controlled trials have been published, many physicians think that this treatment promotes unusually rapid resolution of these illnesses.

EDTA

Ethylenediamine tetraacetic acid (EDTA) is a synthetic amino acid used by some practitioners to treat atherosclerosis. Although EDTA is not an orthomolecular therapy, it is being mentioned here, because many physicians who use orthomolecular therapy also use EDTA.

In the 1950s, it was observed that some patients receiving EDTA for the treatment of lead poisoning experienced unexpected improvement in angina pectoris. Other reports of improvement in patients with atherosclerotic disease soon followed, and EDTA therapy eventually became a popular (though controversial) alternative to bypass surgery.

Although EDTA is known to chelate lead and other metals, its mechanism of action against atherosclerotic disease is not well understood. EDTA does influence lipid metabolism, free-radical production, platelet adhesion, blood coagulation, and prostaglandin synthesis (71). However, none of these actions can adequately explain the observation that the effects of EDTA persist long after the treatment is discontinued.

Physicians who use EDTA believe that it is safe and often dramatically effective in reversing cardiovascular diseases, particularly when administered according to a well-defined protocol and along with lifestyle modifications and various nutritional supplements (72). Chappell et al. presented a meta-analysis of 51 practice-outcome reports (73, 74). Of a total of 24,000 patients treated, 88% showed objective evidence of improvement.

However, in three small randomized trials in patients with peripheral vascular disease who received various lifestyle and nutritional recommendations, EDTA was not significantly more effective than placebo (75–77). Each of these studies has been severely criticized, and one is under investigation by the Dutch courts. To date, there have been no controlled trials of EDTA therapy in patients with coronary artery disease, the condition for which it is most frequently used (78–80).

Thus, a discrepancy exists between the often dramatic effects that practitioners have reported and documented and the results from controlled trials. Large, well-designed clinical trials are therefore urgently needed. If EDTA therapy is, indeed, effective, then it would represent a safer and less expensive alternative to bypass surgery. A complete chapter on EDTA, including its pharmacology and clinical use, and a review of the published research will appear in *Textbook of CAM*, to be published next year.

Other Uses of Orthomolecular Medicine

Published research suggests that many other medical conditions may respond to orthomolecular treatments. These conditions include hypertension, diabetes mellitus, diabetic neuropathy and retinopathy, infertility, rheumatoid arthritis, carpal tunnel syndrome, acne vulgaris, herpes simplex, seborrheic dermatitis, premenstrual syndrome, menorrhagia, cervical dysplasia, fibrocystic breast disease, attention deficit hyperactivity disorder, peptic ulcer, alcoholism, sickle cell disease, Parkinson's disease, anxiety, and tardive dyskinesia. There is also evidence that nutritional treatments might delay the progression of multiple sclerosis, amyotrophic lateral sclerosis, and AIDS (20).

Toxicity

Although nutrients and related compounds are generally quite safe, orthomolecular medicine is not without risk. Large doses of vitamin A, niacin, niacinamide, vitamin B$_6$, zinc, selenium, and certain amino acids have been reported to cause toxic effects. Recently, beta-carotene supplementation was found to increase the risk of lung cancer in cigarette smokers. (For details on the safety and adverse effects of specific nutrients, see Chapter 7 in this book.)

Physicians practicing orthomolecular medicine must be familiar with the adverse effects of nutrients, as well as the dosage ranges at which these effects can develop. In addition, a working knowledge of drug-nutrient and nutrient-nutrient interactions is essential. However, when nutrients are administered with appropriate precautions, the incidence of severe toxicity resulting from nutritional therapy is extremely low.

ORGANIZATION

Training

Currently there are no accredited training programs that certify physicians in the practice of orthomolecular medicine. Practitioners typically become self-trained in this field by reading the medical literature and attending seminars on the subject. A four-day professional workshop, "Nutritional Therapy in Medical Practice," is presented annually by Alan R. Gaby, MD, and Jonathan V. Wright, MD (20). The American Holistic Medical Association and the American College for Advancement in Medicine hold annual and semiannual conventions, respectively, which include various topics related to nutritional therapy and orthomolecular medicine. Naturopathic medical schools require extensive training in nutrition, which includes many aspects of orthomolecular medicine.

Reimbursement Status

Reimbursement for orthomolecular treatments is variable. Evaluation-and-management services are generally reimbursed the same as in conventional medicine. In most cases, nutrients and intravenous therapies are not considered "usual and customary" and are therefore not covered. However, some third-party payers do pay for such treatments or evaluate them on a case-by-case basis. A few medical insurance companies are now offering plans that reimburse for many types of alternative medicine, including nutrients and intravenous therapies.

Relations with Conventional Medicine

There is no official relationship between orthomolecular medicine and conventional medicine. However, a growing number of medical schools are offering courses and continuing education seminars that include various aspects of this discipline.

PROSPECTS FOR THE FUTURE

Practitioners are gradually incorporating more nutritional and orthomolecular treatments into their practices. Hundreds of such practitioners have conscientiously tried these treatments and have been impressed with their effectiveness.

Published research and the clinical experience of many physicians suggest that more widespread application of orthomolecular medicine could improve the safety and effectiveness of medical care while simultaneously reducing costs. Although many of the treatments that show promise have not been subjected to controlled clinical trials, they could easily be tested if research funding were available. By testing the most promising orthomolecular treatments, the practice of medicine might be changed dramatically, with enormous implications for the public health.

REFERENCES

1. Pauling L. Orthomolecular psychiatry. Science 1968;160:265–271.

2. Jancin B. Amino acid defect causes 20% of atherosclerosis in CHD. Family Pract News 1994:7.

3. Pauling L. Vitamin C, the common cold and the flu. San Francisco: W. H. Freeman and Company, 1976.

4. Committee on Dietary Allowances. Recommended Dietary Allowances, 9th rev ed., National Academy of Sciences, Washington, DC, 1980:1.

5. Murata A. Virucidal activity of vitamin C for prevention and treatment of viral diseases. In: Hasegawa T, ed. Proc First Int Congr IAMS, Science Council of Japan, 1975.

6. Sirsi M. Antimicrobial action of vitamin C on *M. tuberculosis* and some other pathogenic organisms. Indian J Med Sci 1952;6:252–255.

7. Rawal BD, McKay G, Blackhall MI. Inhibition of *Pseudomonas aeruginosa* by ascorbic acid acting singly and in combination with antimicrobials: in vitro and in vivo studies. Med J Aust 1974; 1:169–174.

8. Palazzo A, Cobe HM, Ploumis E. The effect of pyridoxine on the oral microbial populations. NY State Dent J 1959;25:303–307.

9. Murthy MSR, Farooqui S, Talwar HS, et al. Effect of pyridoxine supplementation on recurrent stone formers. Int J Clin Pharmacol Ther Toxicol 1982;20:434–437.

10. Steiner M, Anastasi J. Vitamin E: an inhibitor of the platelet release reaction. J Clin Invest 1976; 57:732–737.

11. Okayama H, Okayama M, Aikawa T, et al. Treatment of status asthmaticus with intravenous magnesium sulfate. J Asthma 1991;28:11–17.

12. Benedict CR, Anderson GH, Sole MJ. The influence of oral tyrosine and tryptophan feeding on plasma catecholamines in man. Am J Clin Nutr 1983;38:429.

13. Das UN. Beneficial effect of eicosanpentaenoic and docosahexaenoic acids in the management of systemic lupus erythematosus and its relationship to the cytokine network. Prostaglandins Leukotrienes Essential Fatty Acids 1994;51:207–213.

14. Nierenberg DW, Stukel TA, Baron JA, et al. Determinants of increase in plasma concentration of beta-carotene after chronic oral supplementation. Am J Clin Nutr 1991;53:1443–1449.

15. Baggio E, Gandini R, Plancher AC, et al. Italian multicenter study on the safety and efficacy of coenzyme Q_{10} as adjunctive therapy in heart failure (interim analysis). Clin Invest 1993;71:S145-S149.

16. Azuma J, Sawamura A, Awata N, et al. Double-blind randomized crossover trial of taurine in congestive heart failure. Curr Ther Res 1983;34: 543–557.

17. Frustaci A, Caldarulo M, Schiavoni G, et al. Myocardial magnesium content, histology, and antiarrhythmic response to magnesium infusion. Lancet 1987;2:1019.

18. Coleman M, Steinberg G, Tippett J, et al. A preliminary study of the effect of pyridoxine administration in a subgroup of hyperkinetic children: a double-blind crossover comparison with methylphenidate. Biol Psychiatry 1979;14:741–751.

19. A workshop titled "Nutritional Therapy in Medical Practice" is presented annually by Alan R. Gaby, MD, and Jonathan V. Wright, MD, and is available on audiocassette tape (with reference materials). For information, contact Wright-Gaby Seminars, 515 W. Harrison St., Suite 200, Kent, WA, 98032; 253-854-4900, ext. 166.

20. Hanaki Y, Sugiyama S, Ozawa T, Ohno M. Ratio of low-density lipoprotein cholesterol to ubiquinone as a coronary risk factor. N Engl J Med 1991;325:814–815.

21. Littarru GP, Ho L, Folkers K. Deficiency of coenzyme Q_{10} in human heart disease. Part I. Int J Vitam Nutr Res 1972;42:291–305.

22. Langsjoen PH, Langsjoen PH, Folkers K. Long-term efficacy and safety of coenzyme Q_{10} therapy for idiopathic dilated cardiomyopathy. Am J Cardiol 1990;65:521–523.

23. Morisco C, Trimarco B, Condorelli M. Effect of coenzyme Q_{10} in patients with congestive heart failure: a long-term multicenter randomized study. Clin Invest 1993;71:S134-S136.

24. Azari J, Brumbaugh P, Barbeau A, Huxtable R. Taurine decreases lesion severity in the hearts of cardiomyopathic hamsters. Can J Neurol Sci 1980;7:435–440.

25. Azuma J, Takihara K, Awata N, et al. Beneficial effect of taurine on congestive heart failure induced by chronic aortic regurgitation in rabbits. Res Commun Chem Pathol Pharmacol 1984;45:261–270.

26. Azuma J, Hasegawa H, Sawamura A, et al. Taurine for treatment of congestive heart failure. Int J Cardiol 1982;2:303–304.

27. Kaufman W. The common form of joint dysfunction: its incidence and treatment. Brattleboro, VT: E.L. Hildreth Co., 1949.

28. Kaufman W. The use of vitamin therapy to reverse certain concomitants of aging. J Am Geriatr Soc 1955;11:927–936.

29. Jonas WB, Rapoza CP, Blair WF. The effect of niacinamide on osteoarthritis: a pilot study. Inflamm Res 1996;45:330–334.

30. Rashad S, Revel P, Hemingway A, et al. Effect of non-steroidal anti-inflammatory drugs on the course of osteoarthritis. Lancet 1989;2:519–522.

31. D'Ambrosio E, Casa B, Bompani R, et al. Glucosamine sulphate: a controlled clinical investigation in arthrosis. Pharmatherapeutica 1981;2:504–508.

32. Pujalte JM, Llavore EP, Ylescupidez FR. Double-blind clinical evaluation of oral glucosamine sulphate in the basic treatment of osteoarthritis. Curr Med Res Opin 1980;7:110–114.

33. Vaz AL. Double-blind clinical evaluation of the relative efficacy of glucosamine sulphate in the management of osteoarthritis of the knee in outpatients. Curr Med Res Opin 1982;8:145–149.

34. Muller-Fabbender H, Bach GL, Haase W, et al. Glucosamine sulfate compared to ibuprofen in osteoarthritis of the knee. Osteoarthritis Cartilage 1994;2:61–69.

35. Reichelt A, Forster KK, Fischer M, et al. Efficacy and safety of intramuscular glucosamine sulfate in osteoarthritis of the knee. A randomised, placebo-controlled, double-blind study. Arzneimittelforsch 1994;44:75–80.

36. Drovanti A, Bignamini AA, Rovati AL. Therapeutic activity of oral glucosamine sulfate in osteoarthrosis: a placebo-controlled double-blind investigation. Clin Ther 1980;3:260–272.

37. Vogel RI, Fink RA, Frank O, Baker H. The effect of topical application of folic acid on gingival health. J Oral Med 1978;33(1):20–22.

38. Vogel RI, Fink RA, Schneider LC, et al. The effect of folic acid on gingival health. J Periodontol 1976;47:667–668.

39. Nakamura R, Littarru GP, Folkers K, Wilkinson EG. Study of CoQ$_{10}$-enzymes in gingiva from patients with periodontal disease and evidence for a deficiency of coenzyme Q$_{10}$. Proc Natl Acad Sci U S A 1974;71:1456–1460.

40. Hansen IL, Iwamoto Y, Kishi T, Folkers K. Bioenergetics in clinical medicine. IX. Gingival and leucocytic deficiencies of coenzyme Q$_{10}$ in patients with periodontal disease. Res Commun Chem Pathol Pharmacol 1976;14:729–738.

41. Wilkinson EG, Arnold RM, Folkers K. Bioenergetics in clinical medicine. VI. Adjunctive treatment of periodontal disease with coenzyme Q$_{10}$. Res Commun Chem Pathol Pharmacol 1976;14:715–719.

42. Ellis FR, Nasser S. A pilot study of vitamin B12 in the treatment of tiredness. Br J Nutr 1973;30:277–283.

43. Hicks JT. Treatment of fatigue in general practice: a double-blind study. Clin Med 1964;January: 85–90.

44. Shaw DL Jr, Chesney MA, Tullis IF, Agersborg HPK. Management of fatigue: a physiologic approach. Am J Med Sci 1962;243:758–769.

45. Formica PE. The housewife syndrome: treatment with the potassium and magnesium salts of aspartic acid. Curr Ther Res 1962;4:98–106.

46. Lyon ES, Borden TA, Ellis JE, Vermeulen CW. Calcium oxalate lithiasis produced by pyridoxine deficiency and inhibition with high magnesium diets. Invest Uro 1966;4:133.

47. Thind SK, et al. Role of vitamin B6 in oxalate metabolism in urolithiasis. Am J Clin Nutr 1979;32(6):(Abstract).

48. Johansson G, Backman U, Danielson BG, et al. Effects of magnesium hydroxide in renal stone disease. J Am Coll Nutr 1982;1:179–185.

49. Prien EL, Gershoff SN. Magnesium oxide-pyridoxine therapy for recurrent calcium oxalate calculi. J Urol 1974;112:509–512.

50. Cohen L, Kitzes R. Infrared spectroscopy and magnesium content of bone mineral in osteoporotic women. Isr J Med Sci l981;17:1123–1125.

51. Sojka JE, Weaver CM. Magnesium supplementation and osteoporosis. Nutr Rev 1995;53:71–74.

52. Hart JP, Shearer MJ, Klenerman L, et al. Electrochemical detection of depressed circulating levels of vitamin K1 in osteoporosis. J Clin Endocrinol Metab 1985;60:1268–1269.

53. Vermeer C, Gijsbers BLMG, Craciun AM, et al. Effects of vitamin K on bone mass and bone metabolism. J Nutr 1996;126:1187S–1191S.

54. Strause L, Saltman P, Smith KT, et al. Spinal bone loss in postmenopausal women supplemented with calcium and trace minerals. J Nutr 1994;124: 1060–1064.

55. Eaton-Evans J, McIlrath EM, Jackson WE, et al. Copper supplementation and bone-mineral density in middle-aged women. Proc Nutr Soc 1995; 54:191A.

56. Gaby AR. Preventing and reversing osteoporosis. Rocklin, CA: Prima Publishing, 1994.

57. Gaby AR, Wright JV. Nutrients and osteoporosis. J Nutr Med 1990;1:63–72.

58. Osmond H, Hoffer A. Massive niacin treatment in schizophrenia. Review of a nine-year study. Lancet 1962;1:316–320.

59. Kanofsky JD, Kay SR, Lindenmayer JP, Seifter E. Ascorbate: an adjunctive treatment for schizophrenia. J Am Coll Nutr 1989;8:425.

60. Wright JV. Interview with Abram Hoffer; Nutrition and Healing, September, 1994 (1-800-528-0559).

61. Chouinard G, Young SN, Annable L, Sourkes TL. Tryptophan-nicotinamide, imipramine and their combination in depression. Acta Psychiatr Scand 1979;59:395–414.

62. Gelenberg AJ, Wojcik JD, Growdon JH, et al. Tyrosine treatment of depression. Am J Psychiatry 1980;137:622–623.

63. Buist RA. The therapeutic predictability of tryptophan and tyrosine in the treatment of depression. Int Clin Nutr Rev 1983;3(2):1–3.

64. van Tiggelen CJM, Peperkamp JPC, Tertoolen HJFW. Assessment of vitamin B_{12} status in CSF. Am J Psychiatry 1984;141:136.

65. Crook TH, Tinklenberg J, Yesavage J, et al. Effects of phosphatidylserine in age-associated memory impairment. Neurology 1991;41:644–649.

66. Salvioli G, Neri M. L-acetylcarnitine treatment of mental decline in the elderly. Drugs Exp Clin Res 1994;20:169–176.

67. Birkmayer JGD. Coenzyme nicotinamide adenine dinucleotide. New therapeutic approach for improving dementia of the Alzheimer type. Ann Clin Lab Sci 1996;26:1–9.

68. To request a copy of the intravenous nutrient protocol, send a self-addressed stamped envelope to the Wright/Gaby Nutrition Institute, P.O. Box 21535, Baltimore, MD 21282.

69. Skobeloff EM, Spivey WH, McNamara RM, Greenspan L. Intravenous magnesium sulfate for the treatment of acute asthma in the emergency department. JAMA 1989;262:1210–1213.

70. Mauskop A, Altura BT, Cracco RQ, Altura BM. Intravenous magnesium sulphate relieves migraine attacks in patients with low serum ionized magnesium levels: a pilot study. Clin Sci 1995;89: 633–636.

71. Halstead BM, Rozeman TC. The scientific basis of EDTA chelation therapy. 2nd ed. Landrum, SC: TRC Publishing, 1997.

72. Rozema TC. The protocol for safe and effective administration of EDTA and other chelating agents for vascular disease, degenerative disease, and metal toxicity. J Adv Med 1997;10:5–100.

73. Chappell LT, Stahl JP. The correlation between EDTA chelation therapy and improvement in cardiovascular function: a meta-analysis. J Adv Med 1993;6:139–160.

74. Chappell Lt, Stahl JP, Evans R. EDTA chelation treatment for vascular disease: a meta-analysis using unpublished data. J Adv Med 1994;7:131–142.

75. Van Rij AM, Solomon C, Packer SGK, Hopkins WG. Chelation therapy for intermittent claudication: a double-blind, randomized, controlled trial. Circulation 1994;90:1194–1199.

76. Sloth-Nielson J, Guldager B, Mouritzen C, et al. Arteriographic findings in EDTA chelation therapy on peripheral arteriosclerosis. Am J Surg 1991;162:122–125.

77. Guldager B, Jelnes R, Jorgensen SJ, et al. EDTA treatment of intermittent claudication–a double-blind, placebo controlled study. J Int Med Res 1992;231:261–267.

78. (UVVU) CoSD. Conclusions concerning complaints in connection with trial of EDTA versus placebo in the treatment of arteriosclerosis. Copenhagen, Denmark: Danish Research Council, 1994.

79. Jonas WB. Meta-analysis of EDTA chelation: math that doesn't matter. J Adv Med 1994;7:109–112.

80. Jonas WB. Effectiveness of EDTA chelation therapy. Circulation 1995;92:1352.

CHAPTER 28

HOMEOPATHY

Edward H. Chapman

BACKGROUND

Homeopathy is a unique approach to healing that uses extremely dilute medicines to trigger a person's innate capacity to heal. Homeopathy is based on *the law of similars*, the observation that medicines can produce in healthy people the same symptoms they cure in the sick. Homeopathy approaches the whole patient in a systematic manner, using naturally occurring substances to restore health on physical, emotional, and mental levels. The homeopathic approach is dramatic by nature of the small amount of medicine used—often beyond the concentration that scientists can measure in molecules. However, an effect of those minimal doses can be demonstrated. The controversy about homeopathy centers around this apparent action of microdoses. The advantage of low doses is that the side effects and costs are minimal.

History and Development

The law of similars was first articulated in Germany by Samuel Hahnemann in 1796. His observations and discussion of this healing system were described in the *Organon of the Medical Art*, first published in 1810 (1). Five subsequent editions were printed during his career, the sixth and last in 1842, the year before his death. His method engendered both antagonism and enthusiasm among his colleagues in the medical profession. A committed group of students, the most famous of which in Europe was Clemens Baron von Boenninghausen, complemented the discoveries of their mentor with their own written works and provings (tests on healthy individuals) of new medicines. Other Hahnemann students emigrated to the New World, where homeopathy flourished throughout the rest of the nineteenth century (2).

Hans Graham was the first homeopathic physician to come from Europe to the United States. His arrival in 1825 was soon followed by Constantine Hering, who in 1844 helped to found the America Institute of Homeopathy (AIH) to promote the practice of homeopathy. The AIH is the oldest national medical organization and continues to represent the interests of homeopathic physicians to government, the public, and the insurance industry. Homeopathy flourished in the late 1800s. Developments instituted by a number of American practitioners remain essential to homeopathic practice today. James Tyler Kent authored *Lectures on Homeopathic Philosophy* (3), *Lectures on Homeopathic Materia Medica* (4), and *Kent's General Repertory* (5). The repertory (an index used to help select medications for a patient) changed the way homeopathy was practiced and forms the basis of computerized repertorization systems used today. Many of the original provings of Hahnemann and his disciples were repeated and new substances were also tested. These provings, together with toxicologic and clinical observations of the medicines, were compiled in *materia medicas*. The most famous of these are *The Encyclopedia of Pure Materia Medicas* by Timothy F. Allen, MD (6), and *Guiding Symptoms* by Constantine Hering (7), both of which are used daily by modern homeopaths.

A contentious relationship existed between homeopathic and the allopathic physicians since the nineteenth century. The code of ethics of the American Medical Association (AMA), founded in 1846, was designed to prevent medical practitioners from associating with homeopaths (8).

No one can be a regular practitioner, or fit associate in consultation, whose practice is based on an exclusive dogma, to the rejection of the accumulated experience of the profession, and of the aids actually furnished by anatomy, physiology, pathology, and organic chemistry (9).

Around 1900, 8% of American physicians' practices included homeopathy, and there were twenty homeopathic medical schools (9), including Boston University, Hahnemann Medical School, New York Medical School, and University of Michigan. With the changes in medical education catalyzed by the Flexner report in 1910 and the discovery of antimicrobials, the popularity of homeopathy took a steep decline. Hahnemann Medical School issued its last homeopathic diploma in 1950. However, since the late 1970s, there has been a resurgence of interest prompted by the widespread experience of the limitations of the current conventional medical model: costs, side effects, depersonalization, and ineffectiveness in treating many chronic and acute conditions. Currently in the United States, there are an estimated 500 medical or osteopathic physicians who use homeopathy as a primary modality, and many more who use homeopathy on a limited basis. There are another 1000 practitioners of homeopathy who have other licences (e.g., NP, PA, RN-C, LicAc, DC). Extrapolation of data in a January, 1993, *New England Journal of Medicine* (10) report suggested that 2.5 million Americans used homeopathic medicines; of these, about one third actually visited homeopaths in 1990.

HOMEOPATHY AS AN INTERNATIONAL MEDICINE

According to the World Health Organization (WHO), homeopathy is the second most used health care system in the world. Throughout India, most of Eastern and Western Europe, and Central and South America, homeopathy enjoys public popularity, government recognition, and support. In France, 36% of the population uses homeopathic medicines (11), 68% of French physicians consider homeopathic medicines effective, 32% use it in their practice, and all pharmacies carry the medicines. Data from the French social security system (12) have shown that the total costs per homeopathic physician yearly, including fees, indemnities, laboratory tests, and medications, is 46% lower than that of their allopathic colleagues. Homeopaths spend more time with patients, so fees per consultation are 35% higher; but the average number of consultations is lower by 25%. Additional cost reductions are noted in laboratory examinations (20%), per diem indemnities (50%), and prescription costs (23%), leading to an overall 9% reduction of costs per procedure.

In Germany, 20% of physicians use homeopathic medicines. In Great Britain, 42% of physicians refer patients to homeopaths, and homeopathy is reimbursed by the National Health Service. In Scotland, 20% of general practitioners have taken a postgraduate course in homeopathy. In the Netherlands, 45% of physicians consider the medicines effective (13).

HOMEOPATHY IN PRIMARY CARE

Increasing numbers of families choose homeopathy as their preferred method of primary care, seeking a safe, effective treatment that easily adapts to self-care. Many patients come to homeopaths after finding conventional treatments an unsatisfactory solution for their specific complaint. Based on a survey of AIH members in 1992 (14), 82% of patients seen by homeopaths in the United States seek care for chronic complaints, compared with 48% of the conventional primary care population. The top 10 diagnoses treated by homeopaths surveyed were asthma, depression, otitis media, allergic rhinitis, headache, psychological complaints, allergy, dermatitis, arthritis, and high blood pressure.

The majority of physicians using homeopathy have training in family practice, primary care pediatrics, or general internal medicine, and have supplemented their standard education with the study of homeotherapeutics. Most continue to practice in an outpatient setting in their primary care role. As their homeopathic expertise develops, many physicians and allied health providers function as specialists, seeing patients referred for homeopathic treatment of specific problems.

Principal Concepts

An approach to healing based on the law of similars can be clearly differentiated from conventional medicine. Most modern drugs either inhibit the growth of identified infectious agents, suppress specific processes in the body, or counteract disturbances of physiology. The processes held responsible for the observed pathology and/or changes in function are measured by cellular or biochemical markers. Homeopaths have coined the term *allopathy* [*allos* is Greek for opposite] to describe those treatments that oppose the underlying physiological disturbance of the disease process. Allopathy is most effective when the underlying infectious agent or physiology of the disease process is understood, and the drug is targeted at a known biochemical pathway.

Replacement therapy is a second approach used in modern medicine and is appropriate to diseases of an endocrine nature in which the glands are hypofunctioning, or to nutritional conditions in which the specific vitamins, minerals, or amino acids are lacking or poorly absorbed. Again, this system assumes a knowledge of the disturbed physiology.

Isopathy, a third conventional approach, has many parallels to homeopathy. Isopathy uses smaller or attenuated doses of the actual substances responsible for disease to induce a resistance in the organism to developing the actual disease. Examples of isopathy are allergy desensitization and immunization. Although the production of protective antibodies in immuniza-

tion is understood, the mechanism by which desensitization works is less well known; it depends on complex feedback loops within the immune system.

LAW OF SIMILARS

The law of similars, as used in homeopathy, is based on empirical observations. A medicinal substance given to healthy people provokes a reproducible set of symptoms on mental, emotional, and physical levels. The process by which homeopathic medicines are tested on healthy volunteers is referred to as *proving* (from the German *prüfung*, which means "test"). The resemblance of the proving symptoms of a medicine to the symptoms of a patient renders the patient uniquely sensitive to that medicine's action. An appropriately selected dose of the similar, homeopathically prepared medicine is capable of stimulating the innate curative responses in the body. This curative response occurs with minimal side effects, and often leads to the long-lasting resolution of both acute and chronic symptoms as well as the underlying functional disturbance from which they arise.

Although treatment by similars may be conceptually challenging to modern clinicians and scientists, it may account for the paradoxical action of a number of drugs used in conventional medicine. For example, psychostimulants (e.g., Ritalin) produce many of the same symptoms in otherwise healthy people that they help to control in patients with attention deficit hyperactivity disorder. Digitalis can produce any arrhythmia that it can treat, depending on the dose. The effects of these drugs are well documented, but their mechanism of action is not well understood.

THE MINUTE DOSE

In addition to the law of similars, other aspects of homeopathic theory are controversial. The most significant controversy surrounds the minute dose of the medicine. Some modern pharmacists jokingly refer to the "homeopathic dose," by which they mean a dose too small to have an effect. In homeopathy, the principle of the minimum dose states that one should use the smallest dose and lowest frequency of repetition possible. All good medical practice would agree with this principle. But homeopaths have taken the idea of the minimum dose to a degree that defies any verified law of physics or biochemistry. Homeopathic medicines are prepared by process of serial dilution and agitation. The concentration of the diluted medicine is often so dilute that no molecules are measurable. Furthermore, homeopathic medicines are classically given in single doses at intervals ranging from minutes to months.

TOTALITY OF SYMPTOMS

In addition to the law of similars and the minimum dose principle, there is a third way that the homeopathic model differs from the conventional medical model. The homeopath tries to comprehend the *totality of symptoms*. The homeopath views the signs and symptoms of illness as a representation of the organism's attempt to heal itself. These symptoms, rather than being viewed as an enemy, become the window into the healing efforts of the organism. To apply homeopathy, the physician does not need to know the underlying pathophysiology involved. Hahnemann went so far as to state that "diseases are not mechanical or chemical alterations of the material substance of the organism . . . . They are solely spirit-like, dynamic mistunements of life" (1). Hahnemann believed it is impossible to know the hidden causes of disease, and that fully knowing the "deviations . . . felt by the patient himself, perceived by those around him, or observed by the physician himself" were all that is needed to cure a disease (1).

In other words, disease exists on a dynamic or energetic level before the appearance of measurable and observable changes. This concept is similar to the *chi* in acupuncture, which describes an organized energy system in the body that causes all physical events to occur. Disease is, first, the disruption of the energy of the system. That disruption is experienced through signs and symptoms. Molecular and tissue changes occur from the energetic disruption. In practice, what is curable by homeopathy is known through the signs and symptoms displayed by the organism to the observing physi-

cian. These dynamic changes can be cured only by dynamic medicine. Dynamic medicines affect the energy system, or the *vital force,* active in the body. When the energy is balanced, the signs and symptoms of the disruption resolve spontaneously. Homeopathic medicine communicates information to this system that assists autoregulation.

Conventional medicine attempts to know disease by understanding what is clinically observable and by knowledge of the hidden pathophysiologic disturbances of the organism. Categorization of disease proceeds by defining what is common in people with a given condition, and then through objective measures: pathology specimens, biochemical markers, radiologic images, and electrophysiology. The unique characteristics of the patient are less important. This perspective has led to a therapeutic system that treats conditions rather than patients; it is often described by patients as depersonalized.

Homeopaths emphasize the characteristic, or individualizing, subjective symptoms of the patient (i.e., the totality of symptoms). The medical diagnosis of the patient carries less importance to the homeopathic prescription than the patient's temperament or the sensations experienced and reported by the patient or observers. Homeopaths describe a *state of the patient* that needs to be cured; they describe this as synonymous with the state produced in the provings by the most similar homeopathic medicine. Therefore, patients with a single diagnosis may receive any medicine in the homeopathic *materia medica;* and patients with disparate conditions (e.g., migraine headaches, acute pharyngitis) may receive the same medication.

Modern homeopathic physicians, with their conventional training in the pathophysiologic basis of disease, operate simultaneously in two world views, recognizing the strengths and limitations of both. Surgery is needed when mechanical disturbances are present or the results of an underlying disease process have led to physical changes that are beyond the abilities of the organism to repair. Conventional replacement therapies are essential at times when the body's own sources have become inadequate. Allopathic medications are often lifesaving in acute disease; however, in many acute conditions, they are overused, and in chronic disease may lead to side effects that occasionally rival the severity of the underlying disease process.

THE HOMEOPATHIC PHARMACY

The preparation of homeopathic medicines follows guidelines defined in the Homeopathic Pharmacopoeia Convention of the United States (HPCUS), with oversight by the FDA. The HPCUS was grandfathered into the original Food, Drug and Cosmetic Act of 1938 and was also written into the Medicare Act in 1965. With few exceptions, homeopathic preparations are in the over-the-counter classification, although the HPCUS was included in the 1970 Controlled Substances Act. Forty-five percent of homeopathic medicines are sold through health food stores.

The modern terminology for the process of producing a homeopathic medicine is *serially agitated dilution* (SAD). Classical homeopathic texts refer to it as *potentization*, referring to the observation that the more dilute the substance, the more powerful and specific its effects are on the human organism. Homeopathic medicines are manufactured from substances of plant, mineral, animal, or even disease origin. The preparation of each medicine is specified in monographs approved by the HPCUS.

Preparation of a Homeopathic Medicine

The original substance is initially dissolved in pharmaceutical alcohol. One part of this solution is mixed with nine (decimal, D, or X) or ninety-nine (centesimal, C, or CH) parts of distilled water or pharmaceutical alcohol and vigorously agitated, or succussed. This process of serial dilution and agitation is carried out until the desired potency is achieved. The dilution of typical low potency remedies range from 6X (10^{-6}) to 12C (10^{-24}), intermediate potencies from 30X (10^{-30}) to 200C (10^{-400}), and high potencies from 1000C or 1M (10^{-2000}) to 100M or CM ($10^{-100,000}$). Substances that are insoluble in water or alcohol are initially triturated—ground in a mortar and pestle—and then serially diluted using lactose in a manner parallel to the liquid method. At the concentration at which the lactose mixture becomes soluble, preparation continues using alcohol dilution. The solution in which the medicines are prepared may be used directly, sprayed on sugar pellets of various sizes, or mixed with lactose and pressed into a tablet form.

A standard dose of a homeopathic medicine is 1 to 5 pellets, taken sublingually, with nothing else in the mouth for 10 minutes before or after the dose. The dose is repeated when the action of the first dose is exhausted; this can range from minutes to years, depending on the response. During the time a patient is using homeopathy or the action of the homeopathic dose is continuing, many practitioners recommend that certain exposures, thought to be antidotal to many homeopathic drugs, be avoided. These recommendations vary but include avoiding coffee, strong aromatic oils such as camphor and mint, invasive dental work, exposure to electromagnetic fields, MRIs, electric blankets, and ultrasound.

A discussion of the extraordinary dilutions used in homeopathic medicine is given context by referring to the concept of Avogadro's number from basic chemistry. Avogadro's number is the theoretical number of atoms or molecules in a mole, or the gram molecular weight of a given substance. For example, a mole of sodium, with a gram molecular weight of 22.99, and platinum, with a gram molecular weight of 195, both have the same number of molecules (6.02 $\times 10^{23}$). Therefore, at a dilution of 12C or 24X (10^{-24}), the probability of there being a molecule of the original substance in the solution is 1:10. Given the high level of dilution, the activity of homeopathic medicines is thought to follow from properties of the solvent water conferred to it by the original substance, not the molecules themselves. For the scientist grounded in concepts of chemistry and molecular biology, the observation that medicines that contain no molecules could have biological activity defies all logic, and is frankly unbelievable. But this is precisely what homeopathic proponents claim and is increasing demonstrated in controlled trials (15).

Although evidence of the biological activity of SADs is accumulating, the mechanism of action of these medicines is speculative. Theoretical explanations have revolved around the "memory of water" and a subtle energy system in the living biological systems that can perceive and respond to the information encoded in a homeopathic solution. The physicist Callinan (16) suggests that the process of succussion (i.e., agitation of the solution) produces energy storage in the bonds of the diluent in the infrared spectrum that downloads in contact with the water in living systems. Perhaps the information then spreads like "liquid crystal" through the body water, modifying receptor sites or enzyme action. Proponents refer to the observation that nuclear magnetic resonance (NMR) spectroscopy (17) of solutions containing homeopathic medicines differ from the control solvent that has been similarly diluted and succussed.

The recent discovery of I_E structures in water may be the clearest evidence to date of a mechanism of action of homeopathic medicines (18, 19). I_E structures are crystalline-like structures of water molecules generated in response to electrical dipoles surrounding ions or proteins in solution. They have a circular symmetry and are measurable by ultraviolet transmission; they are also visualized by electronmicroscopy and atomic force microscopy. At ion concentrations below 10^{-7}, these structures become stable and when exposed to shearing forces, break apart into three nanometer fragments, but then reaggregate into more stable structures that are capable of self-replication in more dilute solutions, despite the absence of the original polar molecule. The form that these aggregates take is determined by the electrical field of the original polar solute around which they formed. The shape of these aggregates may contain information that is communicated to highly specific receptor sites on cell surfaces, antibodies, and so on.

The extraordinary implications of the homeopathic theory challenges the molecular biological model. Publication of the results of homeopathic trials has led to several angry exchanges in the scientific press, the most notable being the publication of Benveniste's finding that human basophils degranulated in the presence of antiserum directed against immunoglobulin E (IgE) at dilutions of 10^{-120} (20). More recently, after *Pediatrics* published research on the homeopathic treatment of childhood diarrhea (21), the journal later printed a five-page critique (22). Subsequent letters pointed out that the opinions of these critics reflected lack of knowledge of research design and basic homeopathic principles as well as reflecting a philosophical and political bias (23).

The current evidence for the action of homeopathic medicines in a clinical (15) and laboratory setting (24) are summarized in two meta-analyses. A number of high-quality clinical trials have demonstrated the efficacy of homeopathic medicines, but none has ever been independently replicated. Proponents accept this as adequate information for practice. Skeptics say such extraordinary claims require objective evidence for a mechanism of action. Both critics and proponents agree that more high-quality clinical and laboratory research is needed.

HOMEOPATHIC PROVINGS

Some of the first double-blind, placebo-controlled experiments in human subjects were performed by homeopaths to test their medicine on healthy subjects. Provings provide the data on which knowledge of the different homeopathic medicines is based. Standardization in the methodology of provings is a subject of significant effort among homeopathic physicians and researchers (25).

Provings begin by interviewing healthy volunteers, or *provers*, to assess their state of health and record for a period of time their baseline symptoms in a diary. The homeopathic medicine is prescribed to each prover in potency for several days or until symptoms begin to develop. The prover records in detail the symptoms that develop, including any new thoughts, feelings, changes in sleep, dreams, food cravings and aversions, physical sensations, eruptions, and discharges.

At the end of the proving, each subject is interviewed by the master prover, who is ideally blinded to the substance being proven. The experience of multiple provers is synthesized by the master prover with input from the provers. A picture of the remedy arises from these discussions of the proving experience. Key symptoms are indexed for possible addition to the repertory. The provings are published in journals or electronic media, making them readily accessible to prescribing physicians. The ability to archive and retrieve video images on digital media has made a far richer experience of the provings accessible than the written *materia medicas* of the past could capture.

The provings lead to a detailed understanding of the effect of homeopathic substances in human beings. Although allopathic drug testing focuses on biochemical and physiologic effects, disease-based therapeutic indications, and side effects, homeopathic provings generate a list of the detailed symptoms experienced across all organ systems. The provers are used as an instrument through which the symptoms of the medicine are expressed and can be used in healing the sick.

The goal in the development of allopathic medicines is the "magic bullet"—i.e., a drug with very specific therapeutic effects and a narrow range of untoward effects. The side effect profile of any medicine is an undesirable but necessary byproduct of this therapeutic system. In homeopathy, these symptoms, side effects, are valued; the experiences of provers tell the homeopath the therapeutic indications of the medicine.

Materia Medica

The knowledge of the remedies gained from provings is supplemented by clinical experience. Symptoms that are cured by a specific remedy in multiple patients are added to the *materia medica* of that remedy. The database of symptoms for some of the better known homeopathic remedies often require 80 or 90 pages of written text. Access to this information has been dramatically altered by computers. The current database of the homeopathic *materia medica* includes information for approximately 2500 remedies and consumes approximately 700 megabytes. Programs specifically written to as-

sist homeopathic practice have had a profound effect on the quality of homeopathic prescribing over the past two decades, significantly contributing to the renaissance of homeopathy in this same period.

PROVIDER-PATIENT INTERACTIONS

At first, the patient-physician interaction appears substantially the same in homeopathy as in conventional medicine. The physician sits with the patient, obtains a history, examines the patient, and then prescribes a medicine. However, as seen from the previous discussion, the clinical and pharmacological databases, the underlying assumptions about illness, and thought processes used for decision-making differ substantially. For the homeopathic practitioner, mastery of both the data and approach to the patient can be both refreshing and challenging, and this process is one in which the patient feels at home. The enhanced attention to the individual is welcomed by patients and may have an important role in homeopathy's popularity.

Homeopathic Approaches: Complex and Classical Homeopathy

Two important styles of practice have evolved in the application of homeopathic medicines to clinical medicine—classical and complex homeopathy. Classical homeopaths use a single medicine prescribed for the totality of symptoms. The second approach, complex homeopathy, uses medicines with a combination of ingredients designed to treat a specific condition. To the classical homeopath, the complex approach is not homeopathy, but instead the allopathic use of homeopathically prepared medicines (i.e., prescribing medicine based on pathological or diagnosis-based criteria).

COMPLEX HOMEOPATHY

Complex homeopathy refers to the use of several medicines simultaneously to achieve relief of a disease state. A number of medicines known to be commonly used in a specific condition are combined into a single formulation. This pragmatic approach was developed by the homeopathic pharmaceutical industry, bypassing the need for the extensive evaluation required in the classical approach. The underlying assumptions about the medicines are similar to what has already been presented, but the need for individualization is limited to that of a conventional, diagnosis-driven, approach. The assumption of the complex approach is that one of the elements of the formulation will be the similar remedy. Preparations are designed and labeled for specific clinical entities (e.g., teething, restless children, sinusitis, fever, earache). Few of these products have undergone rigorous testing under blinded, controlled clinical trials.

Combination medicines represent 85% of the over-the-counter homeopathic drug market in the United States. They are popular among physicians and the lay public because the prescription process is based on a familiar model of disease. For example, a medicine labeled for a sore throat is intended to be used on any sore throat. The combination versus single prescription has its parallel in conventional pharmacy. Physicians tend to prescribe a single medicine or several individual medicines. The over-the-counter market more often uses combinations of ingredients. Compounds are developed with a rationale based on the known benefit of the individual ingredients in a specific diagnosis. The complex approach in homeopathy has been most developed in France and Germany. Only a few of these preparations have been subjected to controlled clinical trials and are usually published in proprietary journals. Some complex homeopathic preparations have demonstrated benefit in a number of diagnoses, under controlled trial conditions.

The complex homeopathic approach has also been adopted by a group of practitioners who diagnose physiologic disturbance using instruments derived from electroacupuncture. These instruments, when placed on acupuncture points, measure disturbances of energy systems, which can then be corrected by placing homeopathic preparations in the circuit. Practitioners using this method often prescribe combinations of medicines based on this individualized testing.

CLASSICAL HOMEOPATHY

In classical homeopathy, patient evaluation has five major components:

1. An interview in which the "totality" of the person's mental, emotional, and physical symptoms is understood.
2. Appropriate physical examinations and diagnostic studies.
3. Analysis of the patient's data using homeopathic methods, often with the assistance of computers.
4. Selection and prescription of the most similar, single remedy, given in minute and infrequent doses.
5. Regular follow-up visits to assess the effect of the prescription and determine if the medication should be repeated, changed, or allowed to complete its action without further assistance.

To know what is to be cured has a context in homeopathy that differs considerably from the diagnosis-driven approach of allopathic therapeutics. Homeopathy considers the whole person—mental, emotional, and physical. In addition to understanding the patient's medical condition in all aspects, the homeopath must come to know them as people: their loves, hates, passions, interests, fears, anxieties, dreams, biorhythms, and reactions to temperature, climate, and food. These characteristics are synthesized into a picture, a "totality," that describes the person's unique response to life and how that defines the person's freedom to express and interact, or as Hahnemann expressed, "to achieve the higher purposes of human existence."

The typical interview between a classic homeopath and a new patient may take $1\frac{1}{2}$ hours. The homeopath listens to the spontaneous story of the patient with as few interruptions as possible, paying attention to what the patient says, how he or she says it, and the recurrent themes presented. The expression of the patient's story provides a picture of the way in which innate nature or past experiences has led him or her to filter and interpret experiences. Fears, anxieties, and dreams often provide important information into the unconscious processes that motivate the person's reactions to life events; this is what homeopaths refer to as the mental-emotional picture of the patients. Next in importance are the patient's "generalities." For example:

- Temperature reaction
- Biorhythms
- Responses to environment, storms, climate, other people, sound, and light
- Food cravings and aversions

Final emphasis is placed on the details of the physical symptoms that characterize the patient's disorder (e.g., the side of the body involved, the pattern of radiation of a pain, the modalities that aggravate or ameliorate each symptom, and the relation of one symptom to another).

The homeopath will give priority to those symptoms that have the most profound effect on the patient's physical, social, and occupational functioning. Two factors are considered in this assessment: the importance of the organ system involved and the intensity of symptoms. A mental symptom of severe depression would take priority over a mild skin rash, whereas a severe exfoliative dermatitis would be more important to the patient than a simple, mild phobia.

Homeopathy assumes that disease has a chronic nature and progresses inward within the organism over time. For example, atopy, which presents as eczema in infancy, may progress to asthma by early childhood. Syphilis or Lyme disease progress from the skin to the central nervous system. As a disease progresses inward, it affects more and more vital organ systems with increasing influence over the person's functioning. A cure reverses this process. Known as Hering's law, under homeopathic influence, a cure proceeds from within to without, from top down, from more recent to older expressions of the disease process. For example, under homeopathic treatment, asthma may resolve with the temporary return of a eczema that may have been suppressed with topical steroids earlier in life.

The past history, or biopathography, is the unfolding of the patient's internal disturbance over his or her lifetime. The various disorders of the patient, although representing a number of seemingly unrelated diagnoses in an allopathic context, are all covered by the symptomatology of a single homeopathic medicine. Referred to as a *constitutional* remedy, this medicine covers the totality of the patient's symptoms. A constitutional remedy is contrasted with a medicine prescribed for an acute, circumscribed focus that often has a clear external etiology.

In homeopathy, family history is significant, and not only in the standard medical assessment of risk for inherited illnesses. Homeopaths refer to inherited patterns of disease as *miasms*. The family history often gives a picture of the formative external influence that may have shaped the patient's response to life. In pediatric cases, the child may often share the same remedy as the mother or father. The correct prescription in these cases may include symptoms that the mother experienced in pregnancy. In the interview, the homeopath notes who comes to the interview with the designated patient and the quality of the interactions with family members present.

When a patient is seen for the first time for a chronic complaint, the homeopath uses the data gained from the interview, extracting a set of symptoms that characterize the case. Each of the symptoms is then considered in context of what homeopathic medicines have produced these symptoms in provings or reliably cured them in clinical cases. *Repertorization* is the process by which homeopaths hone in on the most similar remedy. Repertories are printed or computerized indexes of symptoms organized by organ system. Each entry, or *rubric*, is a symptom followed by a list of those remedies that have either produced in their provings or healed in accumulated clinical experience that specific symptom.

For example, the rubric "HEAD, PAIN; LOCALIZATION; Forehead; middle; frontal sinuses from chronic coryza" contains five medicines: **Silica**, *Arsenium album*, *Kali-bichromicum*, *Sanguinaria*, and *Thuja occidentalis*. The remedies in rubrics are listed in four grades—grade one (plain type) has the weakest association and grade four (bold capitals) the strongest.

The process of repertorization leads to the selection of several remedies that may cover the symptoms of the case. Comparative study of the *materia medica* of these remedies helps to select the one most appropriate remedy. *Materia medicas* vary in style. Some contain only the original symptoms from the provings, some include cured clinical symptoms, and some contain discussions of the remedy synthesized from clinical experience of various authors. From this study of options, a single remedy is selected for administration to the patient. Brief examples of this process of remedy selection are given to illustrate these concepts.

THERAPY AND OUTCOMES

Treatment Options

In addition to the professional practice of homeopathy, the over-the-counter status of all but a few homeopathic medicines means that homeopathy is widely available for self-prescribing. Eisenberg estimated that only 30% of the people in his sample who used homeopathy sought professional advice. Sales of homeopathic medicines have grown by 15 to 20% yearly over the last decade. Homeopathic pharmacies do only a small percentage of their business in single remedies, most of which are sold to professionals. The bulk of their sales are in combination products, self-prescribed according to the labeling of these products. Unfortunately, the labeling of both single-remedy and combination products, required by FDA regulations, has limitations (26).

If a patient is seeking to use homeopathy for chronic complaints or serious acute problems, it is generally advised that a homeopathic professional be consulted. Evaluating the abilities of a homeopath may be difficult, but, like choosing any physician, board certification is an important consideration. Medical physicians with homeopathic board certification are designated by the initials DHt, naturopaths as DHANP, and other professions (e.g., nurses, physician's assistants, acupuncturists) as CCH. Lists of practitioners are maintained and made available to the public by the National Center for Homeopathy and the boards themselves.

Description of Treatments

A CHRONIC CASE

A woman in her mid-40s presents with a diagnosis of fibrositis. She has tried many different therapies and is resisting the prescription of an antidepressant to relieve her pain. She has sore muscles, especially near the joints at their tendinous insertions. The muscles feel stiff and contracted, almost like spasms. The pains are worse on first motion or rest. The pain causes her to be in constant motion, during which time she feels well, until she becomes exhausted and eventually in more pain by this prolonged exertion. Her sleep is disturbed by the pains, and she always wakes at 3 am feeling restless. Her pains are relieved by a hot shower and aspirin. These symptoms are a constant presence in her day-to-day life. She feels tired and sore most of the time, but she tries not to let this limit her work, family life, or general lifestyle.

Her life is dedicated to the care of children. Her husband, a psychologist, states that she has visible physiologic stress response to any circumstance in which issues of injustice are involved. She is self-employed as a day-care director, which her husband again remarks is a statement of her issues around authority, arising from a dictatorial stepmother. Her own mother died when she was 2 years old. Her father did not process the grief, nor allow her to, but insisted that she go on with her life. Her father remarried. She became very concerned with the well-being of her younger siblings and never felt bonded to her stepmother. Her first conscious experience with death was when her paternal grandfather died. For years he would come and talk with her in dreams. She has tremendous fears that whenever someone in her family is late something bad has happened.

Symptom Chosen

The symptoms chosen for analysis by the homeopath try to capture the unique characteristics of this person. Symptoms are listed in homeopathic references called repertories, indexed by body part. The symptoms are indexed in repertories in association with a list of remedies known to have produced that symptom (in

MIND; DREAMS; dead; people, of; relatives (K1237,SIII 276) (10) : caust., ferr., fl-ac., hydrog., kali-c., mag-c., mag-s., pitu-a., rheum, sars.

MIND; ANXIETY; others, for (K7, SI 86)(Anxiety; friends at home, about)(Cares; others) (27) : acon., *ambr.*, androc., *arg-n.*, *ars.*, aur., bar-c., *calc-p.*, carb-v., *carc.*, caust., chel., cocc., *dulc.*, *ferr.*, fl-ac., hep., **Manc.**, merc., naja, nat-c., *nux-v.*, perh., ph-ac., *phos., staph., sulph.*

MIND; INJUSTICE, cannot support (SI 633) (16) : calc., calc-p., caust., dros., ign., kali-i., mag-m., med., merc., nat-m., nux-v., phos., sep., *staph.*, sulph., verat.

MIND; FEAR; happen; something will; family, to, or to him (Anxiety; family, about his) (7) : ars., calc., caust., phos., psor., sep., tub.

EXTREMITY PAIN; GENERAL; motion, on; amel. (K1045) (38) : agar., ang., *arg.*, arist-cl., *aur.*, bell-p., caust., cham., chin., *con.*, dig., *dulc., ferr.*, hed., iod., *kali-c.*, kali-i., kali-p., **Kali-s.**, lach., *lyc.*, mag-c., *med.*, merc., *mur-ac., nat-s.*, psor., **Puls.**, **Pyrog.**, *rat.*, **Rhod.**, **Rhus-t.**, *ruta*, sep., thuj., *tub., valer., zinc.*

EXTREMITIES; CONTRACTION of muscles and tendons (K966) (52) : acon., acon-c., ant-c., *ars.*, bar-c., *bell.*, bry., **Calc.**, canth., carb-v., carbn-s., **Caust.**, cedr., cimx., **Coloc.**, con., *crot-c., crot-h., cupr.*, eupi., ferr., ferr-m., **Graph.**, *guai.*, hydr-ac., hydrc., jatr., kali-ar., *kali-i.*, **Lyc.**, mang., *merc.*, mill., mur-ac., *nat-c., nat-m.*, nux-v., oena., op., ph-ac., *phos., plb.*, prot., *ruta*, **Sec.**, *sep., sil.*, still., stram., sulph., syph., vib.

GENERALITIES; AFTERNOON, one pm. - six pm.; four pm. (K1342, SII 7) (43) : *aesc.*, alum., anac., *apis*, ars., arum-t., cact., calc-p., carb-v., *caust., cedr.*, cench., chel., *chin-s.*, cob., *coloc.*, gels., *hell.*, hep., ip., kali-c., lachn., **Lyc.**, mag-m., mang., meli., merc-s., mur-ac., nat-m., nat-s., nit-ac., nux-m., *nux-v.*, phos., plat., puls., rhus-t., sabad., sep., stront-c., sulph., verb., zinc.

FIGURE 28.1. Rubrics of chronic case.

provings) or cured it (in clinical practice). Each symptom with its associated remedies is called a rubric. Each rubric first lists the symptom in the language of the patient, followed by the page number in standard printed references (K = *Kent's Repertory*, S = *Synthetic*). The remedies are abbreviated in alphabetical order. In this woman's case the following rubrics were chosen from MacRepertory (26), a computerized repertory program (Fig. 28.1).

Repertorization

A repertorization program graphs the patient's symptoms against the associated homeopathic medicines (Fig. 28.2). This repertorization graphically displays the strength of the association in four grades. The rubric is listed on the left. The abbreviated names of the remedies are listed across the top. Below them are the weighted scores for each matched rubric and the total number of matched rubrics. In this case, a single remedy contained all seven symp-

toms selected and had a clearly higher intensity score. Selection of the proper rubrics for repertorization requires extensive knowledge of homeopathic principles in chronic cases.

Selected Materia Medica of Causticum

Causticum was chosen as the remedy that best characterized this patient's mental, emotional, and physical symptoms. The homeopathic *materia medicas* are composed of the verbatim proving symptoms of patients, clinician observations of specific symptoms repeatedly cured by the medicine, or clinicians' descriptions of the characteristics of patients who have responded to a remedy. The following statements were taken from materia medica texts of Causticum:

Emotional: ailments from grief [many or long]. Fear something will happen. Internal suffering, kept in. Suffers from injustice in society. Actually helps the oppressed and the poor, not only talks about it. Being strongest

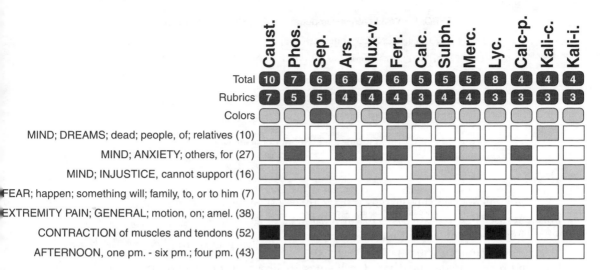

	Caust.	Phos.	Sep.	Ars.	Nux-v.	Ferr.	Calc.	Sulph.	Merc.	Lyc.	Calc-p.	Kali-c.	Kali-i.
Total	10	7	6	6	7	6	5	5	5	8	4	4	4
Rubrics	7	5	5	4	4	4	3	4	4	3	3	3	3
Colors													
MIND; DREAMS; dead; people, of; relatives (10)													
MIND; ANXIETY; others, for (27)													
MIND; INJUSTICE, cannot support (16)													
FEAR; happen; something will; family, to, or to him (7)													
EXTREMITY PAIN; GENERAL; motion, on; amel. (38)													
CONTRACTION of muscles and tendons (52)													
AFTERNOON, one pm. - six pm.; four pm. (43)													

FIGURE 28.2. Repertorization of chronic case. The patient's symptoms are listed to the left; abbreviations of remedies across the top. The intensity of the correlation between the remedy and symptom is graded from one (lowest) to four (highest): white, (0); pale shade, (1); dark shade, (2); and solid, (3). The row named *Rubrics* indicates the number of rubrics matched for each remedy. The row named *Total* indicates the total score for each remedy. The top remedy is *Causticum*.

member of that group, the one who is the most capable of putting up a fight, he regards a threat to any one member of that group as a threat to himself. If he doesn't forestall the threat, it would affect the whole group and he will be weakened (27).

Mental: Immovable points of view, indifference to dictates of conscience. Weakness of memory with the characteristic feeling as if he had forgotten something [has to go back and check].

Extremities: Sensation as if muscles and tendons were too short. Restless legs in the evening and at night, in bed.

Follow-Up

The patient was scheduled to return to the homeopath in 6 weeks and told to call in the interim if she had questions or reactions to the treatment. She was given a single dose of Causticum 1M (10^{-2000}), to be taken after stopping coffee intake for 3 to 4 days. She was in a 2-week break from school, and she was glad because she felt tired for 3 days after taking the dose. Her pains were somewhat increased during that time, initially in her legs. As the leg pain gradu-

ally improved, there was a temporary intensification of her shoulder and neck pain, which had been the original area of symptoms. Despite this, she was able to sleep longer without being awakened. She remarked with some wonder that after taking the remedy she was unusually weepy. Gradually her energy improved and after 6 weeks she reported feeling better than she had in years. Emotionally she feels "lighter" and was able to not go to work on her days off, demonstrating the improvement in the general mental and emotional state of the patient. Over the next 6 months she saw the homeopath twice, and her condition continued to progress. The remedy was repeated once 4 months later when, after her dentist replaced an old amalgam filling, her muscle pain began to worsen. After 6 months she was well, with only occasional pain when she overexerted herself.

AN ACUTE CASE

A 10-year-old boy with a sore throat of two-days duration is brought to a homeopath by his parents. He walks into the office holding a cup half full of saliva. His cervical glands are visibly swollen, his breath is fetid, his tongue is coated

THROAT; SWALLOWING; impeded (K468)(difficult)(impossible) (50)

MOUTH; INDENTED; Tongue (K406) (38)

MOUTH; ODOR; putrid (K409) (107)

MOUTH; SALIVATION; pains, during (12)

FEVER; CHILL; with (K1284)(Chilliness) (92)

FEVER; PERSPIRATION; heat, with (K1289) (96)

FIGURE 28.3. Rubrics of acute case.

white and indented, and his pharynx is red with purulent discharge in the tonsils. He is feverish, with chills and profuse perspiration at night. Streptococcal antigen test is positive. The rubrics and repertorization are detailed in Figures 28.3 and 28.4, respectively.

Selected Materia Medica of Mercury

The following are symptoms from the published *materia medica* of mercury:

Salivation (not a strong symptom in deep mental states), especially at night in sleep

Sensitivity to heat or cold

Metallic taste in mouth

Strong halitosis

Offensive perspiration all over the body that aggravates

Swollen glands anywhere on the body

Recurrent or acute otitis media

Green, thick nasal discharge or sputum from throat

Aphthae and ulcerations on tongue, mouth, and throat

Imprinted teeth on tongue

Pharyngitis

The prescription for the child is *Mercurius vivus*, 1M (10^{-2000}). Within 20 minutes, he is swallowing more easily, and by the next day he is asymptomatic. His symptoms and clinical

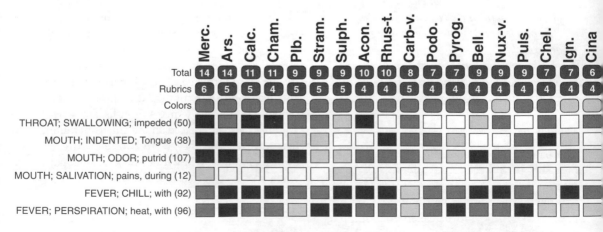

FIGURE 28.4. Repertorization of acute case. The patient's symptoms are listed to the left; abbreviations of remedies are across the top. The intensity of the correlation between the remedy and symptom is graded from one (lowest) to four (highest): white, (0); pale shade, (1); dark shade, (2); and solid, (3). The row named *Rubrics* indicates the number of rubrics matched for each remedy. The row named *Total* indicates the total score for each remedy. The top remedy is *Mercurius*.

examination normalized and rapid strep test became nonreactive in 48 hours. No repetition of the dose was required.

TREATMENT EVALUATION

In homeopathy, outcomes are seen in a broader context than in allopathic medicine. The similar remedy appears to act by focusing and strengthening the innate healing powers of the whole person, rather than by attacking or suppressing a specific disease process or symptom. Consequently, patients describe homeopathic treatment as having positive effects not only in terms of the symptoms of the presenting complaint or disease, but in improved vitality and mental and emotional well-being.

The evaluation of a homeopathic prescription is scheduled at an interval appropriate to the urgency of the case and the patient's needs. In acute cases, the duration may be minutes to hours. In chronic cases, the interval is usually 4 to 6 weeks. In the latter case, the interview usually takes 20 to 30 minutes, during which time the key complaints of the patients are reviewed. Each symptom is assessed: Has the intensity diminished or increased? Was there an aggravation of symptoms after taking the initial dose? Were there changes in secondary complaints, general energy, sense of well-being, or mental and emotional symptoms? The ideal response often begins with a brief period of aggravation, followed by a decrease in the primary symptoms with simultaneous improvements in mental and emotional functioning. Curative responses may include a temporary return of old symptoms, which gradually clear in a specified order—i.e., from recent to the older, and from vital to more superficial organ systems.

The task of the homeopathic prescriber at follow-up interviews is to determine whether the remedy has acted, if the action is continuing, and if the remedy needs to be repeated, changed, or left to continue its action without further intervention. The remedy is seen as a catalyst to a healing process that, once initiated, has its own pace and direction as dictated by the innate wisdom of the organism. If this process is continuing satisfactorily, no other intervention is needed (regardless of whether the period of response is minutes or months). The remedy is repeated only when the response has ceased or shown signs of relapsing.

USE OF THE SYSTEM FOR TREATMENT

Homeopathic physicians are often asked what homeopathy is "good for" and what conditions respond well to this approach. Most classically trained homeopaths will respond that homeopathy does not treat diagnoses, but treats people who are sick. A patient with almost any condition can be helped by homeopathy, whether it be an upper respiratory infection, attention deficit disorder, or cancer. Whether, given specific circumstances, it is cost-effective or the most appropriate approach, or whether there are data to support the use of homeopathy in a given condition is another matter. There are relatively few conditions for which homeopathic treatment has been studied in a rigorous manner. Until data have been accumulated, the following guidelines may be helpful.

Homeopathy stimulates the body's functional capacities. Functional illnesses that have not progressed to the point of irreversible tissue change are more amenable to the influence of homeopathic medicines than those with fixed pathology. A diabetic who has no islet cells, or a patient with advanced Alzheimer's or Parkinson's disease in which neuronal elements have been destroyed, would not be expected to respond significantly. However, a patient with Type II diabetes, a patient with ulcerative colitis, or a patient with mild traumatic brain injury each has functional disturbances with reversible tissue changes and may respond well to homeopathy. When the body can heal, homeopathy can play a role.

The urgency of the situation, the availability of specific treatments with known efficacy, and the risk of using or foregoing the use of conventional therapies are other factors that influence the decision to use homeopathy. A child with acute bacterial meningitis should be treated with the appropriate antibiotic, whereas a child with viral meningitis could be helped by homeopathy. Furthermore, the choice does not need to be "either/or." Homeopathic medicines can be used in conjunction with conventional medical treatment. Whereas the substitution of homeopathy for conventional medicines in cases such as attention deficit disorder or asthma may be disastrous, simultaneous use of the appropriate homeopathic medicine may eventually lead to improved function and often to a reduction or even discontinuation of conventional medicines. The simultaneous use of two therapeutic systems should involve professionals versed in both systems.

ORGANIZATION

Training

There is growing interest in homeopathic training among conventional physicians, especially among the primary care specialties (28). The Council for Homeopathic Education (CHE), founded in 1982, accredits homeopathic training programs. The CHE currently lists more than 30 programs that offer some training and education in homeopathy. Most are postgraduate programs, offering didactic instruction with additional supervised clinical experience. The only undergraduate programs are part of the three naturopathic colleges, which are in Seattle, WA, Portland, OR, and Phoenix, AZ. Training and education necessary for a primary care physician to use homeopathic medicines confidently in acute situations in practice would be about 60 to 100 hours; for a specialist, 1000 hours with an additional supervised clinical experience.

Licensure

Most physicians practice homeopathy under their conventional license and are accepted within their community as an important resource. A small number of physicians have been harassed by their licensing board for using homeopathy. Connecticut, Nevada, and Arizona have separate homeopathic medical boards.

Alaska, New York, North Carolina, and Washington have laws prohibiting censure of a physician solely because he or she practices an unconventional therapy. In North Carolina, this law was passed in response to a decision of the North Carolina Board of Medicine to prohibit a physician from practicing homeopathy. The courts upheld the Board's right to make this decision. The legislature overrode the Board after public protest.

Other professions also practice homeopathy. Many professional groups have been licensed to diagnose and prescribe within guidelines that arise from the scope of training of the specific profession. Medical and osteopathic physicians, podiatrists, dentists, chiropractors, acupuncturists, naturopaths, oriental medical doctors, nurse practitioners, and physician's assistants have been given power by states to prescribe homeopathic medicine. In most states, pharmacists (and, in some, dieticians and cosmetologists, too) may also administer prescribing advice for over-the-counter homeopathic products.

Certification

The current certification in homeopathy for physicians is available at two levels: a Primary Care Certificate in Homeotherapeutics, and a Diplomate in Homeotherapeutics (DHt). A primary care certificate in homeopathy can be obtained through study at either a postgraduate or graduate level, integrated into other primary care teaching programs. This certification requires 60 to 100 hours of training in homeotherapeutics and a written exam. Training and certification at the level of a diplomate in homeotherapeutics is required for treatment of chronic disease or complex pathology. Certification at the diplomate level requires proof of comprehensive didactic and clinical training, as well as 3 years of clinical practice. Both exams offered by the American Board of Homeotherapeutics were developed according to international standards for certification of homeopathic specialists. Naturopathic physicians are certified by the Homeopathic Association of Naturopathic Physicians (DHANP). All other homeopathic practitioners can be certified by the Council for Homeopathic Certification.

Other than in the three naturopathic colleges, graduate programs in homeotherapeutics do not exist at this time. Most practicing homeopathic physicians are already certified in a primary care specialty (e.g., family practice, internal medicine, pediatrics) or a subspecialty. For them, homeopathy represents a second specialization that complements their existing training. Comprehensive homeopathic training programs take from 1 to 4 years to complete, usually on a part-time basis. Most candidates obtain clinical supervision during their early years of training and practice.

Legal Status

The Homeopathic Pharmacopoeia of the United States was included in the 1938 Food and Drug Act and is referenced in the definition of *drugs* in every state. Homeopathic medicine is part of the 1965 Medicare Act. Practitioners use homeopathy within the scope of their conventional license. The over-the-counter status of the medicines has spurned an active self-help study group network supported by the National Center for Homeopathy.

A recent deluge of articles in the medical press has criticized homeopathy to the point of suggesting it be banned. Most of these articles come from authors who are members of the National Council Against Health Fraud. Frustrated by the FDA's lack of response to their petition requesting review of the regulations governing the dispensing of homeopathic products, they used the media to make their point. This group has further directed their frustration to the courts, bringing law suits against both dispensing and manufacturing pharmacies, claiming fraudulent advertising of homeopathic products.

The heart of the criticism is that homeopathic products are being allowed on the over-the-counter market with labels that suggest efficacious treatment for a variety of complaints, ranging from restless children to immune dysfunction. The critics claim this situation represents a double standard within the over-the-counter market—i.e., homeopathic products are not required to demonstrate clinical efficacy whereas conventional drugs are. The homeopathic defense is that homeopathic products, unlike conventional medical products, are safe, have been used successfully for 200 years, and that the public should be free to choose as long as there is no risk.

The FDA, by providing waivers for Phases One and Two studies of the homeopathic medicines used in an NIH-funded clinical trial on mild traumatic brain injury, accepted the clinical safety of homeopathic medicines. Researchers were permitted to go directly to a Phase Three, or efficacy, trial. Within the homeopathic community, many professionals share the concerns about products being marketed with labeling that suggests efficacy for clinical syndromes, without the support of at least Phase Four clinical trials. Equally inappropriate is the labeling of single homeopathic medications with indications. These conditions imposed by the FDA stem from a lack of appreciation of homeopathic principles.

Reimbursement Status

Most insurance companies reimburse homeopathic physician services as they would any other conventional physician. Recent correspondence between the American Institute of Homeopathy and various Medicare carriers has confirmed that physicians may be reimbursed for homeopathic services if coded within the standard evaluation and management codes. Some insurance companies, including Champus and several state Medicaid or Blue Shield plans, have refused to pay for homeopathic medicine although they will pay for physician services. Managed care networks and HMOs have generally not included homeopaths on their rosters as specialists. Whereas physicians in HMOs routinely refer patients to homeopaths, the HMO rarely reimburses patients for those services. Recent state laws (e.g., in Washington) forcing insurance companies to include naturopathic physicians as primary care providers have led to local experiments by insurers to pay for homeopathic care.

PROSPECTS FOR THE FUTURE

Preliminary research into the efficacy and cost effectiveness of homeopathy suggests that this system of therapy will be increasingly used in the primary care setting and as a referral for many chronic complaints in which effective conventional medical treatment does not exist or in which adverse effects make alternatives attractive. For example, experts in infectious disease are seeking to learn more about homeopathy in conditions such as otitis media, in which it is known that antibiotics are overprescribed and antibiotic resistance is becoming a significant public health risk. Recent research into the treatment of mild traumatic brain injury suggests that homeopathy may play a significant role in the recovery from neurologic trauma, an area in which conventional therapies have limited efficacy.

Advocates believe that homeopathy should be included in the prescribing skills of all primary care professionals. Its low cost, absence of adverse effects, applicability to self-care, and potential to improve the health of patients make it the therapy of choice in most common primary care problems. The recognition of homeopathy will increase with quality clinical research and education of primary care physicians about the value of homeopathy in both acute and chronic disease.

REFERENCES

1. Hahnemann S. In: O'Reilly WB, ed. Organon of the medical art. Redmond, WA: Birdcage Books, 1996.
2. Coulter HL. Divided legacy: a history of the schism in medical thought. Volume III. Science and ethics in American medicine. Washington, DC: McGrath Pulishing Co., 1973:1800-1914.
3. Kent JT. Lectures on homeopathic philosophy. Memorial edition. Chicago: Ehrhart & Karl, 1929.
4. Kent JT. Lectures on homeopathic materia medica. 4th ed. Philadelphia: Boericke & Tafel, 1956.
5. Kent JT. In: Kunzli von Fimmelsberg J, ed. Kent's rerporium genrale. Berg, Germany: Barthel & Barthel Publishing, 1987.
6. Allen, TF. The encyclopedia of pure materia medicia. A record of the positive effects of drugs upon healty human organism. Indian edition. New Delhi: B. Jain Publishers, 1982.
7. Hering C. The guiding symptoms of our materia medica. Indian Edition. New Delhi: B. Jain Publishers, 1972.
8. Ernst E, Kaptchuk T. Homeopathy revisited. Arch Intern Med 1996;159:2162-2164.
9. Rothstein WG. American physicians in the 19th century. Baltimore, MD: Johns Hopkins University Press, 1984.
10. Eisenberg DM, Kesser RC, Foster C, et al. Unconventional medicine in the United States. New Engl J Med 1993;328:4,246–252.
11. Homeopathy in the USA, 1995–1996. The American Homeopathic Pharmaceutical Association, Box 174, Norwood, PA 10974.
12. Social Security Statistics, CNAM 61, French Government Report, 1/91.
13. Ullman D. Discovering homeopathy: medicine for the 21st century. Berkeley, CA: North Atlantic Books, 1991.
14. Jacobs J, Crothers D, Chapman E. A comparison of practice patterns between physicians practicing homeopathic medicine and a national survey of conventional physicians. Survey by the American Institute of Homeopathy, 1992.
15. Linde K, Clausius N, Ramirez G, et al. Are the clinical effects of homeopathy placebo effects? A meta-analysis of placebo-controlled trials. Lancet 1997;350:834–843.
16. Reilly DT, Taylor MA, McSharry C, Atkinson T. Is homeopathy a placebo response? Controlled trial of homeopathic potency, with pollen in hayfever as model. Lancet 1986;2:881–885.
17. Demangeat JL, Demangeat C, Gries P, et al. Modifications des temps de relaxation RMN a 4MHz du solvant dans les tres hautes dilutions salines de silice/lactose. J Med Nucl Biophy 1992;16:135–145.
18. Lo SY. Anomalous state of ice. Modern Physics Letters B 1996;10(19):909–919.
19. Lo SY. Physical properties of water with I_E structures. Modern Physics Letters B 1996;10(19):921–930.
20. Poitevin B, Davenas E, Benveniste J. In vitro immunological degranulation of human basophils is modulated by lung histamine and apis mellifica. Br J Clin Pharmacol 1988;25:439–444.
21. Jacobs J, Jimenez ML, Gloyd SS, et al. Treatment of acute diarrhea with homeopathic medicine: a randomized clinical trial in Nicaragua. Pediatrics 1994;93(5):719–725.
22. Sampson W, London W. Homeopathic treatment of diarrhea. Pediatrics 1995;96:961–964.
23. Letters. Pediatrics 1996;97(5):776–779.

24. Linde K, Jonas W, Melchart D, et al. Critical review and meta-analysis of serially agitated dilutions in experimental toxicology. Hum Exp Toxicol 1994;13:481–492.

25. Riley D. Homeopathic drug provings. J Am Inst Homeopathy 1996;89(4):206–210.

26. Warkentin D. MacRepertory. Fairfax, CA: Kent Homeopathic Associates, 1988.

27. Sankaran R. The substance of homeopathy. Bombay, India: Homeopathic Medical Publishers, 1994:171.

28. Berman B, Singh BK, Lao L, et al. Physicians' attitudes towards complementary or alternative medicine: a regional survey. J Am Board Fam Pract 1995;8(5):361–366.

29. Chapman E. President's message: its time to take the high road. J Am Inst Homeopathy 1996;88(4);172–176.

CHAPTER 29

NUTRITIONAL BIOTHERAPY

Keith I. Block

> I will apply dietetic measures for the benefit of the sick according
>
> to my ability and judgment. . . .
>
> The Hippocratic Oath

INTRODUCTION

Nutritional medicine involves therapeutic application of dietary and nutritional modifications to reestablish bodily harmony. During the twentieth century, an explosion of scientific findings on the nutritional influences on disease–from epidemiologic, biochemical, and animal investigations–has occurred. The role and importance of dietary fats, proteins, carbohydrates, some minerals, and many vitamins were established in the early part of this century. Recently, many other vitamins, trace elements, and accessory factors have been discovered to have important roles in human health. Some of these "non-nutritive" substances, such as fibers and phytochemicals, have been identified as bioactive agents or *biological response modifiers* (BRMs) from the plant world. These substances modulate key disease-related mechanisms, such as immune function, oxidative stress, homeostasis, inflammatory activity, and hormonal balances.

By applying a mechanism-based perspective in nutrition science, researchers have increasingly shown methods for the nutritional exploitation of host mechanisms that modulate disease processes. Recognition that disease processes can be modulated through noninvasive biochemical methods has helped the development of the complementary medical discipline known as *nutritional biotherapy*. Nutritional biotherapy is the clinical use of diet and nutrition to influence host–disease relationships as well as the relationships between nutritional biochemistry and standard treatment.

Nutritional biotherapy takes advantage of our rapidly expanding knowledge of the ability of nutrients to modulate key biochemical processes. For example, in classical nutrition science, dietary fats are primarily viewed as a rich source of calories and modifier of membrane fluidity. As a biotherapeutic agent, fats modulate cell-signaling mechanisms and the synthesis of specific hormones, eicosanoids, and cytokines, all of which modulate immune and cardiovascular functions as well as tumor growth-regulatory pathways.

Nutritional biotherapy bridges complementary and conventional care. This emergent field consists of three major areas of clinical application:

1. **Prescriptive dietetics:** the selective use of foods and diets specifically designed for different diseases, depending on many individual factors.

2. **Nutritional pharmacology:** the supplemental use of specific vitamins, minerals, phytochemicals, and botanicals (herbal or plant-derived substances), which are tailored to the individual.
3. **Nutrition support:** the use of intravenous, or parenteral, nutrition (e.g., when there is a compromised gastrointestinal tract) or orally modified formulas (enteral nutrition), when a general diet cannot be consumed. Nutritional support is primarily aimed at malnourished patients who cannot consume food in its original form.

Each dimension of nutritional biotherapy, or some combination thereof, may be incorporated into a complementary treatment plan, depending on the clinical situation. In most cases, prescriptive dietetics is the first area of attention for the complementary practitioner and is generally the safest in the context of nutritional assessments and monitoring. Nutritional pharmacology has garnered considerable interest from researchers and complementary practitioners in recent years and remains the focus of intense debate. Nutritional support has been well accepted by conventional physicians for many years; however, with few exceptions, complementary practitioners have rarely delved into this area of nutritional biotherapy.

Prescriptive dietetics and nutritional pharmacology can be delineated further into two general subcategories: *therapeutic strategies* and *prophylactic strategies*.

Therapeutic strategies address biochemical imbalances or physiological disturbances (e.g., the mode of functioning of organs and tissues caused by organic diseases). The physical state of the tissues or organs can be either improved or worsened by the particular nutritional biotherapy approach. In some cases, the results are palliative rather than curative (e.g., bland, low-protein diets used to alleviate peptic ulcer and inflammatory bowel disorders). In other cases, a complementary approach to illness has emerged. For example, after the life-prolonging success of hemodialysis and transplantation, there has been an interest in low-protein diets for patients with chronic renal disease. High-fiber regimens are almost routinely recommended for patients who are constipated or overweight. Low-fat and nonaromatic foods are now frequently prescribed for patients suffering from nausea.

Prophylactic strategies are aimed at preventing the expression of a particular disease-related genotype and enabling patients to enjoy reasonably good health if they select foods and food preparation methods within certain parameters. The concept also applies to preventive therapeutics, referring to the use of noninvasive interventions to prolong the success of a standard medical therapy by adding a specific biomodulation effect (e.g., reducing serum cholesterol, lowering blood pressure, or enhancing insulin sensitivity) and thus reducing the relapse rate. These strategies may be either specifically tailored to the individual or, as occurs in the conventional medical setting, based on general guidelines for health maintenance.

HISTORY AND BACKGROUND OF NUTRITIONAL MEDICINE

The history of nutritional medicine dates back 2,500 years to the medical systems of ancient China and Greece. The oldest of medical texts, Chi Po's *Yellow Emperor's Classic of Internal Medicine*, recognized food selection and proper cooking as the cornerstone of prevention and relief of illness. In ancient Greece, Hippocrates frequently emphasized the primacy of cereal grains and vegetables in *The Book of Nutriment*, in which he wrote, "Let food be thy medicine, and medicine thy food." In the twelfth century, the famous Rabbinic scholar and Jewish physician Moses Maimonides formulated a broad dietary philosophy and addressed potential therapeutic applications of foods and food combinations, as well as the order of foods eaten in a meal. Each of these recommendations was deemed to have a specific health impact, while other points of dietary advice were related to relief of specific disorders.

Early in the twentieth century, dental surgeon Weston Price performed fieldwork among the Indians of North America, the Eskimos, the Polynesians, and the Australian Aborigines. In his 1945 publication *Nutrition and Physical Degeneration*, Price reported no trace of various degenerative diseases among these populations. During this same period, Drs. Dennis Burkitt and Hugh Tral suggested that diseases common in industrial countries but rare in Africa might be due in part to low dietary fiber intake, as Tral documented in *Western Diseases: Their Emergence and Prevention*. More recently, biochemist T. Colin Campbell conducted an extensive survey of dietary and mortality characteristics of 65 counties in rural China. Campbell's international research team concluded that the higher the intake of high-fat, high-protein diets, the higher the incidence and mortality from "Western diseases"; conversely, plant-based diets were strikingly protective against such diseases (1).

Expert recommendations for health-promoting diets have largely followed suit. *Healthy People 2000*, a report issued by the United States Public Health Service and 22 expert working groups, recommends increasing "complex carbohydrate and fiber-containing foods in the diets of adults to 5 or more daily servings for vegetables (including legumes) and fruits, and to 6 or more daily servings for grain products" (2). To justify these and other guidelines, *Healthy People 2000* draws substantiation from sources such as *The Surgeon General's Report on Nutrition and Health* (3), the *National Research Council's Diet and Health* (4), and the *USDA's Dietary Guidelines for Americans* (5). However, these recommendations focus on prevention, not treatment. Nevertheless, dietary prevention guidelines may prove beneficial to the long-range management of many chronic diseases, with the exception of cancer. (Malignant diseases as a single group exhibit a far more complex histologic and pathological character and thus more personally tailored diet therapy compared with diabetes, heart disease, and other chronic disorders.)

The development of nutritional biotherapy as a complementary medical discipline has been guided by the interplay between nutritional research and the clinical–medical communities. This interaction, catalyzed by Linus Pauling, Roger Williams, Max Gerson, Emanuel Revici,

Kedar Prasad, Ranjit Chandra, and Jeffrey Bland, has expanded the purview of nutritional biotherapy, taking it beyond the correction of nutrient imbalances toward modulating specific disease processes by nutritional means.

Biochemist Roger Williams conducted intensive studies of biochemical individuality (6). In his 1950 *Lancet* paper, "The Concept of Genetotrophic Disease," Williams defined genetotrophic disease as

> "one in which the genetic pattern of the individual calls for an augmented supply of a particular nutrient (or nutrients), for which there develops, as a result, a nutritional deficiency. Partial genetic blocks somewhere in the metabolic machinery are probably commonplace in the inheritance of individuals and explain to a considerable degree why each person possesses a characteristic and distinctive metabolic pattern. . . ." (7).

Williams' postulation regarding inherited or acquired partial enzymatic blocks, with diminished adaptive competency at the level of enzyme synthesis and regulation, explains why the resultant functional defect may raise the body's requirement for a particular food factor or set of factors (8). Thus, clinical situations that benefit from nutritional modulation may often involve conditional deficiencies of these nutrients—that is, deficiencies triggered by disease or other external factors—despite the normal provision of the nutrient that appears deficient.

Currently there is a resurgence of interest in nutritional medicine among physicians throughout the world. The medical community recognizes that successful long-range management of chronic disease requires a biologically-based approach that is grounded in an understanding of the biochemical synergisms and antagonisms that influence disease progression. Heart disease, diabetes, hypertension, cancer, and obesity are all, to varying degrees, responsive to dietary interventions that modulate essential pathological mechanisms. The use of dietary interventions provides a complement to standard medical care. For two decades, we have been coupling nutrients, botanicals, and other bioactive agents with standard medical treatments of cancer and other degenerative diseases. This approach, although still in an early stage, raises provocative possibilities for diminishing untoward effects and improving the efficacy of standard medical care.

PRINCIPAL CONCEPTS OF NUTRITIONAL BIOTHERAPY

Several principles of nutritional biotherapy must be understood for its effective clinical implementation. These principles include:

1. A core dietary regimen.
2. Dietary fat as a separate food.
3. Variety and meaningful quantification.
4. Individual nutritional tailoring.
5. Safe and appropriate supplementation.
6. The complementary nature of nutrition with medical care.

Description of Principal Concepts

This chapter illustrates the application of nutritional biotherapy by describing the approach and rationale we take in our clinic. However, our approach is similar in its principal concepts and approach to many other programs around the world, as we describe later in the chapter.

CORE DIETARY REGIMEN

The Block Integrative Nutritional Therapy (BINT) program, developed over a 20-year period at our Evanston clinics, uses a core diet upon which all individual adjustments are made. The core diet is plant-based, composed of 50 to 70% complex carbohydrates, 10 to 25% fat, and the remaining percent composed of protein. These criteria are individually tailored to meet the needs of those diagnosed with or recovering from illness. An initial goal is to reduce and eventually eliminate meat, dairy, and refined sugars, while obtaining more daily calories from complex carbohydrates (e.g., whole grains and grain products, vegetables, fruits). The primary sources of protein are vegetable proteins (from soy products and other legumes) and cold-water fish. White-flesh poultry without the skin is acceptable as a transitional item and is used to replace meat normally eaten for protein content.

Because of individual health and personal differences, the BINT program provides three levels of core diet:

The transitional level, which allows limited use of many of the food items generally found on the BINT "avoid list," such as eggs, poultry, and wild game.

The maintenance level, which uses the diet structured around the standard exchange lists (see concept 3). The participant does not eat any of the "avoid list" foods and adheres to portions adjusted to meet individual needs.

The therapeutic level, which represents the maintenance level with special and individualized adjustments based on the patient's medical needs. For example, a patient suffering from bleeding colitis will be advised to consume minimal roughage. Some hypertensive individuals would restrict salt intake more aggressively. Diabetics may need to increase fiber intake beyond the usual level of intake for nondiabetics. With an improved or greatly stabilized physical condition, or with clinically confirmed reversal of the disease, the BINT program may then be shifted back to the maintenance level.

DIETARY FAT AS A SEPARATE FOOD GROUP

In the BINT program, we begin teaching patients ways to reduce their fat intake by identifying fat as one of five food groups:

1. Whole grains and grain products.
2. Vegetables.
3. Fruits.
4. Fats.
5. Protein.

Fats are obtained primarily from nuts, seeds, and oils. Protein is provided by both plant and lean animal sources, or legumes and fish, respectively. Cold-water fish or supplemental fish oils help ensure the proper balance of omega-3 to omega-6 fatty acids, which in turn helps lower the risk of chronic inflammatory disorders and immune dysfunction. The optimal range for dietary fat intake is likely to be between 10 and 20% of total calories, with the exception of infants and small children, who could benefit from a higher level of fat intake (25 to 35%), with increased emphasis on omega-3 fatty acids.

VARIETY AND MEANINGFUL QUANTIFICATION

Variety is an important element in developing a health-promoting diet for long-range use. Rather than consume daily servings of the same food from each of the major food groups, one should choose a variety of foods within each group. To provide this dietary variety in a prescriptive yet meaningful way, the BINT program employs the concept of dietary exchange, referring to a food serving that can be exchanged, or traded, for other foods within the same grouping. The BINT exchange lists the five food groups mentioned previously. Each food, with its specified portion, grouped on the exchange list has approximately the same amount of carbohydrate, protein, fat, and calories as the other foods within the same group. Because they are approximate nutritional equivalents, any item on a particular exchange list can be exchanged for any other food item within the same exchange list.

The BINT exchange lists are used to develop a meal-based nutritional prescription that is both meaningful and attractive to the patient. An exchange system translates the scientific formula (total calories, percent of protein, percent of carbohydrates) into a tangible, easy-to-use format. With this system, daily meal planning can be carried out readily, and the desired amounts of protein, fat, carbohydrates, and calories can be monitored and can help a patient meet individual nutritional goals. Individuals are free to choose their favorite foods from a list that tells what one exchange is equal to. Usually the exchange formula is converted into a meal plan by dividing it into three meals or into the number of meals a person is consuming. In its usual application, this means 30% for

breakfast, 30% for lunch, 30% for dinner, and 10% for snacks.

INDIVIDUALIZED NUTRITIONAL REGIMENS

The BINT program considers individual tailoring of nutritional biotherapy protocols an essential part of designing the nutritional approach best suited for each patient's care. Biochemical individuality provides the primary rationale for individual tailoring. Optimal nutrient doses vary from individual to individual and from one disease state to the next. Therefore, the recommended daily allowances (RDAs) are average requirements that are generally inapplicable in nutritional biotherapy. Variations of 20-fold or more in individual requirements may occur, depending on the patient's genetics, biochemistry, and physiological state. Therefore, nutritional biotherapy is concerned with issues such as subclinical micronutrient deficiencies, conditional deficiencies, synergistic supplement combinations, and the need for supraphysiologic doses of one or more micronutrients. The existence of subtle, subclinical deficiency states have been frequently observed in our clinics and are widely reported. These biochemical alterations are targeted on an individual basis. The issue of nutritional requirements being both conditional and individualized becomes even more critical when treating complex, heterogeneous diseases such as cancer.

RATIONAL SUPPLEMENTATION

Supplemental use of nutrients, botanicals, and phytochemicals to manage disease constitutes an important aspect of nutritional biotherapy. Most of the focus has been on prevention: supplemental antioxidants may reduce the risk of specific types of cancers and cardiovascular disease; vitamin B_6 may prevent the onset of carpal tunnel syndrome; niacin can lower blood cholesterol levels; and folic acid for women of childbearing age reduces the risk of neural tube defects (9). However, supplemental nutrients may be particularly helpful in the context of psychological stress, metabolic stress (e.g., stress caused by surgery or cachexia), immunological dysfunction, and a polluted environment. Elderly individuals may benefit from supplementation to help malabsorption problems and difficulty in obtaining a balanced diet. Many commonly used medical treatments and certain disease states either cause or are associated with nutritional deficits that warrant careful supplementation (10–12).

Safe dosages have been established for many nutritional agents and compounds; for those that have not been established in human trials, it is possible to extrapolate from animal data to suggest reasonably safe dosage ranges in humans. In general, temporary administration of very high doses of water-soluble vitamins is feasible without causing toxicity. Overdosing is more common with fat-soluble vitamins because they tend to accumulate in adipose tissues. It is important for physicians to understand these toxic thresholds and to advise their patients accordingly. Particularly, in therapeutic situations involving serious illness, patients may be inclined to think that "more is better." Thus, patients should be advised to follow the recommended dosages to avoid adverse effects.

COMPLEMENTARY NUTRITIONAL STRATEGIES

Complementary intervention with standard medical care is another important principle of nutritional biotherapy. In most cases, nutritional strategies are used in an adjuvant or adjunctive fashion—that is, as a complement to standard medical care. However, this requires careful attention to the potential for synergisms and antagonisms between food factors and medical treatments. The known interactions between drugs and nutrients are legion (13, 14). For example, many drugs can adversely affect nutrient absorption, transport, and metabolism (15). Thus, nutritional supplementation can be used to compensate for such drug-based interference. Micronutrients and phytochemicals also may act as enzymatic cofactors in the metabolism of various anticancer drugs as well as some antibiotics, barbiturates, oral contraceptives, calcitonin, and salicylates.

These interactions may not only modulate the activity of the drugs, but also may cause a decrease in micronutrient availability (16). Drugs such as hydralazine, d-penicillamine, and many antituberculosis drugs may adversely af-

fect vitamin B_6 status. Corticosteroids, thiazide diuretics, d-penicillamine, and several other drugs all adversely affect zinc status. Regular use of oral contraceptive pills may lead to excessive losses of vitamins B_1, B_2, B_6, and folic acid (17, 18). Drug-nutrient interactions can affect every area of conventional medicine, especially pharmacology, and they represent the clearest example of a complementary medical application for nutritional biotherapy.

Therapeutically additive or synergistic interactions between drugs and nutrients are useful in determining the true therapeutic potential of those nutrients for modulating chronic disease progression. For example, vitamin C combined with antibiotic therapy has been shown to accelerate recovery among patients suffering from acute sinusitis (both purulent and catarrhal) (19). The nutrient-drug compound copper aspirinate (copper-bound aspirin) may have potent anti-inflammatory effects (20, 21); these beneficial effects may be augmented further by the use of fish oil supplements for the treatment of arthritis (22, 23). Copper aspirinate has also shown antiulcer, anticonvulsant, anticancer, antimutagenic, and radiation damage repair effects and may be used to prevent reperfusion injury (24). Supplemental N-acetylcysteine (NAC), for example, in combination with nitroglycerin and streptokinase in myocardial infarction is associated with significantly less oxidative stress, a trend toward more rapid reperfusion, and better preservation of left ventricular function (25). Similarly, a drug may be ineffective until a nutritional deficiency is corrected. Patients with chronic oral candidiasis may be clinically unresponsive to topical antifungal agents until iron deficiency is reversed (26).

A nutrient or nutrient combination may also be exploited for its ability to mitigate serious and often dose-limiting side effects of a drug. Peripheral neuropathy induced by the antituberculous drug isoniazid can be inhibited by the administration of vitamin B6 in doses of 50 to 100 mg/day (27). The use of appropriate supplements in a group of elderly people has been shown to improve antibody responsiveness to the influenza virus vaccine (28). The elderly also show greater tolerance toward antituberculous drugs, isoniazid, rifampicin, and pyrazinamide, when simultaneously treated with anti-oxidant supplements (29).

BASIC PRINCIPLES IN NUTRITIONAL ASSESSMENT

The physician should ensure that all patients, regardless of their particular diagnoses, are adequately nourished, either by the actual provision of nutrients or by counseling them in their dietary choices. Normal nutritional requirements vary greatly from one individual to the next, based on past diet, biochemical individuality (and/or individual physiology), age, gender, activity levels, current medications, and disease state. Nutritional needs for a particular nutrient or food factor may increase or decrease over time in response to disease processes and conventional treatments. Complementary medical practitioners should also assure appropriate aspects of the conventional medical approach (e.g., choice of specific medications) with nutritional concerns.

The first step in effective nutritional medicine is assessment of the patient's current nutritional status. Protein-calorie malnutrition is quite prevalent in hospital patients and has been shown to cause longer lengths of stay, higher costs, and increased rates of morbidity and mortality. In fact, when malnutrition is among the diagnoses as a complication or a comorbidity factor and treatment is provided, there is generally a corresponding increase in the reimbursement for the care of the patient. Conditions resulting from protein and calorie malnutrition include cachexia (lean-tissue wasting, which resembles marasmus) and a kwashiorkor-like syndrome, or a combination of these two syndromes. Detection of these conditions should lead to aggressive nutritional adjustments which, in turn, contribute to an improved prognosis and quality of life for the patient.

The nutritional assessment methods used by complementary medical practitioners are the same as, or may even be more comprehensive than, those used by conventional physicians. They involve the ABCDs of nutritional assessment, which stands for anthropometric, biochemical, clinical, and dietary assessment.

In anthropometric assessment, weight is considered in relation to height, and changes in weight are recorded with successive visits and compared with usual weight and reference weight to determine percent-change over time. Body Mass Index (BMI) can be calculated from this and used in risk factor assessment if needed. Biochemical studies include the standard laboratory measures of albumin, transferrin, and prealbumin, as well as vitamin and electrolyte levels, red cell counts and indices, and other aspects of the complete blood count. Clinical assessment includes consideration of nutrition-related problems and risk factors, such as anorexia and nausea, as well as potential treatment–nutrient interactions. A physical examination that looks at evidence of nutrient inadequacies is done (see Chapter 27). Past and present dietary habits are evaluated based on standard questions issued by dietitians.

Within the BINT program, we also incorporate more sophisticated forms of laboratory testing to provide evidence of suboptimal or inadequate nutrition (Fig. 29.1). These tests include measures of antioxidant-micronutrient and antioxidant-phytochemical status, DNA oxidation, and essential fatty acids, immune detoxification, hormonal levels, and, when appropriate, other relevant analyses. In most cases, testing will reveal inadequate nutrition in an individual, even in the absence of clinical findings of classical deficiency syndromes. Because of the high cost of comprehensive nutritional testing, however, it is helpful to apply a disease-related, mechanism-based perspective to each case, focusing on those particular nutritional issues that are most likely to impact the particular disorder in question. A detailed description of the use of nutritionally focused biochemical testing is beyond the scope of this chapter. Interested readers are referred to the courses and literature by Jeffrey Bland, Jonathan Wright, Alan Gaby, and others (see Appendix A).

A SURVEY OF DIETS USED IN COMPLEMENTARY MEDICINE

Within complementary medicine, many different diets and supplementation regimens are

NUTRITION NOTE: INITIAL ASSESSMENT

Name: _____ Date: _____

S: Appetite: _____

_____

_____

O: M/F _____ Age: _____ Birthdate: _____

Medical Diagnosis and Treatment Plan: _____

_____

_____

Nutrition Related Problems/Risk Factors:

☐ Carcinoma ☐ Anorexia/Appetite Change ☐ Obesity
☐ Fever ☐ Nausea ☐ Weight Loss
☐ Infection/Sepsis ☐ Vomiting ☐ NPO/TF/TPN
☐ GI Disorder ☐ Diarrhea ☐ Clear Liquids >3 Days
☐ Surgery ☐ Constipation ☐ Drug/Nutrient Interaction
☐ Chemotherapy ☐ Dysphagia ☐ Food Allergy/Intolerance
☐ Radiation Therapy ☐ Taste Alterations ☐ Compulsive Eating Disorder
☐ Diabetes ☐ Chewing Difficulty ☐ Other

Anthropometrics:

Ht. _____ Wt. _____ Wt. hx _____

Usual Wt. _____ IBW _____ %IBW _____ Adjusted wt. for obesity _____ kg.

Body Composition Analysis _____ %fat _____ %LDM

Laboratory:

Date: _____ Alb. _____ Chol/TG _____

Mg _____ Ca _____ TPRO _____ H/H _____

Other: _____

Medications: _____

Vit/Min: _____

A: _____

_____

_____

_____

Diet Hx reveals: _____

Exercise Hx reveals: _____

Visceral protein stores: ☐ AlbuminN/A ☐ intact ☐ mildly depleted ☐ moderately depleted ☐ severely depleted

Nutritional status assessed as:

☐ noncompromised ☐ at risk ☐ mildly compromised ☐ moderately compromised ☐ severely compromised

Secondary to:

Estimated nutritional needs: Kcal _____ Pro _____

Exchange pattern Rx: _____ Kcal _____ Grain _____ Vegetable _____ Protein _____ Fruit _____ Fat

P: Recommendations/Treatment Plan _____

_____

_____

_____

_____

_____

☐ Keep food diary   ☐ Recommend follow up q _____ wks/mons. _____

FIGURE 29.1. BINT assessment chart.

thought to affect disease processes. Some diets claim to help stop or reverse disease progression; others may help keep disease in remission. The following is a description of the major diets embraced by complementary practitioners.

These diets may be categorized into three basic groups:

1. High-fiber, high-carbohydrate, low-fat diets.
2. High-protein, low-carbohydrate diets.
3. Diets of variable nutrient composition.

A difficulty that many of these approaches face is the lack of a way to meaningfully translate percentages into food quantities and proportions.

High-Fiber, High-Carbohydrate, Low-Fat Diets

MACROBIOTIC DIET

Macrobiotics is a philosophy of eating that originated in Japan with the teachings of Sagen Ishitsuka, MD, and his pupil George Ohsawa. Two of Ohsawa's students, Michio Kushi and Herman Aihara, introduced macrobiotics to the West as a dietary principle that accounts for differing climatic and geographical considerations, as well as a wide variety of individual factors. The so-called Standard Macrobiotic Diet consists of 50 to 60% whole grains, 20 to 25% vegetables, 5 to 10% beans and sea vegetables (typically combined), and 5% vegetable soups. Other foods, such as nuts and seeds, fruits, and fish are consumed on an occasional basis. Red meat, dairy, sugar, and raw fruits are generally avoided. Each person's dietary needs vary according to level of activity, gender, age, climate, season, and various individual factors.

PRITIKIN DIET

Founded by Nathan Pritikin, the Pritikin program is a low-fat, low-cholesterol, low-sodium, high-complex-carbohydrate diet (5 to 10% fat, 10 to 15% protein, and 80% carbohydrate) combined with regular aerobic exercise. The diet is similar to the macrobiotic diet, but with more rigid emphasis on restricting fat intake, as well as the inclusion of low-fat dairy products

and greater variety in choices of animal products. Protein consumption is limited to 3.5 ounces of lean meat a day to reduce total fat and cholesterol intake, because most animal products have high levels of fat and cholesterol. Pritikin himself followed the diet throughout his adult life.

THE WAIANAE DIET

This program was designed by Hawaiian physician Terry Shintani, MD, MPH, in response to the disproportionately high rates of chronic disease among "westernized" native Hawaiians. The diet—which contains less than 10% fat; 12 to 15% protein; 75 to 78% carbohydrate—consists of traditional Hawaiian foods (e.g., fish, seaweed, bread, fruit, yams, sweet potatoes.) All foods are served either raw or steamed in a manner that approximates ancient styles of cooking. A "transition diet" provides palatable alternatives for those unaccustomed to Hawaiian cuisine. This culturally sensitive dietary program, which includes social support and community-based health education, has demonstrated impressive results in weight management. It is also likely to elicit high adherence among people of the same ethnic background.

GERSON DIET

Developed by Austrian physician Max Gerson in the early 1900s, this vegetarian diet consists mainly of raw vegetables and fruit juices, raw calf liver juice (now largely discontinued because of the chemical residues now found in calves), and coffee enemas to stimulate bile elimination. The latter is said to expel toxins accumulated from manifestations of illness and dissolving tumor masses. The program initially includes a period of juice fasting and enemas, after which patients are placed on a low-sodium, high-potassium diet. A modified and more comprehensive Gerson program is used at CHIPSA (Centro Hospitalario Internacional del Pacifico, S.A.) by Gar and Chris Hildenbrand. This program, which is reported to reduce occurrence of malignant melanoma after conventional treatment (30), is easier to follow and is consistent with the standard low-fat, high-fiber dietary pattern.

THE REVERSAL DIET

Developed by Dean Ornish, MD, to reverse the development of atherosclerosis and coronary heart disease, this diet is very similar to the Pritikin Diet. In terms of total calories, the diet is 10 to 12% fat, 70 to 75% carbohydrate, and 15 to 20% protein. Egg whites, nonfat yogurt, and skim milk are allowed as sources of complementary proteins. Additionally, like many other proponents of complementary medicine, Ornish emphasizes the importance of gentle exercises, such as yoga and walking, and of relaxation and visualization techniques to help relieve the body of stress and tension. A recent 5-year follow-up of cardiac patients who follow this program has shown continued regression of coronary lesions that had been reported previously (31).

NEW FOUR FOOD GROUPS DIET

In April 1991, the Physicians Committee for Responsible Medicine (PCRM) proposed the New Four Food Groups: grains, vegetables, fruits, and legumes (eliminating meat and dairy from the old Basic Four). This 100% plant-derived (vegan) diet may be among the most effective weight-loss diets on the market, as cogently argued by PCRM President Neal Barnard, MD, in his book, *Food for Life* (Harmony, 1993). It is not only very low in fat (10% of total calories) and protein (20% of calories), but also very high in complex carbohydrates (70% of calories). Calcium balance is improved because high-protein diets tend to compromise the body's calcium supply.

MCDOUGALL DIET

The McDougall Program, proposed by John A. McDougall, MD, is virtually identical to the PCRM dietary plan (and similar to the Ornish, Pritikin, and Core BINT diets). With McDougall's system, however, a modicum of flexibility is granted for the infrequent (i.e., best to avoid) use of so-called feast foods, such as range-fed beef, organically grown poultry, and fresh fish. The tempered use of such foods may be considered part of a transition to the vegan diet proposed by PCRM. McDougall, who runs a 2-week residential training program for his approach, has documented clinical improvements and reductions in medication in hundreds of patients with chronic illnesses placed on this diet (32).

LIVING FOODS DIET

This diet was introduced by Ann Wigmore of the Hippocrates Institute in Boston. She believed that cooking destroyed many of the enzymes necessary for proper digestion and nutrient assimilation. The diet is composed of wheatgrass juice, fresh and fermented vegetables, fruits, and all variety of sprouted seed, grain, and legume. Although occasional use of raw milk or cheese is permitted, many followers make their own "seed milk" or "seed cheese" from ground, soaked seeds, such as rice or nuts.

COMMENTARY ON HIGH-FIBER, HIGH-CARBOHYDRATE, LOW-FAT DIETS

These diets incorporate a plant-based eating plan, which translates into a high-fiber, low-fat pattern of eating. Nutritional epidemiology has consistently demonstrated that this type of diet is the most likely to lower the incidence of and mortality from chronic diseases Some studies also indicate that a plant-based diet may help increase the prospects of recovery and long-range survival after a diagnosis of cancer, diabetes, or heart disease. Substantial reductions in blood pressure, fasting serum glucose, total plasma cholesterol, and insulin dependency (among diabetics) have been documented following the low-fat, vegetable-based diets outlined in this section. When all fats are markedly restricted, however, deficiencies of omega-3 fatty acids and gamma linoleic acid (an important omega-6) may arise. These fatty acids may exert beneficial effects on the immune, nervous, and cardiovascular systems. Deficiencies in fat-soluble vitamins and gluten hypersensitivity may also develop. Physicians should closely monitor the nutritional status of patients who adhere to low-fat diets (10 to 15% of total calories as fat) without appropriate supplementation.

Vitamin B_{12} deficiency has been documented in rigidly vegan mothers and their nursing infants. Rickets, due to vitamin D deficiency, is also a concern in vegan children in northern climates. Avoidance of supplements and conventional medicine, due to an implicit belief in an "all natural" approach to health, can increase the risk of such complications. For people at risk of developing these deficiencies, vitamin supplements may be needed. Additionally, supplemental eicosapentaenoic acid (EPA) or fish oil may be desirable for patients who avoid fish, because many adults in the United States lack the enzymes that would enable them to convert plant-derived omega-3's (alpha-linolenic acid) into the biologically active compound EPA.

High-Protein, Low-Carbohydrate Diets

ATKINS DIET

Developed by Robert Atkins, MD, this diet emphasizes the consumption of nutrient-dense, unprocessed foods, avoidance of processed or refined carbohydrate foods, and use of nutrient supplements. High-carbohydrate meals (e.g., rice, breads, pasta) are thought to elicit excessive rises in insulin levels, which then result in fat accumulation. In addition, low-protein, low-fat meals tend to leave people less satisfied than meals high in fat and protein, which encourage the body to burn fat for energy. The supplementation component includes a full-spectrum multivitamin and an essential fatty acid formula.

ZONE DIET

The Zone Diet, developed by Barry Sears, PhD, is similar to the Atkins diet—high protein (30%), low carbohydrate (40%), and moderately high fat (30%). Like Atkins, Sears contends that an excess of carbohydrates forces the body to over-secrete insulin, resulting in excess fat accumulation. Sears warns against the use of starchy foods, even high-fiber items such as whole-grain breads and pastas. Only high-fiber fruits and vegetables are allowed.

COMMENTARY ON HIGH-PROTEIN, LOW-CARBOHYDRATE DIETS

The rationale so ardently voiced by proponents of these diets is twofold. First, high-carbohy-

drate diets are thought to decrease insulin sensitivity over time and thus may increase an individual's vulnerability to the "metabolic syndrome" of insulin resistance (obesity, diabetes, hypertension, and cardiovascular disease). However, extensive research documents that high-fiber diets centered around complex carbohydrates increase insulin sensitivity (33), whereas diets relatively high in fat (and/or refined carbohydrates) tend to increase insulin resistance (34, 35). The notion that thin people with elevated insulin levels are at risk is incorrect; these individuals do not, as a rule, have chronically elevated insulin levels. Increased consumption of low-glycemic foods that are high in complex carbohydrates will moderate insulin levels in these individuals in the context of a well-balanced nutritional program.

Second, low-carbohydrate proponents say that high-carbohydrate diets tend to increase blood triglyceride levels. Although it is true that some individuals who follow high-carbohydrate diets may have high triglyceride levels and low HDL cholesterol, low total cholesterol levels require less HDL to remove cholesterol. Increased triglyceride levels in the face of low-fat diets and low serum cholesterol levels are not likely to be important, unless other cardiovascular risk factors are present. Moreover, fish oil supplements (which can be used in selected cases) have been shown clinically to decrease the level of triglycerides and very low-density lipoproteins (VLDL) (36, 37). High triglycerides are often associated with high intake of *refined* carbohydrates, which are not recommended.

The relatively high-protein, high-fat profile of these diets is very appealing to many Americans because of its lenient attitude toward consumption of animal products. Most existing data, however, do not support the use of high-protein, low-carbohydrate diets for the establishment of good health. Rather, epidemiologic studies suggest that such diets, at the fat intake level of 30% of calories, increase the risk of heart disease, osteoporosis, kidney disorders, and various cancers, notably those involving the breast and colorectal tissues. Currently, the scientific literature suggests it is inadvisable for patients already diagnosed with these conditions to use either diet. Elderly patients and patients with renal disease should generally avoid such a regimen, even in the short term.

Diets of Variable Nutrient Composition

BLOOD TYPE-BASED DIET

Peter D'Adamo, MD, drawing from the work of his father, devised a dietary system based on the concept that the ideal diet depends on that aspect of genotype reflected in the blood type. The system consists of four different diets and four different exercise programs, all based on the four ABO blood types. The rationale derives primarily from the in vitro finding that specific lectins, present in many commonly eaten foods, can agglutinate the erythrocytes of certain blood types and exert a diverse range of biological effects. In theory, individuals with certain blood types will be adversely affected by specific lectins, whereas people with other blood types will react to other lectins; avoidance of foods that contain lectins incompatible with one's blood type enables individuals to lose weight, slow the aging process, and prevent common diseases.

KELLEY DIET (METABOLIC TYPES)

Dr. William Donald Kelley, an orthodontist from Texas, developed an anticancer dietary plan that was very similar to the Gerson diet, but with less stringent use of raw plant foods. Kelley developed 10 basic diets with numerous variations, depending on the type of cancer and on certain aspects of the patient's condition. These dietary plans range from vegan to red-meat-based diets. Kelley also recommended regular fasting, colonic irrigation (high enemas), and coffee enemas. Kelley also included pancreatic enzymes in the treatment of cancer patients. One of his students, Nicholas Gonzalez, MD, has subsequently included high levels of nutritional supplementation with micronutrients, amino acids, glandular substances, and digestive enzymes. These programs are individually designed with the goal of modulating sympathetic/parasympathetic imbalances.

AYURVEDIC DIET

Ayurveda, developed centuries ago in India, is the oldest medical system known, and its ancient texts span all the major branches of medicine. The Ayurvedic system of food and herbal selection revolves around the three *doshas*, the innate tendencies that are built into an individual's total make-up. The three *doshas*–*vita*, *pitta*, and *kapha*–manifest in different physical characteristics or metabolic body types. The *dosha* refers to a unique property of the individual that enables one to adapt to one's environment either favorably or unfavorably. Factors such as stress and climate can alter each *dosha*; imbalances in the *doshas* can result in specific diseases. Various foods, herbs, and emotions can either stabilize or disturb the balance of a given *dosha* type. The Ayurvedic system is primarily vegetarian, although meat may be prescribed for certain *doshas* (e.g., one with a predominance of vata) (see Chapter 11 for a detailed description of this system).

NATURAL HYGIENE DIET

First formulated in the early 1800s by Sylvester Graham, this diet has been popularized by Harvey and Marilyn Diamond, authors of *Fit for Life*. A central premise is proper food combinations to maximize digestion. Adherents follow specific rules about digestion, food selection, and usage. For example, fruits and vegetables are never eaten together, nor are protein- and starch-rich foods. Raw, unprocessed foods and freshly squeezed juices are emphasized, as are fresh vegetables, organically grown whenever possible. Occasional use of meat is allowed. Periodic fasting is practiced to remove accumulated toxins from the previous diet or environmental sources.

COMMENTARY ON DIETS OF VARIABLE NUTRIENT COMPOSITION

Several of these systems contain similar components that are part of the shifting paradigm of nutrition. Supporting any regimen that is low in fat and high in fiber, with minimal amounts of animal protein, is consistent with the preponderance of epidemiologic and laboratory data on good health. However, no one has performed the types of studies needed to validate these theories, and in some areas there are grounds for concern. For example, long-term adherence to the high-meat, type O diet (prescribed for more than 40% of the population) may raise the risk of heart disease and several cancers. The potential atherogenicity of this diet may be complicated further by the program's recommendation that type O individuals should avoid supplements of vitamin E and fish oil, both of which may help prevent heart disease. Similarly, one of the 10 diets in the Kelley program calls for raw meat as well as raw meat juices. The resulting high-protein load may cause excessive bone resorption and insulin-like growth factor secretion; also, there is risk of contamination with bacteria, particularly for those people with compromised immune systems.

The primarily vegetarian leaning of the Ayurvedic diet is likely to translate into general health improvements. At this time, however, there are limited published reports of the therapeutic effects of Ayurvedic dietary practices per se. In contrast, a number of studies have been published on the use of Ayurvedic herbal agents as dietary supplements. Similarly, the Natural Hygiene Diet has never been taken seriously by the medical establishment because there is no published evidence that this diet offers health benefits superior to any other low-fat vegetarian plan. The emphasis on proper digestion and food combination may be helpful to people who suffer from intestinal discomfort after eating.

In principle, the lack of cooked, high-fiber foods in a raw-foods regimen might be expected to produce deficiencies in various nutrients, because cooking (in moderation) helps release nutrients from many foods. Juicing and use of organically grown foods can reduce the risk of these deficiencies. There are many anecdotes supporting the use of this approach. In the author's clinical experience, however, raw-foods diets generally tend to be short-lived: adherents tend to increase their intake of energy-rich foods (nuts and nut butters) over time to compensate for the semifasting state, and they eventually switch back to regular consumption of high-calorie foods or cooked foods.

The potential health applications of these dietary approaches remain largely undetermined. Although there are some intriguing associations with blood types, lectins, and diseases, the blood-type theory of dietary selection rests on a set of as yet unsubstantiated assumptions about evolution and physiology. Documentation is scant for Ayurveda as well. This explains why such esoteric-sounding systems are usually shunned and chastised by medical professionals. However, we should remain open to the possibility that these noninvasive systems may have value. Scientific, clinically valid evaluations are needed before judgment can be passed in either direction.

MEDICAL APPLICATIONS OF NUTRITIONAL BIOTHERAPY

The extent of current knowledge on nutritional influences on disease etiology and progression is too vast for a single chapter. The aim of this section is to highlight major areas of clinical relevance whereby nutritional biotherapy may play a role, based on the evidence from nutritional epidemiology, with primary emphasis on clinical trials. The following is a discussion of the efficacy and use of nutritional intervention for four major diseases: cancer, hypertension, coronary heart disease, and diabetes.

Nutritional Biotherapy for Cancer

We have used nutritional biotherapy on two key areas of treatment in cancer: toxicity mitigation and potentiation of standard treatment. With regard to toxicity mitigation, intravenous supplementation with antioxidant nutrients can reduce the damage induced by peroxidation from chemotherapy or radiotherapy (38, 39). Moreover, antioxidants improved the tolerance to chemotherapy and radiation (40). Fat- and water-soluble antioxidants may help alleviate the oxidative stress that accompanies many types of chemotherapy, as well as high-calorie diets, psychological stress, and the aging process (41). Importantly, the results of in vivo studies indicate that antioxidants will not simultaneously protect the tumor or interfere with the results of conventional treatment (42–52).

In the area of potentiating treatment, we now know that additive or synergistic relationships between nutrients and anticancer drugs may increase the therapeutic index, enabling lower doses of the chemotherapy agents to be used without diminishing tumor kill. In most therapeutic situations, the chemotherapy agents act by a direct cytotoxic effect, and the biomodulators simply amplify that effect. In some cases, the drugs may have immunomodulatory properties that synergize with immune-enhancing agents (53). For example, several trials demonstrated that vitamin A acted synergistically with chemotherapy and radiotherapy against metastatic cancers (54–56). When combined with the collagenase inhibitor minocycline (an antiangiogenic agent), beta-carotene significantly enhanced the antitumor activities of several chemotherapy agents both in vitro and in vivo (57). Vitamin C potentiates the anticancer activity of chemotherapy agents in vivo (58) and in vitro (59), particularly when combined with vitamin K (60–64).

Evidence from both randomized and non-randomized trials indicates that laboratory findings may carry over into the clinical realm. Survival and other clinical outcomes for chemotherapy-treated metastatic breast cancer have been improved with adjuvant use of high-dose oral vitamin A (65–70), antioxidant micronutrients and nutriceuticals (including coenzyme Q10) (71–74), L-arginine (75, 76), and folinic acid (the reduced form of the B vitamin, folic acid) (77–81). Low-fat diets may further improve the prognosis of breast cancer patients (82–89), although randomized trials are needed to test this theory. In lung cancer patients, a randomized trial of adjuvant nutrition using high-dose vitamin A led to a significant reduction in tumor recurrences following surgery (90). Other retinoids may hold therapeutic promise for increasing response rates and survival in patients with advanced non-small-cell lung cancer (91–97), although response rates have been relatively low. A preliminary trial of small-cell lung cancer cases found that supple-

mental antioxidants resulted in significant improvements in expected survival (98). Significant prevention of bladder cancer recurrences has been demonstrated in randomized, placebo-controlled trials using vitamin B_6 (99) and various retinoids (100–103) and, more recently, using multiple antioxidants at pharmacological doses versus the RDA for these micronutrients (104).

By far the strongest evidence for the efficacy of adjuvant nutrition, however, has been with various forms of leukemia. For example, clinical trials have demonstrated that all-trans retinoic acid (ATRA, or tretinoin, the acidic form of retinol) induced complete remission rates ranging from 86 to 100% and prolonged survival in acute promyelocytic leukemia patients (APL) (105–111). Patients with refractory or relapsed APL have also shown significant improvements in clinical response rates after ATRA supplementation (112–116). Patients diagnosed with advanced malignant melanoma may benefit by following low-protein, vegetable-rich diets (117, 118) or by supplemental retinoids (119–121). Less well substantiated at this time is the efficacy of adjuvant nutrition for the treatment of pancreatic and prostate cancer and other gastrointestinal cancers, although there are promising preliminary reports.

Nutritional Biotherapy for Hypertension

The standard dietary advice for hypertensive patients consists of salt restriction, weight reduction (for obese patients), and reducing alcohol consumption (122, 123). The first two of these have been shown to interact with each other in an additive fashion (124–126). Additionally, diets rich in fish, fruit, and vegetables have been shown to reverse mild hypertension, to enhance the effects of antihypertensive drugs, and to diminish fatal and nonfatal heart attack and stroke rates (127). Low-fat, plant-based diets are also likely to halt the progression of atherosclerotic and thrombotic disease. Other potentially useful antihypertensive strategies include antioxidant supplementation, cessation of smoking, and adoption of a regular exercise program (128–131). Similar strategies should be implemented in combination with appropriate medication for moderate to more severe forms of hypertension.

The effects of diet on blood pressure have been reviewed elsewhere (132–137). The most compelling data concerning an antihypertensive effect of low-fat, high-fiber diets come from a clinical study of the DASH diet (Dietary Approaches to Stop Hypertension) (138) and from studies of vegetarians (139–147). Additionally, clinical trials and epidemiologic studies have demonstrated antihypertensive effects through seven strategies:

1. Sodium restriction (148–153).
2. Supplemental potassium (154–158).
3. Supplemental magnesium (159–161).
4. Supplemental calcium (162–164); however, this is for women only because of the risk for prostate cancer (165); in older women, calcium should be combined with magnesium to lower the risk of thrombosis (166).
5. Supplemental fish oil (167, 168) (with restricted salt intake).
6. Vegetable oil (169–171).
7. Garlic (172–177).

Nutritional Biotherapy for Coronary Artery Disease (CAD)

Interventional cardiology refers not only to standard treatment (bypass surgery and angioplasty), but also to complementary management of CAD patients. Supplementation with soy protein (178–180), garlic extracts (181–183), coenzyme Q10 (184–186), magnesium (187), vitamin E (ideally with selenium) (188–190), or vitamin C (191–193) have demonstrated a range of beneficial therapeutic effects in the management of CAD patients. Additionally, omega-3 fatty acid supplements, either from fish oil or flaxseed oil, may be useful adjuncts to nutritional protocols for CAD (194–198). In the majority of clinical trials, supplemental use of fish oils significantly decreases the rate of restenosis following coronary angioplasty (199–207).

To date, seven clinical trials have demonstrated that a low-fat diet, usually in conjunction with cholesterol-lowering drugs, can alter coronary lesions and substantially retard CAD progression (208–218). In the highly publicized Lifestyle Heart Trial, Ornish et al. randomized 41 men and women to either usual care or a low-fat diet along with stress management (1 hour per day) and aerobic exercise (3 hours per day) (31). Subjects in the intervention group showed a decrease in average percentage diameter stenosis from 40 to 37.8%, whereas an increase was seen in the control group, 42.7 to 46.1% (p = 0.001) (31). After 4 years, the intervention showed an even greater improvement in stenosis and significant improvement in calculated coronary flow reserve; in contrast, patients in the control group had a further worsening of CAD progression (219, 220). More recent follow-up has demonstrated continued benefits, including CAD regression, with long-term compliance on this program (31), although some have questioned the angiographic criteria used in this study (221).

A larger randomized study (n = 113) in Germany found overall delayed lesion progression in a diet-and-exercise intervention group (n = 56) versus controls (n = 57) (222). CAD progression was significantly retarded in the intervention group (23% versus 48%, p < 0.05), and regression was more pronounced in the intervention group as well (32% versus 17%, p < 0.05) (223). Taken together, these trials suggest that optimal clinical outcomes for CAD treatment may be accomplished through the combined, individually tailored use of cholesterol-lowering drugs, bypass surgery, nutritional interventions, and lifestyle changes, such as exercise and stress management.

Nutritional Biotherapy for Diabetes

Dietary modification is the cornerstone of complementary medical management of diabetes, particularly for noninsulin-dependent or Type II diabetes. Since 1986, the American Diabetes Association has held the position that "medical nutrition therapy is integral to total diabetes care and management" (224). The ideal diet for diabetics is one high in carbohydrate-rich foods that have a low glycemic index, combined with high-fiber content (30 to 40 g/day) (225, 226). Diabetics can greatly reduce their dependency on insulin and improve glucose control by adopting a high-fiber, high-complex-carbohydrate, low-fat diet (227–229). Saturated fats appear detrimental to the course of diabetes (230), whereas both omega-3 polyunsaturates (e.g., fish oils) and monounsaturated fatty acids (from olive oil), combined with vitamin E, may be beneficial to diabetics (231–233). Other nutritional agents that may improve glucose control, insulin sensitivity, and other aspects of diabetes include the following supplements:

Chromium (234–236)

Zinc (237–240)

Magnesium (241–246)

Potassium (247–249)

Vitamin C (250)

Vitamin B6 (pyridoxine) (251–255)

Alpha-lipoic acid (256–263)

In addition to the diet and supplement program, management should include regular exercise and (if the patient is obese) short periods of fasting to reduce tissue resistance to insulin (264).

TRAINING AND QUALITY ASSURANCE IN NUTRITIONAL BIOTHERAPY

Medical training has not kept pace with the rapidly evolving field of nutrition. In general, physicians are inadequately trained in how to use nutrition to prevent and treat illness. In an annual survey by the Association of American Medical Colleges, more than half of medical school graduates consistently reported that their training in nutrition was deficient. Authors of the National Nutrition Monitoring and Related Research Act, passed by Congress in 1990, concluded that the level of physicians' nutrition education could not realistically meet national goals for health promotion and disease prevention.

With few exceptions, United States medical schools expose their students to only the most elementary aspects of nutrition, usually through a biochemistry course. Fewer than 35% of allopathic schools offer a separate nutrition course; schools that do offer this course frequently fail to bridge these teachings into clinical training. At best, medical students learn about vitamin deficiencies that are relatively rare in an affluent society, rather than about the hazards of excess, about important drug-nutrient interactions, or about the nutritional imbalances that may accompany surgery, radiotherapy, and other conventional treatments. In one survey, three of four first-year medical students believed a knowledge of nutrition was important to their career; however, only one in ten felt that way once they reached their third year (265).

In a consensus statement prepared following a 1997 conference sponsored by the American Medical Student Association (AMSA), medical students declared that they lacked sufficient education in three areas: nutrition, research issues, and societal issues in medicine. In response to the call for improved nutrition education, the Washington, D.C.-based Physicians' Committee for Responsible Medicine (PCRM) produced Key Nutrition Issues for Medical Students (Physicians' Committee for Responsible Medicine, [202] 686–2210), which is designed to supplement medical education. This book provides a curriculum guide to key issues related to nutrition biotherapy for cancer, diabetes, heart disease, hypertension, renal disease, osteoporosis, and arthritis. The curriculum also provides study questions for a self-directed learning experience.

In terms of outcomes-based curricular competencies, some medicals schools have begun to incorporate the Physicians' Curriculum in Clinical Nutrition (American Academy of Family Physicians, [800] 274–2237), published by the Society of Teachers of Family Medicine. Like the PCRM guidebook, this curriculum considers key issues in the prevention and treatment of a wide variety of diseases. Section I of the curriculum also explores many issues related to basic care, such as nutritional screening and assessment, nutritional counseling, geriatric care, women's health, obesity, eating disorders, and nutrition support skills. Section II presents issues related to educational program development, patient-care methods (nutrition screening, co-counseling, precepting, chart review), and implementation of a nutrition rotation and nutritional course.

The American Society for Clinical Nutrition (ASCN) recently proposed having at least one physician nutrition specialist (PNS) at every major medical center. To hold this position, the individual would have completed a fellowship in clinical nutrition after residency. The primary function of the PNS would be to provide leadership to the nutrition services team at the hospital and to assist with complex nutritional cases throughout the region. All associated schools of medicine would use the PNS as a role model for physicians in training and for developing and coordinating their nutrition education programs. AMSA recently teamed up with the ASCN to sponsor an internship program that places medical students across the United States to work with authorities in clinical nutrition for 2-month intervals.

The ultimate goal should be to teach all medical students about the interconnectedness between nutrition and health. Dr. Steven Zeissel, nutrition department chair at the University of North Carolina School of Public Health and Medicine, has developed a series of computer-assisted nutrition teaching programs funded, in part, by the National Institutes of Health. This electronic textbook, an interactive CD-ROM system, enables students to interact with a patient on screen along with a guiding physician or role model. With this case-oriented format, students learn practical applications of nutritional biochemistry and appropriate decision making for nutrition-related health problems. Immediate feedback is given to indicate whether the student's chosen nutritional strategy is appropriate. (Note: This program is currently available to medical schools only; see www.med.unc.edu/nutr/nim.)

As of December 1998, the computerized nutrition teaching programs were distributed to 100 medical schools nationwide. Approximately 50 of these schools are using the first 10 modules, which are intended for first- and second-year students. The five modules in the disease series cover issues relevant to the nutritional management of cancer, obesity and cardiovascular disease, diabetes and weight management, anemia, and metabolic stress. The remaining five modules concern the life cycle (maternal and infant health, and nutrition for the second half of life) and special topics (supplements, fortified foods, and sports nutrition).

For physicians who would like to increase their understanding of nutritional medicine issues, postgraduate programs in nutrition are available at many American universities (particularly those which include a school of public health), and excellent programs are increasingly available at medical schools and osteopathic schools as well. The University of Texas Health Science Center at San Antonio has integrated nutrition into all 4 years of training. Most osteopathic medical schools place nutrition in their mission statement. Naturopathic colleges, such as John Bastyr University in Seattle and the National College of Naturopathic Medicine in Portland, also offer comprehensive nutrition programs.

QUALITY ASSURANCE AND PROFESSIONAL COMPETENCY

Currently, quality assurance in the administration of nutritional biotherapy remains a vague, loosely defined concept. This is primarily because there is little or no agreement within the conventional and CAM communities as to the level of nutritional knowledge physicians should have in their clinical practice. For example, the Residency Review Committee for Family Practice has required education in nutrition since 1982. However, a consensus is still lacking as to the core competencies required by a practicing family physician. Many physicians may understand the fundamentals of nutritional biotherapy yet may be ill-equipped to evaluate, manage, and intervene in the nutritional aspects of medical problems. Similarly, they may lack competence to counsel patients on dietary management and prevention of disease.

At the least, physicians should ask patients what they eat and whether they are taking supplemental micronutrients during history-taking. Physicians also should have a substantial grounding in the nutritional literature as it pertains to the management of the major chronic diseases: cancer, heart disease, obesity, diabetes, hypertension, arthritis, osteoporosis, and renal disease. Such knowledge will, in turn, enable them to better integrate information from the medical history (including dietary history), physical examination, and laboratory data used to assess the patient's nutritional status. Dietary and supplementation needs can then be evaluated from a more thoroughly informed nutritional perspective.

If complicated nutritional interventions are needed beyond the initial level of care, or if the physician cannot follow up with patients who are at nutritional risk, he or she should refer them to subspecialists in clinical nutrition. These specialists include registered dietitians or licensed dietitians (RDs and LDs, respectively). The RD is registered to administer medical nutrition care with the Commission on Dietetic Registration, the accrediting body of the American Dietetic Association. Medical nutrition care includes the following three components:

1. Interpreting and recommending nutrient needs relative to medical prescribed diets, including, but not limited to, specialized oral feedings and artificial nutrition (enteral and parenteral formulas).
2. Food, nutrient, and prescription drug interactions.
3. Developing and managing food service operations whose primary function is nutrition care and provision of medical prescribed diets.

The LD is licensed to practice dietetics but cannot make medical differential diagnoses of the health status of an individual.

There is a tendency for physicians to immediately refer patients to clinical nutrition specialists for any nutrition-related complaint or concern. This situation is unfortunate given the many complementary applications of nutritional biotherapy that can accompany conventional medical care. Patients in need of nutritional care should be able to rely on their physicians for the delivery of nutritional screening and a comprehensive assessment (both nutritional status and nutrient intake) as well as counseling on core dietary needs (perhaps using BINT as a reference point). Interactions with the physician should include informed communications, appropriate referral methods, and, whenever possible, advice on testing procedures aimed at elucidating the patient's biochemical individuality.

Mastery of nutritional biotherapy represents an essential but widely undervalued area of proficiency for physicians and, until core competencies in nutritional biotherapy are established, reliability of such skills will likely be questionable. Ideally, physicians actively studying nutritional biotherapy may benefit by observing dietitians in action, and vice versa. In the context of a multifaceted integrative medical team, this should be done in the presence of another clinical nutrition specialist and a psychologist (or behavioral scientist), in order for the practitioner to take cues and offer feedback on improving the clinical delivery of nutritional biotherapy.

REIMBURSEMENT STATUS

Nutritional agents and other dietary supplements do not call for the same level of rigorous testing as investigational drugs, according to the 1994 Dietary Supplement, Health and Education Act. This may help explain why prescriptions for nutritional supplements and other nonpatentable agents are not covered by insurance unless there is evidence of illness induced by a nutritional deficiency. The lack of coverage seems surprising given that dietary modifications or nutritional supplementation can lower overall health care costs.

It is also generally not efficient for medical doctors to spend the needed time for patient education on nutritional issues. Lack of reimbursement, along with time constraints imposed by the managed care economy, are among the primary reasons that physicians today do not typically offer nutritional guidance.

The cost of dietary supplements, including nutrients, botanicals, and phytochemicals, is generally much lower than pharmaceutical drugs. Most of these natural substances are available over the counter; many are now sold in pharmacies and health food stores. This trend has worked to the advantage of naturopathic physicians. In Connecticut and Washington, naturopathic physicians enjoy 100% coverage mandated by state law. Therefore, in those states, nutritional supplements are fully covered for prescriptions written by naturopathic physicians, some of whom work side by side with allopathic practitioners. Although many insurance companies have begun to cover naturopathic medicine per se in recent years, allopathic physicians still cannot obtain coverage for their patients' dietary supplements unless there is evidence of a nutritional deficiency to warrant supplementation from the perspective (albeit outmoded) of the insurance company.

Impact on Conventional Medicine and Medical Costs

Complementary applications of nutritional biotherapy may translate into considerable reductions in treatment costs as well as reductions in overall disease burden and suffering. On the most basic level, there is the problem of malnutrition among hospitalized patients, a problem that often goes unrecognized. Other than patients with AIDS, patients with advanced cancer have the highest prevalence of malnutrition of any hospitalized group, and nearly half these patients die from malnutrition-related complications (266, 267). The prevalence of protein-calorie malnutrition in hospitalized cancer patients is approximately 30 to 50% (268, 269). A 1998 study of hospitalized patients attending the surgical and internal medicine units of a major hospital in Buenos Aires found that many patients suffered from either low body mass index (BMI), excessive weight loss during hospitalization, or being overweight (270). Prompt nutrition assessment and appropriate nutrition intervention are needed to improve clinical outcomes and help lower the cost of health care, and further study is needed on the cost-effectiveness of comprehensive nutritional biotherapy programs.

The disease burden may also be attenuated by combining nutrition with standard medical care in a complementary fashion. For example, in a randomized, double-blind prospective trial of 43 recipients of bone marrow transplants at Brigham and Women's Hospital in Boston, glutamine supplementation significantly reduced the length of hospital stay (by 7 days) and thus the overall cost of postoperative care. For the glutamine-supplemented group, hospital charges were $21,095 less on a per-patient basis compared with charges for patients who received standard therapy. Rates of both positive microbial cultures and clinical infection were also significantly lower among the glutamine recipients. Room and board charges were over $10,000 less per patient for the glutamine-supplemented group (p = 0.02) due to reduced hospital stay (271). Another randomized clinical trial yielded similar outcomes (272). Patients receiving glutamine perioperatively also show more sustained vigor postoperatively compared with nonsupplemented patients (273).

Additionally, appropriate nutritional guidance may lead to broad-based improvements in the control of many chronic diseases. In a cross-sectional study in California, 27,766 Seventh-day Adventists answered questions on diet, exercise, medications, use of health services, and prevalence of disease (274). About half the group (55%) were vegetarians. Nonvegetarian males and females had statistically higher rates of coronary heart disease, stroke, hypertension, diabetes, diverticulosis, rheumatoid arthritis, and rheumatism compared with their vegetarian counterparts. Nonvegetarians also had higher rates of drug and chemical allergies. Compared with vegetarian women, nonvegetarian women reported significantly more overnight hospitalizations and surgeries in the previous year (p < 0.001), and nonvegetarian men reported more overnight hospitalizations and x-rays (p < 0.01). In addition, medication use was higher (115% versus 70%) in nonvegetarian women and was more than double in nonvegetarian men. These findings, along with other studies briefly mentioned in this chapter, suggest that a vegetarian diet and lifestyle modification may result in major decreases in the prevalence of chronic diseases, resulting in a reduced reliance on medications and health services.

A major limitation of the cross-sectional design of large observational studies, however, is its inability to detect the temporal direction of cause and effect. For example, if an individual adopted a more nonvegetarian diet when he or she became ill, this could influence the findings like that reported in this study. However, the Seventh-day Adventist population advocates vegetarianism as the optimal diet, based on their philosophy of health. When illness occurs, it is more likely that the affected individuals would alter their diet in accord with this philosophy (toward vegetarianism) and so may actually underestimate the true protective effect of vegetarianism against chronic disease.

The same study did not detect higher rates of cancer for nonvegetarian Seventh-day Adventists. However, a cancer-preventive effect of vegetarian diets has been demonstrated in previous studies of this population (275–277). One study showed an orderly dose-response relationship between fatal prostate cancer and increasing intakes of animal products (milk, cheese, eggs, and meat) among Seventh-day Adventists (278). Results from another study of this population suggested that adopting a vegetarian diet early in life was of decisive importance with regard to eventual disease-related mortality; making dietary changes later in life had a smaller effect on the risk of eventually dying from chronic disease (279).

Overall, these and other studies suggest a lower morbidity burden in people who follow a vegetarian diet. Advocating a vegetarian diet may be an effective way to reduce health care costs, primarily through reductions in the number of hospitalizations, frequency of sick leave, and expenditures for medication and health services. Ideally we should work toward shifting medical resources away from treating life-threatening illnesses to patient education and the management of chronic diseases.

PROSPECTS FOR THE FUTURE

The ancient notion that diet and nutrition have an important influence on health has evolved into the complex, multidisciplinary science of nutrition. Today, the notion that diet has an etiological role in cancer and other chronic diseases is well accepted. It is estimated that about half the diseases a primary care physician sees have a nutrition-related cause, and at least five of the top ten causes of death in the United States are linked to diet. Nutrition has been established as a major factor in the prevention and reversal of diabetes, hypertension, and heart disease. Substantial evidence also suggests that nutritional interventions can improve cancer survival and lessen the toxic effects of standard anticancer therapy, thus improving quality of life (280).

One of the areas in which nutritional biotherapy could have a profound impact is medical care for the elderly, many of whom are already in crisis because of increased disease burden and limited resources for medical care coverage in this population. By the year 2020, 20% of the United States population will be aged 65 years or older, and the greatest increase in numbers over the next two decades will be among those 85 years of age or older. This is expected to place an extraordinary burden on medical services. Nutritional biotherapy may effectively address disease-related processes associated with aging. For example, aging is associated with impaired immune responses and an increase in infection-related morbidity. Randomized placebo-controlled trials have demonstrated that modest supplementation with vitamins and minerals significantly improve immunity and decrease the risk of infection in old age (281, 282). Another example is that high potassium intake, either from diet or supplements, significantly lowered the risk of stroke. Men who took potassium supplements were 69% less likely to suffer a stroke compared with men who did not take supplements in the first 2 years of the study (283).

By fostering healthy aging, nutritional practitioners can improve the cost-effectiveness of health care delivery. Bland (1998) contends that nutritional pharmacology may biochemically modify some of the primary physical aspects of unhealthy aging; for example, chronic inflammation and oxidative stress, altered mitochondrial function, increased protein glycation (glycosylation), defects in methylation, poor detoxification capacity, and impaired immunocompetence (284). Nutritional–pharmacological strategies may also be applied effectively to mental health problems, ranging from learning disability and behavioral disorders in children to the cognitive and emotional disorders that afflict millions of adults and elderly persons (285). In addition, fitness training, stress management, cognitive restructuring, ergonomic adjustments, and counseling on a life-affirming lifestyle may reinforce the health-promoting benefits of a comprehensive nutritional program.

Another ongoing development is the explosion of new nutritional agents by the purveyors of nutritional pharmacology. Studies of tocotrienols, a form of vitamin E, indicate that these compounds may potentiate tamoxifen's therapeutic effects on breast cancer (286). Other forms of vitamin E, including gamma-tocopherol and tocopheryl succinate, may also hold similar promise for an improved therapeutic index in the complementary medical setting. Additionally, retinoids (vitamin A compounds) are now widely used in the treatment of cancers of the lung, breast, ovary, and bladder, as well as basal cell carcinoma, squamous cell carcinoma, melanoma, cutaneous T-cell lymphoma, and acute promyelocytic leukemia. Many of these agents are now considered part of standard cancer care, and yet they clearly fulfill a complementary role by serving as differentiators and immune modulators (287).

In the coming decades, the focus of nutritional biotherapy will move beyond primary prevention to encompass the adjuvant treatment and long-range management (including secondary and tertiary prevention) of chronic diseases. In this regard, nutritional modulation of standard treatments and of pathological mechanisms offer exciting possibilities for a more innovative and functional form of medicine. Considered on its own, nutritional biotherapy should never be labeled a cure for any of the major degenerative diseases. However, if properly implemented within the context of integrative medicine and complementary care strategies, nutritional biotherapy will become an increasingly valuable adjunct to primary medical treatment strategies.

REFERENCES

1. Campbell TC, Junshi C. Diet and chronic degenerative diseases: perspectives from China. Am J Clin Nutr 1994;59(5 Suppl):1153S–1161S.
2. Department of Health and Human Services. Healthy People 2000. 1990. The baseline data source of this recommendation is the Continuing Survey of Food Intakes by Individuals, CSFII, USDA.
3. Department of Health and Human Services. The Surgeon General's report, 1988.
4. National Research Council. Diet and health: implications for reducing chronic disease risk. Washington, D.C.: National Academy Press, 1989.
5. U.S. Dept. of Agriculture and U.S. Dept. of Health and Human Services. Dietary guidelines for Americans. Washington, D.C.: The Departments, 1990.
6. Williams RJ. Biochemical individuality: the basis for the genetotrophic concept. Austin & London: University of Texas Press, 1977.
7. Williams RJ, Beerstecher E, Berry LJ. The concept of genetotrophic disease. Lancet 1950; 287–289.
8. Davies S. Scientific and ethical foundations of nutritional and environmental medicine. Part II. Further glimpses of "the higher medicine." J Nutr Environ Med 1995;5:5–11.
9. Reynolds RD. Vitamin supplements: current controversies. J Am Coll Nutr 1994;13(2):118–126.
10. Stewart AS. Medical applications of nutrition. In: 1986: a year in nutritional medicine. 2nd ed. New Canaan, CT: Keats Publishing, 1986:333–358.
11. Bland JS. The nutritional effects of free radical pathology. In: 1986: a year in nutritional medicine. 2nd ed. New Canaan, CT: Keats Publishing, 1986:293–322.
12. Werbach MR. Illnesses and the effects of nutrients, toxics and environmental sensitivities. In: Nutritional influences on illness. New Canaan, CT: Keats Publishing, 1988:3–448.
13. Roe DA. Effects of drugs on vitamin needs. Ann N Y Acad Sci 1992;669:156–163.
14. Roe DA. Drug-food and drug-nutrient interactions. J Environ Pathol Toxicol Oncol 1985; 5(6):115–135.

15. Roe DA. Drug effects on nutrient absorption, transport, and metabolism. Drug–Nutrient Interactions 1985;4(1–2):117–135.
16. Filiberti R, Giacosa A, Brignoli O. High-risk subjects for vitamin deficiency. Eur J Cancer Prev 1997;6(suppl 1):S37–S42.
17. Tonkin SY. Oral contraceptives and vitamin status. In: Briggs MH, ed. Vitamins in human biology and medicine. Boca Raton, FL: CRC Press, 1980:29–64.
18. Stewart AS. Medical applications of nutrition. In: 1986: a year in nutritional medicine. 2nd ed. New Canaan, CT: Keats Publishing, 1986:333–358.
19. Nikolaev MP, Logunov AI, Tsyrulnikova LG, Dzhalilov DS. Clinical and biochemical aspects in the treatment of acute maxillary sinusitis with antioxidants. Vestn Otorinolaringol 1994;1: 22–26.
20. Sorenson JR. Antiinflammatory, analgesic, and antiulcer activities of copper complexes suggest their use in a physiologic approach to treatment of arthritic diseases. Basic Life Sci 1988; 49:591–594.
21. Sorenson JR. Copper complexes offer a physiological approach to treatment of chronic diseases. Prog Med Chem 1989;26:437–568.
22. Cathcart ES, Gonnerman WA, Leslie CA, Hayes KC. Dietary n-3 fatty acids and arthritis. J Intern Med Suppl 1989;225(731):217–223.
23. Leslie CA, Conte JM, Hayes KC, Cathcart ES. A fish oil diet reduces the severity of collagen induced arthritis after onset of the disease. Clin Exp Immunol 1988;73(2):328–332.
24. Sorenson JR, Soderberg LS, Chidambaram MV, et al. Bioavailable copper complexes offer a physiologic approach to treatment of chronic diseases. Adv Exp Med Biol 1989;258:229–234.
25. Arstall MA, Yang J, Stafford I, et al. N-acetylcysteine in combination with nitroglycerin and streptokinase for the treatment of evolving acute myocardial infarction. Safety and biochemical effects. Circulation 1995;92(10):2855–2862.
26. Wells RS, Higgs JM, Macdonald A, et al. Familial chronic muco-cutaneous candidiasis. J Med Genet 1972; 9(3):302–310.
27. Laurence DR, Bennett PN. Drugs used in tuberculosis. In: Clinical pharmacology. London: Churchill Livingstone, 1980:272–277.
28. Chandra RK, Puri S. Nutritional support improves antibody response to influenza virus vaccine in the elderly. BMJ 1985;291:705–706.
29. Walubo A. Smith PJ. Folb PI. Oxidative stress during antituberculous therapy in young and elderly patients. Biomed Environ Sci 1995; 8(2):106–113.
30. Hildenbrand G, Cavin S. Five-year survival rates of melanoma patients treated by diet therapy after the manner of Gerson: a retrospective review. Altern Therap Health Med 1995;1(4):29–37.
31. Ornish D, Scherwitz LW, Billings JH, et al. Intensive lifestyle changes for reversal of coronary heart disease. JAMA 1998;280:2001–2007.
32. McDougall J, Litzau K, Haver E, et al. Rapid reduction of serum cholesterol and blood pressure by a twelve-day, very low fat, strictly vegetarian diet. J Am Coll Nutr 1995;14:491–496.
33. Levine R. Monosaccharides in health and disease. Ann Review Nutr 1986;6:211–224.
34. Rupp H. Insulin resistance, hyperinsulinemia, and cardiovascular disease. The need for novel dietary prevention strategies. Basic Res Cardiol 1992; 87(2):99–105.
35. Grimditch GK. Barnard RJ. Hendricks L. Weitzman D. Peripheral insulin sensitivity as modified by diet and exercise training. Am J Clin Nutr 1988;48(1):38–43.
36. Harris WS, Connor WE, Alam N, Illingworth DR. Reduction of postprandial triglyceridemia in humans by dietary n-3 fatty acids. J Lip Res 1988;29(11):1451–1460.
37. Connor WE. Effects of omega-3 fatty acids in hypertriglyceridemic states. Semin Thromb Hemost 1988;14(3):271–284.
38. Clemens MR, Muller F, Ladner CI, Gey KF. Vitamine bei hochdosierter Chemo- und Strahlentherapie. Z Ernahrungswiss 1992;31:110–120.
39. Clemens MR. Vitamins and therapy of malignancies. Therapeutische Umschau 1994;51(7): 483–488.
40. Jaakkola K, Lahteenmaki P, Laakso J, et al. Treatment with antioxidant and other nutrients in combination with chemotherapy and irradiation in patients with small-cell lung cancer. Anticancer Res 1992;12(3):599–606.
41. Anonymous. Free radicals and breast cancer. Environ Health Perspect 1996;104(8):821.
42. Fujita K, Shinpo K, Yamada K, et al. Reduction of adriamycin toxicity by ascorbate in mice and guinea pigs. Cancer Res 1982;42(1):309–316.
43. Kobrinsky NL, Hartfield D, Horner H, et al. Treatment of advanced malignancies with high-dose acetaminophen and N-acetylcysteine rescue. Cancer Invest 1996;14(3):202–210.
44. Okunieff P. Interactions between ascorbic acid and the radiation of bone marrow, skin, and tumor. Am J Clin Nutr 1991;54(6 Suppl):1281S–1283S.

45. Pritsos CA, Sokoloff M, Gustafson DL. PZ-51 (Ebselen) in vivo protection against adriamycin-induced mouse cardiac and hepatic lipid peroxidation and toxicity. Biochem Pharmacol 1992; 44(4):839–841.

46. Schmitt-Graff A, Scheulen ME. Prevention of adriamycin cardiotoxicity by niacin, isocitrate or N-acetyl-cysteine in mice. A morphological study. Pathol Res Pract 1986;181(2):168–174.

47. Pinto J, Raiczyk GB, Huang YP, Rivlin R. New approaches to the possible prevention of side effects of chemotherapy by nutrition. Cancer 1986;48:1911–1914.

48. Myers CE, McGuire W, Young R. Adriamycin: amelioration of toxicity by alpha-tocopherol. Cancer Treat Rep 1976;60(7):961–962.

49. Shimpo K, Nagatsu T, Yamada K, et al. Ascorbic acid and adriamycin toxicity. Am J Clin Nutr 1991;54(6 Suppl):1298S–1301S.

50. Sugiyama S, Yamada K, Hayakawa M, Ozawa T. Approaches that mitigate doxorubicin-induced delayed adverse effects on mitochondrial function in rat hearts; liposome-encapsulated doxorubicin or combination therapy with antioxidant. Biochem Mol Biol Int 1995;36(5):1001–1007.

51. Shinozawa S, Gomita Y, Araki Y. Protective effects of various drugs on adriamycin (doxorubicin)-induced toxicity and microsomal lipid peroxidation in mice and rats. Biol Pharm Bull 1993;16(11):1114–1117.

52. Shinozawa S, Kawasaki H, Gomita Y. Effect of biological membrane stabilizing drugs (coenzyme Q10, dextran sulfate and reduced glutathione) on adriamycin (doxorubicin)-induced toxicity and microsomal lipid peroxidation in mice. Japn J Cancer Res 1996;23(1):93–98.

53. Tursz T. Combination of BRMs with chemotherapy. Am J Med 1995;99(suppl 6A):56S–58S.

54. Israel L, Hajji O, Grefft-Alami A, et al. Vitamin A augmentation of the effects of chemotherapy in metastatic breast cancers after menopause. Randomized trial in 100 patients. Ann Med Intern 1985;136(7):551–554.

55. Komiyama S, Kudoh S, Yanagita T, Kuwano M. Synergistic combination therapy of 5-fluorouracil, vitamin A, and cobalt-60 radiation for head and neck tumors—antitumor combination therapy with vitamin A. Auris Nasus Larynx 1985; 12(suppl 2):S239–S243.

56. Komiyama S, Hiroto I, Ryu S, et al. Synergistic combination therapy of 5-fluorouracil, vitamin A and cobalt-60 radiation upon head and neck tumors. Oncology 1978;35(6):253–257.

57. Teicher BA, Schwartz JL, Holden SA, et al. In vivo modulation of several anticancer agents by beta-carotene. Cancer Chemother Pharmacol 1994;34(3):235–241.

58. Meadows GG, Pierson HF, Abdallah RM. Ascorbate in the treatment of experimental transplanted melanoma. Am J Clin Nutr 1991;54(6 Suppl):1284S–1291S.

59. Kurbacher CM, Wagner U, Kolster B, et al. Ascorbic acid (vitamin C) improves the antineoplastic activity of doxorubicin, cisplatin, and paclitaxel in human breast carcinoma cells in vitro. Cancer Lett 1996;103(2):183–189.

60. Taper HS, de Gerlache J, Lans M, Roberfroid M. Non-toxic potentiation of cancer chemotherapy by combined C and K3 vitamin pre-treatment. Int J Cancer 1987;40(4):575–579.

61. Noto V, Taper HS, Jiang YH, et al. Effects of sodium ascorbate (vitamin C) and 2-methyl-1,4-naphthoquinone (vitamin K3) treatment on human tumor cell growth in vitro. I. Synergism of combined vitamin C and K3 action. Cancer 1989;63(5):901–906.

62. Gilloteaux J, Jamison JM, Venugopal M, et al. Scanning electron microscopy and transmission electron microscopy aspects of synergistic antitumor activity of vitamin C–vitamin K3 combinations against human prostatic carcinoma cells. Scanning Microsc 1995;9(1):159–173.

63. De Loecker W, Janssens J, Bonte J, Taper HS. Effects of sodium ascorbate (vitamin C) and 2-methyl-1,4-naphthoquinone (vitamin K3) treatment on human tumor cell growth in vitro. II. Synergism with combined chemotherapy action. Anticancer Res 1993;13(1):103–106.

64. Taper HS, Roberfroid M. Non-toxic sensitization of cancer chemotherapy by combined vitamin C and K3 pretreatment in a mouse tumor resistant to oncovin. Anticancer Res 1992;2(5):1651–1654.

65. Boccardo F, Canobbio L, Resasco M, et al. Phase II study of tamoxifen and high-dose retinyl acetate in patients with advanced breast cancer. J Cancer Res Clin Oncol 1990;116(5):503–506.

66. Recchia F, Sica G, de Filippis S, et al. Interferon-beta, retinoids, and tamoxifen in the treatment of metastatic breast cancer: a phase II study. J Interferon Cytokine Res 1995;15(7):605–610.

67. Israel L, Hajji O, Grefft-Alami A, et al. Vitamin A augmentation of the effects of chemotherapy in metastatic breast cancers after menopause. Randomized trial in 100 patients. Ann Intern Med 1985;136(7):551–554.

68. Recchia F, Rea S, Corrao G, et al. Sequential chemotherapy, beta interferon, retinoids and ta-

moxifen in the treatment of metastatic breast cancer. A pilot study. Eur J Cancer 1995;31A(11): 1887–1888.

69. Recchia F, Rea S, Pompili P, et al. Beta-interferon, retinoids and tamoxifen as maintenance therapy in metastatic breast cancer. A pilot study. Clinica Terapeutica 1995;146(10):603–610.

70. Recchia F, Frati L, Rea S, et al. Minimal residual disease in metastatic breast cancer: treatment with IFN-beta, retinoids, and tamoxifen. J Interferon Cytokine Res 1998;18(1):41–47.

71. Lockwood K, Moesgaard S, Hanioka T, Folkers K. Apparent partial remission of breast cancer in 'high risk' patients supplemented with nutritional antioxidants, essential fatty acids and coenzyme Q10. Mol Aspects Med 1994;15(Suppl):231–240.

72. Lockwood K, Moesgaard S, Folkers K. Partial and complete regression of breast cancer in patients in relation to dosage of coenzyme Q10. Biochem Biophysi Res Comm 1994;199(3):1504–1508.

73. Lockwood K, Moesgaard S, Yamamoto T, Folkers K. Progress on therapy of breast cancer with vitamin Q10 and the regression of metastases. Biochem Biophys Res Comm 1995;212(1):172–177.

74. Folkers K, Brown R, Judy WV, Morita M. Survival of cancer patients on therapy with coenzyme Q10. Biochem Biophys Res Comm 1993;192(1): 241–245.

75. Brittenden J, Heys SD, Miller I, et al. Dietary supplementation with L-arginine in patients with breast cancer (4 cm) receiving multimodality treatment: report of a feasibility study. Br J Cancer 1994;69(5):918–921.

76. Heys SD, Sarkar TK, Ah-See AK, et al. Multimodality treatment in the management of locally advanced breast cancer. J R Coll Surg Edinb 1993;38(1):9–15.

77. Nole F, de Braud F, Aapro M, et al. Phase I-II study of vinorelbine in combination with 5-fluorouracil and folinic acid as first-line chemotherapy in metastatic breast cancer: a regimen with a low subjective toxic burden. Ann Oncol 1997;8(9):865–870.

78. Parnes HL, Abrams JS, Tait N, et al. Phase I/II study of cyclophosphamide, doxorubicin, fluorouracil, and leucovorin for treatment of metastatic adenocarcinoma. J Natl Cancer Inst 1991;83(14):1017–1020.

79. Hainsworth JD, Jolivet J, Birch R, et al. Mitoxantrone, 5-fluorouracil, and high dose leucovorin (NFL) versus intravenous cyclophosphamide, methotrexate, and 5-fluorouracil (CMF) in first-line chemotherapy for patients with metastatic

breast carcinoma: a randomized phase II trial. Cancer 1997;79(4):740–748.

80. Ribas A, Albanell J, Sole-Calvo LA, et al. Cyclophosphamide, methotrexate, and chronic oral tegafur modulated by folinic acid in the treatment of patients with advanced breast carcinoma. Cancer 1998;82(5):878–885.

81. Klaassen U, Wilke H, Weyhofen R, et al. Phase II study with cisplatin and paclitaxel in combination with weekly high-dose 24 h infusional 5-fluorouracil/leucovorin for first-line treatment of metastatic breast cancer. Anticancer Drugs 1998;9(3):203–207.

82. Gregorio DI, Emrich LJ, Graham S, et al. Dietary fat consumption and survival among women with breast cancer. J Natl Cancer Inst 1985;75(1): 37–41.

83. Nomura AM, Marchand LL, Kolonel LN, et al. The effect of dietary fat on breast cancer survival among Caucasian and Japanese women in Hawaii. Breast Cancer Res Treat 1991;18(Suppl 1):S135–S141.

84. Sopotsinskaia EB, Balitskii KP, Tarutinov VI, et al. Experience with the use of a low-calorie diet in breast cancer patients to prevent metastasis. Vopr Onkol 1992;38(5):592–599.

85. Holm LE, Nordevang E, Hjalmar ML, et al. Treatment failure and dietary habits in women with breast cancer. J Natl Cancer Inst 1993; 85(1):32–36.

86. Rohan TE, Hiller JE, McMichael AJ. Dietary factors and survival from breast cancer. Nutr Cancer 1993;20(2):167–177.

87. Jain M, Miller AB, To T. Premorbid diet and the prognosis of women with breast cancer. J Natl Cancer Inst 1994;86(18):1390–1397.

88. Zhang S, Folsom AR, Sellers TA, et al. Better breast cancer survival for postmenopausal women who are less overweight and eat less fat. The Iowa Women's Health Study. Cancer 1995; 76(2):275–283.

89. Jain M, Miller AB. Tumor characteristics and survival of breast cancer patients in relation to premorbid diet and body size. Breast Cancer Res Treat 1997;42(1):43–55.

90. Pastorino U, Infante M, Maioli M, et al. Adjuvant treatment of stage I lung cancer with high-dose vitamin A. J Clin Oncol 1993;11(7):1216–1222.

91. Thiruvengadam R, Atiba JO, Azawi SH. A phase II trial of a differentiating agent (tRA) with cisplatin-VP 16 chemotherapy in advanced non-small cell lung cancer. Invest New Drugs 1996;14(4):395–401.

92. Meyskens FL Jr, Gilmartin E, Alberts DS, et al. Activity of isotretinoin against squamous cell cancers and preneoplastic lesions. Cancer Treat Rep 1982;66(6):1315–1319.

93. Friedland D, Luginbuhl W, Meehan L, et al. Phase II trial of all-trans retinoic acid in metastatic non-small cell lung cancer. Proc ASCO 1994; 6:712.

94. Arnold A, Ayoub J, Douglas L, et al. Phase II trial of 13-cis-retinoic acid plus interferon-alpha in non-small-cell lung cancer. J Natl Cancer Inst 1994;86(4):306–309.

95. Roth AD, Abele R, Alberto P. 13-cis-retinoic acid plus interferon-alpha: a phase II clinical study in squamous cell carcinoma of the lung and the head and neck. Oncology 1994;51(1):84–86.

96. Uphouse W, Oishi N, Berenberg J, et al. Treatment of advanced non-small cell lung cancer with 13-cis-retinoic acid. Proc ASCO 1987;6:712.

97. Grunberg SM, Itri LM. Phase II study of isotretinoin in the treatment of advanced non-small cell lung cancer. Cancer Treat Rep 1987;71(11):1097–1098.

98. Jaakkola K, Lahteenmaki P, Laakso J, et al. Treatment with antioxidant and other nutrients in combination with chemotherapy and irradiation in patients with small-cell lung cancer. Anticancer Res 1992;12(3):599–606.

99. Byar D, Blackard C. Comparisons of placebo, pyridoxine, and topical thiotepa in preventing recurrence of stage I bladder cancer. Urology 1977;10(6):556–561.

100. Alfthan O, Tarkkanen J, Grohn P, et al. Tigason (etretinate) in prevention of recurrence of superficial bladder tumors. A double-blind clinical trial. Eur Urol 1983;9(1):6–9.

101. Studer UE, Biedermann C, Chollet D, et al. Prevention of recurrent superficial bladder tumors by oral etretinate: preliminary results of a randomized, double blind multicenter trial in Switzerland. J Urol 1984;131(1):47–49.

102. Yoshida O, Miyakawa M, Watanabe H, et al. Prophylactic effect of etretinate on the recurrence of superficial bladder tumors—results of a randomized control study. Hinyokika Kiyo 1986;32(9): 1349–1358.

103. Studer UE, Jenzer S, Biedermann C, et al. Adjuvant treatment with a vitamin A analogue (etretinate) after transurethral resection of superficial bladder tumors. Final analysis of a prospective, randomized multicenter trial in Switzerland. Eur Urol 1995;28(4):284–290.

104. Lamm DL, Riggs DR, Shriver JS, et al. Megadose vitamins in bladder cancer: a double-blind clinical trial. J Urol 1994;151(1):21–26.

105. Fenaux P, Le Deley MC, Castaigne S, et al. Effect of all transretinoic acid in newly diagnosed acute promyelocytic leukemia. Results of a multicenter randomized trial. European APL 91 Group. Blood 1993;82(11):3241–3249.

106. Tallman MS, Andersen JW, Schiffer CA, et al. All-trans-retinoic acid in acute promyelocytic leukemia. N Engl J Med 1997;337(15):1021–1028.

107. Latagliata R, Avvisati G, Lo Coco F, et al. The role of all-trans-retinoic acid (ATRA) treatment in newly-diagnosed acute promyelocytic leukemia patients aged > 60 years. Ann Oncol 1997;8(12):1273–1275.

108. Tallman MS, Andersen JW, Schiffer CA, et al. All-trans-retinoic acid in acute promyelocytic leukemia. N Engl J Med 1997;337(15):1021–1028.

109. Kanamaru A, Takemoto Y, Tanimoto M, et al. All-trans retinoic acid for the treatment of newly diagnosed acute promyelocytic leukemia. Japan Adult Leukemia Study Group. Blood 1995; 85(5):1202–1206.

110. Frankel SR, Eardley A, Heller G, et al. All-trans retinoic acid for acute promyelocytic leukemia. Results of the New York Study. Ann Intern Med 1994;120(4):278–286.

111. Fenaux P, Le Deley MC, Castaigne S, et al. Effect of all transretinoic acid in newly diagnosed acute promyelocytic leukemia. Results of a multicenter randomized trial. European APL 91 Group. Blood 1993;82(11):3241–3249.

112. Thomas X, Anglaret B, Thiebaut A, et al. Improvement of prognosis in refractory and relapsed acute promyelocytic leukemia over recent years: the role of all-trans retinoic acid therapy. Ann Hematol 1997;75(5–6):195–200.

113. Ohno R, Ohnishi K, Takeshita A, et al. All-trans retinoic acid therapy in relapsed/refractory or newly diagnosed acute promyelocytic leukemia (APL) in Japan. Leukemia 1994;8(Suppl3):S64–S69.

114. Cortes JE, Kantarjian H, O'Brien S, et al. All-trans retinoic acid followed by chemotherapy for salvage of refractory or relapsed acute promyelocytic leukemia. Cancer 1994;73(12):2946–2952.

115. Ohno R, Yoshida H, Fukutani H, et al. Multiinstitutional study of all-trans-retinoic acid as a differentiation therapy of refractory acute promyelocytic leukemia. Leukemia Study Group of the Ministry of Health and Welfare. Leukemia 1993;7(11):1722–1727.

116. Liang R, Chow WS, Chiu E, et al. Effective salvage therapy using all-trans retinoic acid for relapsed

and resistant acute promyelocytic leukemia. Anti-cancer Drugs 1993;4(3):339–340.

117. Hildenbrand GL, Hildenbrand LC, Bradford K, Cavin SW. Five-year survival rates of melanoma patients treated by diet therapy after the manner of Gerson: a retrospective review. Altern Therap Health Med 1995;1(4):29–37.

118. Demopoulos HB. Effects of reducing the phenyl-alanine-tyrosine intake of patients with advanced malignant melanoma. Cancer 1966;19(5):657–664.

119. Rustin GJ, Dische S, de Garis ST, Nelstrop A. Treatment of advanced malignant melanoma with interferon alpha and etretinate. Eur J Cancer Clin Oncol 1988;24(4):783–784.

120. Triozzi PL, Walker MJ, Pellegrini AE, Dayton MA. Isotretinoin and recombinant interferon alfa-2a therapy of metastatic malignant melanoma. Cancer Invest 1996;14(4):293–298.

121. Fierlbeck G, Schreiner T, Rassner G. Combina-tion of highly purified human leukocyte interferon alpha and 13-cis-retinoic acid for the treatment of metastatic melanoma. Cancer Immunol Immu-nother 1995;40(3):157–164.

122. The Joint National Committee on Detection, Evaluation, and Treatment of High Blood Pres-sure. The fifth report of the Joint National Com-mittee on Detection, Evaluation, and Treatment of High Blood Pressure (JNC V). Arch Intern Med 1993;153:154–183.

123. Working Group on Primary Prevention of Hyper-tension. National High Blood Pressure Education Program Working Group report on primary pre-vention of hypertension. Arch Intern Med 1993;153:186–208.

124. Gillum RF, Prineas RJ, Jeffery RW, et al. Non-pharmacologic therapy of hypertension: the inde-pendent effects of weight reduction and sodium restriction in overweight borderline hypertensive patients. Am Heart J 1983;105(1):128–133.

125. Stamler R, Stamler J, Grimm R, et al. Nutritional therapy for high blood pressure. Final report of a four-year randomized controlled trial–the Hy-pertension Control Program. JAMA 1987;257(11):1484–1491.

126. Prineas RJ. Clinical interaction of salt and weight change on blood pressure level. Hypertension 1991;17(1 Suppl):I143–I149.

127. Beilin LJ. Non-pharmacological management of hypertension: optimal strategies for reducing car-diovascular risk. J Hypertens Suppl 1994;12(10):S71–S81.

128. Efstratopoulos AD, Voyaki SM. Effect of anti-oxidants on acute blood pressure response to

smoking in normotensives and hypertensives. J Hypertens Suppl 1993;11(Suppl 5):S112–S113.

129. Tse WY, Maxwell SR, Thomason H, et al. Antiox-idant status in controlled and uncontrolled hyper-tension and its relationship to endothelial damage. J Hum Hypertens 1994;8(11):843–849.

130. Lavie CJ, Milani RV, Ventura HO, et al. Car-diac rehabilitation, exercise training, and pre-ventive cardiology research at Ochsner Heart and Vascular Institute. Tex Heart Inst J 1995;22(1):44–52.

131. Barnard RJ, Wen SJ. Exercise and diet in the prevention and control of the metabolic syn-drome. Sports Med 1994;18(4):218–228.

132. McKnight JA, Moore TJ. The effects of dietary factors on blood pressure. Compr Ther 1994;20(9):511–517.

133. Oberman A, Wassertheil-Smoller S, Langford HG, et al. Pharmacologic and nutritional treat-ment of mild hypertension: changes in cardiovas-cular risk status. Ann Intern Med 1990;112(2):89–95.

134. Moore TJ, McKnight JA. Dietary factors and blood pressure regulation. Endocrinol Metab Clin North Am 1995; 24(3):643–655.

135. Beilin LJ. Non-pharmacological management of hypertension: optimal strategies for reducing car-diovascular risk. J Hypertens Suppl 1994;12(10):S71–S81.

136. Stein PP, Black HR. The role of diet in the genesis and treatment of hypertension. Med Clin North Am 1993;77(4):831–847.

137. McCarron DA, Henry HJ, Morris CD. Human nutrition and blood pressure regulation: an integrated approach. Hypertension 1982;4(5 Pt 2):III2–III13.

138. Appel LJ, Moore TJ, Obarzanek E, et al. A clinical trial of the effects of dietary patterns on blood pressure. DASH Collaborative Research Group. N Engl J Med 1997;336(16):1117–1124.

139. Beilin LJ. Vegetarian and other complex diets, fats, fiber, and hypertension. Am J Clin Nutr 1994;59(5 Suppl):1130S–1135S.

140. Rouse IL, Armstrong BK, Beilin LJ. Vegetarian diet, lifestyle and blood pressure in two religious populations. Clin Exp Pharmacol Physiol 1982;9(3):327–330.

141. Melby CL, Goldflies DG, Hyner GC, Lyle RM. Relation between vegetarian/nonvegetarian diets and blood pressure in black and white adults. Am J Public Health 1989;79(9):1283–1288.

142. McCarron DA, Oparil S, Resnick LM, et al. Com-prehensive nutrition plan improves cardiovascular

risk factors in essential hypertension. Am J Hypertens 1998;11(1 Pt 1):31–40.

143. McDougall J, Litzau K, Haver E, et al. Rapid reduction of serum cholesterol and blood pressure by a twelve-day, very low fat, strictly vegetarian diet. J Am Coll Nutr 1995;14(5):491–496.

144. Sacks FM, Donner A, Castelli WP, et al. Effect of ingestion of meat on plasma cholesterol of vegetarians. JAMA 1981;246(6):640–644.

145. Appel LJ, Moore TJ, Obarzanek E, et al. A clinical trial of the effects of dietary patterns on blood pressure. DASH Collaborative Research Group. N Engl J Med 1997;336(16):1117–1124.

146. Margetts BM, Beilin LJ, Vandongen R, Armstrong BK. Vegetarian diet in mild hypertension: a randomized controlled trial. Br Med J (Clin Res Ed) 1986;293(6560):1468–1471.

147. Rouse IL, Beilin LJ, Mahoney DP, et al. Nutrient intake, blood pressure, serum and urinary prostaglandins and serum thromboxane B2 in a controlled trial with a lacto-ovo-vegetarian diet. J Hypertens 1986; 4(2):241–50

148. Anonymous. Intersalt: an international study of electrolyte excretion and blood pressure. Results for 24 hour urinary sodium and potassium excretion. Intersalt Cooperative Research Group. BMJ 1988; 297(6644):319–328.

149. Whelton PK, Appel LJ, Espeland MA, et al. Sodium reduction and weight loss in the treatment of hypertension in older persons: a randomized controlled trial of nonpharmacologic interventions in the elderly (TONE). TONE Collaborative Research Group JAMA 1998;279(11):839–846.

150. Gillum RF, Prineas RJ, Jeffery RW, et al. Nonpharmacologic therapy of hypertension: the independent effects of weight reduction and sodium restriction in overweight borderline hypertensive patients. Am Heart J 1983;105(1):128–133.

151. Stamler R, Stamler J, Grimm R, et al. Nutritional therapy for high blood pressure. Final report of a four-year randomized controlled trial–the Hypertension Control Program. JAMA 1987; 257(11):1484–1491.

152. Prineas RJ. Clinical interaction of salt and weight change on blood pressure level. Hypertension 1991;17(1 Suppl):I143-I149.

153. Cappuccio FP, Markandu ND, Carney C, et al. Double-blind randomized trial of modest salt restriction in older people. Lancet 1997; 350(9081):850–4

154. Whelton PK, He J, Cutler JA, et al. Effects of oral potassium on blood pressure. Meta-analysis of randomized controlled clinical trials. JAMA 1997;277(20):1624–1632.

155. Fotherby MD, Potter JF. Long-term potassium supplementation lowers blood pressure in elderly hypertensive subjects. Int J Clin Pract 1997; 51(4):219–222.

156. Langford HG. Dietary potassium and hypertension: epidemiologic data. Ann Intern Med 1983;98(5 Pt 2):770–772.

157. Sorof JM, Forman A, Cole N, et al. Potassium intake and cardiovascular reactivity in children with risk factors for essential hypertension. J Pediatr 1997;131(1 Pt 1):87–94.

158. Hoes AW, Grobbee DE, Lubsen J. Sudden cardiac death in patients with hypertension. An association with diuretics and beta-blockers? Drug Saf 1997;16(4):233–241.

159. Geleijnse JM, Witteman JC, den Breeijen JH, et al. Dietary electrolyte intake and blood pressure in older subjects: the Rotterdam Study. J Hypertens 1996;14(6):737–741.

160. Witteman J, Stampfer MJ. Prospective study of nutritional factors, blood pressure, and hypertension among US women. Hypertension 1996; 27(5):1065–1072.

161. Ozono R, Oshima T, Matsuura H. Systemic magnesium deficiency disclosed by magnesium loading test in patients with essential hypertension. Hypertens Res 1995;18(1):39–42.

162. McCarron DA. Role of adequate dietary calcium intake in the prevention and management of salt-sensitive hypertension. Am J Clin Nutr 1997;65(2 Suppl):712S–716S.

163. Witteman JC, Willett WC, Stampfer MJ, et al. A prospective study of nutritional factors and hypertension among U.S. women. Circulation 1989;80(5):1320–1327.

164. McCarron D, Morris C. Blood pressure response to oral calcium in persons with mild to moderate hypertension. Ann Intern Med 1985;103:825–829.

165. Giovannucci E, Rimm EB, Wolk A, et al. Calcium and fructose intake in relation to risk of prostate cancer. Cancer Res 1998;58(3):442–447.

166. Seelig MS. Interrelationship of magnesium and estrogen in cardiovascular and bone disorders, eclampsia, migraine and premenstrual syndrome. J Am Coll Nutr 1993;12(4):442–458.

167. Bonaa KH, Bjerve KS, Straume B, et al. Effect of eicosapentaenoic and docosahexaenoic acids on blood pressure in hypertension. A population-based intervention trial from the

Tromso study. N Engl J Med 1990;322(12): 795–801.

168. Cobiac L, Nestel PJ, Wing LM, Howe PR. A low-sodium diet supplemented with fish oil lowers blood pressure in the elderly. J Hypertens 1992;10(1):87–92.

169. Iacono JM, Dougherty RM, Puska P. Dietary fats and the management of hypertension. Can J Physiol Pharmacol 1986;64(6):856–862.

170. Puska P, Iacono JM, Nissinen A, et al. Controlled, randomized trial of the effect of dietary fat on blood pressure. Lancet 1983;1:1–5.

171. Puska P, Nissinen A, Pietinen P, Iacono J. Role of dietary fat in blood pressure control. Scand J Clin Lab Invest Suppl 1985;176:62–69.

172. Kendler BS. Garlic (Allium sativum) and onion (Allium cepa): a review of their relationship to cardiovascular disease. Prev Med 1987; 16(5):670–685.

173. Orekhov AN, Grunwald J. Effects of garlic on atherosclerosis. Nutrition 1997;13(7–8):656–663.

174. Auer W, Eiber A, Hertkorn E, et al. Hypertension and hyperlipidaemia: garlic helps in mild cases. Br J Clin Pract Suppl 1990;69:3–6.

175. Vorberg G, Schneider B. Therapy with garlic: results of a placebo-controlled, double-blind study. Br J Clin Pract Suppl 1990;69:7–11.

176. McMahon FG, Vargas R. Can garlic lower blood pressure? A pilot study. Pharmacotherapy 1993;13(4):406–407.

177. Anonymous. The effect of essential oil of garlic on hyperlipemia and platelet aggregation—an analysis of 308 cases. Cooperative Group for Essential Oil of Garlic. J Trad Chinese Med 1986;6(2): 117–120.

178. Anderson JW, Johnstone BM, Cook-Newell ME. Meta-analysis of the effects of soy protein intake on serum lipids. N Engl J Med 1995;333(5): 276–282.

179. Bakhit RM, Klein BP, Essex-Sorlie D, et al. Intake of 25 g of soybean protein with or without soybean fiber alters plasma lipids in men with elevated cholesterol concentrations. J Nutr 1994;124(2): 213–222.

180. Clarkson TB, Anthony MS, Williams JK, et al. The potential of soybean phytoestrogens for postmenopausal hormone replacement therapy. Proc Soc Exp Biol Med 1998;217(3):365–368.

181. Warshafsky S, Kamer RS, Sivak SL. Effect of garlic on total serum cholesterol. A meta-analysis. Ann Intern Med 1993;119(7 Pt 1):599–605.

182. Silagy C, Neil A. Garlic as a lipid lowering agent—a meta-analysis. J Roy Coll Phys Lond 1994; 28(1):39–45.

183. Kendler BS. Garlic (Allium sativum) and onion (Allium cepa): a review of their relationship to cardiovascular disease. Prev Med 1987;16(5): 670–685.

184. Rizzon P, Iliceto S, Marangelli V. Metabolic approach to myocardial ischemia: a novel therapeutic strategy for patients with coronary artery disease. Cardiologia 1995;40(10):717–720.

185. Greenberg SM, Frishman WH. Coenzyme Q10: a new drug for myocardial ischemia? Med Clin North Am 1988;72(1):243–258.

186. Greenberg SM, Frishman WH. Coenzyme Q10: a new drug for myocardial ischemia? Med Clin North Am 1988;72(1):243–258.

187. Roth A, Eshchar Y, Keren G, et al. Effect of magnesium on restenosis after percutaneous transluminal coronary angioplasty: a clinical and angiographic evaluation in a randomized patient population. A pilot study. The Ichilov Magnesium Study Group. Eur Heart J 1994;15(9):1164–1173.

188. Stampfer MJ, Hennekens CH, Manson JE, et al. Vitamin E consumption and the risk of coronary disease in women. N Engl J Med 1993;328:1444–1449.

189. Rimm EB, Stampfer MJ, Ascherio A, et al. Vitamin E consumption and the risk of coronary heart disease in men. N Engl J Med 1993;328:1450–1456.

190. Stephens NG, Parsons A, Schofield PM, et al. Randomized controlled trial of vitamin E in patients with coronary disease: Cambridge Heart Antioxidant Study (CHAOS). Lancet 1996; 347:781–786.

191. Tomoda H, Yoshitake M, Morimoto K, Aoki N. Possible prevention of postangioplasty restenosis by ascorbic acid. Am J Cardiol 1996;78(11): 1284–1286.

192. Levine GN, Frei B, Koulouris SN, et al. Ascorbic acid reverses endothelial vasomotor dysfunction in patients with coronary artery disease. Circulation 1996;93(6):1107–1113.

193. Vita JA, Keaney JF Jr, Raby KE, et al. Low plasma ascorbic acid independently predicts the presence of an unstable coronary syndrome. J Am Coll Cardiol 1998;31(5):980–986.

194. Connor WE. Do the n-3 fatty acids from fish prevent deaths from cardiovascular disease? Am J Clin Nutr 1997;66(1):188–189.

195. Harris WS, Connor WE, Alam N, Illingworth DR. Reduction of postprandial triglyceridemia in humans by dietary n-3 fatty acids. J Lipid Res 1988;29(11):1451–1460.

196. Connor WE. Effects of omega-3 fatty acids in hypertriglyceridemic states. Semin Thromb Hemost 1988;14(3):271–284.

197. Braden GA, Knapp HR, FitzGerald GA. Suppression of eicosanoid biosynthesis during coronary angioplasty by fish oil and aspirin. Circulation 1991;84(2):679–685.

198. Von Schacky C. Prophylaxis of atherosclerosis with marine omega-3 fatty acids: a comprehensive strategy. Ann Intern Med 1988;107:890–899.

199. Ilsley CD, Nye ER, Sutherland W, et al. Randomized placebo-controlled trial of maxepa and aspirin/persantin after successful coronary angioplasty. Aust N Z J Med 1987;17(4):559. (Suppl 2).

200. Milner MR, Gallino RA, Leffingwell A, et al. High-dose omega-3 fatty acid supplementation reduces clinical restenosis after angioplasty. Circulation 1988;78(Supp II):634.

201. Slack JD, Pinkerton CA, Van Tassel J, et al. Can oral fish oil supplement minimize restenosis after percutaneous transluminal coronary angioplasty? J Am Coll Cardiol 1987;9(2):64A (Suppl A).

202. Milner MR, Gallino RA, Leffingwell A, et al. Usefulness of fish oil supplements in preventing clinical evidence of restenosis after percutaneous transluminal coronary angioplasty. Am J Cardiol 1989;64(5):294–299.

203. Dehmer GJ, Popma JJ, van den Berg EK, et al. Reduction in the rate of early restenosis after coronary angioplasty by a diet supplemented with n-3 fatty acids. N Engl J Med 1988;319(12):733–740.

204. Bairati I, Roy L, Meyer F. Double-blind, randomized, controlled trial of fish oil supplements in prevention of recurrence of stenosis after coronary angioplasty. Circulation 1992;85(3):950–956.

205. Nye ER, Ablett MB, Robertson MC, et al. Effect of eicosapentaenoic acid on restenosis rate, clinical course and blood lipids in patients after percutaneous transluminal coronary angioplasty. Aust N Z J Med 1990;20(4):549–552.

206. Mehta VY, Jorgensen MB, Raizner AE, et al. Spontaneous regression of restenosis: an angiographic study. J Am Coll Cardiol 1995;26(3):696–702.

207. O'Connor GT, Malenka DJ, Olmstead EM, et al. A meta-analysis of randomized trials of fish oil in prevention of restenosis following coronary angioplasty. Am J Prev Med 1992;8(3):186–192.

208. Brensike JF, Kelsey SF, Passamani ER. National Heart, Lung, and Blood Institute Type II Coronary Intervention Study: design, methods, and baseline characteristics. Control Clin Trials 1982;3:91–111.

209. Brensike JF, Levy RI, Kelsey SF. Effects of therapy with cholestyramine on progression of coronary arteriosclerosis: results of the NHLBI Type II Coronary Intervention Study. Circulation 1984;69:313–324.

210. Blankenhorn DH, Nessim SA, Johnson RL. Beneficial effects of combined colestipol-niacin therapy on coronary atherosclerosis and coronary venous bypass grafts. JAMA 1987;257:3233–3240.

211. Blankenhorn DH, Johnson RL, Nessim SA. The Cholesterol Lowering Atherosclerosis Study (CLAS): design, methods, and baseline results. Control Clin Trials 1987;8:354–387.

212. Cashin-Hemphill L, Mack WJ, Pogoda JM. Beneficial effects of coletipol-niacin on coronary atherosclerosis: a 4-year follow-up. JAMA 1990;264:3013–3017.

213. Arntzenius AC, Kromhout D, Barth JD. Diet, lipoproteins, and the progression of coronary atherosclerosis: the Leiden Intervention Trial. N Engl J Med 1985;312:805–811.

214. Arntzenius AC. Diet, lipoproteins and the progression of coronary atherosclerosis. The Leiden Intervention Trial. Drugs 1986;31(Suppl 1):61–65.

215. Haskell WL, Alderman EL, Fair JM, et al. Effects of intensive multiple risk factor reduction on coronary atherosclerosis and clinical cardiac events in men and women with coronary artery disease. The Stanford Coronary Risk Intervention Project (SCRIP). Circulation 1994;89(3):975–990.

216. Watts GF, Lewis B, Brunt JN, et al. Effects on coronary artery disease of lipid-lowering diet, or diet plus cholestyramine, in the St Thomas' Atherosclerosis Regression Study (STARS). Lancet 1992;339(8793):563–569.

217. Watts GF, Jackson P, Burke V, Lewis B. Dietary fatty acids and progression of coronary artery disease in men. Am J Clin Nutr 1996;64(2):202–209.

218. Kane JP, Malloy MJ, Ports TA, et al. Regression of coronary atherosclerosis during treatment of familial hypercholesterolemia with combined drug regimens. JAMA 1990;264(23):3007–3012.

219. Gould KL, Ornish D, Kirkeeide R, et al. Improved stenosis geometry by quantitative coronary arteriography after vigorous risk factor modification. Am J Cardiol 1992;69(9):845–853.

220. Gould KL, Ornish D, Scherwitz L, et al. Changes in myocardial perfusion abnormalities by positron emission tomography after long-term, intense risk factor modification. JAMA 1995;274(11):894–901.

221. Flynn MK, Spann L, Sullivan MJ. Risk factor interventions and delayed progression of atherosclerosis. In: Rubin GS, Calff RM, O'Neill WW, et al, eds. Interventional cardiovascular medicine: principles and practice. New York: Churchill-Livingstone, 1994:108.

222. Schuler G, Hambrecht R, Schlierf G, et al. Regular physical exercise and low-fat diet. Effects on progression of coronary artery disease. Circulation 1992;86(1):1–11.

223. Niebauer J, Hambrecht R, Velich T, et al. Predictive value of lipid profile for salutary coronary angiographic changes in patients on a low-fat diet and physical exercise program. Am J Cardiol 1996;78(2):163–167.

224. Anonymous. Nutrition recommendations and principles for people with diabetes mellitus. Diabetes Care 1994;17(5):519–530.

225. Anderson JW, Geil PB. New perspectives in nutrition management of diabetes mellitus. Am J Med 1988;85(5A):159–165.

226. Smith U. Carbohydrates, fat, and insulin action. Am J Clin Nutr 1994;59(Suppl 3):686S–689S.

227. Anderson JW, Smith BM, Geil PB. High-fiber diet for diabetes. Safe and effective treatment. Postgrad Med 1990;88(2):157–161, 164, 167–168.

228. Anderson JW. Recent advances in carbohydrate nutrition and metabolism in diabetes mellitus. J Am Coll Nutr 1989;8 (Suppl):61S–67S.

229. Anderson JW, Gustafson NJ, Bryant CA, Tietyen-Clark J. Dietary fiber and diabetes: a comprehensive review and practical application. J Am Diet Assoc 1987;87(9):1189–1197.

230. Uusitupa MI. Early lifestyle intervention in patients with non-insulin-dependent diabetes mellitus and impaired glucose tolerance. Ann Med 1996;28(5):445–449.

231. Berry EM. Dietary fatty acids in the management of diabetes mellitus. Am J Clin Nutr 1997;66(4 Suppl):991S–997S.

232. Parillo M, Rivellese AA, Ciardullo AV, et al. A high-monounsaturated-fat/low-carbohydrate diet improves peripheral insulin sensitivity in non-insulin-dependent diabetic patients. Metabolism 1992;41(12):1373–1378.

233. Berry EM. Dietary fatty acids in the management of diabetes mellitus. Am J Clin Nutr 1997;66(4 Suppl):991S–997S.

234. Anderson RA, Cheng N, Bryden NA, et al. Elevated intakes of supplemental chromium improve glucose and insulin variables in individuals with type 2 diabetes. Diabetes 1997;46(11):1786–1791.

235. Offenbacher EG, Pi-Sunyer FX. Beneficial effect of chromium-rich yeast on glucose tolerance and blood lipids in elderly subjects. Diabetes 1980;29(11):919–925.

236. Wilson BE. Gondy A. Effects of chromium supplementation on fasting insulin levels and lipid parameters in healthy, non-obese young subjects. Diabetes Res Clin Pract 1995;28(3):179–184.

237. Faure P, Roussel A, Coudray C, et al. Zinc and insulin sensitivity. Biol Trace Elem Res 1992;32:305–310.

238. Sprietsma JE, Schuitemaker GE. Diabetes can be prevented by reducing insulin production. Med Hypotheses 1994;42(1):15–23.

239. Engel ED, Erlick NE, Davis RH. Diabetes mellitus: impaired wound healing from zinc deficiency. J Am Podiatr Med Assoc 1981; 71(10):536–544.

240. Agren MS, Stromberg HE, Rindby A, Hallmans G. Selenium, zinc, iron and copper levels in serum of patients with arterial and venous leg ulcers. Acta Derm Venereol 1986;66(3):237–240.

241. Paolisso G, Scheen A, D'Onofrio F, Lefebvre P. Magnesium and glucose homeostasis. Diabetologia 1990;33(9):511–514.

242. Srivastava VK, Chauhan AK, Lahiri VL. The significance of serum magnesium in diabetes mellitus. Indian J Med Sci 1993;47(5):119–123.

243. Grafton G, Baxter MA. The role of magnesium in diabetes mellitus. A possible mechanism for the development of diabetic complications. J Diabetes Complications 1992;6(2):143–149.

244. Grafton G, Bunce CM, Sheppard MC, et al. Effect of Mg2+ on Na(+)-dependent inositol transport. Role for Mg2+ in etiology of diabetic complications. Diabetes 1992;41(1):35–39.

245. White JR Jr, Campbell RK. Magnesium and diabetes: a review. Ann Pharmacother 1993;27(6):775–780.

246. Tosiello L. Hypomagnesemia and diabetes mellitus. A review of clinical implications. Arch Intern Med 1996;156(11):1143–1148.

247. Plavinik FL, Rodrigues CI, Zanella MT, Ribeiro AB. Hypokalemia, glucose intolerance, and hyperinsulinemia during diuretic therapy. Hypertension 1992;19(2 Suppl):II26–II29.

248. Thai AC, Husband DJ, Gill GV, Alberti KG. Management of diabetes during surgery. A retro-

spective study of 112 cases. Diabetes Metab 1984;10(2):65–70.

249. Pezzarossa A, Taddei F, Cimicchi MC, et al. Perioperative management of diabetic subjects. Subcutaneous versus intravenous insulin administration during glucose-potassium infusion. Diabetes Care 1988;11(1):52–58.

250. Eriksson J, Kohvakka A. Magnesium and ascorbic acid supplementation in diabetes mellitus. Ann Nutr Metab 1995;39(4):217–223.

251. Rogers KS, Mohan C. Vitamin B6 metabolism and diabetes. Biochem Med Metab Biol 1994;52(1):10–17.

252. Editorial. Vitamin B6 and diabetes. Lancet 1976;1(7963):788–789.

253. Spellacy WN, Buhi WC, Birk SA. Vitamin B6 treatment of gestational diabetes mellitus: studies of blood glucose and plasma insulin. Am J Obstet Gynecol 1977;127(6):599–602.

254. Rose DP, Leklem JE, Brown RR, Linkswiler HM. Effect of oral contraceptives and vitamin B6 deficiency on carbohydrate metabolism. Am J Clin Nutr 1975;28(8):872–878.

255. Adams PW, Wynn V, Folkard J, Seed M. Influence of oral contraceptives, pyridoxine (vitamin B6), and tryptophan on carbohydrate metabolism. Lancet 1976;1(7963):759–764.

256. Packer L, Witt EH, Tritschler HJ. Alpha-lipoic acid as a biological antioxidant. Free Radical Biol Med 1995;19(2):227–250.

257. Roy S, Sen CK, Tritschler HJ, Packer L. Modulation of cellular reducing equivalent homeostasis by alpha-lipoic acid. Mechanisms and implications for diabetes and ischemic injury. Biochem Pharmacol 1997;53(3):393–399.

258. Ziegler D, Hanefeld M, Ruhnau KJ, et al. Treatment of symptomatic diabetic peripheral neuropathy with the anti-oxidant alpha-lipoic acid. A 3-week multicentre randomized controlled trial (ALADIN Study). Diabetologia 1995;38(12):1425–1433.

259. Ziegler D, Gries FA. Alpha-lipoic acid in the treatment of diabetic peripheral and cardiac autonomic neuropathy. Diabetes 1997;46(Suppl 2):S62–S66.

260. Jacob S, Henriksen EJ, Tritschler HJ, et al. Improvement of insulin-stimulated glucose-disposal in type 2 diabetes after repeated parenteral administration of thioctic acid. Exp Clin Endocrinol Diabetes 1996;104(3):284–288.

261. Strodter D, Lehmann E, Lehmann U, et al. The influence of thioctic acid on metabolism and function of the diabetic heart. Diabetes Res Clin Pract 1995;29(1):19–26.

262. Kilic F, Handelman GJ, Serbinova E, et al. Modelling cortical cataractogenesis 17: in vitro effect of a-lipoic acid on glucose-induced lens membrane damage, a model of diabetic cataractogenesis. Biochem Mol Biol Int 1995;37(2):361–370.

263. Packer L. Antioxidant properties of lipoic acid and its therapeutic effects in prevention of diabetes complications and cataracts. Ann N Y Acad Sci 1994;738:257–264.

264. McCarty MF. Maturity-onset diabetes mellitus—toward a physiological appropriate management. Med Hypotheses 1981;7(10):1265–1285.

265. Barnard ND. Key nutrition issues for medical students. Washington, DC: Physicians Committee for Responsible Medicine 1997:3.

266. Blackburn GL. Total parenteral nutrition. (Associate Professor of Surgery, Harvard Medical School.) Adjuvant Nutrition in Cancer Treatment Symposium. CTCA/American College of Nutrition. Tampa, Florida. September 19, 1995.

267. Torosian MH, Daly JM. Nutritional support in the cancer-bearing host. Cancer 1986;58:1915–1929.

268. Copeland EM, Daly JM, Dudrick SJ. Nutrition as an adjunct to cancer treatment in the adult. Cancer Res 1977;37:2451–2456.

269. Mullen JL, Gertner MH, Buzby GP, et al. Implications of malnutrition in the surgical patient. Arch Surg 1979;114:121–125.

270. Wyszynski DF, Crivelli A, Ezquerro S, Rodriguez A. Assessment of nutritional status in a population of recently hospitalized patients. Medicina 1998;58(1):51–57.

271. MacBurney M, Young LS, Ziegler TR, Wilmore DW. A cost-evaluation of glutamine-supplemented parenteral nutrition in adult bone marrow transplant patients. J Am Diet Assoc 1994;94(11):1263–1266.

272. Ziegler TR, Young LS, Benfell K, et al. Clinical and metabolic efficacy of glutamine-supplemented parenteral nutrition after bone marrow transplantation. A randomized, double-blind, controlled study. Ann Intern Med 1992;116(10):821–828.

273. Young LS, Bye R, Scheltinga M, et al. Patients receiving glutamine-supplemented intravenous feedings report an improvement in mood. JPEN J Parenter Enteral Nutr 1993;17(5):422–427.

274. Knutsen SF. Lifestyle and the use of health services. Am J Clin Nutr 1994;59(5 Suppl):1171S–1175S.

275. Mills PK, Beeson WL, Phillips RL, Fraser GE. Cancer incidence among California Seventh-Day

Adventists, 1976–1982. Am J Clin Nutr 1994;59(5 Suppl):1136S–1142S.

276. Fraser GE, Beeson WL, Phillips RL. Diet and lung cancer in California Seventh-day Adventists. Am J Epidemiol 1991;133(7):683–693.

277. Snowdon DA. Animal product consumption and mortality because of all causes combined, coronary heart disease, stroke, diabetes, and cancer in Seventh-day Adventists. Am J Clin Nutr 1988;48(3 Suppl):739–748.

278. Snowdon DA, Phillips RL, Choi W. Diet, obesity, and risk of fatal prostate cancer. Am J Epidemiol 1984;120(2):244–250.

279. Fonnebo V. Mortality in Norwegian Seventh-Day Adventists 1962–1986. J Clin Epidemiol 1992;45(2):157–167.

280. Block KI. Adjuvant nutrition and nutritional pharmacology in cancer treatment: the emerging role of nutritional biotherapy in complementary oncology. Unpublished manuscript [under consideration for publication in the Archives of Internal Medicine for the spring of 1999].

281. Chandra RK. Effect of vitamin and trace-element supplementation on immune responses and infection in elderly subjects. Lancet 1992; 340(8828):1124–1127.

282. Pike J, Chandra RK. Effect of vitamin and trace element supplementation on immune indices in healthy elderly. Int J Vitam Nutr Res 1995;65(2):117–121.

283. Ascherio A, Rimm EB, Hernan MA, et al. Intake of potassium, magnesium, calcium, and fiber and risk of stroke among US men. Circulation 1998;98:1198–1204.

284. Bland JS. The use of complementary medicine for healthy aging. Altern Therap Health Med 1998;4(4):42–48.

285. Bland JS. Psychoneuro-nutritional medicine: an advancing paradigm. Altern Therap Health Med 1995;1(2):22–27.

286. Guthrie N, Gapor A, Chambers AF, et al. Inhibition of proliferation of estrogen receptor-negative MDA-MB-435 and -positive MCF-7 human breast cancer cells by palm oil tocotrienols and tamoxifen, alone and in combination. J Nutr 1997;127(3):544S–548S.

287. Bollag W. The retinoid revolution. Overview. FASEB Journal 1996;10(9):938–939.

CHAPTER 30

MEDITATION AND MINDFULNESS

Michael J. Baime

BACKGROUND

General Considerations

Meditation is one of the oldest and most widely practiced mind–body therapies. An increasing enthusiasm for meditation as a therapeutic tool in Western medicine accompanies a new understanding of the mind's role in health and disease. A large body of knowledge suggests that subjective experience, quality of life, and psychosocial variables play a central role in health and healing. Depression, anxiety, personality traits, social support, and spirituality have all been associated with disease incidence and outcomes (1). This association has been proven strikingly in ischemic heart disease (2–4), and there is intriguing evidence to suggest that the outcomes of diseases as dramatic as cancer (5) and as prevalent as the common cold (6) are influenced by psychosocial variables. These variables, which are largely subjective and difficult to measure except by self-report, are also difficult to influence by traditional Western medical approaches. Psychotherapy and psychotropic medications provide a tremendous benefit when they are indicated, but they are inappropriate, unavailable, or unacceptable for many patients. Meditation has been shown to improve some of the psychological and social variables associated with a poor outcome of many diseases. Meditation reduces stress, anxiety, and depression, and enhances quality of life.

Evidence that the mind has a meaningful role in health maintenance and disease recovery has fueled interest in meditation as a medical treatment. Meditation has been used as primary therapy to treat specific diseases, as adjunctive therapy in comprehensive treatment plans, and as means of improving the quality of life of individuals with chronic or debilitating illnesses. Meditation can teach patients how to cope more successfully with the stresses of illness and treatment (1). The extent to which the improvement of psychosocial variables will cure illness or prevent disease is unknown, but there is suggestive evidence and much ongoing research. A recent report to the National Institutes of Health on alternative medicine concluded the following:

> More than 30 years of research, as well as the experiences of a large and growing number of individuals and health care providers, suggests that meditation and similar forms of relaxation can lead to better health, higher quality of life, and lowered health care costs. ... Most important, meditation techniques offer the potential of learning how to live in an increasingly complex and stressful society while helping to preserve health in the process. Given their low cost and demonstrated health benefits, these simple mental technologies may be some of the best candidates among the alternative therapies for widespread inclusion in medical practice and for investment of medical resources (7).

The interest in meditation in health care has grown as our Western health care system has progressively emphasized and valued technology and procedures. This emphasis often results in treatments that depersonalize the personal aspects of illness and healing that accompany all disease. The objective, mechanistic approach of Western medicine may not always address a patient's anxiety about his or her illness. It is natural for people to fear pain, disfigurement, and death when they become ill. Anxiety can be heightened by many routine medical procedures. For example, a hypertensive patient may be full of apprehension from a simple blood pressure determination. This accounts for the phenomenon of white-coat hypertension, a well-described syndrome in which the patient's blood pressure is elevated only when a doctor or health-care professional measures it (8). Stress or anxiety may become particularly distressing when an individual faces chronic illness that affects quality of life (e.g., persistent pain, diagnosis of cancer, heart attack). In the time-pressured environment of modern medicine, it is difficult for most health care practitioners to fully address these concerns. Many busy clinicians do not have the training, tools, or time to help their patients cope with the stresses of their illness or of their lives in general. Patients can experience a demoralizing and frightening loss of control because of the intrinsic uncertainties of illness or the impersonal external demands of the health care system. Meditation practice can provide patients with self-directed and self-administered tools for cultivating mental and physical relaxation that helps return autonomy and control to the patient.

Definition

Meditation techniques originated as spiritual practices within traditional religious contexts, such as the contemplative reveries of the Jesuits or the Buddhist practice of sitting meditation. Most of the meditation techniques discussed in this chapter originated in the 3,000-year-old yogic practices of India (9). Over the centuries, hundreds of techniques have evolved. The original goal of these techniques was to lead the practitioner to a more absolute, unconditional, or sacred state of consciousness. In some tradi-

tional Eastern cultures, the full expression of this state of mind is termed *enlightenment*. There is, however, nothing inherently religious or spiritual about meditation. Meditation can be taken from its traditional cultural or religious setting and used as a tool to improve health and quality of life. The same techniques that are used to promote personal or spiritual growth may be directed toward the relief of stress and physical discomfort.

Meditation techniques all share a structured mental process that steadies and deepens awareness by bringing it to rest on a stable focus. This process may be accomplished by resting the attention:

1. On a **physical sensation, such as breathing**; this is used as a focus in some forms of traditional Buddhist or mindfulness meditation.
2. On a **thought or word** that is silently repeated; this is used in some yoga practices and in transcendental meditation (TM).
3. On an **external object**, such as a candle's flame or a statue.
4. To the **process of attention itself**, as in some Tibetan Buddhist traditions.

By intentionally directing and regulating attention, the meditator modifies the functioning of the mind and its relationship to the body. The individual learns to rest the awareness in the present moment without struggle or wandering. This cessation of struggle is often experienced as deep mental and physical relaxation.

Types of Meditation

The literature on meditation distinguishes between *mindfulness* and *concentrative* meditation. Mindfulness meditation exemplifies the tradition of expansive, or opening-up, techniques (11). These techniques cultivate a meditative resting of the entire field of attention, including all sensory and mental contents. This meditation contrasts with concentrative, or restrictive, meditation, which directs awareness to a single thought or sensation, such as a *mantra*, to the exclusion of all else. In practice, however, these theoretical types of meditation may be similar

(10, 11). The most widely taught form of mindfulness meditation uses breathing as focus for the attention, just as concentrative meditation uses an object or a thought. In mindfulness meditation, the meditator is taught to allow sensations, thoughts, and emotions to arise and fade without provoking a mental or psychological reaction. Similarly, in concentrative meditation, when thoughts and emotions arise, the meditator is advised to gently direct the attention back to the object of concentration without suppression or struggle. One meditation researcher has concluded that "the more common versions of meditation, such as Transcendental Meditation and Zen (a mindfulness meditation tradition), use an integrated approach, i.e., they combine concentration and mindfulness elements, with the former tending to dominate—especially in the earlier stages. However, with increased adeptness, mindfulness plays a greater role"(11).

Individuals who practice meditation regularly have significant reductions in anxiety and depression; these reductions have been documented with many commonly used psychometric tools. There is also evidence that the regular practice of meditation improves a person's functional status and quality of life. Meditation has been shown to significantly reduce the number of somatic symptoms reported by a broad range of patients with medical diagnoses. Meditation also benefits individuals without acute medical illness or stress. People who meditate regularly report that they feel more confident and more in control of their lives. They say that their relationships with others are improved and that they experience more enjoyment and appreciation of life (12, 13).

MINDFULNESS MEDITATION

Mindfulness meditation has its origins in traditional Buddhist meditation. It was introduced into the medical setting by Jon Kabat-Zinn, who founded The Stress Reduction Clinic at the University of Massachusetts Medical Center in 1979. Since that time, Kabat-Zinn has been instrumental in promoting the use of meditation as a treatment in Western medicine. Mindfulness meditation has been used in medical centers and hospital-based stress management programs throughout the United States. It is integrated easily into the allopathic medical system and is now taught in several medical schools and hospitals.

Mindfulness teaches its practitioners to cultivate a nonjudgmental state of openness and relaxation that can be maintained throughout activity. In formal mindfulness meditation, practitioners are taught to place their attention on a simple event, such as **breathing**, and to stabilize and evenly rest the awareness in the present moment. Mindfulness is the practice of resting steadily with "the clear and single-minded awareness of what actually happens *to* us and in us at the successive moments of perception" (14). During this meditation, wandering thoughts and shifts in attention are noticed as they occur without the individual suppressing, resisting, or commenting on them. Mindfulness meditation cultivates "an intentionally non-reactive, non-judgmental moment-to-moment awareness of a changing field of objects" (15). Informal meditation practice, described as the application of mindfulness outside of formal meditation sessions, is also emphasized. Meditators are taught to rest their awareness on any event that occurs. This is said to cultivate both a balanced equanimity and a more full and rich experience of life. Kabat-Zinn says:

> The key to mindfulness is not so much what you choose to focus on but the quality of the awareness that you bring to each moment. It is this investigative, discerning observation of whatever comes up in the present moment that is the hallmark of mindfulness and differentiates it most from other forms of meditation. The goal of mindfulness is for you to be more aware, more in touch with life and with whatever is happening in your own body and mind at the time it is happening— that is, the present moment. By fully accepting what each moment offers, you open yourself to experiencing life much more completely and make it more likely that you will be able to respond effectively to any situation that presents itself (16).

Mindfulness meditation provides cognitive learning as well as relaxation. Meditators are taught to recognize the repetitive patterns of their stressful thoughts and emotions and to inquire into them. Discovering that the thoughts and feelings accompanying stress reactions are often maladaptive or inaccurate leads one to more adaptive and skillful responses to stress.

TRANSCENDENTAL MEDITATION (TM)

TM is one of the most widely practiced forms of meditation in the West; somewhere between 2 and 4 million individuals have been taught the technique (17, 18). Numerous research studies have been performed to investigate its efficacy, and much of what is known about the physiology of meditation comes from the study of TM. TM has its origins in the Vedic tradition of India and was introduced to the West by Maharishi Mahesh Yogi. In TM, the meditator sits with his or her eyes closed for 20 minutes, twice a day, and effortlessly attends to a syllable or word (i.e., a *mantra*). Whenever thoughts or distractions arise, the attention is directed back to the *mantra*. One report states that TM ". . . is said to allow the individual to experience increasingly refined levels of mental activity until a state of 'pure consciousness' is experienced in which the mind is fully alert, yet completely silent and settled. This distinctive experience of 'restful alertness' has been distinguished from the aroused state of ordinary waking and the restful but inert state of sleep . . . " (19). The late Charles Alexander, a prominent TM researcher, writes that "during TM, ordinary waking mental activity is said to settle down, until even the subtlest thought is transcended and a completely unified wholeness of awareness beyond the division of subject and object is experienced. In this silent, self-referential state of pure wakefulness, consciousness is fully awake to itself alone with no objects of thought or perception" (18).

TM proponents claim that this state of rest and relaxation is more profound than that of other meditation techniques. The TM program now teaches another technique: the TM-Siddhi program. This more active form of meditative yoga also has its roots in Vedic tradition. More recently, Maharishi Mahesh Yogi has also recommended Ayurvedic medicine, the traditional health care system of India, and has promoted the use of Ayurvedic food supplements and products as a complement to TM (20).

PRINCIPAL CONCEPTS

Despite many theories, it is difficult to demonstrate how meditation works (just as it is often difficult to determine the mechanism through which many common medical treatments confer their beneficial effect). The development of the tradition of meditation has been largely empirical. Meditation is practiced because it produces a subjective effect that is valued by the meditator. Techniques that are subjectively beneficial have been handed down from teacher to student. Each generation of meditators refines these techniques and then passes them to the next generation. The meditation techniques that are being adapted for use in health care are the result of several thousand years of progressive development and refinement. These techniques are extremely sophisticated tools for working with experience and consciousness, but their evolution has been guided by subjective experience rather than objective medical data. Because of the largely subjective nature of meditation, it has been viewed with skepticism by medical scientists (21). An organized, scientific investigation of the physiological effects of meditation practice has only begun during the last 30 years. Well-designed clinical research into the benefits of meditation is just beginning to emerge. Meditation may have unique benefits that distinguish it from other self-regulation strategies, such as biofeedback or progressive relaxation (10).

Common Benefits of Meditation

Practitioners of all types of meditation consistently report some common effects. All forms of meditation generate a state of deep relaxation.

This relaxation appears to be different from that induced by other more active or physical methods of relaxation, such as exercise or progressive muscle relaxation. Another frequently reported benefit is a sense of psychological balance or equanimity. Meditation cultivates an emotional stability that allows the meditator to experience intense emotions fully while simultaneously maintaining perspective on them. As described in the tradition of mindfulness meditation, "the practitioner of bare attention [i.e., mindfulness] becomes able to contain any reaction: making space for it, but not completely identifying with it because of the concomitant presence of nonjudgmental awareness" (22). TM also describes the development of this type of emotional balance and suggests that it is a consequence of the deep relaxation that meditation provides.

Some types of meditation—particularly, mindfulness meditation and TM—claim to enhance psychological insight or understanding. Through the sustained application of nonjudgmental awareness, the mediator sees repetitive patterns of behavior and cognition more clearly. In mindfulness meditation, individuals are taught to experience and explore thoughts and feelings as events that are allowed to occur without invoking habitual patterns of response; this allows the meditator to gain insight into the nature of their involuntary habitual reactions. Kabat-Zinn writes that the "element of constant inquiry characteristic of mindfulness practice, promoted not through thinking but through bare attending and a continual non-discursive questioning about what one is actually experiencing, lays the foundation for such insight to arise"(15). Although insight is not emphasized as strongly in TM as in other types of meditation, enhancement of autonomy and freedom from unhealthy patterns of behavior are frequently described. One prominent investigator of TM writes that "meditators become better able to see another person's perspective, yet they cannot easily be swayed by social pressure to do something which they judge to be wrong" (Orme-Johnson D. Summary of Scientific Research on Maharishi's Transcendental Meditation and TM-Siddhi program. Unpublished material.).

Meditation and Stress Management

Meditation reduces more than just the stress of illness. Chronic stress is one of the most widespread maladies of our culture. Although life has undeniably always been stressful, present-day culture has its own unique stressors and demands. Many people think that these demands are more than they can reasonably manage. The relentless pace of time-pressured activity may be continuous, and unceasing activity and tension may become so deeply ingrained that a person may have difficulty relaxing when he or she has a moment to rest. Meditation has been used for a millennia as a way to calm and stabilize the mind. Initially, formal meditation periods provide a respite from the speed and turmoil of everyday life. Later, the meditator learns to remain in a state of relaxation even in the midst of activity or stressful surroundings. Meditators consistently report that they can handle difficult situations more easily as they become more adept at meditation. Ultimately, the path of meditation becomes a larger journey toward greater psychological stability and health. The initial need to deal with a stressful medical condition may be subsumed into the larger goal of learning to cope more skillfully with all of the stresses of life. A participant in the author's meditation-based stress management program states that:

> I was sent here because I had a heart attack and I was afraid that my Type-A personality would cause another. I was shocked to find that there were more important things to face. I had spent years running away from my family and myself and really from everything that I cared for most. I worked harder and enjoyed myself less. Here I found that the most important question was not whether I would die from heart disease but if I could live more fully and appreciate it while I was still alive. This is the most important message that I could ever hear–that it is possible for me to live fully and enjoy my life. Meditation has taught me how. This program should not be called stress management. It should be called life manage-

ment. The fact that my experience of stress has been reduced is almost insignificant in comparison to all else that has happened to me through this class.

PHYSIOLOGY OF MEDITATION

Western medical science began an organized study of the physiological changes associated with meditation in the early 1960s, and by 1970 there was a growing body of evidence that meditation alters physiology as well as the psyche (23). In some cases, specific findings varied among early studies and among different meditation techniques (24), although it was apparent that the physiological state produced during meditation differs from that which occurs during rest (25). Subsequent research has clarified many of these differences and has begun to show a consistent set of physiological changes that accompany meditation. It is hypothesized that meditation creates a unique physiological state that maintains a high level of central nervous system functioning and alertness while simultaneously allowing for deep rest and relaxation (26). Meditation affects many different physiological systems, and these biological changes provide part of the theoretical rationale for the use of meditation as a medical treatment.

Metabolism

Most studies have found that metabolic rate, respiration, and oxygen consumption decrease during meditation and that these changes are more marked than those that occur during other types of rest. One representative study documented a 50% decline in respiratory rate and a 40% decrease in oxygen consumption during meditation in experienced meditators (27). This study also describes brief periods of complete respiratory cessation that correlate with the meditators' report of peak meditative intensity. Another report documented that three Buddhist monks were able to vary oxygen consumption markedly using different advanced Tibetan Buddhist meditative techniques: oxygen con-

sumption decreased as much as 64% and, during a different meditative practice that attempts to increase "inner heat," increased as much as 61% (28).

Endocrinology

There is compelling evidence that the neuroendocrine system is significantly influenced by meditation. The effects of meditation on the pituitary–adrenal axis are particularly well studied. Numerous studies show an acute decrease in cortisol secretion during meditation (29–31), and a recent preliminary study found that meditators had reduced cortisol, thyroid-stimulating hormone, and growth hormone secretion in response to an experimental stress (32). Other research has shown alterations in concentrations of beta-endorphin and corticotropin-releasing hormone (33), melatonin (34), dehydroepiandrosterone sulfate (DHEA-S) (35), and gamma aminobutyric acid (GABA) (36).

Central Nervous System

Extensive research has explored electroencephalogram (EEG) changes during meditation. Most of this work shows increases in high-voltage theta wave burst activity and frontal alpha wave coherence in tracings obtained during meditation. EEG phase coherence, a measure of simultaneous phase EEG activity at different cortical locations, is also increased during meditation and may be associated with some of the subjective experiences of meditation (27); however, the significance of these changes is unknown. Functional brain scanning, a newer technique that directly measures brain activity or central nervous system blood flow, has been used to quantify changes in regional brain function during meditation. Meaningful changes in the activation of focal brain regions have been documented during meditation (37, 38). Research into the physiology of perception in meditators has also found changes in sensitivity to stimuli and in sensory evoked potentials (39–41).

Autonomic Nervous System

It has been difficult to demonstrate a consistent effect from meditation on autonomic nervous system function. There is little evidence for a reproducible effect on heart rate that differs significantly from other types of rest. However, galvanic skin resistance seems to increase reliably during meditation, suggesting decreased sympathetic activity (26). A recent preliminary study found that meditators experienced no changes in circulating catecholamines but did experience significant decreases in beta-adrenergic receptors (42). Another study found decreases in autonomic activation among inexperienced meditators but increased activation in more proficient meditators (43). This disparity possibly explains some of the inconsistent results in other studies.

Clinical Research

Research on meditation as a medical therapy has been complicated by some of the same problems confronting research of other alternative and complementary therapies: although the prospective, randomized, placebo-controlled double-blind study is the gold standard of clinical research, it may not be optimal for the investigation of meditation and similar mind–body therapies. It is difficult to create a suitable placebo for a meditation-based intervention, especially when a research design requires using a blinded control group that cannot be told if it is receiving the active treatment. It is difficult to design a convincing placebo that can be presented as meditation. An interesting study that investigated biofeedback and cognitive therapy for vascular headache prescribed "pseudomeditation" as a placebo control and found that this placebo became an active relaxation condition that provided a significant therapeutic benefit (44).

It can be argued that meditation works by the same mechanism as does the placebo effect. This point does not diminish the effect of meditation, but rather suggests that treatments that enhance the mind's capacity to heal the body (with low cost and little risk) may provide meaningful clinical benefits. A placebo may be an effective treatment because it provides a focus

through which the mind can affect the body; meditation may provide or heighten the same benefit.

Even if a suitable placebo can be devised, it may be difficult to randomize participants to a nontreatment group. Individuals who will commit the time and effort to practice meditation regularly are usually convinced of its benefits and may not consent to be part of an untreated control group. The cultivation of a regular meditation practice demands more active participation from the patient than do most medical treatments. Some studies compare meditators to a demographically similar nonmeditating control population; but even when this is done prospectively, significant differences in lifestyle or personality between two such groups are likely. These differences weaken the findings of any such comparison.

USE OF THE SYSTEM FOR TREATMENT

Major Indications

PAIN

Despite the inherent challenges of designing conclusive clinical studies of meditation, there is a considerable amount of evidence that details the medical benefits of meditation practice. In general, meditation practice decreases the number of physical symptoms reported by patients with a wide variety of medical conditions (Fig. 30.1). Meditation is a generally accepted therapy for chronic pain (45, 46). A recent Technology Assessment Statement of the National Institutes of Health reviewed the evidence for the use of different relaxation treatments for chronic pain, including meditation, autogenic training, and progressive muscle relaxation. The statement concluded that, "The evidence is strong for the effectiveness of this class of techniques in reducing chronic pain in a variety of medical conditions" (47).

PSYCHOTHERAPY

Meditation has long been used as a psychological therapy, and some of the earliest proponents

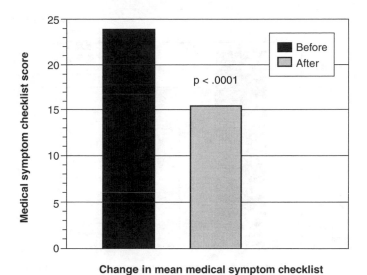

FIGURE 30.1. Change in medical symptoms following completion of a hospital-based meditation program. (Adapted with permission from Kabat-Zinn J. Mindfulness meditation. In: Haruki Y, Ishii Y, Suzuki M, eds. Comparative and psychological study on meditation. The Netherlands: Eburon, 1996:161–170.)

of meditation in the West were psychologists. During a lecture at Harvard University in the early 1900s, the renowned psychologist William James is said to have recognized a visiting Buddhist monk in the audience and exclaimed, "Take my chair! You are better equipped to lecture on psychology than I. This is the psychology everyone will be studying twenty-five years from now" (48). Although his prediction was premature, in the last 20 years many clinicians have reviewed the use of meditation as an adjunct to psychotherapy and explored its psychotherapeutic benefits (49–58). A recent book by Epstein explores the uses of mindfulness meditation in psychotherapy. He examines meditation from the perspective of Western psychology and claims that "the meditative practices of bare attention, concentration, mindfulness, and analytic inquiry speak to issues that are at the forefront of contemporary psychodynamic concern; they are not about seeking some otherworldly abode . . . . I hope to make clear how potent a force they can be in conjunction with more traditional Western psychotherapies" (59).

Other researchers have noted that Eastern psychology provides a fresh perspective on the nature of mind and its workings. At a symposium sponsored by Harvard Medical School, Daniel Goleman remarked:

> Buddhist psychology offers modern psychology the opportunity for genuine dialogue with a system of thought that has evolved outside of conceptual systems that have spawned contemporary psychology. Here is a fully realized psychology that offers the chance for a complementary view of many of the fundamental issues of modern psychology: the nature of mind; the limits of human potential for growth; the possibilities for mental health; the means for psychological change and transformation (60).

Clinical research into the psychotherapeutic benefits of meditation clearly suggests that regular meditation results in decreased anxiety (61–66) and depression (66–68) (Fig. 30.2).

The insight resulting from mindfulness meditation is similar to what is described during cognitive therapy, in which patients are taught to objectively see their thoughts and feelings to learn where cognitive and emotional distortions arise (69). Some therapists have suggested that

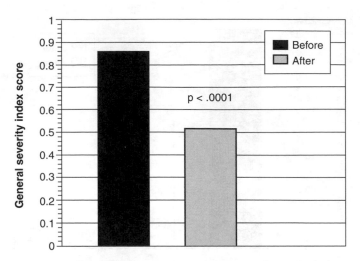

FIGURE 30.2. Measures of psychological distress before and after completion of a hospital-based meditation program. (Adapted with permission from Kabat-Zinn J. Mindfulness meditation. In: Haruki Y, Ishii Y, Suzuki M, eds. Comparative and psychological study on meditation. The Netherlands: Eburon, 1996:161–170.)

the antidepressant effects of cognitive therapy can be maintained with meditation (70). Meditation also has similarities to the process of psychodynamic psychotherapy (71).

HYPERTENSION AND CARDIOVASCULAR DISEASE

Meditation has long been recommended as an effective treatment for hypertension, but controversy exists over the magnitude of the benefit it provides. Some studies have documented only small decreases in blood pressure as compared with medication (72–74). Much of the published research has inadequate study design and sample size. One recent review identified more than 800 published studies and concluded that only 26 were well-designed enough to be useful (72). Despite these methodological problems, most of the studies show reductions in blood pressure with meditation (75, 76). Antihypertensive drugs are clearly more effective than meditation, but because of the high prevalence of hypertension, even a relatively small treatment benefit could be expected to have a meaningful impact on both public health and the overall cost of medical care. Meditation is likely

to be a highly cost-effective and efficacious treatment of mild hypertension when the risks and cost of pharmacological treatment outweigh the benefits. It might also be a useful adjunct to drug treatment.

Meditation, in conjunction with standard medical care, has been used to treat coronary artery disease. One recent study documented a significant decrease in exercise-induced cardiac ischemia measured with standard treadmill exercise testing (Fig. 30.3) (77). Dean Ornish and his group at the University of California have demonstrated significant regression of coronary artery stenoses as measured by both coronary angiography and positron emission tomography with a lifestyle regimen that included at least 1 hour of stress management, including meditation, daily (78–80). Preliminary findings suggest that cardiovascular mortality in the elderly is also decreased by meditation (81). Accumulating data about the psychosocial factors associated with coronary heart disease have fueled interest in this area (82). Many studies are ongoing, and much can be learned regarding the role of meditation and other mind–body interventions in the treatment of heart disease during the next decade.

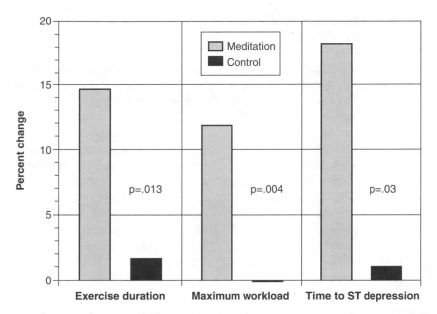

FIGURE 30.3. Exercise duration, workload, and time of onset of ST segment changes after 6 to 8 months of meditation. (Adapted with permission from Zamarra JW, Schneider RH, Besseghini I, et al. Usefulness of the transcendental meditation program in the treatment of patients with coronary artery disease. Am J Cardiol 1996;77:867–870.)

OTHER INDICATIONS

Meditation has been studied as a treatment for many other diseases, but in most areas the studies are too small or too few to allow meaningful conclusions. Numerous case reports have documented regression of various cancers with intensive meditation, but there are no well-designed prospective clinical trials. An investigation of the use of meditation for the treatment of breast cancer is currently underway at the University of Massachusetts (Kabat-Zinn J, personal communication). A small prospective study used stress-management techniques that included meditation for a group of HIV-positive men, and improvements were found in T-cell counts as well as in several psychological measures of well-being (83). One study found that meditation decreased the symptoms of fibromyalgia, a difficult-to-treat syndrome of chronic pain and fatigue, and reported significant improvement in over one-half of participants (84).

Meditation has been reported to improve function or reduce symptoms in patients with several neurological diseases, including epilepsy in patients resistant to standard treatment (85, 86) as well as patients with Parkinsonism (87) and patients with multiple sclerosis who experience fatigue (88).

Adverse Effects

A few reports describing deleterious psychological effects of meditation have been published. There is no prospective study of the adverse effects of meditation, although in the face of the millions of individuals who practice meditation regularly, such problems seem uncommon. Individuals with severe preexisting psychopathology, such as schizophrenia, are probably at the highest risk of experiencing adverse effects; one report suggests that meditation precipitated acute psychotic breaks in patients with chronic schizophrenia (89). Episodes of depersonalization are also reported, although they may not create any problems for the individual; it is difficult to interpret them outside of the context of the individual's experience (90, 91).

Shapiro canvassed 27 participants of an intensive meditation retreat and found that, although subjects reported many more beneficial than negative effects, 63% of them had experienced at least one adverse effect at some time. Adverse effects were described as including "increased awareness of negative qualities and emotions within myself"; increased disorientation, "such as becoming aware of how low my self image is, how often I get down on myself"; addiction to meditation; and boredom or pain. The same study found that 92% of the subjects reported positive effects, including "greater happiness and joy; more positive thinking; more self confidence; better ability to get things done; better problem solving . . . more relaxed; less stressed" (92). Finally, one researcher reported an increased incidence of what were described as "complex partial epileptic-like signs" in regular meditators, although symptoms included "profound meaning from reading poetry/prose" and "religious phenomenology" (93). Thus, it is plausible that individuals predisposed to such experiences are more likely to pursue meditation in the first place. In general, most proponents of meditation in a medical setting would not recommend meditation to individuals with severe personality disorders, psychotic disorders, or severe depression (especially with suicidal ideation or intent) unless concomitant psychotherapeutic or medical treatment is obtained.

ORGANIZATION

Training and Credentialing

One of the challenges caused by the more widespread use of meditation in health care is the lack of formal credentialing or licensure for meditation instructors. There are many traditions of meditation, and individuals with widely varying degrees of training and experience teach meditation in many different contexts. Although this means that there are numerous opportunities to learn how to meditate, there is no consensus about what constitutes the necessary training for a meditation teacher. There is no certification for Western instructors who wish to teach meditation as a medical or mind–body therapy. Traditional religions or organizations, such as Buddhism or TM, that include medita-

tion as a core component of their activity have specific requirements for formal training and explicit credentialing for new teachers. Usually, extensive experience and a high level of expertise are required for authorization as a teacher within such traditions, but such teachers may not have extensive experience with medical patients.

At the University of Pennsylvania Program for Stress Management, we suggest that an individual have at least 10 years of personal practice and formal instruction in mindfulness meditation before receiving additional training to teach meditation. For individuals with appropriate training, we have offered a 4- to 6-month internship that addresses some of the specific issues which arise when meditation is practiced as a medical therapy. Our teachers are also expected to spend at least 2 weeks out of each year in intensive meditation retreats. There are exceptions to these guidelines, but we encourage individuals with less experience to work wholeheartedly to deepen their own practice and study.

The Stress Reduction Clinic at the University of Massachusetts also provides several types of professional training programs. Five- to seven-day residential programs are offered at sites throughout the United States. These programs are highly experiential and require no previous training or experience. Further study is also available at a Professional Internship Program held at its Massachusetts clinic. These programs are not intended to certify that a participant is qualified to teach meditation. They provide basic training in the practice and principles of mindfulness meditation and explore how it might be applied to an individual's own personal or professional situation. Jon Kabat-Zinn's book *Full Catastrophe Living* details the University of Massachusetts program and is an excellent introduction to the use of mindfulness meditation in medicine.

Reimbursement

Because meditation is not considered to be a medical procedure or intervention by most insurers, it is often not reimbursed by medical insurance. Providers of medical or psychological treatment can teach patients about meditation as part of a routine patient encounter and then bill for the service provided. Many patients simply opt to pay for additional meditation training themselves. Various groups are engaged in ongoing discussions with third-party payers and HMOs, and these groups expect increasing numbers of insurers to pay for meditation as a medical treatment for selected patients. Ongoing research documenting the benefits of meditation will encourage this trend.

PROSPECTS FOR THE FUTURE

The presentation of meditation has evolved to meet the needs of each culture it has entered. Meditation is entering Western medicine as a secular and scientifically validated medical therapy. In keeping with the inclinations and goals of Western culture, meditation will be used because of its practical and concrete benefits. Meditation will likely be shown to be an efficacious treatment for many medical problems and an effective way to decrease health care costs and utilization. Ultimately, however, meditation will be practiced here for the same reason that it has flourished in so many cultures for thousands of years—because it helps people to feel better and to enjoy life more fully.

REFERENCES

1. Achterberg J, Dossey L, Gordon JS, et al. Mind–body interventions. In: Alternative medicine: expanding medical horizons. A report to the National Institutes of Health on alternative medical systems and practices in the United States. Washington, DC: U.S. Government Printing Office, 1995: 3–43.
2. Lesperance F, Frasure-Smith N. Negative emotions and coronary heart disease: getting to the heart of the matter. Lancet 1996; 347:414–415.
3. Karasek RA, Theorell T, Schwartz JE, et al. Job characteristics in relation to the prevalence of myocardial infarction in the US Health Examination Survey (HES) and the Health and Nutrition Examination Survey (HANES). Am J Public Health 1988;78:910–918.
4. Ruberman W, Weinblatt E, Goldberg JD, Chaudhary BS. Psychosocial influences on mortality after myocardial infarction. N Engl J Med 1984; 311:552–559.
5. Creagan ET. Attitude and disposition: do they make a difference in cancer survival? Mayo Clin Proc 1997;72:160–164.
6. Cohen S, Tyrrell DA, Smith AP. Psychological stress and susceptibility to the common cold. N Eng J Med 1991;325:606–612.
7. Achterberg, J, Dossey L, Gordon JS, et al. Mind–body interventions. In: Alternative medicine: expanding medical horizons. Washington, DC: US Government Printing Office, 1995:16.
8. Pickering T, James G, Boddie C, et al. How common is white coat hypertension? JAMA 1988; 259:225–228.
9. Eliade M. Yoga: immortality and freedom. 2nd ed. Princeton: Princeton University Press, 1969.
10. Shapiro DHJ. Overview: clinical and physiological comparison of meditation with other self-control strategies. Am J Psychiatry 1982;139:267–274.
11. DelMonte M. Constructivist view of meditation. Am J Psychotherapy 1987;41:286–298.
12. Kabat-Zinn J. Mindfulness meditation. In: Haruki Y, Ishii Y, Suzuki M, eds. Comparative and psychological study on meditation. The Netherlands: Eburon, 1996:161–170.
13. Baime MJ, Baime RV. Stress management using mindfulness meditation in a primary care general internal medicine practice. J Gen Int Med 1996; 11(S1):131.
14. Thera N. The heart of Buddhist meditation. New York: Samuel Weiser, 1962:30.
15. Kabat-Zinn J, Ohm Massion A, Herbert JR, Rosenbaum E. Meditation. In: Holland J, ed. Textbook of psycho-oncology. New York: Oxford University Press, In press.
16. Kabat-Zinn J. Mindfulness meditation: health benefits of an ancient Buddhist practice. In: Goleman D, Gurin J, eds. Mind–body medicine. Yonkers, NY: Consumer Reports Books, 1993:262–263.
17. Achterberg, J, Dossey L, Gordon JS, et al. Mind–body interventions. In: Alternative medicine: expanding medical horizons. Washington DC: US Government Printing Office, 1995:14.
18. Alexander CN. Transcendental meditation. Encyclopedia of psychology. 2nd ed. New York: John Wiley & Sons, 1994:545.
19. Alexander CN, Swanson GC, Rainforth MV, et al. Effects of the TM program on stress reduction, health and employee development: a prospective study in two occupational settings. Anxiety, Stress, and Coping 1993;6:245–261.

20. Sharma HM, Alexander CN. Maharishi ayurveda: research review. Complement Med Int 1996;3(2): 17–28.

21. Shimano ET, Douglas DB. On research in Zen. Am J Psychiatry 1975;132:1300–1302.

22. Epstein M. Thoughts without a thinker. New York: Basic Books, 1995:111.

23. Wallace RK. Physiological effects of transcendental meditation. Science 1970;167:1751–1754.

24. Woolfolk RL. Psychophysiological correlates of meditation. Arch Gen Psychiatry 1975:32:1326–1333.

25. Dillbeck MC, Orme-Johnson DW. Physiological differences between transcendental meditation and rest. Am Psychol 1987;42:879–881.

26. Jevning R, Wallace RK, Beidebach M. The physiology of meditation: a review. A wakeful hypometabolic integrated response. Neurosci Biobehav Rev 1992;16:415–424.

27. Farrow JT, Hebert R. Breath suspension during the transcendental meditation technique. Psychosom Med 1982;44:133–153.

28. Benson H, Malhotra MS, Goldman RF, et al. Three case reports of the metabolic and electroencephalographic changes during advanced Buddhist meditation techniques. Behav Med 1990;16:90–95.

29. Jevning R, Wilson AF, Davidson JM. Adrenocortical activity during meditation. Horm Behav 1978; 10:54–60.

30. Michaels RR, Parra J, McCann DS, Vander AJ. Renin, cortisol, and aldosterone during transcendental meditation. Psychosom Med 1979;41: 50–54.

31. Sudsuang R, Chentanez V, Veluvan K. Effect on Buddhist meditation on serum cortisol and total protein levels, blood pressure, pulse rate, lung volume and reaction time. Physiol Behav 1991;50: 543–548.

32. MacLean CR, Walton KG, Wenneberg SR, et al. Altered responses of cortisol, GH, TSH and testosterone to acute stress after four months' practice of transcendental meditation (TM). Ann N Y Acad Sci 1994;746:381–384.

33. Harte JL, Eifert GH, Smith R. The effects of running and meditation on beta-endorphin, corticotropin-releasing hormone and cortisol in plasma, and on mood. Biol Psychol 1995;40:251–265.

34. Massion AO, Teas J, Hebert JR, et al. Meditation, melatonin and breast/prostate cancer: hypothesis and preliminary data. Med Hypotheses 1995;44: 39–46.

35. Glaser JL, Brind JL, Vogelman JH, et al. Elevated serum dehydroepiandrosterone sulfate levels in practitioners of the Transcendental Meditation (TM) and TM-Sidhi programs. J Behav Med 1992;15:327–341.

36. Elias AN, Wilson AF. Serum hormonal concentrations following transcendental meditation—potential role of gamma aminobutyric acid. Med Hypotheses 1995;44:287–291.

37. Herzog H, Lele VR, Kuwert T, et al. Changed pattern of regional glucose metabolism during yoga meditative relaxation. Neuropsychobiology 1990–91;23:182–187.

38. Newberg AB, Baime MJ, d'Aquili EG, et al. HMPAO-SPECT imaging during intense Tibetan Buddhist meditation. Presented at the Annual Meeting of the Society of Biological Psychiatry, 1995; Miami, FL.

39. Becker DE, Shapiro D. Physiological responses to clicks during Zen, Yoga, and TM meditation. Psychophysiology 1981;18:694–699

40. Brown D, Forte M, Dysart M. Visual sensitivity and mindfulness meditation. Percept Mot Skills 1984;58:775–784.

41. McEvoy TM, Frumkin LR, Harkins SW. Effects of meditation on brainstem auditory evoked potentials. Int J Neurosci 1980;10:165–170.

42. Mills PJ, Schneider RH, Hill D, et al. Beta-adrenergic receptor sensitivity in subjects practicing transcendental meditation. J Psychosomat Res 1990; 34:29–33.

43. Corby JC, Roth WT, Zarcone VPJ, Kopell BS. Psychophysiological correlates of the practice of Tantric Yoga meditation. Arch Gen Psychiatry 1978;35:571–577.

44. Blanchard EB, Appelbaum KA, Radnitz CL, et al. A controlled evaluation of thermal biofeedback and thermal biofeedback combined with cognitive therapy in the treatment of vascular headache. J Consult Clin Psychol 1990;58:216–224.

45. Integration of Behavioral and Relaxation Approaches into the Treatment of Chronic Pain and Insomnia. National Institutes of Health Technology Assessment Statement. Oct 16–18, 1995: 1–34.

46. Kabat-Zinn J, Lipworth L, Burney R. The clinical use of mindfulness meditation for the self- regulation of chronic pain. J Behav Med 1985;8: 163–190.

47. Integration of Behavioral and Relaxation Approaches into the Treatment of Chronic Pain and Insomnia. National Institutes of Health Technology Assessment Statement. Oct 16–18, 1995:9.

48. Fields R. How the swans came to the lake: a narrative history of Buddhism in America. Boulder: Shambhala Publications, 1981:135.

49. Kutz I, Borysenko JZ, Benson H. Meditation and psychotherapy: a rationale for the integration of dynamic psychotherapy, the relaxation response, and mindfulness meditation. Am J Psychiatry 1985;142:1–8.

50. Goleman D. Meditation and consciousness: an Asian approach to mental health. Am J Psychotherapy 1976;30:41–54.

51. Shapiro DHJ. Overview: clinical and physiological comparison of meditation with other self-control strategies. Am J Psychiatry 1982;139:267–274.

52. DelMonte M. Constructivist view of meditation. Am J Psychotherapy 1987;41:286–298

53. Craven JL. Meditation and psychotherapy. Can J Psychiatry 1989;34:648–653.

54. Kutz I, Leserman J, Dorrington C, et al. Meditation as an adjunct to psychotherapy. An outcome study. Psychother Psychosom 1985;43:209–218.

55. Bogart G. The use of meditation in psychotherapy: a review of the literature. Am J Psychotherapy 1991;45:383–412.

56. Carpenter JT. Meditation, esoteric traditions—contributions to psychotherapy. Am J Psychotherapy 1977;31:394–404.

57. Shapiro DHJ, Giber D. Meditation and psychotherapeutic effects. Self-regulation strategy and altered state of consciousness. Arch Gen Psychiatry 1978;35:294–302.

58. Delmonte MM. Meditation, the unconscious, and psychosomatic disorders. Int J Psychosom 1989;36:45–52.

59. Epstein M. Thoughts without a thinker. New York: Basic Books, 1995:8.

60. Goleman D. A western perspective. In: Goleman D, Thurman R, eds. MindScience: an East-West dialogue. Boston: Wisdom Publications, 1991:4.

61. Miller JJ, Fletcher K, Kabat-Zinn J. Three-year follow-up and clinical implications of a mindfulness meditation-based stress reduction intervention in the treatment of anxiety disorders. Gen Hosp Psychiatry 1995;17:192–200

62. Gaylord C, Orme-Johnson D, Travis F. The effects of the transcendental meditation technique and progressive muscle relaxation on EEG coherence, stress reactivity, and mental health in black adults. Int J Neurosci 1989;46:77–86.

63. Kabat-Zinn J, Massion AO, Kristeller J, et al. Effectiveness of a mediation-based stress reduction program in the treatment of anxiety disorders. Am J Psychiatry 1992;149:936–943.

64. Goldberg RJ. Anxiety reduction by self-regulation: theory, practice, and evaluation. [Review]. Ann Intern Med 1982;96:483–487.

65. Puryear HB, Cayce CT, Thurston MA. Anxiety reduction associated with meditation: home study. Percept Mot Skills 1976;42:527–531.

66. Smith WP, Compton WC, West WB. Meditation as an adjunct to a happiness enhancement program. J Clin Psychol 1995;51:269–273.

67. Teasdale JD, Segal Z, Williams JM. How does cognitive therapy prevent depressive relapse and why should attentional control (mindfulness) training help? Behav Res Therap 1995;33:25–39.

68. Baime MJ, Baime RV. Stress management using mindfulness meditation in a primary care general internal medicine practice. J Gen Intern Med 1966;11(S1):131.

69. Beck AT, Rush AJ, Shaw BF, Emery G. Cognitive therapy of depression. New York: Guilford Press, 1979.

70. Teasdale JD, Segal Z, Williams JM. How does cognitive therapy prevent depressive relapse and why should attentional control (mindfulness) training help? Behav Res Therap 1995;33:25–39.

71. Epstein M. Thoughts without a thinker. New York: Basic Books, 1995.[4]

72. Eisenberg DM, Delbanco TL, Berkey CS, et al. Cognitive behavioral techniques for hypertension: are they effective? Ann Intern Med 1993;118:964–972

73. Silverberg DS. Non-pharmacological treatment of hypertension. J Hypertens Suppl 1990;8:S21–S26.

74. Mathias CJ. Management of hypertension by reduction in sympathetic activity. Hypertension 1991;17(3):69–74.

75. Alexander CN, Schneider RH, Staggers F, et al. Trial of stress reduction for hypertension in older African Americans. II. Sex and risk subgroup analysis. Hypertension 1996;28:228–237.

76. Schneider RH, Staggers F, Alexander CN, et al. A randomised controlled trial of stress reduction for hypertension in older African Americans. Hypertension 1995;26:820–827.

77. Zamarra JW, Schneider RH, Besseghini I, et al. Usefulness of the transcendental meditation program in the treatment of patients with coronary artery disease. Am J Cardiol 1996;77:867–870.

78. Ornish DM, Brown SE, Scherwitz LZ, et al. Can lifestyle changes reverse atherosclerosis? Lancet 1990;336:129–133.

79. Gould KL, Ornish D, Kirkeeide R, et al. Improved stenosis geometry by quantitative coronary arteriography after vigorous risk factor modification. Am J Cardiol 1992;69:845–853.

80. Gould KL, Ornish D, Scherwitz L, et al. Changes in myocardial perfusion abnormalities by positron emission tomography after long-term, intense risk factor modification. JAMA 1996;274:894–901.

81. Alexander C, Barnes V, Schneider R, et al. A randomized controlled trial of stress reduction on cardiovascular and all-cause mortality in the elderly: results of 8 and 15 year follow-ups. Presented at the 36th Annual Conference on Cardiovascular Disease Epidemiology and Prevention; March 13–16, 1996; San Francisco, CA.

82. Kabat-Zinn J. Psychosocial factors: their importance and management. In: Ockene IS, Ockene JK, eds. Prevention of coronary heart disease. Boston: Little, Brown & Co., 1992:300–333.

83. Taylor DN. Effects of a behavioral stress-management program on anxiety, mood, self- esteem, and T-cell count in HIV positive men. Psychol Rep 1995;76:451–457.

84. Kaplan KH, Goldenberg DL, Galvin-Nadeau M. The impact of a meditation-based stress reduction program on fibromyalgia. Gen Hosp Psychiatry 1993;15:284–289.

85. Deepak KK, Manchanda SK, Maheshwari MC. Meditation improves clinicoelectroencephalographic measures in drug-resistant epileptics. Biofeedback Self Regulation 1994;19:25–40.

86. Panjwani U, Gupta HL, Singh SH, et al. Effect of Sahaja yoga practice on stress management in patients of epilepsy. Ind J Physiol Pharmacol 1995;39:111–116.

87. Szekely BC, Turner SM, Jacob RG. Behavioral control of L-dopa induced dyskinesia in Parkinsonism. Biofeedback Self Regulation 1982; 7:443–447.

88. Freal JE, Kraft GH, Coryell JK. Symptomatic fatigue in multiple sclerosis. Arch Phys Med Rehabil 1984;65:135–138.

89. Walsh R, Roche L. Precipitation of acute psychotic episodes by intensive meditation in individuals with a history of schizophrenia. Am J Psychiatry 1979; 136;1085–1086.

90. Castillo RJ. Depersonalization and meditation. Psychiatry 1990;53:158–168.

91. Kennedy RBJ. Self-induced depersonalization syndrome. Am J Psychiatry 1976;133:1326–1328.

92. Shapiro DHJ. Adverse effects of meditation: a preliminary investigation of long-term meditators. Int J Psychosom 1992;39:62–67.

93. Persinger MA. Transcendental meditation and general meditation are associated with enhanced complex partial epileptic-like signs: evidence for "cognitive" kindling? Percept Mot Skills 1993;76:80–82.

ORGANIZATIONS AND SUGGESTED READINGS

The following organizations are main sources of information for each complementary and alternative medicine category covered in this book. These organizations range from large, long-established organizations to small organizations with limited staff. Please note that the scope and degree of assistance that these organizations can provide may therefore vary considerably.

Acupuncture

ORGANIZATIONS

The American Academy of Medical Acupuncture (AAMA)
5820 Wilshire Boulevard, Suite 500
Los Angeles, CA 90036
tel: (323) 937-5514   fax: (323) 937-0959
e-mail: medicalacupuncture@windseye.com

American Association of Oriental Medicine (AAOM)
433 Front Street
Catasauqua, PA 18032
tel: (610) 433-2448   fax: (610) 264-2768
e-mail: aaom1@aol.com
website: www.aaom.org

National Acupuncture and Oriental Medicine Alliance (NAOMA)
14637 Starr Road SE
Olalla, WA 98359
tel: (253) 851-6896   fax: (253) 851-6883
website: www.acuall.org

SUGGESTED READING

Helms JM. Acupuncture energetics: a clinical approach for physicians. Berkeley: Medical Acupuncture Publishers, 1995.

Stux G, Pomeranz B. Acupuncture: textbook and atlas. Berlin: Springer-Verlag, 1987.

Ayurveda

ORGANIZATIONS

The Ayurvedic Institute
Post Office Box 23445
Albuquerque, NM 87192
tel: (505) 291-9698   fax: (505) 294-7572
website: www.ayurveda.com

The College of Maharishi Vedic Medicine
1603 North Fourth Street
Fairfield, IA 52556
tel: (515) 472-8477

SUGGESTED READING

Frawley D. Ayurvedic healing. Salt Lake City: Morson Publishing, 1989.

Lad V. The science of self-healing. Santa Fe: Lotus Press, 1986.

Morrison JH. The book of Ayurveda: a holistic approach to health and longevity. New York: Simon & Schuster, 1995.

Svoboda RE. Ayurveda: life, health and longevity. London: Penguin, 1992.

Svoboda RE. The hidden secret of Ayurveda. Pune, India: 1980; reprint, Albuquerque, NM: The Ayurvedic Press, 1994.

Behavioral Medicine

ORGANIZATIONS

Academy of Psychosomatic Medicine
5824 North Magnolia
Chicago, IL 60660
tel: (773) 784-2025   fax: (773) 784-1304
e-mail: APsychMed@aol.com
website: www.apm.org

Society of Behavioral Medicine
7611 Elmwood Avenue, Suite 201
Middleton, WI 53562
tel: (608) 827-7267 fax: (608) 831-5122
e-mail: sbm@tmahq.com
website: www.sbmweb.org

SUGGESTED READING

Goleman D, Gurin J, eds. Mind-body medicine: how
    to use your mind for better health. New York: Con-
    sumer Reports Books, 1993.
Hafen BQ, Karren KJ, Frandsen KJ, Smith NL. Mind/
    body health: the effects of attitudes, emotions, and
    relationships. Boston: Allyn and Bacon, 1996.
Lehrer PM, Woolford RL, eds. Principles and practice
    of stress management. 2nd ed. New York: Guilford
    Press, 1993.
Sobel DS, Ornstein R. The healthy mind, healthy body
    handbook. Los Altos, CA: DR Press, 1996.
Tunks E, Bellissimo A. Behavioral medicine: concepts
    and procedures. New York: Pergamon Press, 1991.

Biofeedback

ORGANIZATIONS

Association for Applied Psychophysiology and
    Biofeedback (AAPB)
10200 West 44th Avenue, Suite 304
Wheat Ridge, CO 80033-2840
tel: (303) 422-8436   fax: (303) 422-8894
e-mail: aapb@resourcenter.com

Biofeedback Certification Institute of America
    (BCIA)
10200 West 44th Avenue, Suite 310
Wheat Ridge, CO 80033-2840
tel: (303) 420-2902   fax: (303) 422-8894
e-mail: bcia@resourcenter.com

SUGGESTED READING

Cram JR, Kasman GS, with Holtz J. Introduction to
    surface electromyography. Gaithersburg, MD:
    Aspen Publishers, 1997.

Kasman GS, Cram JR, Wolf SL. Clinical applications
    in surface electromyography. Gaithersburg, MD:
    Aspen Publishers, 1997.
Schwartz MS, et al. Biofeedback: a practitioner's guide.
    New York: Guilford Press, 1995.
Shellenberger R, Amar P, Schneider C, Turner J. Clini-
    cal efficacy and cost effectiveness of biofeedback
    therapy. Wheat Ridge, CO: Association for Applied
    Psychophysiology and Biofeedback, 1994.
Striefel S. Practice guidelines and standards for providers
    of biofeedback and applied psychophysiological ser-
    vices. Wheat Ridge, CO: Association for Applied
    Psychophysiology and Biofeedback, 1998.

Chiropractic

ORGANIZATIONS

American Chiropractic Association (ACA)
1701 Clarendon Boulevard
Arlington, VA 22209
tel: (703) 276-8800   fax: (703) 243-2593
e-mail: AmerChiro@aol.com
website: www.amerchiro.org

International Chiropractic Association (ICA)
1110 North Glebe Road, Suite 1000
Arlington, VA 22201
tel: (703) 528-5000 or 1-800-423-4690
fax: (703) 528-5023
website: www.chiropractic.org

Foundation for Chiropractic Education and
    Research (FCER)
704 East Fourth Street
Des Moines, IA 50309
tel: (515) 282-7118   fax: (515) 282-3347
e-mail: fcernow@aol.com

National Board of Chiropractic Examiners
    (NBCE)
901 54th Avenue
Greeley, CO 80634
tel: (970) 356-9100   fax: (970) 356-6134
e-mail: nbce@nbce.org
website: www.nbce.org

SUGGESTED READING

Bergmann TF, Peterson DH, Lawrence DJ. Chiroprac-
    tic technique: principles and procedures. New York:
    Churchill Livingstone, 1993.
Gatterman M. Foundations of chiropractic: subluxa-
    tion. St. Louis: Mosby Year Book, 1997.

Haldeman S. Principles and practice of chiropractic. 2nd ed. Norwalk, CT: Appleton and Lange, 1992.

Leach RA. The chiropractic theories: principles and clinical applications. Baltimore: Williams & Wilkins, 1994.

Redwood D. Contemporary chiropractic. New York: Churchill Livingstone, 1998.

Diet Therapy

ORGANIZATIONS

American Dietetic Association
216 West Jackson Boulevard
Chicago, IL 60606
tel: (312) 899-0040   fax: (312) 899-1712
website: www.eatright.org

American Society of Clinical Nutrition
9650 Rockville Pike, Suite L3300
Bethesda, MD 20814
tel: (301) 530-7038   fax: (301) 571-8303
email: secretar@ascn.faseb.org
website: www.faseb.org/ascn

Center for Science in the Public Interest
1875 Connecticut Ave. N.W. Ste. 300
Washington, D.C. 20009-5728
tel: (202) 332-9110 (Nutrition Action Newsletter)

NOHA
Nutrition for Optimal Health Association, Inc.
P.O. Box 1380
Winnetka, IL 60093
tel: (847) 835-5030

SUGGESTED READING

Alpers D. Manual of nutritional therapeutics. Little-Brown, 1995.

Brody T. Nutritional biochemistry, 2nd ed. San Diego: Academic Press, Inc., 1999.

Eschleman M. Introductory nutrition and nutrition therapy. Philadelphia: Lippincott, 1996.

Mahan LK. Krause's food, nutrition and diet therapy. Philadelphia: WB Saunders, 1996.

McDougall JA. McDougall medicine. Piscataway, NJ: New Century Publishers, 1986.

Ornish D. Dr. Dean Ornish's program for reversing heart disease. New York: Ballantine, 1992.

Peckenpaugh, NJ. Nutrition Essentials and Diet Therapy. Saunders, W.B., 1999.

Holistic Nursing

ORGANIZATION

American Holistic Nurses' Association (AHNA)
Post Office Box 2130
Flagstaff, AZ 86003
tel: (520) 526-2196 or (800) 278-AHNA
fax: (520) 526-2752
e-mail: AHNA-flag@flaglink.com
website: www.ahna.org

Nurse Healers–Professional Associates International, Inc. (NH-PAI, Inc.)
1211 Locust Street
Philadelphia, PA 19107
tel: (215) 545-8079   fax: (215) 545-8107
email: nhpa@nursecominc.com
website: www.therapeutic-touch.org

SUGGESTED READING

Dossey B, Keegan L, Guzzetta C, Kolkmeier L. Holistic nursing: a handbook for practice. Gaithersburg, MD: Aspen Publishers, 1995.

Guzzetta C. Essential readings in holistic nursing. Gaithersburg, MD: Aspen Publishers, 1998.

McMahon R, Pearson A, eds. Nursing as therapy. 2nd ed. Cheltenham, UK: Stanley Thornes, Ltd., 1998.

Nurse's Handbook of Alternative & Complementary Therapies. Springhouse, PA: Springhouse Corp., 1998.

Watson J. Postmodern nursing, the emergence of transpersonal caring-healing. Edinburgh, Scotland: Churchill Livingstone (Harcourt-Brace), 1999.

Homeopathy

ORGANIZATIONS

American Board of Homeotherapeutics
801 North Fairfax Street, Suite 306
Alexandria, VA 22314
tel: (703) 548-7790   fax: (703) 548-7792
e-mail: nchinfo@igc.org

American Institute of Homeopathy
801 North Fairfax Street, Suite 306
Alexandria, VA 22314
tel: (703) 548-7790   fax: (703) 548-7792

Council for Homeopathic Education (CHE)
3 Main Street
Chatham, NY 12037
tel: (518) 392-7975   fax: (518) 392 6456
e-mail: ched@igc.org

The National Center for Homeopathy
801 North Fairfax Street, Suite 306
Alexandria, VA 22314
tel: (703) 548-7790   fax: (703) 548-7792
e-mail: nchinfo@igc.org
website: www.homeopathic.org

Suggested Reading

Bellavite P, Signorini A. Homeopathy: a frontier in medical science. (Steele A, translator.) Berkeley: North Atlantic Books, 1995.

Castro M. The complete book of homeopathy. London: St. Martins Press, 1990.

Hahnemann S. Organon of the medical art. O'Reilly WB, ed. Redmond, WA: Birdcage Books, 1996.

Jonas WB, Jacobs J. Healing with homeopathy: the complete guide. New York: Warner Books, 1996.

Kayne SB. Homeopathic pharmacy: an introduction and handbook. Edinburgh: Churchill Livingstone, 1997.

Hypnotherapy

Organizations

The American Society of Clinical Hypnosis
2200 East Devon Avenue, Suite 291
Des Plaines, IL 60018
tel: (847) 297-3317   fax: (847) 297-7309

Society for Clinical and Experimental Hypnosis
2201 Haeder Road, Suite 1
Pullman, WA 99163
tel: (509) 332-7555   fax: (509) 332-5907
e-mail: sceh@pullman.com

American Board of Psychological Hypnosis
5410 Connecticut Avenue, NW, Suite 112
Washington, D.C. 20015
tel: (202) 363-8008
e-mail: hjwain@erols.com

Suggested Readings

Bowers KS. Hypnosis for the seriously curious. Monterey, CA: Brooks/Cole, 1976.

Fromm E, Nash MR, eds. Contemporary hypnosis research. New York: Guilford Press, 1992.

Hilgard ER. Hypnotic susceptibility. New York: Harcourt-Brace and World, Inc., 1965.

Rhue JW, Lynn SJ, Kirsch I, eds. Handbook of clinical hypnosis. Washington, D.C.: American Psychological Association, 1993.

Spiegel H, Spiegel D. Trance and treatment: clinical uses of hypnosis. Washington, D.C.: The American Psychiatric Press, 1978.

Wickramasekera I. Clinical behavioral medicine: some concepts and procedures. New York: Plenum, 1988.

Massage

Organizations

American Massage Therapy Association
820 Davis Street, Suite 100
Evanston, IL 60201-4444
tel: (847) 864-0123   fax: (847) 864-1178
email: info@inet.amtamassage.org
website: www.amtamassage.org

Associated Bodywork and Massage Professionals
28677 Buffalo Park Road
Evergreen, CO 80439-7347
tel: (303) 674-8478 or (800) 458-2267
fax: (303) 674 0859
e-mail: expectmore@abmp.com
website: www.abmp.com

International Association of Massage Therapy
3000 Connecticut Avenue, NW, Suite 308
Washington, D.C. 20008

Suggested Reading

Beck M. A theory and practice of therapeutic massage. New York: Milady, 1988.

Chaitlow LJ. Soft tissue manipulation. Wellingborough: Thorsons, 1988.

Field T. Touch. Boston: Harvard University Press, 1997.

Hollis N. Massage for therapists. Oxford: Blackwell, 1987.

Vickers A. Massage and aromatherapy. London: Chapman & Hall, 1996.

Meditation and Mindfulness

Organizations

Insight Meditation Society
1230 Pleasant Street
Barre, MA 01005
tel: (978) 355-4378   fax: (978) 355-6398
website: www.dharma.org

Shambhala International
1084 Tower Road
Halifax, NS B3H 2Y5 Canada
tel: (902) 420-1118   fax: (902) 423-2750
e-mail: info@shambhala.org

Transcendental Meditation program
National referral number: (888) LEARN TM
   (532-7686)
e-mail: info@tm.org
website: www.tm.org

Mind/Body Medical Institute
Department of Medicine
Beth Israel Deaconess Medical Center
110 Francis St, Suite 1A
Boston, MA 02215
tel: (617) 632-9530   fax: (617) 632-7383
e-mail: Mind/Body_Medical_
   Institute@bidmc.harvard.edu
website: www.med.harvard.edu/programs/mind
body

The Center for Mindfulness in Medicine,
   Health Care and Society
Stress Reduction Clinic
University of Massachusetts Memorial Health
   Care
55 Lake Avenue North
Worcester, MA 01655
tel: (508) 856-2656   fax: (508) 856-1977
e-mail: jon.kabat-zinn@banyan@ummed.edu

SUGGESTED READING

Advances: The Journal of Mind-Body Health For sub-
   scription information, contact: The Fetzer Institute,
   9292 West KL Avenue, Kalamazoo, MI 49009, tel:
   (616) 375-2000.
Austin JH. Zen and the brain: toward an understanding
   of meditation and consciousness. Boston: MIT
   Press, 1998.
Kabat-Zinn J. Full catastrophe living: using the wisdom
   of your body & mind to face stress, pain & illness.
   The Program of the Stress Reduction Clinic at the
   University of Massachusetts Medical Center: Dell
   Publishing, 1990.
Gunaratana, The Venerable H. Mindfulness in plain
   English. Somerville, MA: Wisdom Publications,
   1993.
Trungpa C. Shambhala: The sacred path of the warrior.
   San Francisco: Shambhala Publications, 1995.

Native American Medicine

ORGANIZATIONS

American Indian Science & Engineering Society (AISES)
5661 Airport Boulevard
Boulder, CO 80301-2339
tel: (303) 939-0023   fax: (303) 939-8150
e-mail: aiseshq@spot.colorado.edu
website: www.colorado.edu/aises

The Buffalo Trust
Post Office Box 89
Jemez Springs, NM 87025-0089
tel: (505) 829-3635   fax: (505) 829-3450
email: natachee@aol.com

Cultural Survival
96 Mount Auburn Street
Cambridge, MA 02138
tel: (617) 441-5400   fax: (617) 441-5417
e-mail: csinc@cs.org
website: www.cs.org

Diné College, Office of Continuing Education
Post Office Box 731
Tuba City, AZ 86045
tel: (520) 283-6321   fax: (520) 283-4590
email: nccce@crystal.ncc.cc.nm.us

SUGGESTED READING

Beck PV, Walters AL. The Sacred: ways of knowledge,
   sources of life. Tsaile (Navajo Nation), AZ: Navajo
   Community College Press, 1977.
Cohen KS. Honoring the medicine: Native American
   healing. New York: Ballantine, 1999.
Krippner S, Welch P. Spiritual dimensions of healing.
   New York: Irvington Publishers, 1992.
Lyon WS. Encyclopedia of Native American healing.
   New York: WW Norton, 1996.
Vogel VJ. American Indian medicine. Norman: Univer-
   sity of Oklahoma Press, 1970.

Naturopathy

ORGANIZATIONS

Council on Naturopathic Medical Education
   (CNME)
Post Office Box 11426
Eugene, OR 97440-3626
tel: (541) 687-7183 or (541) 484-6028
e-mail: dir@cnme.org
website: www.cnme.org

American Association of Naturopathic
   Physicians (AANP)
601 Valley Street, Suite 105
Seattle, WA 98109-4229
tel: (206) 298-0126   Referral Line: (206) 298-
   0125
website: www.naturopathic.org

NPLEX (Naturopathic Physicians Licensing Examination)
Post Office Box 69657
Portland, OR 97201
tel: (503) 250-9141 fax
e-mail: 73422.3360@compuserve.com
has information about licensing examination and
   scoring only

Suggested Reading

Kirchfeld F, Boyle W. Nature doctors. East Palestine,
   OH: Buckeye Naturopathic Press, 1994.
Lininger S, Wright J, Austin S, et al. The natural phar-
   macy. Rocklin, CA: Prima, 1998.
Marz R. Medical nutrition from Marz: textbook in
   clinical nutrition. Portland, OR: Omni Press, 1997.
Murray MT. Natural alternatives to over the counter
   prescription drugs. New York: William Morrow,
   1994.
Murray MT, Pizzorno JE. Encyclopedia of natural med-
   icine. Rocklin, CA: Prima, 1998.
Pizzorno JE. Total wellness. Rocklin, CA: Prima, 1996.
Pizzorno JE, Murray MT. Textbook of natural medicine. New York: Churchill Livingstone, 1998.
Sullivan A. A path to healing. New York: Doubleday, 1998.

Orthomolecular Therapy

Organizations

American Holistic Medical Association
6728 Old McLean Village Drive
McLean, VA 22101
tel: (703) 556-9245   fax: (703) 556-8729
e-mail: ahma@degnon.org
website: www.holisticmedicine.org

American College for Advancement in
   Medicine
23121 Verdugo Drive, Suite 204
Laguna Hills, CA 92653
tel: (800) LEAD-OUT   fax: (949) 455-9679
e-mail: acam@acam.org
website: www.acam.org

Suggested Reading

Gaby A, Wright J. Nutritional therapy in medical prac-
   tice. (Audiotapes and reference manual.) For infor-
   mation, e-mail: gaby@halcyon.com.
Murray M. Encyclopedia of nutritional supplements.
   Rocklin, CA: Prima Publications, 1996.
Werbach M. Nutritional influences on illness. 2nd ed.
   Tarzana, CA: Third Line Press, 1996.

Osteopathy

Organizations

American Osteopathic Association (AOA)
142 East Ontario Street
Chicago, IL 60611
tel: (312) 202-8000 or (800) 621-1773
fax: (312) 202-8200
website: www.am-osteo-assn.org

American Academy of Osteopathy
3500 DePauw Boulevard, Suite 1080
Indianapolis, IN 46268
tel: (317) 879-1881   fax: (317) 879-0563
email: aaomm@aol.com
website: www.aao.medguide.net

The Cranial Academy
8202 Clearvista Parkway, Suite 9D
Indianapolis, IN 46256
tel: (317) 594-0411   fax: (317) 594-9299
email: CranAcad@aol.com

Suggested Reading

DiGiovanna E, Schiowitz S. An osteopathic approach
   to diagnosis and treatment. Philadelphia: JB Lippin-
   cott, 1991.
Kuchera W, Kuchera M. Osteopathic principles in prac-
   tice. 2nd Re-revised ed. Columbus, OH: Greyden
   Press, 1994.
Magoun H, ed. Osteopathy in the cranial field. 1st ed.
   Kirksville, MO: Journal Printing Co., 1951. (Re-
   printed by Sutherland Cranial Teaching Foun-
   dation)
Still AT. Osteopathy: research and practice. Seattle:
   Eastland Press, 1992.
Ward R, ed. Foundations for osteopathic medicine.
   Baltimore: Williams & Wilkins, 1997.
Sources for Books:
All volumes available from Health Resources Press, 1359
   Alderton Lane, Silver Spring, MD 20906.
Books by A.T. Still are obtainable from the American
   Academy of Osteopathy.

Phytomedicine

Organizations

American Botanical Council
Post Office Box 144345
Austin, TX 78714
tel: (512) 331-8868   fax: (512) 926-2345
website: www.herbalgram.org

Herb Research Foundation
1007 Pearl Street, Suite 200
Boulder, CO 80302
tel: (303) 449-2265   fax: (303) 449-7849
website: www.herbs.org

Suggested Reading

Blumenthal M, Busse WR, Goldberg A, et al, eds. The Complete German Commission E Monographs: the therapeutic guide to herbal medicines. American Botanical Council, 1998.

Brinker F. Herb contraindications and drug interactions. Sandy, OR: Eclectic Medical Publications, 1997.

Bruneton J. Pharmacognosy, phytochemistry, medicinal plants. Paris: Lavoisier Publishers, 1995.

deSmet PAGM, Keller K, Hansel R, Chandler RF. Adverse effects of herbal drugs. Berlin: Springer-Verlag, 1997.

Schulz V, Hansel R, Tyler VE. Rational phytotherapy, a physician's guide to herbal medicine. Berlin: Springer-Verlag, 1997.

Wichtl M. Herbal drugs and phytopharmaceuticals. Norman Bisset, ed. Stuttgart: Medpharm Scientific Publishers, 1994.

Qigong

Organizations

The Qigong Institute
East-West Academy of Healing Arts
450 Sutter Street, Suite 2104
San Francisco, CA 94108
tel/fax: (650) 323-1221
website: www.healthy.net/qigonginstitute

Qigong Research and Practice Center
Post Office Box 1727
Nederland, CO 80466
tel/fax: (303) 258-0971

ZuYie Tai Chi Center
GiaYie, Taiwan
tel: 05-236-3583   fax: 05-235-0018

Tao and Zen Research Center
5910 Amboy Road
Staten Island, NY 10309
tel: (718) 967-4624   fax: (718) 356-1922

Suggested Reading

Chiang WC. Yin Si Tzu's meditation method for health. Taipei, China: Jian Shan Mei, 1964. (In Chinese.)

Cohen KS. The way of Qigong: the art and science of Chinese energy healing. New York: Ballantine, 1997.

Fang CY. The complete work of Chinese Qigong. Chielin, China: Chielin Science and Technology Publishing, 1989. (In Chinese.)

Zorn FH. Chi Gong Ho. Longevity, June 1994.

Yang JM. The root of Chinese Chi Gung. Jamaica Plain, MA: Yang's Martial Arts Association (YMAA), 1996.

Spiritual Healing

Organizations

Barbara Brennan School of Healing
Post Office Box 2005
East Hampton, NY 11937
tel: (516) 329-0951   fax: (516) 324-9745
e-mail: bbshoffice@barbarabrennan.com

Healing Touch International
12477 West Cedar Drive, Suite 202
Lakewood, CO 80228
tel: (303) 989-7982
e-mail: HTIheal@aol.com
website: www.healingtouch.net

LeShan Healing
315 East 68th Street, Box 9G
New York, NY 10021

Nurse Healers–Professional Associates
   International, Inc. (NH-PAI)
1211 Locust Street
Philadelphia, PA 19107
tel: (215) 545-8079   fax: (215) 545-8107
email: nhpa@nursecominc.com
website: www.therapeutic-touch.org

SUGGESTED READING

Benor DJ. Healing research volumes I-IV. Southfield, MI: Vision Publications, 1999.

Brennan B. Hands of light. New York: Bantam, 1993.

Gerber R. Vibrational medicine: new choices for healing ourselves. Santa Fe, NM: Bear & Co., 1988.

LeShan L. The medium, the mystic and the physicist: toward a general theory of the paranormal. New York: Ballantine, 1974.

The Qigong Institute. Qigong database. East-West Academy of Healing Arts. (Available from: The Qigong Institute, 450 Sutter Street, Suite 2104, San Francisco, CA 94108, tel/fax: (415) 323-1221, www.healthy.net/qigonginstitute)

Tibetan Medicine

ORGANIZATIONS

Tibet House
22 West 15th Street
New York, NY 10011
tel: (212) 807-0563   fax: (212) 807-0565
e-mail: mail@tibethouse.com

The Center for Meditation and Healing
Columbia Presbyterian/Eastside
16 East 60th Street, Suite 400
New York, NY 10021
tel: (212) 326-8435 fax: (212) 326-8590
e-mail: loizzoj@cpmail-nz.cis.columbia.edu

SUGGESTED READING

Clark B. The quintessence tantras of Tibetan medicine. Ithaca, NY: Snow Lion Publications, 1995.

Clifford T. Tibetan Buddhist medicine and psychiatry: the diamond healing. York Beach, ME: Samuel Weiser, Inc., 1984.

Kunzang J, Rechung Rinpoche. Tibetan medicine. Berkeley and Los Angeles: University of California Press, 1973.

Wangyal T. Wonders of the natural mind: the essence of Dzogchen in the Native Bon Tradition of Tibet. Barrytown, NY: Station Hill Press, 1993.

Yeshi Donden. Health through balance: an introduction to Tibetan medicine. Ithaca, NY: Snow Lion Publications, 1986.

Traditional Chinese Medicine

ORGANIZATIONS

Accreditation Commission for Acupuncture and Oriental Medicine
1010 Wayne Avenue, Suite 1270
Silver Spring, MD 20910
tel: (301) 608-9680   fax: (301) 608-9576

American Association of Oriental Medicine (AAOM)
433 Front Street
Catasauqua, PA 18032
tel: (610) 433-2448   fax: (610) 264-2768
e-mail: aaom1@aol.com
website: www.aaom.org

Council of Colleges of Acupuncture and Oriental Medicine (CCAOM)
8403 Colesville Road, Suite 370
Silver Spring, MD 20910
tel: (301) 608-9175

National Acupuncture and Oriental Medicine Alliance (NAOMA)
14637 Starr Road SE
Olalla, WA 98359
tel: (253) 851-6896   fax: (253) 851-6883

SUGGESTED READING

Beinfield H, Korngold E. Between heaven and earth: a guide to Chinese medicine. New York: Ballantine Books, 1991.

Kaptchuk TJ. The web that has no weaver. New York: Congdon & Weed, Inc., 1983.

Liu J, Gordon P. Chinese dietary therapy. New York: Churchill Livingstone, 1995.

Maciocia G. The foundations of Chinese medicine: a comprehensive text for acupuncturists and herbalists. New York: Churchill Livingstone, 1989.

Stux G, Pomeranz B. Acupuncture: textbook and atlas. New York: Springer-Verlag, 1987.

INDICATIONS AND PRECAUTIONS CHART WITH CLINICAL TRIALS

This chart lists the most common conditions seen by physicians in primary care and the complementary or alternative medicine (CAM) systems or modalities described in this book for them. It also allows you to know, at a single glance, the number of clinical trials that have been done for a condition in each CAM modality.

Column one lists the top 130 conditions seen in primary care. Column two lists the CAM systems or modalities described for that condition in this book. Column three lists the location of those descriptions. Column four lists the location of any precautions described for the CAM modality listed in this book. Column five lists the number of controlled clinical trials listed in the Cochrane Complementary Medicine Field Group's database of clinical trials as of the end of 1998.

When you are faced with a question about a particular clinical condition and complementary medicine, the following steps are suggested. First, look at column five to see if a possible evidence-based medicine (EBM) approach to addressing the problem is possible. The more controlled clinical trials there are for that modality, the more likely you can use current research to help guide clinical decisions. The prinicples described in Chapter 4 on EBM can then be applied. Summaries of many of the studies listed in column five can be accessed through the Cochrane collaboration database or at the NIH National Center for Complementary and Alternative Medicine's website at www.altmed.od.nih.gov/NCCAM.

Information in this book about the condition and selected CAM modality use and precautions are at the chapter listed under columns 3 and 4, respectively. This chart provides indications for the possible use of these practices according to the expert authors of these chapters. Any use of CAM must be done in the context of proper medical care. These descriptions should not be used as definitive recommendations for the use of these practices and should not be the practitioner's sole source of information nor substitute for proper clinical judgment.

CONDITION	SYSTEM/MODALITY DESCRIBED FOR THIS CONDITION IN THIS BOOK	CHAPTER FOR INDICATION	PRECAUTIONS DESCRIBED FOR THIS SYSTEM/MODALITY IN THIS BOOK	NUMBER OF KNOWN CLINICAL TRIALS (#) FOR THIS CONDITION IN THIS SYSTEM/MODALITY
Acne	1. Ayurveda	1. ch 11	1. ch 11	Aromatherapy (1) Ayurveda (1) Biofeedback (1) Diet Therapy (1) Homeopathy (1) Naturopathy (2) Phytomedicine (5) Traditional Chinese Medicine (1)
Addiction (see specific drug)	1. Acupuncture 2. Ayurveda 3. Hypnotherapy 4. Native American Medicine 5. Tibetan Medicine 6. Traditional Chinese Medicine	1. ch 19 2. ch 11 3. ch 25 4. ch 13 5. ch 14 6. ch 12	1. ch 19 2. ch 11 3. ch 25 6. ch 12	Acupuncture (1) Aromatherapy (1)
Alcoholism	1. Megavitamin and Orthomolecular Therapy 2. Phytomedicine	1. ch 27 1. ch 20	1. ch 27 2. ch 20	Acupuncture (12) Ayurveda (1) Behavioral Medicine (4) Biofeedback (6) Electric Stimulation (8) Holistic Nursing (1) Homeopathy (1) Hypnosis (5) Imagery (1) Meditation (10) Megavitamin and Orthomolecular (2) Naturopathy (8) Psychotherapy (4) Relaxation (8) Spiritual Healing (1) Traditional Chinese Medicine (2)
Allergy	1. Ayurveda 2. Hypnotherapy 3. Megavitamin and Orthomolecular Therapy 4. Naturopathy	1. ch 11 2. ch 25 3. ch 27 4. ch 17	1. ch 11 2. ch 25 3. ch 27	Acupuncture (1) Thymus Extract (1)

Condition	Therapies			Reported (number of studies)
Alzheimer's Disease	1. Ayurveda 2. Naturopathy 3. Phytomedicine	1. ch 11 2. ch 17 3. ch 20	1. ch 11 3. ch 20	Aromatherapy (1) Electric Stimulation (3) Holistic Nursing (1) Massage (4) Megavitamin and Orthomolecular (8) Naturopathy (8) Phytomedicine (3)
Amblyopia	1. Osteopathy	1. ch 16	1. ch 16	Acupuncture (1) Biofeedback (1) Megavitamin and Orthomolecular (1)
Amyotropic Lateral Sclerosis	1. Megavitamin and Orthomolecular Therapy	1. ch 27	1. ch 27	Biofeedback (1) Diet Therapy (1) Electric Stimulation (2) Thymus Extract (1)
Angina	1. Naturopathy 2. Megavitamin and Orthomolecular Therapy 3. Osteopathy 4. Phytomedicine	1. ch 17 2. ch 27 3. ch 16 4. ch 20	2. ch 27 3. ch 16 4. ch 20	Acupuncture (7) Biofeedback (1) Diet Therapy (1) Electric Stimulation (14) Homeopathy (2) Lasers (1) Meditation (1) Megavitamin and Orthomolecular (8) Music Therapy (1) Naturopathy (16) Phytomedicine (22) Psychotherapy (1) Relaxation (1) Traditional Chinese Medicine (4)

continued

CONDITION	SYSTEM/MODALITY DESCRIBED FOR THIS CONDITION IN THIS BOOK	CHAPTER FOR INDICATION	PRECAUTIONS DESCRIBED FOR THIS SYSTEM/MODALITY IN THIS BOOK	NUMBER OF KNOWN CLINICAL TRIALS (#) FOR THIS CONDITION IN THIS SYSTEM/MODALITY
Anxiety	1. Acupuncture 2. Ayurveda 3. Behavioral Medicine 4. Biofeedback 5. Hypnotherapy 6. Massage 7. Meditation 8. Megavitamin and Orthomolecular Therapy 9. Phytomedicine 10. Qigong 11. Spiritual Healing	1. ch 19 2. ch 11 3. ch 26 4. ch 24 5. ch 25 6. ch 22 7. ch 30 8. ch 27 9. ch 20 10. ch 23 11. ch 21	1. ch 19 2. ch 11 4. ch 24 5. ch 25 6. ch 22 7. ch 30 8. ch 27 9. ch 20 10. ch 23 11. ch 21	Acupuncture (14) Acupressure (1) Art Therapy (1) Ayurveda (1) Behavioral Medicine (86) Biofeedback (57) Chiropractic (3) Dance Therapy (1) Electric Stimulation (16) Homeopathy (6) Hypnosis (67) Imagery (33) Massage (27) Meditation (49) Music Therapy (25) Naturopathy (4) Holistic Nursing (13) Psychotherapy (54) Phytomedicine (19) Relaxation (184) Spiritual Healing (5) Traditional Chinese Medicine (1)
Arrhythmia	1. Osteopathy	1. ch 16	1. ch 16	Acupuncture (1) Electric Stimulation (9) Megavitamin and Orthomolecular (1) Naturopathy (4) Phytomedicine (10) Reflexology (1) Traditional Chinese Medicine (1)
Arthralgia	1. Acupuncture	1. ch 19	1. ch 19	Electric Stimulation (1)
Arthritis	1. Ayurveda 2. Biofeedback 3. Phytomedicine 4. Qigong 5. Traditional Chinese Medicine	1. ch 11 2. ch 24 3. ch 20 4. ch 23 5. ch 12	1. ch 11 2. ch 24 3. ch 20 4. ch 23 5. ch 12	Acupuncture (19) Anthroposophy (1) Ayurveda (3) Behavioral Medicine (4) Biofeedback (4)

Dance Therapy (1)
Electric Stimulation (9)
Homeopathy (17)
Hypnosis (2)
Imagery (2)
Lasers (4)
Massage (1)
Naturopathy (65)
Megavitamin and Orthomolecular (17)
Music (1)
Phytomedicine (18)
Psychotherapy (6)
Qigong (1)
Relaxation (13)
Spiritual Healing (1)
Tibetan Medicine (1)
Traditional Chinese Medicine (2)

Asthma

1. Acupuncture	1. ch 19	1. ch 19
2. Ayurveda	2. ch 11	2. ch 11
3. Behavioral Medicine	3. ch 26	4. ch 24
4. Biofeedback	4. ch 24	5. ch 25
5. Hypnotherapy	5. ch 25	6. ch 22
6. Massage	6. ch 22	7. ch 27
7. Megavitamin and Orthomolecular Therapy	7. ch 27	8. ch 16
8. Osteopathy	8. ch 16	9. ch 20
9. Phytomedicine	9. ch 20	10. ch 12
10. Traditional Chinese Medicine	10. ch 12	

Acupuncture (36)
Aromatherapy (1)
Behavioral Medicine (10)
Biofeedback (10)
Chiropractic (2)
Diet Therapy (9)
Electric Stimulation (8)
Homeopathy (12)
Hypnosis (17)
Imagery (2)
Lasers (3)
Massage (2)
Meditation (3)
Megavitamin and Orthomolecular (22)
Music (1)
Naturopathy (22)
Phytomedicine (23)
Psychotherapy (15)
Relaxation (35)
Thymus Extract (2)
Traditional Chinese Medicine (4)

continued

CONDITION	SYSTEM/MODALITY DESCRIBED FOR THIS CONDITION IN THIS BOOK	CHAPTER FOR INDICATION	PRECAUTIONS DESCRIBED FOR THIS SYSTEM/MODALITY IN THIS BOOK	NUMBER OF KNOWN CLINICAL TRIALS (#) FOR THIS CONDITION IN THIS SYSTEM/MODALITY
Atherosclerosis	1. Naturopathy	1. ch 17		Ayurveda (1) Diet Therapy (2) Electric Stimulation (3) Lasers (1) Megavitamin and Orthomolecular (3) Naturopathy (6) Ozone Therapy (1) Phytomedicine (4) Tibetan Medicine (1)
Attention Deficit Disorder	1. Biofeedback 2. Megavitamin and Orthomolecular Therapy 3. Osteopathy	1. ch 24 2. ch 27 3. ch 16	1. ch 24 2. ch 27 3. ch 16	Acupuncture (1) Behavioral Medicine (1) Biofeedback (5) Diet Therapy (6) Homeopathy (1) Massage (2) Megavitamin and Orthomolecular (1) Music Therapy (1) Naturopathy (12) Phytomedicine (2) Relaxation (5)
Back Pain	1. Ayurveda 2. Chiropractic	1. ch 11 2. ch 15	1. ch 11 2. ch 15	Acupuncture (45) Aromatherapy (2) Behavioral Medicine (19) Biofeedback (12) Chiropractic (53) Electric Stimulation (55) Homeopathy (1) Hypnosis (5) Imagery (1) Lasers (4) Massage (16) Megavitamin and Orthomolecular (2) Naturopathy (8) Orthopedic Manipulation (54) Osteopathy (11) Phytomedicine (5) Psychotherapy (4) Relaxation (16) Traditional Chinese Medicine (1)

Condition				
Bell's Palsy	1. Osteopathy	1. ch 16	1. ch 16	
Benign Prostatic Hypertrophy	1. Phytomedicine	1. ch 20	1. ch 20	Naturopathy (1) Phytomedicine (39)
Bowel Dysfunction	1. Acupuncture	1. ch 19	1. ch 19	
Bronchitis	1. Acupuncture 2. Ayurveda	1. ch 19 2. ch 11	1. ch 19 2. ch 11	Acupuncture (1) Aromatherapy (3) Electric Stimulation (7) Homeopathy (1) Imagery (1) Lasers (1) Naturopathy (2) Phytomedicine (13) Thymus Extract (2)
Bulimia	1. Massage	2. ch 22	2. ch 22	Behavioral Medicine (2) Dance Therapy (1) Hypnosis (7) Naturopathy (1)
Burns	1. Massage	1. ch 22	1. ch 22	Acupuncture (1) Behavioral Medicine (1) Electric Stimulation (4) Homeopathy (2) Hypnosis (6) Massage (1) Music Therapy (1) Naturopathy (3) Phytomedicine (6) Relaxation (1)
Bursitis	1. Chiropractic	1. ch 15	1. ch 15	Acupuncture (1) Orthopedic Manipulation (1)

continued

CONDITION	SYSTEM/MODALITY DESCRIBED FOR THIS CONDITION IN THIS BOOK	CHAPTER FOR INDICATION	PRECAUTIONS DESCRIBED FOR THIS SYSTEM/MODALITY IN THIS BOOK	NUMBER OF KNOWN CLINICAL TRIALS (#) FOR THIS CONDITION IN THIS SYSTEM/MODALITY
Cancer	1. Acupuncture 2. Behavioral Medicine 3. Biofeedback 4. Hypnotherapy 5. Massage 6. Meditation 7. Naturopathy 8. Osteopathy 9. Phytomedicine 10. Qigong 11. Spiritual Healing 12. Traditional Chinese Medicine	1. ch 19 2. ch 26 3. ch 24 4. ch 25 5. ch 22 6. ch 30 7. ch 17 8. ch 16 9. ch 20 10. ch 23 11. ch 21 12. ch 12	1. ch 19 3. ch 24 4. ch 25 5. ch 22 6. ch 30 8. ch 16 9. ch 20 10. ch 23 11. ch 21 12. ch 12	Acupuncture (3) Behavioral Medicine (2) Electric Stimulation (13) Homeopathy (1) Hypnosis (5) Imagery (1) Massage (1) Megavitamin and Orthomolecular (8) Naturopathy (10) Phytomedicine (25) Psychotherapy (2) Relaxation (2) Spiritual Healing (1) Thymus Extract (37) Traditional Chinese Medicine (2)
Cardiovascular Disease	1. Behavioral Medicine 2. Meditation 3. Megavitamin and Orthomolecular Therapy 4. Qigong	1. ch 26 2. ch 30 3. ch 27 4. ch 23	2. ch 30 3. ch 27 4. ch 23	Acupuncture (2) Aromatherapy (1) Behavioral Medicine (1) Electric Stimulation (3) Homeopathy (1) Hypnosis (1) Massage (1) Naturopathy (17) Phytomedicine (18) Relaxation (4) Traditional Chinese Medicine (1)
Carpal Tunnel Syndrome	1. Acupuncture 2. Megavitamin and Orthomolecular Therapy 3. Osteopathy 4. Traditional Chinese Medicine	1. ch 19 2. ch 27 3. ch 16 4. ch 12	1. ch 19 2. ch 27 3. ch 16 4. ch 12	Chiropractic (1) Megavitamin and Orthomolecular (3) Naturopathy (3) Osteopathy (1)
Cervical Dysplasia	1. Megavitamin and Orthomolecular Therapy	1. ch 27	1. ch 27	Megavitamin and Orthomolecular (1) Naturopathy (1)

Condition	Therapies	Chapters	Approaches
Chronic Fatigue Syndrome	1. Acupuncture 2. Massage 3. Megavitamin and Orthomolecular Therapy	1. ch 19 2. ch 22 3. ch 27	Behavioral Medicine (2) Homeopathy (2) Naturopathy (4) Phytomedicine (1) Relaxation (1)
Claudication	1. Phytomedicine	1. ch 20	EDTA Chelation (2) Electric Stimulation (4) Lasers (2) Megavitamin and Orthomolecular (7) Naturopathy (17) Phytomedicine (20) Tibetan Medicine (7)
Colitis	1. Osteopathy	1. ch 16	Electric Stimulation (1) Naturopathy (1)
Colitis, Ulcerative	1. Acupuncture	1. ch 19	Behavioral Medicine (1) Biofeedback (1) Diet Therapy (8) Hypnosis (1) Naturopathy (15) Phytomedicine (7) Relaxation (3) Thymus Extract (1) Traditional Chinese Medicine (3)
Common Cold	1. Ayurveda 2. Megavitamin and Orthomolecular Therapy 3. Traditional Chinese Medicine	1. ch 11 2. ch 27 3. ch 20 4. ch 12	Aromatherapy (2) Homeopathy (4) Megavitamin and Orthomolecular (2) Naturopathy (6) Phytomedicine (6)
Congestive Heart Failure	1. Naturopathy 2. Megavitamin and Orthomolecular Therapy	1. ch 17 2. ch 27	Acupuncture (1) Biofeedback (2) Electric Stimulation (3) Imagery (1) Megavitamin and Orthomolecular (3) Naturopathy (7) Phytomedicine (17) Relaxation (1) Traditional Chinese Medicine (1)

continued

CONDITION	SYSTEM/MODALITY DESCRIBED FOR THIS CONDITION IN THIS BOOK	CHAPTER FOR INDICATION	PRECAUTIONS DESCRIBED FOR THIS SYSTEM/MODALITY IN THIS BOOK	NUMBER OF KNOWN CLINICAL TRIALS (#) FOR THIS CONDITION IN THIS SYSTEM/MODALITY
Constipation	1. Ayurveda 2. Native American Medicine 3. Phytomedicine 4. Tibetan Medicine	1. ch 11 2. ch 30 3. ch 20 4. ch 14	1. ch 11 3. ch 20	Acupuncture (1) Art Therapy (1) Biofeedback (11) Electric Stimulation (3) Massage (1) Megavitamin and Orthomolecular (2) Naturopathy (2) Phytomedicine (16) Relaxation (2)
Coronary Artery Disease	1. Meditation	1. ch 30	1. ch 30	
Dementia	1. Megavitamin and Orthomolecular Therapy 2. Phytomedicine	1. ch 27 2. ch 20	1. ch 27 2. ch 20	Acupuncture (3) Aromatherapy (2) Holistic Nursing (1) Homeopathy (1) Megavitamin and Orthomolecular (2) Music Therapy (2) Naturopathy (3) Phytomedicine (13) Relaxation (4) Traditional Chinese Medicine (2)
Depression	1. Acupuncture 2. Behavioral Medicine 3. Massage 4. Meditation 5. Megavitamin and Orthomolecular Therapy 6. Phytomedicine 7. Qigong 8. Spiritual Healing	1. ch 19 2. ch 26 3. ch 22 4. ch 30 5. ch 27 6. ch 20 7. ch 23 8. ch 21	1. ch 19 3. ch 22 4. ch 30 5. ch 27 6. ch 20 7. ch 23 8. ch 21	Acupuncture (8) Acupressure (3) Art Therapy (1) Ayurveda (1) Behavioral Medicine(13) Biofeedback (10) Chiropractic (1) Dance Therapy (1) Electric Stimulation (11) Holistic Nursing (4) Hypnosis (8) Imagery (7) Light Therapy (2) Massage (9)

			Meditation (6)
			Music Therapy (4)
			Naturopathy (1)
			Megavitamin and Orthomolecular (1)
			Phytomedicine (33)
			Psychotherapy (13)
			Relaxation (27)
			Spiritual Healing (2)

Condition	Therapies			Reference list
Diabetes	1. Ayurveda	1. ch 11	1. ch 11	Acupuncture (4)
	2. Behavioral Medicine	2. ch 26	3. ch 24	African Medicine (1)
	3. Biofeedback	3. ch 24	4. ch 22	Ayurveda (2)
	4. Massage	4. ch 22	6. ch 27	Biofeedback (6)
	5. Naturopathy	5. ch 17		Diet Therapy (3)
	6. Megavitamin and Orthomolecular Therapy	6. ch 27		Electric Stimulation (5)
				Homeopathy (2)
				Hyponosis (2)
				Imagery (1)
				Massage (2)
				Megavitamin and Orthomolecular (2)
				Naturopathy (15)
				Phytomedicine (33)
				Psychotherapy (1)
				Reflexology (1)
				Reflexation (8)
				Spiritual Healing (1)
				Traditional Chinese Medicine (3)
Disc Disease	1. Acupuncture	1. ch 19	1. ch 19	
	2. Chiropractic	2. ch 15	2. ch 15	
Dysmenorrhea	1. Acupuncture	1. ch 19	1. ch 19	Acupunture (5)
				Behavioral Medicine (2)
				Biofeedback (1)
				Chiropractic (1)
				Electric Stimulation (8)
				Homeopathy (2)
				Imagery (1)
				Megavitamin and Orthomolecular (1)
				Naturopathy (1)
				Orthopedic Manipulation (2)
				Osteopathy (1)
				Phytomedicine (2)

continued

CONDITION	SYSTEM/MODALITY DESCRIBED FOR THIS CONDITION IN THIS BOOK	CHAPTER FOR INDICATION	PRECAUTIONS DESCRIBED FOR THIS SYSTEM/MODALITY IN THIS BOOK	NUMBER OF KNOWN CLINICAL TRIALS (#) FOR THIS CONDITION IN THIS SYSTEM/MODALITY
Eczema	1. Ayurveda 2. Hypnotherapy 3. Naturopathy 4. Phytomedicine 5. Traditional Chinese Medicine	1. ch 11 2. ch 25 3. ch 17 4. ch 20 5. ch 12	1. ch 11 2. ch 25 4. ch 20 5. ch 12	Behavioral Medicine (1) Diet Therapy (6) Homeopathy (1) Naturopathy (11) Phytomedicine (12) Thymus Extract (3)
Edema	1. Ayurveda 2. Megavitamin and Orthomolecular Therapy	1. ch 11 2. ch 27	1. ch11 2. ch 27	Acupuncture (6) Electric Stimulation (7) Homeopathy (7) Massage (7) Naturopathy (2) Phytomedicine (13)
Epilepsy	1. Biofeedback 2. Meditation 3. Osteopathy	1. ch 24 2. ch 30 3. ch 16	1. ch 24 2. ch 30 3. ch 16	Acupuncture (3) Behavioral Medicine (1) Biofeedback (9) Diet Therapy (1) Electric Stimulation (44) Hypnosis (1) Meditation (3) Megavitamin and Orthomolecular (3) Naturopathy (7) Phytomedicine (8) Relaxation (6) Traditional Chinese Medicine (1)
Fibrocystic Breast Disease	1. Megavitamin and Orthomolecular Therapy	1. ch 27	1. ch 27	Acupuncture (1) Diet Therapy (1) Homeopathy (1) Megavitamin and Orthomolecular (1) Naturopathy (3) Phytomedicine (1)

Fibrositis, Fibromyalgia	1. Homeopathy 2. Hypnotherapy 3. Massage 4. Meditation 5. Megavitamin and Orthomolecular Therapy 6. Traditional Chinese Medicine	1. ch 28 2. ch 25 2. ch 25 3. ch 22 3. ch 22 4. ch 30 4. ch 30 5. ch 27 5. ch 27 6. ch 12 6. ch 12	Acupuncture (4) Behavioral Medicine (1) Biofeedback (2) Chiropractic (1) Electric Stimulation (1) Homeopathy (4) Massage (2) Meditation (1) Naturopathy (1) Relaxation (5)
Gastritis	1. Acupuncture	1. ch 19 1. ch 19	Acupuncture (2) Electric Stimulation (3) Homeopathy (1) Megavitamin and Orthomolecular (2) Naturopathy (3) Phytomedicine (12) Traditional Chinese Medicine (1)
Gastroenteritis	1. Acupuncture	1. ch 19 1. ch 19	
Gastroesophageal Reflux	1. Osteopathy	1. ch 16 1. ch 16	Relaxation (1)
Gout	1. Ayurveda	1. ch 11 1. ch 11	Homeopathy (1) Phytomedicine (1) Traditional Chinese Medicine (1)
Head Injury	1. Osteopathy	1. ch 16 1. ch 16	

continued

CONDITION	SYSTEM/MODALITY DESCRIBED FOR THIS CONDITION IN THIS BOOK	CHAPTER FOR INDICATION	PRECAUTIONS DESCRIBED FOR THIS SYSTEM/MODALITY IN THIS BOOK	NUMBER OF KNOWN CLINICAL TRIALS (#) FOR THIS CONDITION IN THIS SYSTEM/MODALITY
Headache	1. Acupuncture 2. Biofeedback 3. Chiropractic 4. Hypnotherapy 5. Meditation 6. Naturopathy 7. Osteopathy 8. Phytomedicine 9. Spiritual Healing	1. ch 19 2. ch 24 3. ch 15 4. ch 25 5. ch 30 6. ch 17 7. ch 16 8. ch 20 9. ch 21	1. ch 19 2. ch 24 3. ch 15 4. ch 25 5. ch 30 7. ch 16 8. ch 20 9. ch 21	Acupuncture (31) Aromatherapy (4) Behavioral Medicine (17) Biofeedback (54) Chiropractic (6) Electric Stimulation (19) Holistic Nursing (2) Homeopathy (5) Hypnosis (18) Imagery (4) Lasers (3) Massage (3) Meditation (3) Naturopathy (5) Orthopedic Manipulation (5) Osteopathy (1) Phytomedicine (5) Psychotherapy (9) Relaxation (63) Traditional Chinese Medicine (5)
Heart Disease (ischemia, angina)	1. Meditation 2. Traditional Chinese Medicine	1. ch 30 2. ch 12	1. ch 30 2. ch 12	Acupuncture (4) Behavioral Medicine (4) Biofeedback (5) Electric Stimulation (9) Homeopathy (1) Massage (2) Meditation (2) Music Therapy (2) Naturopathy (6) Phytomedicine (19) Relaxation (12) Spiritual Healing (2) Thymus Extract (5) Traditional Chinese Medicine (2)
Heartburn	1. Tibetan Medicine	1. ch 14	1. ch 12	Phytomedicine (1)

Condition				
Hemorrhoid	1. Acupuncture	1. ch 19	1. ch 19	Electric Stimulation (1) Naturopathy (3) Phytomedicine (3) Relaxation (1)
Hepatitis	1. Acupuncture 2. Megavitamin and Orthomolecular Therapy 3. Osteopathy 4. Phytomedicine	1. ch 19 2. ch 27 3. ch 16 4. ch 20	1. ch 19 2. ch 27 3. ch 16 4. ch 20	Acupuncture (1) Ayurveda (2) Homeopathy (1) Megavitamin and Orthomolecular (2) Naturopathy (3) Phytomedicine (32) Thymus Extract (10) Traditional Chinese Medicine (1)
Hives	1. Ayurveda	1. ch 11	1. ch 11	
HIV and AIDS	1. Acupuncture 2. Massage 3. Meditation 4. Megavitamin and Orthomolecular Therapy	1. ch 19 2. ch 22 3. ch 30 4. ch 27	1. ch 19 2. ch 22 3. ch 30 4. ch 27	Acupuncture (2) Behavioral Medicine (3) Biofeedback (1) Diet Therapy (3) Homeopathy (3) Hypnosis (1) Massage (2) Meditation (1) Megavitamin and Orthomolecular (5) Naturopathy (1) Phytomedicine (5) Psychotherapy (3) Relaxation (5) Thymus Extract (7)
Hypercholesterolemia	1. Ayurveda 2. Phytomedicine	1. ch 11 2. ch 20	1. ch 11 2. ch 20	Ayurveda (1) Diet Therapy (15) Homeopathy (1) Meditation (1) Megavitamin and Orthomolecular (5) Naturopathy (28) Phytomedicine (20) Qigong (1) Relaxation (1)
Hyperglycemia	1. Biofeedback	1. ch 24	1. ch 24	

continued

CONDITION	SYSTEM/MODALITY DESCRIBED FOR THIS CONDITION IN THIS BOOK	CHAPTER FOR INDICATION	PRECAUTIONS DESCRIBED FOR THIS SYSTEM/MODALITY IN THIS BOOK	NUMBER OF KNOWN CLINICAL TRIALS (#) FOR THIS CONDITION IN THIS SYSTEM/MODALITY
Hyperkinesis	1. Megavitamin and Orthomolecular Therapy 2. Osteopathy 3. Phytomedicine 4. Qigong	1. ch 27 2. ch 16 3. ch 20 4. ch 23	1. ch 27 2. ch 16 3. ch 20 4. ch 23	Acupuncture (2) Biofeedback (3) Diet Therapy (8) Electric Stimulation (2) Naturopathy (9) Relaxation (2)
Hypertension	1. Ayurveda 2. Biofeedback 3. Chiropractic 4. Hypnotherapy 5. Meditation 6. Naturopathy 7. Megavitamin and Orthomolecular Therapy 8. Phytomedicine 9. Qigong	1. ch 11 2. ch 24 3. ch 15 4. ch 25 5. ch 30 6. ch 17 7. ch 27 8. ch 20 9. ch 23	1. ch 11 2. ch 24 3. ch 15 4. ch 25 5. ch 30 7. ch 27 8. ch 20 9. ch 23	Acupuncture (15) Anthroposophy (1) Behavioral Medicine (23) Biofeedback (61) Diet Therapy (14) Electric Stimulation (18) Homeopathy (7) Hypnosis (9) Imagery (4) Massage (1) Meditation (15) Megavitamin and Orthomolecular (6) Osteopathy (2) Naturopathy (31) Phytomedicine (47) Psychotherapy (7) Qigong (6) Relaxation (96) Spiritual Healing (2) Traditional Chinese Medicine (6)
Hypoglycemia	1. Biofeedback	1. ch 24	1. ch 24	
Ileus	1. Osteopathy	1. ch 16	1. ch 16	
Impotence	1. Acupuncture	1. ch 19	1. ch 19	Acupuncture (1) Behavioral Medicine (1) Biofeedback (2) Electric Stimulation (5) Hypnosis (2) Phytomedicine (3) Relaxation (1)

Condition				
Indigestion	1. Ayurveda	1. ch 11	1. ch 11	
Infertility, Female	1. Acupuncture 2. Megavitamin and Orthomolecular Therapy 3. Osteopathy	1. ch 19 2. ch 27 3. ch 16	1. ch 19 2. ch 27 3. ch 16	Acupuncture (5) Electric Stimulation (6) Homeopathy (3) Megavitamin and Orthomolecular (2) Naturopathy (4) Phytomedicine (2) Traditional Chinese Medicine (2)
Infertility, Male	1. Acupuncture	1. ch 19	1. ch 19	Acupuncture (2) Homeopathy (1) Megavitamin and Orthomolecular (2) Naturopathy (4) Phytomedicine (3) Traditional Chinese Medicine (1)
Inflammatory Bowel Disease	1. Naturopathy	1. ch 17		Behavioral Medicine (1) Diet Therapy (3) Naturopathy (3) Relaxation (2)
Influenza/Viral Syndrome	1. Acupuncture 2. Megavitamin and Orthomolecular Therapy 3. Osteopathy 4. Phytomedicine 5. Spiritual Healing 6. Tibetan Medicine	1. ch 19 2. ch 27 3. ch 16 4. ch 20 5. ch 21 6. ch 14	1. ch 19 2. ch 27 3. ch 16 5. ch 21 6. ch 12	Homeopathy (11) Magavitamin and Orthomolecular (1) Naturopathy (1) Phytomedicine (4) Thymus Extract (1) Traditional Chinese Medicine (1)
Insomnia	1. Acupuncture 2. Biofeedback 3. Hypnotherapy 4. Massage 5. Phytomedicine 6. Traditional Chinese Medicine	1. ch 19 2. ch 24 3. ch 25 4. ch 22 5. ch 20 6. ch 12	1. ch 19 2. ch 24 3. ch 25 4. ch 22 5. ch 12	Acupuncture (2) Aromatherapy (2) Behavioral Medicine (15) Biofeedback (6) Electric Stimulation (2) Homeopathy (1) Hypnosis (7) Meditation (6) Music Therapy (1) Psychotherapy (1) Relaxation (22)
Irritable Bladder	1. Acupuncture	1. ch 19	1. ch 19	

continued

CONDITION	SYSTEM/MODALITY DESCRIBED FOR THIS CONDITION IN THIS BOOK	CHAPTER FOR INDICATION	PRECAUTIONS DESCRIBED FOR THIS SYSTEM/MODALITY IN THIS BOOK	NUMBER OF KNOWN CLINICAL TRIALS (#) FOR THIS CONDITION IN THIS SYSTEM/MODALITY
Irritable Bowel Syndrome	1. Acupuncture 2. Biofeedback 3. Hypnotherapy	1. ch 19 2. ch 24 3. ch 25	1. ch 19 2. ch 24 3. ch 25	Acupuncture (1) Aromatherapy (4) Ayurveda (1) Behavioral Medicine (3) Biofeedback (2) Diet Therapy (3) Homeopathy (3) Hypnosis (5) Meditation (1) Naturopathy (4) Phytomedicine (9) Psychotherapy (7) Relaxation (8)
Jaundice	1. Ayurveda	1. ch 11	1. ch 11	
Kidney Stones	1. Ayurveda 2. Naturopathy 3. Megavitamin and Orthomo-lecular Therapy	1. ch 11 2. ch 17 3. ch 27	1. ch 11 3. ch 27	Acupuncture (2) Electric Stimulation (4) Phytomedicine (1)
Leukemia	1. Native American Medicine	2. ch 13		Behavioral Medicine (2) Electric Stimulation (1) Homeopathy (1) Hypnosis (3) Imagery (1) Megavitamin and Orthomolecular (2) Naturopathy (3) Phytomedicine (4) Relaxation (2) Spiritual Healing (1) Thymus Extract (1) Traditional Chinese Medicine (2)

Condition			
Low Back Pain	1. Chiropractic 2. Massage 3. Osteopathy 4. Traditional Chinese Medicine	1. ch 15 2. ch 22 3. ch 16 4. ch 12	Acupuncture (24) Behavioral Medicine (11) Biofeedback Chiropractic (37) Electric Stimulation (22) Homeopathy (1) Hypnosis (1) Lasers (3) Massage (8) Naturopathy (6) Orthopedic Manipulation (34) Osteopathy (6) Psychotherapy (3) Relaxation (8)
Lupus Erythematosus	1. Naturopathy	1. ch 17	Thymus Extract (5)
Macular Degeneration	1. Phytomedicine	1. ch 20	Electric Stimulation (1) Megavitamin and Orthomolecular (2) Naturopathy (2) Phytomedicine (1)
Malaise/Fatigue	1. Massage 2. Naturopathy 3. Megavitamin and Orthomolecular Therapy 4. Phytomedicine 5. Qigong	1. ch 22 2. ch 17 3. ch 27 4. ch 20 5. ch 23	Art Therapy (1) Behavioral Medicine (2) Biofeedback (3) Electric Stimulation (14) Homeopathy (2) Hypnosis (2) Imagery (1) Meditation (1) Megavitamin and Orthomolecular (1) Naturopathy (6) Osteopathy (1) Phytomedicine (6)
		1. ch 22 3. ch 27 5. ch 23	
Menstrual Irregularity/Disorder	1. Megavitamin and Orthomolecular Therapy	1. ch 27	Acupuncture (2) Homeopathy (1) Light Therapy (1)

continued

CONDITION	SYSTEM/MODALITY DESCRIBED FOR THIS CONDITION IN THIS BOOK	CHAPTER FOR INDICATION	PRECAUTIONS DESCRIBED FOR THIS SYSTEM/MODALITY IN THIS BOOK	NUMBER OF KNOWN CLINICAL TRIALS (#) FOR THIS CONDITION IN THIS SYSTEM/MODALITY
Menopausal Symptoms	1. Phytomedicine	1. ch 20	1. ch 20	Acupuncture (3) Behavioral Medicine (2) Biofeedback (2) Homeopathy (3) Megavitamin and Orthomolecular (1) Naturopathy (1) Osteopathy (3) Phytomedicine (6) Relaxation (4)
Migraine Headache	1. Ayurveda 2. Biofeedback 3. Hypnotherapy 4. Naturopathy 5. Megavitamin and Orthomolecular Therapy 6. Phytomedicine 7. Traditional Chinese Medicine	1. ch 11 2. ch 24 3. ch 25 4. ch 17 5. ch 27 6. ch 20 7. ch 12	1. ch 11 2. ch 24 3. ch 25 5. ch 27 6. ch 20 7. ch 12	Acupuncture (22) Behavioral Medicine (22) Biofeedback (59) Chiropractic (1) Diet Therapy (9) Electric Stimulation (14) Homeopathy (6) Hypnosis (10) Imagery (3) Meditation (1) Megavitamin and Orthomolecular (3) Music Therapy (1) Naturopathy (11) Phytomedicine (4) Psychotherapy (7) Relaxation (50) Traditional Chinese Medicine (1)
Mitral Valve Prolapse	1. Naturopathy	1. ch 17		Biofeedback (1)
Mononucleosis	1. Megavitamin and Orthomolecular Therapy 2. Osteopathy	1. ch 27 2. ch 16	1. ch 27 2. ch 16	

Condition	Therapies			Referenced Therapies (count)
Motion Sickness	1. Biofeedback 2. Phytomedicine	1. ch 24 2. ch 20	1. ch 24 2. ch 20	Acupuncture (3) Behavioral Medicine (1) Biofeedback (4) Electric Stimulation (3) Homeopathy (2) Phytomedicine (2) Relaxation (3)
Multiple Sclerosis	1. Meditation 2. Naturopathy 3. Megavitamin and Orthomolecular Therapy	1. ch 30 2. ch 17 3. ch 27	1. ch 30 3. ch 27	Acupuncture (1) Art Therapy (2) Behavioral Medicine (2) Biofeedback (3) Diet Therapy (12) Electric Stimulation (9) Imagery (2) Massage (2) Meditation (1) Naturopathy (11) Phytomedicine (3) Psychotherapy (3) Reflexology (1) Thymus Extract (1) Tibetan Medicine (1) Traditional Chinese Medicine (1)
Muscle Spasm	1. Acupuncture 2. Massage 3. Traditional Chinese Medicine	1. ch 19 2. ch 22 3. ch 12	1. ch 19 2. ch 22 3. ch 12	Aromatherapy (1) Biofeedback (1) Electric Stimulation (3)
Myocardial Infarction	1. Spiritual Healing	1. ch 21	1. ch 21	Acupuncture (1) Behavioral Medicine (3) Biofeedback (2) Diet Therapy (3) Electric Stimulation (7) Imagery (1) Megavitamin and Orthomolecular (10) Music Therapy (3) Naturopathy (10) Osteopathy (2) Phytomedicine (13) Psychotherapy (1) Relaxation (19) Traditional Chinese Medicine (2)

continued

CONDITION	SYSTEM/MODALITY DESCRIBED FOR THIS CONDITION IN THIS BOOK	CHAPTER FOR INDICATION	PRECAUTIONS DESCRIBED FOR THIS SYSTEM/MODALITY IN THIS BOOK	NUMBER OF KNOWN CLINICAL TRIALS (#) FOR THIS CONDITION IN THIS SYSTEM/MODALITY
Myofascial Pain	1. Biofeedback 2. Chiropractic	1. ch 24 2. ch 15	1. ch 24 2. ch 15	Acupuncture (14) Biofeedback (2) Chiropractic (2) Electric Stimulation (11) Lasers (4) Massage (1) Orthopedic Manipulation (1) Relaxation (1)
Nausea and Vomiting	1. Ayurveda 2. Hypnotherapy 3. Phytomedicine 4. Traditional Chinese Medicine	1. ch 11 2. ch 25 3. ch 20 4. ch 12	1. ch 11 2. ch 25 3. ch 20 4. ch 12	Acupuncture (55) Behavioral Medicine (5) Biofeedback (2) Hypnosis (15) Imagery (3) Megavitamin and Orthomolecular (1) Naturopathy (2) Phytomedicine (19) Psychotherapy (6) Relaxation (13)
Neck Pain	1. Ayurveda 2. Chiropractic 3. Osteopathy 4. Traditional Chinese Medicine	1. ch 11 2. ch 15 3. ch 16 4. ch 12	1. ch 11 2. ch 15 3. ch 16 4. ch 12	Acupuncture (21) Behavioral Medicine (1) Biofeedback (3) Chiropractic (17) Electric Stimulation (9) Lasers (5) Massage (3) Naturopathy (1) Orthopedic Manipulation (13) Osteopathy (3)
Neuritis	1. Osteopathy	1. ch 16	1. ch 16	Acupuncture (1) Biofeedback (1) Electric Stimulation (4)

Condition	Therapies			Other
Obesity	1. Hypnotherapy	1. ch 25	1. ch 25	Acupuncture (5) Ayurveda (1) Behavioral Medicine (7) Diet Therapy (7) Electric Stimulation (1) Homeopathy (1) Hypnosis (14) Megavitamin and Orthomolecular (1) Naturopathy (8) Phythomedicine (2) Psychotherapy (2) Relaxation (5)
Osteoarthritis	1. Chiropractic 2. Naturopathy 3. Megavitamin and Orthomolecular Therapy 4. Traditional Chinese Medicine	1. ch 15 2. ch 17 3. ch 27 4. ch 12	1. ch 15 3. ch 27 4. ch 12	Acupuncture (25) Diet Therapy (1) Electric Stimulation (23) Holistic Nursing (1) Homeopathy (5) Lasers (4) Massage (1) Megavitamin and Orthomolecular (3) Naturopathy (16) Phytomedicine (7) Relaxation (2) Tissue Therapy (8)
Osteoporosis	1. Naturopathy 2. Megavitamin and Orthomolecular Therapy 3. Qigong	1. ch 17 2. ch 27 3. ch 23	2. ch 27 3. ch 23	Megavitamin and Orthomolecular (4) Naturopathy (4) Phytomedicine (2) Thymus Extract (1)
Otitis Media	1. Osteopathy	1. ch 16	1. ch 16	Homeopathy (7) Megavitamin and Orthomolecular (2) Naturopathy (2) Phytomedicine (1)

CONDITION	SYSTEM/MODALITY DESCRIBED FOR THIS CONDITION IN THIS BOOK	CHAPTER FOR INDICATION	PRECAUTIONS DESCRIBED FOR THIS SYSTEM/MODALITY IN THIS BOOK	NUMBER OF KNOWN CLINICAL TRIALS (#) FOR THIS CONDITION IN THIS SYSTEM/MODALITY
Pain from Other Causes	1. Acupuncture	1. ch 19	1. ch 19	Acupuncture (166)
	2. Behavioral Medicine	2. ch 26	3. ch 25	Aromatherapy (6)
	3. Hypnotherapy	3. ch 25	4. ch 22	Behavioral Medicine (22)
	4. Massage	4. ch 22	5. ch 30	Biofeedback (23)
	5. Meditation	5. ch 30	7. ch 16	Chiropractic (9)
	6. Native American Medicine	6. ch 13	8. ch 21	Electric Stimulation (244)
	7. Osteopathy	7. ch 16	9. ch 12	Homeopathy (17)
	8. Spiritual Healing	8. ch 21		Hypnosis (86)
	9. Traditional Chinese Medicine	9. ch 12		Imagery (16)
				Lasers (18)
				Massage (28)
				Meditation (4)
				Megavitamin and Orthomolecular (1)
				Music Therapy (15)
				Naturopathy (17)
				Holistic Nursing (6)
				Orthopedic Manipulation (7)
				Phytomedicine (27)
				Psychotherapy (20)
				Relaxation (60)
				Spiritual Healing (1)
				Traditional Chinese Medicine (5)
Parkinson Disease	1. Ayurveda	1. ch 11	1. ch 11	Aromatherapy (1)
	2. Meditation	2. ch 30	2. ch 30	Ayurveda (1)
	3. Megavitamin and Orthomolecular Therapy	3. ch 27	3. ch 27	Biofeedback (1)
				Electric Stimulation (15)
				Massage (1)
				Megavitamin and Orthomolecular (9)
				Naturopathy (9)
				Phytomedicine (4)
				Relaxation (1)
Peptic Ulcer	1. Chiropractic	1. ch 15	1. ch 15	Diet Therapy (1)
	2. Massage	2. ch 22	2. ch 22	Electric Stimulation (4)
	3. Megavitamin and Orthomolecular Therapy	3. ch 27	3. ch 27	Naturopathy (1)
				Phytomedicine (18)
				Thymus Extract (1)

Condition				
Peripheral Vascular Disease	1. Phytomedicine 2. Tibetan Medicine	1. ch 20 2. ch 14	1. ch 20	EDTA Chelation (1) Electric Stimulation (1) Naturopathy (2)
Pharyngitis, Acute	1. Acupuncture 2. Homeopathy	1. ch 19 2. ch 28	1. ch 19	Acupuncture (1) Naturopathy (2) Phytomedicine (2) Thymus Extract (1)
Plagiocephaly	1. Osteopathy	1. ch 16	1. ch 16	
Plantar Fasciitis	1. Acupuncture	1. ch 19	1. ch 19	Acupuncture (1)
Pneumonia	1. Native American Medicine 2. Osteopathy	1. ch 13 2. ch 16	2. ch 16	Diet Therapy (1) Biofeedback (1) Electric Stimulation (2) Naturopathy (3) Phytomedicine (5) Thymus Extract (1)
Post-traumatic Stress Disorder	1. Ayurveda	1. ch 11	1. ch 11	Behavioral Medicine (1) Hypnosis (2) Meditation (1) Psychotherapy (2) Relaxation (1)
Postherpetic Neuralgia	1. Acupuncture	1. ch 19	1. ch 19	Acupuncture (1) Electric Stimulation (1)
Premenstrual Syndrome	1. Naturopathy 2. Phytomedicine	1. ch 17 2. ch 20	2. ch 20	Behavioral Medicine (1) Biofeedback (1) Chiropractic (1) Diet Therapy (6) Homeopathy (5) Megavitamin and Orthomolecular (10) Naturopathy (16) Phytomedicine (7) Reflexology (1) Relaxation (2)
Prostatitis	1. Acupuncture	1. ch 19	1. ch 19	Biofeedback (2) Electric Stimulation (7)

continued

CONDITION	SYSTEM/MODALITY DESCRIBED FOR THIS CONDITION IN THIS BOOK	CHAPTER FOR INDICATION	PRECAUTIONS DESCRIBED FOR THIS SYSTEM/MODALITY IN THIS BOOK	NUMBER OF KNOWN CLINICAL TRIALS (#) FOR THIS CONDITION IN THIS SYSTEM/MODALITY
Psoriasis	1. Naturopathy	1. ch 17	1. ch 17	Diet Therapy (1) Hypnosis (2) Imagery (5) Meditation (2) Music Therapy (1) Naturopathy (12) Phytomedicine (5) Psychotherapy (5) Thymus Extract (1)
Pulmonary Edema	1. Megavitamin and Orthomolecular Therapy	1. ch 27	1. ch 27	Electric Stimulation (1) Phytomedicine (2)
Pulmonary Sarcoidosis	1. Osteopathy	1. ch 16	1. ch 16	Thymus Extract (1)
Rash	1. Ayurveda	1. ch 11	1. ch 11	
Raynaud's Disease	1. Biofeedback 2. Phytomedicine	1. ch 24 2. ch 20	1. ch 24 2. ch 20	Acupuncture (1) Behavioral Medicine (3) Biofeedback (9) Electric Stimulation (1) Hypnosis (1) Massage (1) Naturopathy (1) Phytomedicine (1) Relaxation (7)
Repetitive Strain Disorder	1. Acupuncture	1. ch 19	1. ch 19	
Rheumatoid Arthritis	1. Acupuncture 2. Ayurveda 3. Behavioral Medicine 4. Biofeedback 5. Naturopathy 6. Megavitamin and Orthomolecular Therapy	1. ch 19 2. ch 11 3. ch 26 4. ch 24 5. ch 17 6. ch 27	1. ch 19 2. ch 11 4. ch 24 6. ch 27	Acupuncture (14) Ayurveda (3) Behavioral Medicine (5) Biofeedback (3) Dance Therapy (1) Diet (38) Electric Stimulation (8) Homeopathy (13) Hypnosis (2) Imagery (2)

Condition	Recommended Therapies	Chapter	Therapies (number of studies)
(continued)			Lasers (4) Massage (1) Megavitamin and Orthomolecular (4) Music Therapy (1) Naturopathy (57) Phytomedicine (14) Psychotherapy (2) Relaxation (12) Thymus Extract (7) Traditional Chinese Medicine (1)
Rhinitis, Allergic	1. Acupuncture	1. ch 19	Acupuncture (2) Homeopathy (1) Naturopathy (1) Phytomedicine (1)
Schizophrenia	1. Megavitamin and Orthomolecular Therapy	1. ch 27	Acupuncture (5) Ayurveda (1) Behavioral Medicine (1) Biofeedback (4) Electric Stimulation (2) Hypnosis (4) Massage (1) Meditation (2) Megavitamin and Orthomolecular (4) Music Therapy (4) Naturopathy (8) Phytomedicine (5) Relaxation (5)
Sciatica	1. Ayurveda	1. ch 11	Acupuncture (6) Chiropractic (1) Electric Stimulation (5) Orthopedic Manipulation (3) Traditional Chinese Medicine (1)
Seizure Disorder	1. Megavitamin and Orthomolecular Therapy	1. ch 27	
Sexual Dysfunction	1. Acupuncture 2. Ayurveda	1. ch 19 2. ch 11	Hypnosis (1)

continued

CONDITION	SYSTEM/MODALITY DESCRIBED FOR THIS CONDITION IN THIS BOOK	CHAPTER FOR INDICATION	PRECAUTIONS DESCRIBED FOR THIS SYSTEM/MODALITY IN THIS BOOK	NUMBER OF KNOWN CLINICAL TRIALS (#) FOR THIS CONDITION IN THIS SYSTEM/MODALITY
Sickle Cell Disease	1. Megavitamin and Orthomolecular Therapy	1. ch 27	1. ch 27	Acupuncture (1) Electric Stimulation (1) Hypnosis (1) Megavitamin and Orthomolecular (1) Naturopathy (1)
Sinusitis, Acute	1. Acupuncture 2. Ayurveda 3. Osteopathy	1. ch 19 2. ch 11 3. ch 13	1. ch 19 2. ch 11 3. ch 16	Aromatherapy (1)
Sinusitis, Chronic	1. Acupuncture 2. Ayurveda 3. Osteopathy	1. ch 19 2. ch 11 3. ch 16	1. ch 19 2. ch 11 3. ch 16	Acupuncture (1) Electric Stimulation (1) Phytomedicine (1) Thymus Extract (1)
Soft Tissue Injury	1. Acupuncture 2. Osteopathy	1. ch 19 2. ch 16	1. ch 19 2. ch 16	Biofeedback (1) Chiropractic (2) Lasers (1)
Sprains and Strains	1. Acupuncture 2. Chiropractic 3. Native American Medicine 4. Osteopathy	1. ch 19 2. ch 15 3. ch 13 4. ch 16	1. ch 19 2. ch 15 4. ch 16	Acupuncture (4) Biofeedback (1) Chiropractic (1) Electric Stimulation (4) Homeopathy (5) Naturopathy (1) Phytomedicine (5) Relaxation (1)
Stroke	1. Biofeedback 2. Native American Medicine 3. Osteopathy 4. Traditional Chinese Medicine	1. ch 24 2. ch 13 3. ch 16 4. ch 12	1. ch 24 3. ch 16 4. ch 12	Acupuncture (13) Ayurveda (2) Behavioral Medicine (1) Biofeedback (8) Electric Stimulation (2) Homeopathy (2) Hypnosis (1) Massage (1) Naturopathy (3) Phytomedicine (5) Relaxation (1) Traditional Chinese Medicine (2)

Condition				
Temporomandibular Joint Syndrome	1. Acupuncture 2. Biofeedback 3. Osteopathy	1. ch 19 2. ch 24 3. ch 16	1. ch 19 2. ch 24 3. ch 16	Acupuncture (1) Behavioral Medicine (6) Biofeedback (19) Chiropractic (1) Electric Stimulation (9) Hypnosis (2) Massage (1) Relaxation (14)
Tendonitis and Tenosynovitis	1. Chiropractic	1. ch 15	1. ch 15	
Tennis Elbow	1. Acupuncture	1. ch 19	1. ch 19	Acupuncture (7) Electric Stimulation (2) Lasers (3) Orthopedic Manipulation (3)
Thoracic Outlet Syndrome	1. Osteopathy	1. ch 16	1. ch 16	Acupuncture (1) Traditional Chinese Medicine (1)
Tinnitus	1. Osteopathy 2. Phytomedicine	1. ch 16 2. ch 20	1. ch 16 2. ch 20	Acupuncture (10) Behavioral Medicine (6) Biofeedback (5) Electric Stimulation (17) Homeopathy (1) Hypnosis (6) Lasers (1) Naturopathy (2) Phytomedicine (5) Psychotherapy (3) Relaxation (7)
Tonsillitis	1. Ayurveda	1. ch 11	1. ch 11	Electric Stimulation (2) Homeopathy (2) Megavitamin and Orthomolecular (1) Naturopathy (2) Phytomedicine (1)
Torticollis	1. Biofeedback	1. ch 24	1. ch 24	Biofeedback (2) Electric Stimulation (1) Relaxation (1)

continued

CONDITION	SYSTEM/MODALITY DESCRIBED FOR THIS CONDITION IN THIS BOOK	CHAPTER FOR INDICATION	PRECAUTIONS DESCRIBED FOR THIS SYSTEM/MODALITY IN THIS BOOK	NUMBER OF KNOWN CLINICAL TRIALS (#) FOR THIS CONDITION IN THIS SYSTEM/MODALITY
Tuberculosis	1. Native American Medicine	1. ch 13		Acupuncture (2) Electric Stimulation (5) Naturopathy (1) Phytomedicine (4) Thymus Extract (4)
Upper Respiratory Infection	1. Phytomedicine	1. ch 20	1. ch 20	Phytomedicine (1) Thymus Extract (4)
Urinary Incontinence	1. Biofeedback	1. ch 24	1. ch 24	Acupuncture (5) Behavioral Medicine (5) Biofeedback (20) Electric Stimulation (51) Naturopathy (1) Phytomedicine (5)
Urticaria	1. Ayurveda 2. Hypnotherapy 3. Megavitamin and Orthomolecular Therapy	1. ch 11 2. ch 25 3. ch 27	1. ch 11 2. ch 25 3. ch 27	Acupuncture (1) Naturopathy (1)
Vertigo	1. Osteopathy 2. Phythomedicine	1. ch 16 2. ch 20	1. ch 16 2. ch 20	Electric Stimulation (1) Homeopathy (1) Phytomedicine (4)
Warts	1. Hypnotherapy	1. ch 25	1. ch 25	Electric Stimulation (1) Homeopathy (5) Hypnosis (4) Imagery (1) Phytomedicine (2)
Whiplash Injury	1. Chiropractic 2. Osteopathy	1. ch 15 2. ch 16	1. ch 15 2. ch 16	Acupuncture (2) Chiropractic (3) Lasers (1) Orthopedic Manipulation (1)

APPELLATIONS

ACR—Advanced Certified Rolfer

AMTA—American Massage Therapy Association

AOBA—American Oriental Bodywork Association

ARNP—Advanced Registered Nurse Practitioner

ATR—Art Therapist Registered

BAMS—Bachelor of Ayurvedic Medicine and Surgery

CA—Certified Acupuncturist

CAMT—Certified Acupressure Massage Therapist

CAT—Certified Acupressure Therapist

CCH—Certified Clinical Hypnotherapist

CFP—Certified Feldenkrais Practitioner

CHt/CHT—Certified Hypnotherapist

CH—Certified Herbalist

CMA—Certified Movement Analyst

CMT—Certified Massage Therapist

CR—Certified Reflexologist or Certified Rolfer

DAc—Diplomate of Acupuncture

DC—Doctor of Chiropractic

DHt—Diplomate in Homeotherapeutics

DHANP—Diplomate of Homeopathic Academy of Naturopathic Physicians

DO—Doctor of Osteopathy

DOM—Doctor of Oriental Medicine

DiplAc—Diplomate in Acupuncture

HHD—Doctor of Holistic Health

HHP—Holistic Health Practitioner

LAc—Licensed Acupuncturist

LicAc—Licensed Acupuncturist

LD—Licensed Dietitian

LM—Licensed Midwife

LMT—Licensed Massage Therapist

MAc—Master of Acupuncture

MASc—Master of Ayurvedic Science

MH—Master Herbalist

MOM—Master of Oriental Medicine

MT—Massage Therapist

NASTAT—North American Society of Teachers of the Alexander Technique

ND—Naturopathic Doctor or Doctor of Naturopathy

NMD—Naturopathic Medical Doctor

NP—Nurse Practitioner

OMD—Oriental Medical Doctor

RAc—Registered Acupuncturist

RD—Registered Dietitian

RDT—Registered Drama Therapist

RMT—Registered Massage Therapist or Registered Music Therapist

RPP—Registered Polarity Practitioner

RPT—Registered Physical Therapist

GLOSSARY

acupressure: the practice of applying pressure to acupuncture points along the body's meridian system to treat disease, relieve pain, and balance the flow of qi in the body.

acupuncture: the practice of inserting needles into specific points along the body's meridian system to treat disease, relieve pain, and balance the flow of qi in the body.

adjustment: a term in chiropractic that refers to the manipulation of joints by the act of applying a controlled dynamic thrust.

Alexander technique: an educational/therapeutic method of expending a minimum of effort to achieve the maximum efficient use of muscles and movement to relieve pain and to improve posture and overall health.

allopathy: a term generally used to describe Western medicine, whereby the treatment of disease is approached by the use of remedies (such as drugs or surgery) that create the opposite effect to those produced by the disease; the opposite of homeopathy, which posits that like cures like.

alpha state: a brain-wave state associated with wakeful relaxation.

amino acids: the chief components of proteins that are either manufactured by the body or supplied to the body through dietary or supplement intake.

applied kinesiology: a diagnostic and therapeutic system that employs the practice of muscle-testing to identify nutritional deficiencies and health problems with the belief that weakness in certain muscles relates to respective imbalances and diseases in the body.

art therapy: a therapeutic method that uses a number of artistic mediums, such as drawing or painting, to help people express themselves and relieve unresolved issues.

atherosclerosis: the disease state caused by the accumulation and calcification of plaques and resultant narrowing on the inner arterial wall.

aura therapy: a therapeutic method that corrects physical, mental, emotional, and spiritual imbalances through the interpretation and manipulation of the luminous, colored energy field that emanates from and surrounds the human body.

auricular therapy: the practice of inserting needles into specific acupuncture points located on the ear that relate to specific parts of the body.

autogenic training and therapy: a method of teaching individuals to recognize the origin of certain mental and physical disorders within themselves and to use that awareness and relaxation for the self-treatment of those disturbances.

autointoxication: a disorder produced by a poison that is generated from within the body.

Avicenna (979–1037 AD): an Arab physician and author of one of the most famous medical texts, the Canon, a compilation of Greco-Arabic medicine that served as a standard in Europe throughout the seventeenth century.

Ayurvedic medicine: Sanskrit for "life" (ayur) and "knowledge" (veda), thus, "the science of life"; one of the oldest known systems of healing, Ayurveda approaches health as the balance of body, mind, emotion, and spirit and uses an understanding of qualities of energy and the application of preventive and corrective treatments such as yoga, meditation, purification regimens, dietary changes, and herbal remedies.

Bach flower remedies: a therapeutic system that uses specially prepared plant infusions to balance physical and emotional disturbances.

bioelectromagnetics: the scientific study of electromagnetic fields and their effects on and interactions with living organisms.

bioenergetics: a therapeutic system that uses breath and body movement to release and transform blocked energy and to restore health.

biofeedback: the use of instrumentation to monitor, amplify, and feed back physiological information, so that a client can learn to change or regulate the process being monitored.

biofield: an energy field permeating and surrounding several inches around the human body that can be manipulated therapeutically to treat illness and restore health and well-being.

bioflavonoids: a naturally occurring group of antioxidant compounds found in fruits that are essential for the assimilation of vitamin C.

biogenesis: a theory proposed by Thomas Huxley that life develops from pre-existing life.

biophoton: a minute emission of electromagnetic energy from living organisms.

birth trauma: a negative psychological imprint resulting from the birth process.

blood purifier: a botanical medicine with an antibiotic action.

blue-green algae: a commercially cultivated algae claimed to have health promoting properties; also known as spirulina.

body-mind medicine: a healing approach that recognizes the connection between the physical and mental/emotional aspects of disease and treats both.

body-mind-spirit: a central concept in holistic medicine that holds that health and healing are functions of a whole and integrated human being on the physical, mental/emotional, and spiritual levels.

bodywork: the use of a wide variety of manipulative therapeutic touching techniques to treat illness and promote health.

botanical medicine: the use of healing remedies derived from plant sources.

calisthenics: a form of exercise that uses a system of rhythmic body movements performed without apparatus.

carminative: a remedy that stimulates the expelling of gas from the alimentary canal to relieve the pain of colic and gripe.

catechu: an extract from the heart wood of the Acacia catechu tree containing catechin, an astringent used for diarrhea.

cellular acidosis: a decrease of alkali in body fluids due to an accumulation of acid metabolites.

chakra: a vortex of physical or spiritual energy associated with the seven vital energy centers of the subtle bodies, according to Indian yogic metaphysics.

chelation: a process describing how certain molecules surround and bind to metal ions and the resulting variety of biochemical alterations that occur.

chelation therapy: use of chelation for purposes of treating atherosclerosis and other chronic degenerative diseases, consisting of a series of intravenous infusions with EDTA (ethylenediaminetetraacetic acid), accompanied by vitamins, minerals, and other supplements.

chi: see qi.

chiropractic medicine: a major school of Western medicine that focuses on the spine as integrally involved in maintaining health, providing primacy to the nervous system as the primary coordinator for function, and thus health, in the body; maintenance of optimal neurophysiological balance in the body is accomplished by correcting structural or biomechanical abnormalities or disrelationships through the use of chiropractic adjustment.

circadian rhythm: biological activity and events that occur in a cycle of approximately twenty-four hours.

clairsentience: the faculty of using touch to discern subtle variations in the biofield that are beyond the range of normal human perception.

clairvoyance: the faculty of discerning information that is beyond the range of normal human perception.

coenzyme Q10: a substance necessary at the cellular level for energy production; levels decrease with the aging process.

colon therapy: the irrigation of the entire large intestine with water to remove toxins and promote regular bowel movements.

color therapy: a therapeutic method that uses color to treat emotional and physical imbalance.

complementary medicine: the use of therapeutic systems and modalities together with conventional treatments to enhance the effectiveness of therapy.

craniosacral system: denotes the brain, spinal cord, cerebrospinal fluid, surrounding membranes, and their relationship within the parasympathetic portion of the autonomic nervous system.

craniosacral therapy: a therapeutic technique developed by William G. Sutherland, DO, that uses very gentle manual pressure applied to the skull, spine, and membranes to restore proper rhythmic flow to the craniosacral system and relieve pain and certain disorders closely related to the skull and spine, such as headache, TMJ, and vertigo.

crystal therapy: a therapeutic method that uses crystals and gems for physical, emotional, and spiritual balance and healing.

cupping: 1. a therapeutic massage technique performed by forming a hollow in the palm of the hand and striking the body with a rhythmic motion. 2. a therapeutic method in Traditional Chinese Medicine that refers to the application of a heated cup over an area of the body, which, as it cools, creates a slight suction on the area that stimulates blood circulation.

dance therapy: a therapeutic method that uses dance and movement to facilitate the expression and release of blocked emotion and stress to promote health and well-being.

dementia: the progressive deterioration of mental function characterized by confusion, impaired judgment and memory, and emotional apathy.

dental amalgam: an alloy of mercury, tin, silver, copper, or zinc that is used for dental fillings.

designer food: food that is fortified with ingredients that prevent disease, such as orange juice supplemented with calcium; also refers to genetically engineered food.

detoxification: the removal of toxins or poisons and their effects from the body.

DHEA (dehydroepiandrosterone): an androgenic steroid produced by the adrenal cortex believed to have an anti-aging effect; recently manufactured synthetically as a dietary supplement.

diathermy: a therapeutic method that uses high-frequency electric currents to generate heat in body tissues.

dietary supplement: a product taken in addition to the diet that supplies nutrients and other substances to promote health or to treat disease.

dietetics: the study and application of diet in the promotion of health and treatment of disease.

dilution: to reduce the potency of a solution.

direct technique: a manipulative technique used to correct an area of the body (such as joint) that is resistant to full range of motion; the area is immobilized and force is applied against the barrier to restore proper function.

DMSO (dimethyl sulfoxide): a by-product of weed-pulp manufacture used as a solvent and as an anti-inflammatory for pain relief in certain medical conditions.

do-in: a therapeutic self-help program used primarily in China and Japan for health maintenance that includes the use of acupressure, breathing, and stretching exercises.

doshas: in Ayurvedic medicine, the three constitution types (vata, pitta, and kapha) that define the physical, emotional, intellectual, and spiritual tendencies that are expressed in an individual; dosha imbalance is believed to cause illness.

electromagnetism: the magnetism produced by a current of electricity.

elimination diet: a method used for identifying food allergies by eliminating specific foods or food types from the diet one at a time.

environmental medicine: a healing approach that looks at the interaction of the environment with the body and determines how exposure and allergy to environmental toxins may be major factors in the development of disease.

enzyme therapy: a therapeutic method that uses botanical supplements and animal enzymes to improve digestive function and promote health.

enzymes: proteins produced by living cells that cause or enhance biochemical reactions in the body.

essential: a necessary substance not manufactured by the body and that must be supplied by the diet.

essential amino acids: the nine amino acids nutritionally required by the body and that must be supplied by the diet because the body does not manufacture them.

essential fatty acids: a nutritionally necessary fatty acid not manufactured by the body, such as linoleic and linolenic acids.

etheric body: the most proximal energy field that surrounds, permeates, and emanates from the physical body.

faith healing: use of faith in God and prayer to heal.

Feldenkrais: a therapeutic method that uses awareness of movement and teaches proper body movement through gentle massage, stretching, and exercise.

feng shui: the practice of analyzing the relationship between the flow of the earth's qi (wind and water) and buildings and rooms and then changing their alignment and placement to harmonious patterns that will enhance the inhabitant's health and well-being.

fixation: in chiropractic, an impedance of motion that inhibits the correct flow of nerve impulses and interferes with the normal state of health.

flavonoids: a group of plant pigments that promote beneficial biological activity in the human body.

flotation therapy: a therapeutic method using sensory deprivation to create a state of deep relaxation by having an individual float in darkness in an enclosed tank filled with salt and mineral water.

free radical: a highly chemically-reactive, unpaired molecule that interacts with nearby molecules and causes cellular damage.

fu zheng: a Chinese herbal therapy used in advanced cancers that uses ginseng and astragalus to extend life expectancy.

functional food: a food or food ingredient that has been altered to provide health benefits by increasing its normal nutrient level.

galvanic skin response: an alteration in the electrical current of the skin caused by physiochemical changes brought on by emotional reactions.

Gestalt therapy: a psychotherapeutic method of increasing an individual's self-awareness and the perception of the mind as a uniform functional configuration that cannot and should not be reduced by splitting it into parts.

glandulars: substances used therapeutically that are made up of freeze-dried animal glands produced in pill form and that provide a hormonal stimulant to improve glandular function.

glucosamine sulfate: a natural amino sugar that occurs in the cellular membranes of joint structures and that is produced as a dietary supplement to treat arthritis.

glycyrrhetinic acid: a vitamin A derivative that is believed to help prevent disease.

heal: to make whole.

herbal medicine: a healing approach that uses medicinal plants singly or in combination to treat disease and as a preventive to promote health and well-being.

hertz (Hz): the unit of frequency that measures cycles per second of electromagnetic radiation.

high sense perception: a diagnostic system that uses clairvoyance and clairsentience as its primary tools.

histamine: a chemical released by the body during an allergic reaction.

holistic medicine: an approach to healing that considers the whole person's body, mind, and spirit, and their interactions in the process of treating disease and promoting health and well-being.

homeopathy: a unique approach to healing that uses extremely dilute medicines to trigger a person's innate capacity to heal; based on the law of similars, the observation that medicines can produce in healthy people the same symptoms they cure in the sick; approaches the whole person in a systemic manner, using naturally occurring substances to restore health on physical, emotional, and mental levels.

humoralism, humorism: an approach that dates back to the Hippocratic school and is based on the belief that disease comes from imbalance among certain body fluids (such as blood, phlegm, and bile) and that restoring their balance promotes health.

hydrosol: a mixture of water and essential oil obtained in the distillation of certain medicinal plant materials used in aromatherapy.

hydrotherapy: the application of water, externally or internally, as a therapeutic method in the treatment of disease.

hypnosis: a form of cognitive information-processing in which a suspension of peripheral awareness and critical analytic cognition can lead to apparently involuntary changes in perception, memory, mood, and physiology.

hypnotherapy: a psychotherapeutic method that uses hypnosis (a trance-like state) to facilitate the relaxation of the conscious mind and make use of a heightened susceptibility to positive suggestion for the diagnosis and treatment of medical and psychological disorders.

hypotension: a condition of subnormal arterial blood pressure; low blood pressure.

indirect technique: a technique of manipulation that involves movement directed away from the area of restricted motion to obtain a state of balanced tension.

iridology: a method of diagnosis that studies changes in the iris as indications of health and disease.

ki: the Japanese term for qi.

kinesiology: a diagnostic method that uses muscle-testing to determine weaknesses that indicate an individual's state of health or imbalance.

lactose-intolerant: a gastrointestinal upset caused by intolerance to milk or other dairy products.

light box: a specially designed box that contains a set of high-intensity broad-spectrum light bulbs and uses a reflective background and diffusing screen to produce a light stronger than ordinary indoor light; used to treat seasonal affective disorder (SAD).

light-emitting diodes (LEDs): a semiconductor diode used primarily as a light source in electronic display, but more recently identified as a phototherapeutic method that can be used to stimulate healing of wounds and other skin conditions.

local healing: a healing method that involves the placement of the practitioner's hands on the client's body.

malabsorption: a defect that interferes with the absorption of nutrients in the gastrointestinal tract.

mandala: a graphic symbol of the universe in a circular design, used in Buddhist and Hindu art.

manipulation: a therapeutic technique that uses the application of manual force in various bodywork modalities such as osteopathy, chiropractic, and massage.

massage: a therapeutic method of manually applying rubbing, stroking, tapping, and kneading to the body (either a particular area or the whole body) for the purpose of treating physical and emotional disorders, increasing blood flow, reducing pain, and promoting relaxation, muscle tension release, and general health and well-being.

materia medica: a written text concerned with the source, preparation, dosage, and administration of substances used medicinally as drugs or in the practice of homeopathy.

medical acupuncture: the therapeutic insertion of solid needles in various combinations and patterns based on a combination of traditional concepts (such as encouraging the flow of qi) and modern concepts (such as recruiting neuroanatomical activities in segmental distributions).

meditation: a technique originally developed as a spiritual discipline that uses intention to direct one's focus on a word or the breath as a means to increase awareness of the present, reduce stress, promote relaxation, and attain personal and spiritual growth.

megadose: a very large dose (usually of vitamins) that surpasses the recommended daily allowance and is used therapeutically to prevent or to treat disease or in nutritional deficiency.

megavitamins: a very large dose of a specific vitamin given for therapeutic or preventive purposes; also known as orthomolecular medicine.

melatonin: a hormone formed by the pineal gland that is involved with the function and balance of the circadian rhythm; manufactured synthetically as a dietary supplement and promoted as a treatment for insomnia and jet lag.

mental healing: the use of conscious intent by a healer to produce a healing effect in another individual.

meridian: in traditional Asian medicine, a circuit that loops throughout the body and carries the vital qi along one of 12 main channels connecting, regulating, and balancing the function of the principle organs and body structures; in acupuncture, specific points along the meridians are used to correct the flow of qi and to restore proper function.

metamorphic technique: a therapeutic method that teaches the use of pressure applied by circular finger movements on the feet, ankles, wrists, hands, and head to promote healing and to balance the body's energies.

metaphysics: the branch of philosophy that investigates the origin and nature of reality and generally refers to that which is outside objective experience.

motion palpation: a diagnostic method that uses passive and active examination of a segmental joint with the hands to determine range of motion.

motor hand: the hand that the practitioner uses to induce passive movement in the subject.

music therapy: a therapeutic method that uses music to help an individual release repressed emotions in the treatment of certain physical and emotional disorders and to promote relaxation, stress reduction, and general health and well-being.

naturopathy: a philosophy and way of life that emphasizes the body's ability to heal itself naturally by living within the laws of nature and by the use of natural foods and medicines that support self-healing mechanisms (such as homeopathy and nutritional therapy); intervention therapies that are noninvasive and have a low incidence of side effects (such as massage and hydrotherapy); proper exercise; fresh air; commitment to improving the quality of the environment, and avoidance of drugs and surgery.

neural therapy: a therapeutic method that uses injection of anesthetics into certain points of the autonomic nervous system and/or acupuncture meridian system to correct disruptions in biological energy and to treat the resulting imbalances that cause certain disorders.

neurotropic injection technique: a therapeutic technique that involves the injection of small amounts (0.5 ml or less) of sterile saline solution into the back muscles near where the nerves enter on either side of the spine to improve nerve function, circulation, relieve pain, and treat a number of other disorders.

nocebo effect: the negative effects of a placebo.

noninvasive: referring to a diagnostic or treatment procedure that does not involve physical penetration of the skin or any body orifice.

nonlocal: an influence that occurs from a distance.

nosode: a minute dosage of substance derived from diseased tissue or body secretions used to induce an immune response and provide immunization against the specific disease from which the remedy was prepared.

nutriceutical: a food- or plant-based supplement used for treatment or prevention of specific medical conditions.

orthomolecular medicine: the adjustment of concentrations of molecules (e.g., vitamins, minerals, amino acids, hormones, and metabolic intermediates) that are normally present in the body for the prevention and treatment of disease.

osteopathy: a complete system of health care that teaches and practices the concepts of the body as a unit that possesses self-protecting and self-regulating mechanisms and that, because its structure and function are reciprocally interrelated, can achieve normalization of function by restoring structural integrity through use of therapeutic (such as osteopathic technique) and diagnostic approaches that effectively, gently, and functionally promote local and systemic homeostasis.

palpation: the art of feeling by hand to determine a variety of parameters governing the health and mobility of the tissues on or near the surface of the body.

parapsychology: the study of extrasensory perception and paranormal psychological phenomena such as clairvoyance and psychokinesis.

pet therapy: a therapeutic approach based on the concept that the loving interaction between a person and pet has positive health benefits and can reduce stress, lower blood pressure, and help alleviate depression and feelings of isolation.

pharmacopoeia: a written text issued by an officially recognized authority that describes the standards for the strength, purity, and formulation of therapeutic agents (drugs, chemicals, and other medical preparations).

pharmafood: a food or nutrient that is used to prevent or treat disease, or improve health.

phytoestrogens: a plant compound with chemical constituents similar to the hormone estrogen.

phytotherapy: the therapeutic application of plants.

placebo: an innocuous substance or treatment that is given for its suggestive effect; a substance or treatment given to the control group in a blinded controlled trial in order to distinguish between effects of the substance or treatment being tested and the effects of suggestion.

polarity: the presence of contrasted energy properties.

polarity therapy: a therapeutic method based on the theory that positive and negative energies flow throughout the body along five predictable pathways and that the flow can be balanced by the placement of the polarity therapist's hands at specific points along the channel to correct certain disorders.

polyunsaturated fats: an oil with double or triple bonds that can bind to hydrogen.

potentized: refers to the preparation of homeopathic remedies whereby a substance is diluted and "succussed," or shaken, to make the remedy more active and effective.

prana: in the yogic tradition, the invisible life force that flows throughout the universe and originates in the body with the breath.

pranayama: in the yogic tradition, a term for breath control.

probiotic: a dietary supplement, such as acidophilus, that enhances and restores the normal balance of bacteria in the intestines.

progestin: a hormone released by the corpus luteum.

psychic healing: healing that occurs from intervention through nonmaterial or paranormal means.

psychoneuroimmunology: the study of the nervous system, brain, and emotional states and how their interaction affects the immune system and the outcome of disease.

psychosomatic medicine: a field of medical research and practice that examines the influence of the mind and emotions on the development of bodily disorders and disease and uses physical and psychological means to treat them.

psychotherapy: a form of treatment that uses verbal communication, or "talk therapy," to gain an awareness, understanding, and resolution of emotional, behavioral, and psychiatric disorders and related physical disorders.

qi (chi, ki): pronounced "chee"; in traditional Asian philosophies, the unified vital life energy that permeates and animates the individual and the universe; in acupuncture, illness is the result of blocked qi.

qigong: a major branch of Traditional Chinese Medicine (TCM); denotes methods used to cultivate, regulate, and harness qi (vital energy) for general self-preservation and health, healing, self-defense, longevity, and, particularly, spiritual development.

recommended daily (or dietary) allowance (RDA): the minimum amount of vitamins and nutrients necessary to maintain health and prevent nutritional deficiency.

reflexology: a therapeutic method that uses manual pressure applied to specific areas, or zones, of the foot that correspond to areas of the body, in order to relieve stress and prevent and treat physical disorders.

Rolfing: a therapeutic method of systematic, deep, gentle muscle massage that is used to realign the body's structure, restore balance, and improve posture; also called structural integration.

seasonal affective disorder (SAD): a depressive mood disorder that recurs especially in winter and spontaneously remits in the spring; characterized by fatigue, morning hypersomnia, weight gain, and carbohydrate craving.

sensing hand: in manual therapies, the hand that senses and assesses changes caused by the motion of the motor hand.

shamanism: a method of healing practiced in traditional cultures, each of which dresses it in rituals and explanatory systems appropriate to its own time, place, and cosmology and which may include the use of meditation, prayer, chanting, and other practices, often in combination with herbalism.

shark cartilage: a dietary supplement derived from the cartilage of sharks and that is used as a cancer treatment due to idea that sharks rarely get cancer; it is believed that this is because of some special protective properties in their cartilage.

Shiatsu: literally, "finger pressure"; a therapeutic massage technique that applies vigorous pressure to specific points on the meridian system to treat medical conditions and to balance one's energy, thus promoting health and well-being.

somatic dysfunction: difficult or impaired function of the somatic system.

sorbitol: a product of glucose and sorbose found in fruits and which can accumulate in diabetics.

sounding the body: a diagnostic and therapeutic method used by a sound healer to analyze an individual's energy frequencies in order to indicate imbalances which can be corrected by the application of sound using either the healer's voice or tuning forks.

spiritual energy: the cosmic or universal vital force that originates from beyond the material level and gives life to physical organisms.

spiritual healing: the systematic, purposeful intervention by one or more persons aiming to help another living being or beings (whether person, animal, plant, or other living system) by means of focused intention, by touch, or by holding the hands near the other being, without application of physical, chemical, or conventional energetic means of intervention.

steroids: a group of organic or synthetic compounds with similar chemical composition, including drugs, hormones, and other bodily substances.

structural exam: a diagnostic technique used by osteopaths that involves an observational and manual (palpation) assessment of a lengthy series of specific factors that reveal a client's condition.

subluxation: the partial dislocation of the bones within a joint, interfering with proper neurophysiological function; realignment of the bones is known as chiropractic adjustment.

t'ai chi ch'uan: an ancient Chinese system of meditative movements used to maintain a healthy mental and physical state.

theosophy: a spiritual philosophy based on the view that knowledge of God and the universe come from intuitive or mystical insight that can lead to self-mastery and self-determination.

thrust: in chiropractic, a gentle, high-velocity, short-amplitude directional force applied manually to an area of the body in order to correct its alignment.

tonic: an herbal preparation used as a restorative and preventive agent to cleanse, invigorate the system, and maintain health.

toning: a therapeutic technique used in sound healing where an individual generates a soft resonant sound to balance the mind and body, promote relaxation, and reduce stress.

Traditional Chinese Medicine: a coherent system of medicine that views the human body as a whole and as a part of nature; while harmony within bodily functions and between the body and nature maintains health, disease occurs when this harmony is disrupted and can be restored by several therapeutic approaches such as Chinese herbal medicine, acupuncture/moxibustion, Tui Na (Chinese massage and acupressure), mind–body exercise, and Chinese dietary therapy.

transcranial electrostimulation: a therapeutic method that uses external electrical stimulation of the brain through the skull.

transcutaneous electrical nerve stimulation (TENS): a therapeutic method in which a low-voltage electrical current is delivered to the nerves by attaching electrodes to the skin in order to relieve pain by stimulating endorphin production.

trigger points: points on the body in the muscles and fascia that are painful when pressed and can be deactivated with trigger point therapy.

vibrational medicine: a system of healing that posits that disease originates from an imbalance or blockage of energy and that certain therapeutic methods such as homeopathy, color, sound, or crystal healing and certain biofield therapies can be used to unblock and balance the energies and restore health and well-being.

vis medicatrix naturae: literally, "the healing power of nature."

visualization therapy: a therapeutic method that uses imagery to correct unhealthy attitudes and views.

yang organs: the hollow outer organs, such as the intestines, spleen, gallbladder, and the skin.

yin and yang: in Chinese philosophy, the two opposite yet complementary dynamic components that make up the body and the universe; yin is the feminine, passive, dark, cold, moist aspect; yang is the active, light, warm, dry aspect; yin and yang blend and balance to maintain a harmonious healthy state in the body, but when unbalanced, the qi becomes disturbed and can result in illness.

yin or yang deficiency: an imbalance in the equilibrium of yin and yang that causes the yin or yang energy to become stagnant; this deficiency gives rise to illness.

yin organs: the dense, internal organs, such as the kidneys, lungs, liver, and bones.

yoga: an ancient Indian philosophy that uses gentle stretching exercises, breath control, and meditation to gain self-mastery and self-realization.

Zen therapy: a spiritual discipline that uses meditative practices to achieve the integration of the body, mind, and spirit and, thus, self-realization and enlightenment.

zone therapy: another term for reflexology.

Index

Page numbers in *italic* indicate figures. Page numbers followed by "t" indicate tables.